Pulmonary Disease
Examination and
Board Review

Pulmonary Disease
Examination and
Board Review

Edited by

Ronaldo Collo Go, MD

Faculty
Division of Pulmonary, Critical Care, and Sleep Medicine
Mount Sinai Beth Israel
New York, New York
and
Crystal Run Health Care
Middletown, New York

New York   Chicago   San Francisco   Athens   London   Madrid   Mexico City
New Delhi   San Juan   Singapore   Sydney   Toronto

ISBN 978-0-07-184529-8
MHID 0-07-184529-1

This book was set in Minion Pro.
The editors were Brian Belval and Christie Naglieri.
The production supervisor was Catherine Saggese.
Project Management was provided by Amit Kashyap, Aptara, Inc.
RR Donnelley was printer and binder.

This book is printed on acid-free paper.

Library of Congress Cataloging-in-Publication Data

Pulmonary disease examination and board review / edited by Ronaldo Collo Go.
     p. ; cm.
   Includes bibliographical references and index.
   ISBN 978-0-07-184529-8 (pbk. : alk. paper)—ISBN 0-07-184529-1 (pbk. : alk. paper)
   I. Go, Ronaldo Collo, editor.
   [DNLM: 1.   Respiratory Tract Diseases—Examination Questions.
2. Pulmonary Medicine—Examination Questions.   WF 18.2]
   RC756
   616.2'40076—dc23

                          2015011040

McGraw-Hill Education books are available at special quantity discounts to use as premiums and sales promotions or for use in corporate training programs. To contact a representative, please visit the Contact Us pages at www.mhprofessional.com

This book is dedicated to:

Evangeline and Benjamin Go
Anna Go, Jean Go, and Juan Truyol
Natalio Collo and Brigida Zapanta Collo
Jose Go and Rosalina Go
Sabina, Esther and the Bediones Family
Truyol Family
Lydia, Rodolfo, Imelda, and the Jovellanos Family
Rosa, Fortunato, and the Garces Family
Go Family
Collo Family
Tabobo Family
May Martin
Our patients

Contents

Contributors

Anthony F. Arredondo, MD
Fellow
Division of Pulmonary, Critical Care, and
    Sleep Medicine
Ronald Reagan UCLA Medical Center
Los Angeles, California

Alfredo Astua, MD
Assistant Professor of Medicine
Division of Pulmonary, Critical Care, and
    Sleep Medicine
Mount Sinai Beth Israel
New York, New York

Lea Azour, MD
Resident
Department of Radiology
Mount Sinai Hospital
New York, New York

Lisa Bajpayee, MD
Resident
Department of Internal Medicine
Boston University Medical Center
Boston, Massachusetts

Michael P. Bergman, MD
Fellow
Division of Pulmonary, Critical Care, and
    Sleep Medicine
Mount Sinai Beth Israel
New York, New York

Aloke Chakravarti, MD
Fellow
Division of Pulmonary, Critical Care, and
    Sleep Medicine
Mount Sinai Beth Israel Medical Center
New York, New York

Matthew Cham, MD
Associate Professor of Radiology and Medicine
Icahn School of Medicine at Mount Sinai
Department of Radiology
Mount Sinai Hospital
New York, New York

Steven Y. Chang, MD, PhD
Associate Clinical Professor of Medicine
Division of Pulmonary, Critical Care, and
    Sleep Medicine
David Geffen School of Medicine at UCLA
Ronald Reagan UCLA Medical Center
Los Angeles, California

George Cheng, MD, PhD
Fellow
Division of Pulmonary and Critical Care Medicine
Massachusetts General Hospital
Boston, Massachusetts

Dong-Seok Daniel Lee, MD
Assistant Professor of Surgery
Department of Thoracic Surgery
Icahn School of Medicine at Mount Sinai
Mount Sinai Hospital
New York, New York

Vikram Dhawan, MD
Fellow
Division of Surgical Critical Care
Mount Sinai Hospital
New York, New York

Corey Eber, MD
Assistant Professor of Radiology
Icahn School of Medicine at Mount Sinai
Department of Radiology
Mount Sinai Hospital
New York, New York

Michael Elias, MD
Fellow
Division of Surgical Critical Care
Mount Sinai Hospital
New York, New York

Oleg Epelbaum, MD
Director
Bronchoscopy and Interventional Pulmonology
Elmhurst Hospital Center
Assistant Professor of Medicine
Icahn School of Medicine at Mount Sinai
New York, New York

Ronald Evans, DO
Fellow
Division of Pulmonary and Critical Care Medicine
Geisinger Medical Center
Danville, Pennsylvania

Jason Filopei, MD
Fellow
Division of Pulmonary, Critical Care, and Sleep Medicine
Mount Sinai Beth Israel
New York, New York

Erik Folch, MD
Assistant Professor of Medicine
Associate Director of Interventional Pulmonology
Beth Israel Deaconess Medical Center
Harvard Medical School
Boston, Massachusetts

Irene Galperin, MD
Director, Pleural Disease Service
Division of Pulmonary and Critical Care Medicine
Lenox Hill Hospital – NSLIJ
Assistant Professor of Medicine
Albert Einstein College of Medicine
New York, New York

Ronaldo Collo Go, MD
Faculty
Division of Pulmonary, Critical Care, and
    Sleep Medicine
Mount Sinai Beth Israel
New York, New York
And
Crystal Run Health Care
Middletown, New York

Daniel Greenblatt Fein, MD
Fellow
Division of Pulmonary, Critical Care, and
    Sleep Medicine
Mount Sinai Beth Israel
New York, New York

Richard Huynh, MD
Fellow
Division of Pulmonary, Critical Care, and
    Sleep Medicine
Ronald Reagan UCLA Medical Center
Los Angeles, California

Omar Ibrahim, MD
Assistant Professor of Medicine
Director of Interventional Pulmonary
Division of Pulmonary and Critical Care Medicine
University of Connecticut School of Medicine
Farmington, Connecticut

Adam Jacobi, MD
Assistant Professor of Radiology
Icahn School of Medicine at Mount Sinai
Department of Radiology
Mount Sinai Hospital
New York, New York

Jimmy Johannes, MD
Fellow
Division of Pulmonary, Critical Care, and
    Sleep Medicine
Ronald Reagan UCLA Medical Center
Los Angeles, California

Colleen Keyes, MD, MPH
Associate Program Director, Combined BIDMC-MGH
    Interventional Pulmonary Fellowship
Division of Pulmonary, Critical Care, and
    Sleep Medicine
Massachusetts General Hospital
Instructor, Harvard Medical School
Boston, Massachusetts

Irene K. Louh, MD, PhD
Fellow
Division of Pulmonary, Allergy, and
    Critical Care Medicine
Columbia University Medical Center
New York, New York

Nagendra Madisi, MD
Fellow
Division of Surgical Critical Care
Mount Sinai Hospital
New York, New York

Amit Mahajan, MD
Cardiac, Vascular, and Surgical Associates
Interventional Pulmonology INOVA Fairfax Hospital
Falls Church, Virginia

Evelyn Mai, MD
Faculty
Division of Pulmonary, Critical Care, and
    Sleep Medicine
Geisinger Medical Center
Danville, Pennsylvania

Adnan Majid, MD
Director, Section of Interventional Pulmonology
Director, Combined BIDMC-MGH Interventional
    Pulmonology Fellowship
Division of Thoracic Surgery and Interventional
    Pulmonology
Beth Israel Deaconess Medical Center
Associate Professor of Medicine
Harvard Medical School
Boston, Massachusetts

Joseph Marchione, MD
Resident
Department of Radiology
Mount Sinai Hospital
New York, New York

Michael Marino, DO
Faculty
Division of Pulmonary, Critical Care, and
    Sleep Medicine
Geisinger Medical Center
Danville, Pennsylvania

Andrew Matragrano, MD
Director of Pulmonary Function Lab
Geisinger Medical Center
Danville, Pennsylvania

Tessy Paul, MD
Fellow
Division of Pulmonary, Critical Care, and
    Sleep Medicine
Ronald Reagan UCLA Medical Center
Los Angeles, California

Luis D. Quintero, DO, MPH
Resident
Department of Internal Medicine
Mount Sinai Beth Israel
New York, New York

Navitha Ramesh, MD
Fellow
Division of Pulmonary, Critical Care, and
    Sleep Medicine
Mount Sinai Beth Israel Medical Center
New York, New York

Abul Ala Syed Rifat Mannan, MD
Resident
Department of Pathology
Mount Sinai St. Luke's Roosevelt Hospital Center
New York, New York

Hilary Robbins, MD
Assistant Professor of Clinical Medicine
Lung Transplant Program
Division of Pulmonary, Allergy, and
    Critical Care Medicine
New York Presbyterian-Columbia
New York, New York

Mary Salvatore, MD
Assistant Professor of Radiology
Icahn School of Medicine at Mount Sinai
Department of Radiology
Mount Sinai Hospital
New York, New York

Amar Anantdeep Singh Sarao, MD
Fellow
Division of Surgical Critical Care
Mount Sinai Hospital
New York, New York

Lori Shah, MD
Assistant Professor of Clinical Medicine
Lung Transplant Program
Division of Pulmonary, Allergy, and Critical Medicine
New York Presbyterian-Columbia
Medical Center
New York, New York

Michael Silverberg, MD
Faculty
Division of Pulmonary, Critical Care, and
Sleep Medicine
Hackensack University Medical Center
Hackensack, New Jersey

Stephen Spindel, MD
Resident
Department of Cardiothoracic Surgery
Mount Sinai Hospital
New York, New York

Roxana Sulica, MD
Director of Pulmonary Hypertension Program
Assistant Professor of Medicine
Icahn School of Medicine at Mount Sinai
Division of Pulmonary, Critical Care, and
Sleep Medicine
Mount Sinai Beth Israel
New York, New York

Sarun Thomas, DO
Fellow
Division of Pulmonary, Critical Care, and
Sleep Medicine
Mount Sinai Beth Israel
New York, New York

Patricia Walker, MD
Co-director of Adult Cystic Fibrosis Center
Acting Chief
Division of Pulmonary, Critical Care, and
Sleep Medicine
Mount Sinai Beth Israel
New York, New York

Brian M. Walsh, DO
Fellow
Division of Pulmonary, Critical Care, and
Sleep Medicine
Geisinger Medical Center
Danville, Pennsylvania

Tisha Wang, MD
Assistant Clinical Professor of Medicine
Fellowship Program Director
Associate Chief of Inpatient Services and Training
Division of Pulmonary, Critical Care, and
Sleep Medicine
David Geffen School of Medicine at UCLA
Ronald Reagan UCLA Medical Center
Los Angeles, California

Stacey Verzosa Weisman, MD
Associate Professor of Radiology
Mount Sinai Health Systems – Beth Israel,
St. Luke's, and Roosevelt Hospitals
New York, New York

Songyang Yuan, MD, PhD
Faculty
Department of Pathology
Mount Sinai Beth Israel Medical Center
New York, New York

Rafael Alba Yunen, MD
Fellow
Division of Surgical Critical Care
Mount Sinai Hospital
New York, New York

Preface

McGraw Hill's *Pulmonary Disease Examination and Board Review* is intended for the resident with an interest in pulmonary disease, the pulmonary fellow, and the pulmonary attending studying for the boards. The idea for the book began with a desire to not only pass the boards but obtain a deeper understanding of pulmonary diseases. For that reason, I have asked physicians from the departments of radiology, pathology, cardiothoracic surgery, pulmonary and critical care to provide a multidisciplinary perspective. The content consists of current diagnostic and therapeutic approaches as well as the fundamentals of medicine such as physiology, microbiology, and cellular immunology. The vignettes simulate clinical dilemmas that may evolve over time to illustrate the clinical course of each pulmonary disease, and present diagnostic confounders and treatment-associated complications.

I am hopeful that this book will reinforce or enhance your knowledge of pulmonary disease and help you pass the pulmonary boards.

Ronaldo Collo Go, MD
Editor
Faculty
Division of Pulmonary, Critical Care, and
Sleep Medicine
Mount Sinai Beth Israel
New York, New York
and
Crystal Run Health Care
Middletown, New York

Preface

McGraw-Hill's Pulmonary Disease Examination and Board Review is intended for the resident with an interest in pulmonary disease, the pulmonary fellow and the pulmonary attending studying for the boards. The idea for the book began with a desire to not only pass the boards but obtain a deeper understanding of pulmonary diseases. For that reason, I have asked physicians from the departments of radiology, pathology, cardiothoracic surgery, pulmonary, and critical care to provide a multidisciplinary perspective. The content consists of current diagnostic and therapeutic approaches as well as the fundamentals of medicine such as physiology, immunology, and cellular immunology. The vignettes stimulate clinical dilemmas that may evolve over time to illustrate the clinical course of each pulmonary disease, and present diagnostic conundrums, and treatment associated complications.

I am hopeful that this book will reinforce or enhance your knowledge of pulmonary disease and help you pass the pulmonary boards.

Ronaldo Collo Go, MD
Editor
Faculty
Division of Pulmonary, Critical Care, and Sleep Medicine
Mount Sinai Beth Israel
New York, New York
and
Crystal Run Health Care
Middletown, New York

The Cell and Immunology

Ronaldo Collo Go MD

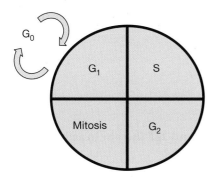

Question 1: What stage of the cell cycle is the first checkpoint for aberrant DNA?

A. G_0
B. Mitosis
C. G_1
D. S
E. G_2

Question 2: Which of the following is responsible for senescence?

A. Telomere
B. Mitochondria
C. Cytokine
D. Integrin
E. tRNA

Question 3: Which of the following confers resistance to tyrosine kinase inhibitors in patients with EGFR mutations?

A. Deletions on exon 19
B. Point mutation in L858R in exon 21
C. V600 mutation

D. p85a mutation
E. T790M point mutation

CASE 2

Human immune system consists of two parts: innate immunity which recognizes pathogen receptor motifs in many microbes and adaptive immunity which involves generation of specific antigen receptors on T and B cells.

Question 1: Which of the following have azurophilic granules?

A. Macrophages
B. Dendritic cells
C. Natural killer cells
D. Neutrophils
E. Eosinophils

Question 2: An important component of the innate immunity is the complement system. Which complement component is responsible for the membrane attack complex?

A. C4 a
B. C3 a
C. C3 b
D. C5 a
E. C5–9

Question 3: Cytokines are proteins that are critical in both innate and adaptive immunity. They function to promote active immune cells and mediate the inflammatory response. Different cytokines have similar functions and each cytokine may have different actions on different cells. Their actions can be autocrine, paracrine, or endocrine. Which cytokine is responsible for the release of eosinophils?

A. IL-5
B. IL-1, IL-6, TNF-alpha
C. IL-2
D. Il-17
E. IL-10

Question 4: Adaptive immunity requires an initial contact with the antigen followed by a more vigorous inflammatory response after re-exposure to the antigen. Bone marrow is the major site for B cells and thymus is the major site for T cells. In the lymph nodes, the T cells are in the deep paracortical areas around B-cell germinal centers. Two important subsets of T cells include the cytotoxic CD8+/MHC Class I and helper CD4+/MHC Class II. Which of the following is true regarding the T-cell receptor (TCR) recognition of an antigen?

A. It is a heterodimer with CD3 subunits.
B. It closely resembles the immunoglobulin heavy and light chains.
C. Diversity is determined by rearrangements of V (variable), D (diversity), and J (joining) regions.
D. TCR recognizes protein antigen peptides which have been "processed" by antigen presenting cells.
E. All of the above.

Question 5: B cells express immunoglobulins on their surface which can recognize unprocessed native antigens and components of activated complement. Which immunoglobulin is found as either a monomer or dimer, with J chain, and has secretory properties?

A. IgG
B. IgA
C. IgM
D. IgD
E. IgE

Question 6: What type of hypersensitivity involves arthus reaction?

A. Type I hypersensitivity reaction
B. Type II hypersensitivity reaction
C. Type III hypersensitivity reaction
D. Type IV hypersensitivity reaction
E. Type V hypersensitivity reaction

Question 7: Which interferon is prominent in granuloma formation in sarcoidosis?

A. Interferon alpha
B. Interferon beta
C. Interferon gamma
D. Interferon alpha and beta
E. All of the above

Question 8: Which Toll-like receptor proteins are associated with gram-negative septic shock?

A. TLR1
B. TLR3
C. TLR4
D. TLR5
E. TLR6

Question 9: Anti-IgE therapy in asthma involves which type of antibody?

A. IgG
B. IgA
C. IgM
D. IgD
E. None of the above

Question 10: Which of the following is profibrotic?

A. TGF-beta
B. Platelet-derived growth factor
C. Insulin-like growth factor
D. Connective tissue growth factor
E. All of the above

Answers

CASE 1

Question 1: C. G_1

The cell cycle leads to duplication and division of one cell into two daughter cells. It consists of two phases: interphase and mitosis. Interphase consists of three events: G_1 is the biosynthetic and growth stage, S phase is where DNA is replicated, and G_2 is continued growth and preparation for karyokinesis, or mitosis. Mitosis is further subdivided into: prophase, metaphase, anaphase, telophase, and cytokinesis. G_0 is a state of senescence where cells stop dividing, sometimes due to nonviable progeny. Progression of the cell cycle is dependent on a heterodimer that consists of cyclin, which is the regulatory unit, and a catalytic unit, cyclin-dependent kinase (CDK). Once activated by cyclin, the CDK phosphorylates and activates or inactivates a target protein.

* *

There are three checkpoints: G_1, G_2, and the metaphase of mitosis. In the G_1 and G_2 phase, P53 acts as a gate keeper and prevents further replication and synthesis of aberrant DNA.[1]

* *

Target cells in lung cancer are the basal bronchial cells and clara cells. Tumor growth is enhanced by evasion of apoptosis through death cell dysregulation via FAS ligand and E2F (Figs. 1–1 and 1–2), cell immortalization via telomerase, epigenetic modification via DNA methylation, and miRNA.[2]

* *

One of the most well-studied risk factors, tobacco, with polycyclic aromatic hydrocarbons and nitrosamines, cause genetic mutations via DNA adducts. Excision of these adducts occurs via nucleotide repair family which includes ERCC1 and XRCC. Persistence of adducts lead to mutations such as in either P53, which is usually not seen in immunohistochemistry because of the short half-life, 14[ARF], RAS, or INKa family. Less than 20% of smokers develop cancer suggesting a genetic predisposition. Polymorphisms in cytochrome P450 1A1 gene, GSTM1 homozygous deletion, polymorphisms in DNA repair gene, and nicotinic receptor polymorphism at chromosome locus 15q25 can predispose a person to lung cancer risk.

Question 2: A. Telomere

Telomeres are repetitive nucleotide sequences, usually TTAGGG, and act as buffers from chromosomal deterioration. Telomeres shorten after each cell division. Telomerase, the enzyme responsible for addition of this nucleotide sequence, has two subunits: hTERT, the reverse transcriptase, and hTR, an RNA that contains telomere template repeat. Stability is dependent on X-chromosome DKC1 gene. Shortened telomeres are perceived as damaged DNA and undergo apoptosis or senescence via P53/ATM pathway.

* *

Telomeres are important in lung diseases. Idiopathic pulmonary fibrosis is the most commonly associated manifestation of telomerase mutations, particularly when involving hTERT, hTR, and DKC1.[3] Besides lung diseases, shortened telomeres cause accelerated aging as seen in aplastic anemia and dyskeratosis congenital (DC). In lung carcinogenesis, these shortened telomeres continue to proliferate because P53 pathway is inactivated. COPD is found as early manifestations in telomerase mutation carriers.

Question 3: E. T790 point mutation

Due to its association with carcinogenesis, one of the most studied growth signaling pathways is EGFR. Ligands bind to the extracellular domains which result in heterodimer or homodimer formation and transphosphorylation. This leads to activation of two sets of downstream signaling: RAS/mitogen-activated protein kinase and P13 K/AKT pathways. Mutations or dysregulation on any component of the pathway cause them to be oncogenes. One of the most common mutations is deletions

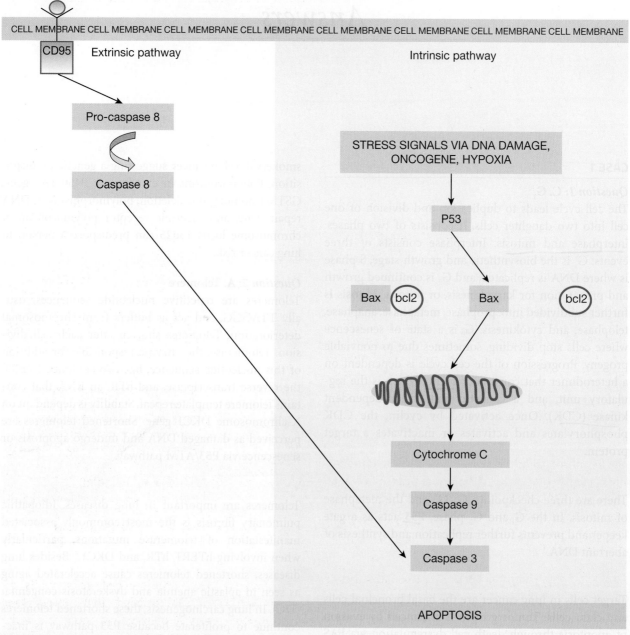

Figure 1–1 There are two pathways leading to apoptosis. The intrinsic pathway involves the P53 system which detects stress signals via DNA damage, oncogene, and hypoxia. This activates the BAX to proceed to increased permeability and release of cytochrome C. The extrinsic pathway involves binding of Fas Ligand and entering the apoptosis pathway via Caspase 3.

on exon 19 and point mutation in L858R in exon 21. KRAS can have missense mutations; BRAF has V600 mutation; and PI3 K has mutations in p85a subunit. Some mutations are sensitive to certain chemotherapies while others render them resistant. For example, primary resistance to TKI to EGFR is secondary to exon 20 insertion mutations and secondary resistance to T790M point mutation.

CASE 2

Question 1: D. Neutrophils
Azurophilic granules contain antimicrobial elements such as myeloperoxidase, phospholipase A2, acid hydrolases, elastase, defensins, proteases, lysozymes, and cathepsin G. They are most closely associated with neutrophils.

**

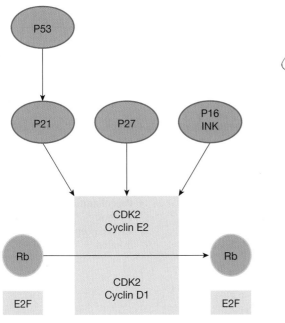

Figure 1–2 Rb Pathway. The retinoblastoma pathway is the downstream pathway for P53 and disrupts G_1 entry to S phase. This is highlighted by phosphorylation of Rb/E2F product, causing dissociation of E2F from Rb. (Reproduced with permission of Brambilla E, Gazdar A. Pathogenesis of lung cancer signalling pathways: roadmap for therapies. *Eur Respir J.* 2009; 33(6):1485–1497.)

The five phases of host defense include: (1) migration of leukocytes to antigen; (2) antigen recognition by innate immunity; (3) antigen recognition by adaptive immunity; (4) inflammatory response; and (5) destruction and removal of particles.

* *

Migration of the leukocyte, such as a neutrophil, involves interaction with endothelial cells and conformational change with their adhesion molecules. The first stage, called attachment and rolling, involves leukocyte leaving the blood stream through the post-capillary venule, mediated by L-selectin molecule. The second stage, firm adhesion with activation-dependent stable arrest, is attachment of leukocyte to high endothelial venules via cytokines. The third stage is the migration of leukocyte to endothelial cells and release of matrix metalloprotenases which digest the subendothelial basement membrane.

Question 2: E. C5–9
The complement system is a cascading series of reactions which results in cell lysis. There are three pathways: classic activation pathway via immune complex, mannose-binding lectin pathway, and alternative pathway.

Effector Cells	
Macrophages	First line of defense of innate immunity Binding LPS APC to T lymphocytes Secretions of IL-1, TNF-a, IL-12, IL-6
Dendritic cells	APC CD83, MHC II, multiple thin membrane projectile Most potent producers of IFN-alpha
Natural killer cells	Surface receptors for Fc of IgG, NCAM-I (CD56), CD8 Dual role: Antibody-dependent cytotoxicity and nonimmune killing of target cells Killing ability is inversely related to levels of MHC I
Granulocytes:	
Neutrophils	Fc receptors for IgG (CD16) and for complement components (C3b and CD35) Secretes azurophilic granules into the surface generating superoxide radicals after stimulation from immune complexes or opsonized bacteria
Eosinophils	Fc receptors of IgG (CD32) Cytotoxic to parasitic infections Contents include major basic protein, eosinophilic cationic protein, neurotoxin and Anti-inflammatory enzymes such as histaminase, arylsulfase, phospholipase D
Basophils	IL-4 High affinity for IgE (FCRI) Release histaminine, eosinophlic chemotactic factor, neutral protease Expresses C3a and C5b receptors

C4a, C3a, and C5a release histamine from basophils and mast cells.[4] C3b and C3bi participate in the phagocytosis by neutrophils and macrophages and participate in the formation of immune complex. C5–9 is the membrane attack complex.

Question 3: A. IL-5
Recognition interleukins and their roles might have therapeutic implications such as in asthma. The normal airway is rich with Th1 cells. In an asthmatic airway, they are rich in Th2 cells.[8] Below is a table that lists selected interleukins, their mechanisms, and associated drugs.[8]

Question 4: E. All of the above
MHC-peptide-TCR is the initiation of an antigen driven immune response. The major histocompatibility complex (MHC), also called human leukocyte antigen

Interleukin	Mechanism	Drugs
IL-1	• Stimulates IL-5 release from smooth muscles and influences eosinophilic recruitment and activation	• Anakinra–inhaled IL-1R antagonist
IL-2	• Promotes effector T-cell and T-reg responses • Secreted by malignancies and its antibodies have been used to suppress rejection in organ transplants	• Daclizumab–antibody against a subunit of IL-2 receptor
IL-5	• Promotes proliferation, differentiation and survival of eosinophils and development of basophils and mast cells	• Mepolizumab and reslizumab are IL-5 antibodies • Benralizumab–antibody against alpha chain of IL-R5
IL-4 IL-13	• Highly involved in allergic reaction and following signaling via STAT6 • Produce IgE • Associated with subepithelial fibrosis and airway remodeling • Fibroblastic	• Lebrikizumab—IL-13 antibody • Pascolizumab—anti-IL-4 antibody • Altrakincept and nuvance–inhaled
IL-6	• Promotes Th2 and Th17 differentiation and Th1 suppression	
IL-8	• Induces migration of neutrophils, monocytes and eosinophils to sites of inflammation	
IL-9	• Role in airway hyperresponsiveness, eosinophilia, and IgE	
IL-10	• Anti-inflammatory and inhibits release of IL-1,IL-6,IL-12, and TNF-alpha • Deactivates macrophages, mast cells, and eosinophils	• Corticosteroids • Vitamin D
IL-12	• Suppress allergies and eosinophilia	
IL-17	• Proinflammatory and released by IL-23 • Secreted by Th17 • Role in neutrophilic asthma and corticosteroid insensitive	• Secukinumab
IL-22	• Acts on nonhematopoietic tissue to secret antimicrobial peptides and maintain cellular integrity	
IL-25	• Causes eosinophilia indirectly by increasing secretion of IL-5	
IL-33	• Released from necrotic cells and leads to Th2 response	

(HLA) complex, is located on chromosome 6 and has a role on antigen specificity and presentation. They have roles in pathogen resistance and autoimmune disease. There are two classes. Class I—HLA-A,-B, and -C—appear to have particular characteristics such as polymorphism and linkage disequilibrium. Recognized by CD8 cells, class I allele has a heavy chain and a nonpolymorphic B_2-microglobulin light chain. Recognized by CD4 cells, class II consists of a heterodimer with amino-terminal domains representing antigen-binding regions.

* *

The association of HLA and sarcoidosis has been well documented, initially with Class I HLA-B8 but more so with Class II HLA, with variable implications.[13] HLA-DQB1*0201 and HLA-DRB1-301 are associated with good prognosis in British and Dutch and in Swedish respectively.[14,15] HLA-DRB1*01 and HLA-DQB1*0501 have been shown to be protective against sarcoidosis.[14]

Other groups of HLA are organ specific such as: HLA-DRB1*12 and HLA-DRB1*14 are associated with lung involvement, HLA-DRB1*04-BQB1*0301 are associated with uveitis, and HLA-DQB1*0601 are associated with cardiac involvement.[13–18]

* *

CD4 helper T cells produce cytokines. Th1 CD4+ aide in cellular killing and help generate opsonizing antibodies that lead to a delayed hypersensitivity response. They secrete IL-2, IFN-gamma, IL-3, TNF-alpha, GM-CSF, and TNF-beta. Th2 CD4+ produce IL3-6, IL-10, and IL-13 that regulate humoral immunity and isotype switching.

* *

CD4 and CD8 regulatory T cells are produced by dendritic cells and suppress immune response, particularly those from self-antigens.

Question 5: B. IgA

Immunoglobulins are products of B cells and mediate humoral response by binding to antigen and promote inactivation or removal of an offending substance. The basic structure consists of two heavy chains, which determine the subtype, and two light chains. Each chain has a constant and variable region. Disulfide bridges link the heavy chains together and the heavy chain to the light chain. The variable regions are also the antibody-binding sites.

IgG	Monomer Mass = 150 kDa 75–85% total Serum Ig Binding Macrophages, neutrophils, lymphocytes Crosses placenta, secondary response
IgA	Monomer, dimer J chain Mass = 150-600 kDa 7–15% total Serum Ig Binding of lymphocytes Secretory
IgM	Pentamer, hexamer J chain Mass = 950–1150 kDa 5–10% total Serum Ig Binding of lymphocytes Primary response, Autoimmune diseases
IgD	Monomer Mass = 175 kDa 0.3 % of total Serum Ig Mature B Cell Marker
IgE	Monomer Mass = 190 kDa 0.019% total Serum Ig Binding of Mast cells, Basophils, and B cells Allergic response, antiparasitic response

Question 6: C. Type III Hypersensitivity Reaction

Type I: immediate hypersensitivity with IgE	Anaphylaxis
Type II: cytotoxic hypersensitivity with IgG or IgM	Hemolytic anemia
Type III: circulating antigen–antibody immune complexes	Serum sickness, arthus reaction
Type IV: delayed hypersensitivity	Contact dermatitis

Question 7: C. Interferon gamma

Interferons are glycoproteins with immunomodulatory properties and act primarily as a response to viral infections but have roles in response to tumor cells, parasites, and bacteria. Type I IFN, which consists of IFN-alpha and IFN-beta, is produced by nucleated cells and Type II IFN-gamma is produced by NK cells and T lymphocytes.

* *

Granulomas form to contain pathogen and limit inflammation. Interferon alpha promotes overexpression of major histocompatibility complex (MHC) II on antigen presenting cell. This leads to increased cytokine release from dendritic cells, IL-12 from monocytes, and interferon gamma from natural killer cells. Treatment with interferon therapy has led to interferon-induced sarcoidosis.[5] This can be seen in interferon alpha therapy for hepatitis C but case reports have suggested the development of sarcoidosis from interferon beta therapy in patient with multiple sclerosis and renal cell carcinoma.[6] The dependence of sarcoidosis on CD4 counts was observed in a retrospective study HIV that showed patients with CD4>200 were more likely to have sarcoidosis than those with CD4<200.[7]

Question 8: C. TLR4

Toll-like receptors initiate the adaptive immune response and have also had roles in the development of septic shock.[12] They are associated with CD14 and are expressed on macrophages, dendritic cells, and B cells. They activate intracellular signaling that lead to bacterial and viral killing. TLR2 and TLR4 have been studied in their role in gram-negative septic shock.

Question 9: A. IgG

Anti-IgE therapy, such as omalizumab, is an IgG antibody that binds to IgE.[9,11] It is recommended for patients with moderate to severe asthma, a total serum IgE 30 to 700 IU/mL, inadequately controlled on high dose–inhaled corticosteroids, and positive skin testing and in vitro testing.[11]

Question 10: E. All of the above

Pulmonary fibrosis consists of an inflammatory state that results in excessive extracellular matrix accumulation and lung architecture distortion. This is a consequence of abnormal re-epithelization and an imbalance between inflammatory molecules, fibrogenetic and antifibrogenic molecules, oxidants and antioxidants, and antivascular and provascular molecules. Sites of epithelial injury show migration and organization of fibroblasts and myofibroblasts into fibrotic foci. Fibroblasts differentiate into myofibroblasts and perpetuate collagen synthesis, and decreased synthesis of tissue inhibitor of metalloproteinase. The following table lists the cells or molecules and their mechanisms in pulmonary fibrosis.[10]

Cells or Molecules	Mechanisms in Pulmonary Fibrosis
Transforming growth factor beta	• Stimulates fibroblast production, myofibroblast differentiation, resistance to apoptosis, and ROS production
Connective tissue growth factor	• Stimulates fibroblast production and ECM production
Platelet growth factor	• Stimulates fibroblast production and chemotaxis
Insulin-like growth factor	• Stimulates fibroblast production
T cells	• Profibrotic via TLR -beta and PDGF • CD8+ T cells associated with worse prognosis
Macrophages	• Overexpression of reactive oxygen species • Profibrotic • Receptors to proteinase
B Cells	• Autoantibodies against periplakin, a component of desmosomes • Overexpression of CD19 • May have some "protective" effects although this remains unclear
Fibrocytes	• Bone marrow derived, they produce collagen and express CD45 (leukocytes) and CD34 (stem cells) • Differentiate to myofibroblasts and contribute to ECM or differentiate into mesenchymal cells • Recruitment dependent on CXCL12, CCL2, CCL3, and IL-10
CD40–CD40 L	• Co-stimulators in the activation of CD4+ cells via CD40L and antigen presenting cell (APC) via CD40 • With IL-4, promotes fibroblasts
Fas–FasL	• Inherent resistance to apoptosis • Cells within fibroblastic foci have minimal or absent expression of Fas
Integrins	• Cell surface molecules involve in adhesion between cell to cell and cell to ECM • Roles in cell migration, growth, and survival

REFERENCES

1. Rom WN, Hay JG, Lee TC, et al. Molecular and genetic aspects of lung cancer. *Am J Respir Crit Care Med.* 2000; 161:1355–1367.

2. Brambilla E, Gazdar A. Pathogenesis of lung cancer signaling pathways: roadway to therapies. *Eur Respir J.* 2009;33(6): 1485–1497.

3. Armanios, M. Telomerase and idiopathic pulmonary fibrosis. *Mutat Res.* 2012;730:52–58.

4. Stone KD, Prussin C, Metcalfe DD. IgE, mast cells, basophils and eosinophils. *J Allergic Clin Immunol.* 2010;125:S73–S80.

5. Marzouk K, Saleh S, Kannass M, et al. Interferon-induced granulomatous lung disease. *Curr Opin Pulm Med.* 2004; 10(5):435–440.

6. Petousi N, Thomas EC. Interferon-B-induced pulmonary sarcoidosis in a 30-year-old woman treated for multiple sclerosis. *J Med Case Reports.* 2012;6:344.

7. Morris DG, Jasmer RM, Huang L, et al. Sarcoidosis following HIV Infection: Evidence for CD4+ lymphocyte dependence. *Chest.* 2003;124:929–935.

8. Garcia G, Taille C, Pierantonio L, et al. Anti-interleukin-5 therapy in severe asthma. *Eur Respir Rev.* 2013;22:251–257.

9. Gibeon D, Menzies-Gow AN. Targeting interleukins to treat severe asthma. *Expert Rev Respir Med.* 2012;6(4):423–429.

10. Todd NW, Lyzina IG, Atamas SP. Molecular and cellular mechanisms of pulmonary fibrosis. *Fibrogenesis Tissue Repair.* 2012;5(11):1–24.

11. Strunk RC, Bloomberg GR. Omalizumab for asthma. *N Engl J Med.* 2006;354:2689–2695.

12. Abbas AK, Lichtman AH. *Basic Immunology.* New York, NY: Saunders; 2010.

13. Inannuzzi MC, Rybicki BA, Teirstein AS. Sarcoidoisis. *N Engl J Med.* 2007;357:2153–2165.

14. Grunewald J, Eklund A. Lofgren's Syndrome. Human Leukocyte Antigen Strongly Influences the Disease. Course. *Am J Respir Crit Care Med.* 2009;179:307–312.

15. Sato H, Grutters JC, Pantelidis P, et al. HLA-DQB1*0201. *Am J Respir Cell Mol Biol.* 2002;27:406–412.

16. Sato H, Woodhead FA, Ahmad T, et al. Sarcoidosis HLA Class II genotype distinguishes differences of clinical phenotype across ethnic groups. *Hum Mol Gen.* 2012;19: 4100–4111.

17. Iannuzzi MC, Maliarik MJ, Poisson LM, et al. Sarcoidosis susceptibility and resistance HLA-DQB1 alleles in African Americans. *Am J Respir Crit Care Med.* 2003;167:1225–1231.

18. Ayyala US, Nair AP, Padilla ML. Cardiac Sarcoidosis. *Clin Chest Med.* 2008;29:493–508.

2
Pulmonary Function Tests

Ronald Evans DO, Ronaldo Collo Go MD, Andrew Matragrano MD, and Paul Simonelli MD, PhD

CASE 1

A 24-year-old woman is being evaluated for chronic cough with a pulmonary function test.

* *

Volume versus Time and Flow versus Time is seen below.

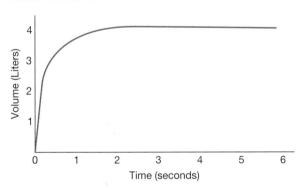

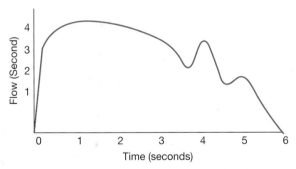

Question 1: **What kind of artifact do you see?**

A. Cough
B. Hesitation
C. Early termination
D. Air leak
E. Glottis closure

Question 2: **Which of the following is part of the reproducibility criteria?**

A. No artifacts
B. Exhalation >6 seconds
C. Two largest values of FVC are within 0.150 L from each other
D. The start is <5% extrapolated volume of FVC
E. Plateau in volume-time curve

CASE 2

A 30-year-old woman, 34 weeks age of gestation with history of asthma comes in for routine follow-up.

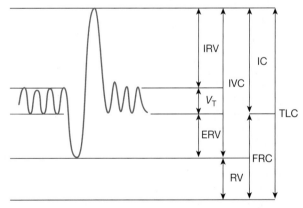

Reproduced with permission from Wanger J, Clausen JL, Coates A, et al. Standardisation of the measurement of lung volumes. *Eur Respir J.* 2005;26(3):511–522.

Question 1: **Which of the following is increased during the third trimester of pregnancy?**

A. V_T and IC
B. IVC
C. FRC, ERV, RV

D. TLC

E. ERV, IRV

Question 2: **Which of the following is primarily measured by body plethysmography and gas dilution techniques?**

A. V_T

B. IVC

C. RV

D. TLC

E. FRC

CASE 3

A 50-year-old man with COPD was referred to your clinic for his pulmonary disease. Pulmonary function tests were ordered as part of the initial evaluation.

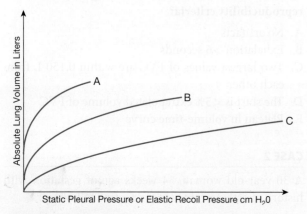

Modified with permission from Hyatt RE, Scanlon PD, Nakamura M. *Interpretation of Pulmonary Function Tests.* 3rd ed. Philadelphia, PA: Wolters-Kluwer/Lipincott Williams & Wilkins; 2008.

Question 1: **In the static pleural pressure versus lung volume graph above, which is more likely to represent this patient?**

A. A

B. B

C. C

D. A and C

E. All of the above

Question 2: **The patient had a single breath nitrogen test and the graph is below. Which portion of the graph illustrates the nonuniform ventilation secondary to his disease?**

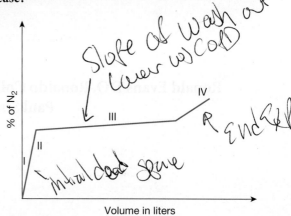

A. I

B. II

C. III

D. IV

E. All of the above

CASE 4

A 24-year-old man who was clinically diagnosed with childhood asthma arrives in clinic for asthma evaluation. He is asymptomatic and has no complaints.

* *

On physical examination, his vital signs are within normal limits, including pulse oximetry of 97% on room air. He appears fit and muscular. His heart and lung examination is normal. Chest x-ray is also normal.

* *

Spirometry performed by his primary care physician prior to specialty consultation is as follows:

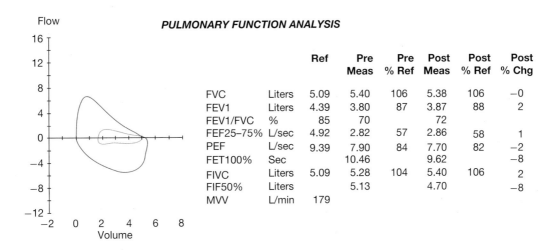

PULMONARY FUNCTION ANALYSIS

		Ref	Pre Meas	Pre % Ref	Post Meas	Post % Ref	Post % Chg
FVC	Liters	5.09	5.40	106	5.38	106	−0
FEV1	Liters	4.39	3.80	87	3.87	88	2
FEV1/FVC	%	85	70		72		
FEF25–75%	L/sec	4.92	2.82	57	2.86	58	1
PEF	L/sec	9.39	7.90	84	7.70	82	−2
FET100%	Sec		10.46		9.62		−8
FIVC	Liters	5.09	5.28	104	5.40	106	2
FIF50%	Liters		5.13		4.70		−8
MVV	L/min	179					

* *

He is sent for a methacholine challenge test as there is a strong need to clarify if he truly has a diagnosis of asthma. Results of the methacholine challenge test are as follows:

	BASELINE		MAX RESPONSE			Post-BD	
	Pred	Actual	% Pred	Actual	% Chng	Actual	% Chng
— SPIROMETRY —							
FVC (L)	5.05	5.20	102	4.38	−15	5.30	+2
FEV₁ (L)	4.20	3.69	87	2.86	−22	3.79	+2
FEF 25–75% (L/sec)	4.45	2.67	59	1.06	−60	2.85	+6
FEF max (L/sec)	9.52	8.73	91	6.34	−27	8.30	−4

Stage	BASELINE	0.031 MG/ML	0.0625 MG/ML	0.125 MG/ML
Dose	0.00000	0.03100	0.06250	0.12500
Does Units	0.00000	0.15500	0.31250	0.62500
C.D.U.s	0.00000	0.15500	0.46750	1.09250
— SPIROMETRY —				
FVC (L)	5.20	5.24	5.15	5.13
% Change	+0	+0	+0	−1
FEV_1 (L)	3.69	3.65	3.58	3.49
% Change	+0	+0	−2	−5
FEF 25–75% (L/sec)	2.67	2.62	2.47	2.28
% Change	+0	−1	−7	−14
FEF max (L/sec)	8.73	8.19	7.69	7.74
% Change	+0	−6	−11	−11

Stage	0.25 MG/ML	0.5 MG/ML	1 MG/ML	2 MG/ML
Dose	0.25000	0.50000	1.00000	2.00000
Dose units	1.25000	2.50000	3.00000	10.00000
C.D.U.s	2.34250	4.84250	9.842S0	19.84250
— SPIROMETRY —				
FVC (L)	5.05	4.93	4.74	4.84
% Change	−2	−5	−8	−6
FEV_1 (L)	3.44	3.28	3.18	3.27
% Change	−6	−10	−13	−11
FEF 25–75% (L/sec)	2.15	1.87	1.68	1.81
% Change	−19	−30	−37	−31
FEF max (L/sec)	7.23	7.55	7.08	7.29
% Change	−17	−13	−18	−16

Stage	4 MG/ML	8 MG/ML	POST-BRONCH
Dose	4.00000	8.00000	0.00000
Dose Units	20.00000	40.00000	0.00000
C.D.U.s	39.84250	79.84250	79.84250
— SPIROMETRY —			
FVC (L)	4.74	4.38	5.30
% Change	−8	−15	+2
FEV_1 (L)	3.13	2.86	3.79
% Change	−15	−22	+2
FEF 25–75% (L/sec)	1.59	1.06	2.85
% Change	−40	−60	+6
FEF max (L/sec)	7.05	6.34	8.30
% Change	−19	−27	−4

Question 1: **What can be said about this patient having a diagnosis of asthma?**

A. The patient absolutely has asthma as evidenced by the >20% decrease in FEV$_1$ during methacholine testing

B. The patient absolutely does not have a diagnosis of asthma as his FEV$_1$ did not fall below 20% until a concentration of 8 mg/mL methacholine

C. The probability of the patient having asthma is borderline due to the methacholine concentration needed to induce a 20% or greater decrease in FEV$_1$, but his lack of asthmatic symptoms give him a low pre-test probability for a diagnosis of asthma

D. PFTs prior to methacholine testing showed a 2% improvement in FEV$_1$ following bronchodilator. This alone shows bronchial responsiveness and proves enough evidence for the diagnosis of asthma in this patient

E. He has asthma as evidenced by the diagnosis he carries from childhood

Question 2: **Which of the following may have interfered with the methacholine challenge testing?**

A. The patient used albuterol inhaler 1 day prior to methacholine testing

B. The patient came to clinic after eating milk and oat cereal for breakfast prior to methacholine testing

C. The patient drank a cup of regular coffee on the way to his methacholine test

D. The patient took 1,000 mg acetaminophen on the morning of his methacholine test

E. He also takes lisinopril for hypertension

CASE 5

A 73-year-old man has recently been diagnosed with COPD and has smoked 1 pack per day for 50 years. He notes his shortness of breath is not limiting his daily activities and he continues doing strenuous manual labor around his home daily. He notes daily symptoms of cough productive of yellow-brown sputum and states he has one to two bouts of "bronchitis" per year, for which he sees his primary care physician and is typically treated with a course of oral antibiotics and oral corticosteroids.

* *

His physical examination is otherwise unremarkable except for a BMI 32 and occasional expiratory wheeze.

* *

Pulmonary function tests are shown below:

	Pre-Bronch			Post-Bronch			
	Actual	**Pred**	**% Pred**	**SD**	**LLN**	**Actual**	**% Chng**
— SPIROMETRY —							
FVC (L)	2.86	3.97	72	0.54	3.08		
FEV$_1$ (L)	1.42	2.88	49	0.45	2.14		
FEV$_1$/FVC (%)	50	73	67	6	63		
FEF 25% (L/sec)	1.61						
FEF 75% (L/sec)	0.27						
FEF 25–75% (L/sec)	0.58	2.12	27	0.92	0.60		
FEF max (L/sec)	3.75	7.56	49	1.33	5.37		
FIVC (L)	2.22						
FIF max (L/sec)	2.71						

(continued)

(*Continued*)

	Pre-Bronch			Post-Bronch			
	Actual	Pred	% Pred	SD	LLN	Actual	% Chng
— LUNG VOLUMES —							
SVC (L)	3.22	3.97	81	0.54	3.08		
IC (L)	2.43	3.12	77				
ERV (L)	0.79	0.85	92				
TGV (L)	5.25	3.54	148	0.72	2.10		
RV (Pleth) (L)	4.46	2.42	184	0.37	1.68		
TLC (Pleth) (L)	7.68	6.66	115	0.79	5.08		
RV/TLC (Pleth)(%)	58	37	157	4	29		
Trapped gas (L)							
— DIFFUSION —							
DLCOunc (mL/min/mm Hg)	15.09	29.49	51	4.83	19.83		
DLCOcor (mL/min/mm Hg)		29.49		4.83	19.83		
DL/VA (mL/min/mm Hg/L)	2.76	4.43	62				
VA (L)	5.47	6.66	82	0.79	5.36		
— AIRWAYS RESISTANCE —							
Raw (cmH$_2$O/L/s)		1.45		0.48	0.66		
Gaw (L/s/cmH$_2$O)		1.03					

● Pred   — Pre

Six-minute walk test results: Walked 372 m in 6 minutes

	SpO$_2$ (%)	Heart Rate	Borg Scale	O$_2$ (L/min)
Baseline	94	94	2	Room air
1 minute	93	99	2	Room air
2 minutes	93	102	3	Room air
3 minutes	93	100	3	Room air
4 minutes	94	104	4	Room air
5 minutes	94	103	4	Room air
6 minutes	93	103	4	Room air
Recovery				
1 minute	94	98	3	Room air
2 minutes	96	93	3	Room air
3 minutes	96	95	2	Room air
4 minutes	95	92	2	Room air
5 minutes	95	92	2	Room air

Question 1: **What does his pulmonary function testing and 6-minute walk test indicate about his lung disease?**

A. His COPD persists but is likely unchanged since previous testing 12 years earlier when the severity was moderate
B. His COPD is severe, lung volumes are suggestive of air trapping, his DLCO is moderately decreased, and there is no evidence of hypoxemia with exertion
C. His COPD is severe, lung volumes are not suggestive of air trapping, his DLCO is moderately decreased, and there is no evidence of hypoxemia with exertion
D. His COPD is very severe, lung volumes are suggestive of air trapping, his DLCO is moderately decreased, and there is no evidence of hypoxemia with exertion
E. His COPD is severe, lung volumes are suggestive of air trapping, his DLCO is severely decreased, and there is no evidence of hypoxemia with exertion

CASE 6

A 68-year-old man with 50 pack-years and quit 11 years ago, obstructive sleep apnea on CPAP, hypertension, GERD, and hypothyroidism presents for evaluation of increasing dyspnea on exertion. He can presently climb less than one flight of stairs before having to rest due to breathlessness. He also notes dyspnea when dressing himself. However, he has no shortness of breath at rest or when lying flat. He denies any occupational, environmental, or chemical exposures.

* *

His physical examination is remarkable for body mass index is 36 kg/m², Mallampati score of II, and bilateral crackles.

* *

His pulmonary function tests, including spirometry, lung volumes, DLCO, and 6-minute walk testing are performed. The results are below:

	Actual	Pred	% Pred	SD	LLN	Actual	% Chng
— SPIROMETRY —							
FVC (L)	2.32	4.12	56	0.53	3.25	2.25	−3
FEV$_1$ (L)	2.00	3.04	65	0.45	2.30	1.96	−2
FEV$_1$/FVC (%)	86	74	116	6	64	87	+1
FEF 25% (L/sec)	5.59					6.90	+23
FEF 75% (L/sec)	0.94					0.75	−20
FEF 25–75% (L/sec)	2.78	2.36	117	0.91	0.86	2.57	−7
FEF max (L/sec)	5.92	8.04	73	1.32	5.86	6.87	+16
FIVC (L)	1.73					1.81	+4
FIF max (L/sec)	3.73					4.10	+10

(continued)

(*Continued*)

	Actual	Pred	% Pred	SD	LLN	Actual	% Chng
— LUNG VOLUMES —							
SVC (L)	2.29	4.12	55	0.53	3.25		
IC (L)	1.79	3.12	57				
ERV (L)	0.50	1.00	50				
TGV (L)	2.70	3.44	78	0.72	2.00		
RV (Pleth) (L)	2.20	2.28	96	0.37	1.54		
TLC (Pleth) (L)	4.48	6.56	68	0.79	4.98		
RV/TLC (Pleth) (%)	49	35	139	4	27		
Trapped gas (L)							
— DIFFUSION —							
DLCOunc (mL/min/mm Hg)	10.76	30.32	35	4.83	20.66		
DLCOcor (mL/min/mm Hg)		30.32		4.83	20.66		
DL/VA (mL/min/mm Hg/L)	3.45	4.62	74				
VA (L)	3.12	6.56	47	0.79	5.26		
— AIRWAYS RESISTANCE —							
Raw (cmH$_2$O/L/s)		1.45		0.48	0.66		
Gaw (L/s/cmH$_2$O)		1.03					
sRaw (cmH$_2$O*s)		<4.76					
sGaw (1/cmH$_2$O*s)		0.20		0.07	0.08		

● Pred — Pre — Post

A 6-minute walk test: Walked 305 m in 6 minutes

	SpO$_2$ (%)	Heart Rate	Borg Scale	O$_2$ (L/min)
Baseline	95	83	2	Room air
1 minute	87	99	3	Room air
2 minutes	79	105	4	Room air
3 minutes	81	95	4	Room air
4 minutes	80	91	3	Room air
5 minutes	78	113	4	Room air
6 minutes	82	99	3	Room air

	SpO$_2$ (%)	Heart Rate	Borg Scale	O$_2$ (L/min)
Recovery				
1 minute	85	73	2	Room air
2 minutes	93	77	1	Room air
3 minutes	95	78	0	Room air
4 minutes	96	74	0	Room air
5 minutes	95	73	0	Room air

Question 1: **What is the major finding in the spirometry and lung volumes?**

A. Restrictive physiology but not true restriction due to the preserved total lung capacity
B. Obstructive lung disease due to the FEV_1 being less than the lower limit of normal
C. True restrictive disease
D. Emphysema due to the low DLCO
E. Normal spirometry

CASE 7

A 20-year-old woman with a past medical history significant for tobacco use (half pack of cigarettes per day for 4 years—quit 1 month prior to presentation), atrial septal defect, and mild intermittent asthma diagnosed clinically (without PFTs) when she was a child presents for evaluation of shortness of breath. Until recently, she has felt that her asthma symptoms were under control and had not used her albuterol inhaler for months. She notes an insidious onset of dyspnea on exertion over the past 1 to 2 years. She mainly has noted difficulty performing her daily aerobic exercise routine due to dyspnea. She notes she has tried her albuterol inhaler with only mild relief of her symptoms. She feels her symptoms only occur with physical exertion and feel different than her previous asthma symptoms.

* *

Physical examination is remarkable for BMI is 24 kg/m² and fixed split S2.

* *

Pulmonary function testing is performed and the results follow.

	Pre-Bronch					Post-Bronch		
	Actual	**Pred**	**% Pred**	**SD**	**LLN**	**Actual**	**% Pred**	**% Chng**
— SPIROMETRY —								
FVC (L)	4.03	3.97	101	0.44	3.24	4.23	106	+4
FEV_1 (L)	2.51	3.45	72	0.37	2.84	3.14	91	+25
FEV_1/FVC (%)	62	86	72	6	76	74	86	+19
FEF 25% (L/sec)	2.60	6.08	42	1.30	3.94	3.32	54	+27
FEF 75% (L/sw)	1.79	2.11	84	0.58	1.15	2.17	102	+21
FEF 25–75% (L/sec)	2.35	3.81	61	0.79	2.51	3.05	79	+29
FEF max (L/sec)	2.70	7.08	38	1.09	5.28	3.42	48	+26
FIVC (L)	2.17					2.17		+0
FIF max (L/sec)	2.58					3.89		+50
FEV_6 (L)	4.03	3.97	101	0.43	3.26	4.23	106	+4
Time to FEF max (sec)	0.355					0.465		+30

• Pred — Pre — Post

Question 1: **What does the flow-volume loop indicate?**

A. Classic obstructive lung disease. Most likely asthma
B. Restrictive physiology with likely "Fingerprinting" in the expiratory limb of the flow-volume loop
C. Variable extrathoracic obstruction
D. Variable intrathoracic obstruction
E. Fixed obstruction

CASE 8

A 50-year-old man with history of COPD and congestive heart failure is sent for cardiopulmonary exercise testing to evaluate his dyspnea. His medications consist of tiotropium, furosemide, metoprolol, lisinopril, and albuterol as needed. Review of prior chest computed tomography shows upper-lobe emphysematous changes with fibrotic changes in the lower lobes. The CPET is aborted for dyspnea.

CPET:

Work Rate	80	65% predicted	SaO_2%	93 Rest	84 Peak
VO_2	1.10	65% predicted	SpO_2%	90 Rest	84 Peak
AT	0.80	N	PaO_2	67 Rest	50 Peak
HR	135	85% predicted	$PaCO_2$	40 Rest	50 Peak
O_2 pulse	8	80% predicted	PO_2 (A–a)	20 Rest	35 Peak
BP	170/80		V_D/V_T	0.45	0.43
V_E	50	120% predicted			
FR	39	N			
V_E/VCO_2					
at AT	44				
RER	1				

(continued)

(*Continued*)

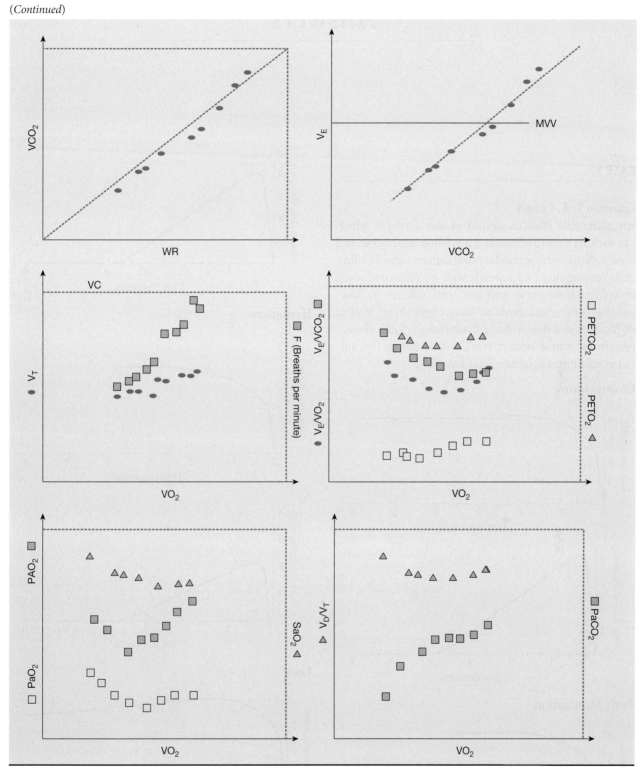

Modified with permission from American Thoracic Society; American College of Chest Physicians. ATS/ACCP Statement on cardiopulmonary exercise testing. *Am J Respir Crit Care Med.* 2003;167(2):211–277.

Question 1: What contributes to his exercise intolerance?

A. COPD

B. CHF

C. Interstitial lung disease

D. Psychogenic

E. None of the above

Answers

CASE 1

Question 1: A. Cough

An acceptable effort is devoid of any artifacts, which can include abnormalities in the volume-time curve and flow-volume curve secondary to cough or variable effort, early termination (<6 seconds with no plateau reached in volume-time curve and low total volume in flow-volume curve), leak (volume-time curve drops instead of plateaus and flow-volume backtracks), glottis closure (an abrupt stop in both curves), and hesitation (the initial exhalation is delayed or not forceful).

Glottis closure

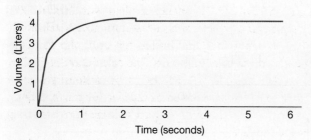

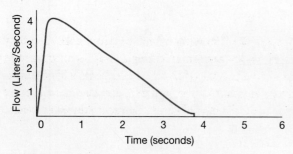

Early termination

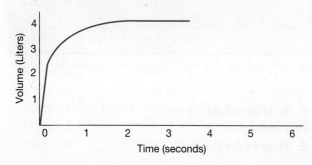

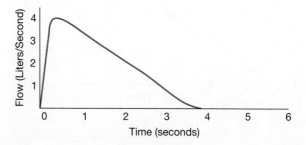

Hesitation

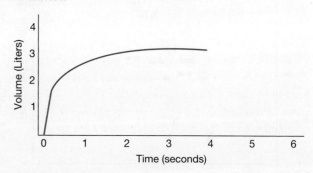

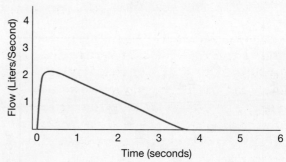

Leak

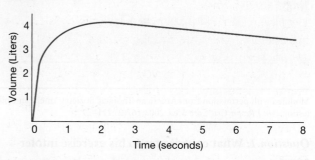

20

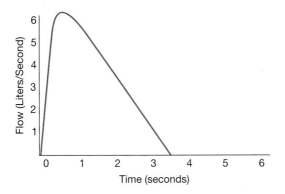

exhaled]/[concentration of alveolar nitrogen]) with small corrections for remaining concentration of alveolar nitrogen and nitrogen produced by body tissues.[2]

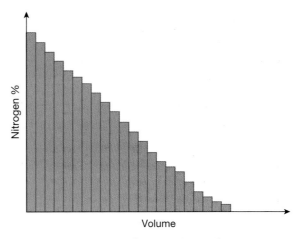

Modified with permission from Wanger J, Clausen JL, Coates A, et al; ATS/ERS Task Force. Standardisation of the measurement of lung volumes. *Eur Respir Jl.* 2005;26(3):511–522.

* *

Another gas dilution technique is the closed circuit helium dilution. Spirometer is filled with 20% to 30% oxygen, air and helium is added until 10% is achieved.[2] Patient rebreathes the spirometer until the He concentration is in equilibrium. The calculation is FRC = (% Helium$_{initial}$ − % Helium$_{final}$) × system volume% Helium$_{final}$.[2] Adjustments are made for 100 mL for helium lost in the blood and dead-space volume from breathing valve and filter.

* *

In body plethysmography, volume from both communicating and noncommunicating airways is accounted for. The patient is placed in a box and pants with hands on cheek, against a closed shutter. Decreases in cabinet volume are indirectly related to thoracic volume increase.[2]

CASE 3

Question 1: A. A

Resistance is the pressure required to flow 1 L/S in and out of the lung.[3] It has a reciprocal relationship with conductance and is less in larger airways compared to smaller airways. It is measured in two ways: (1) obtaining the pleural pressure indirectly via a small balloon catheter at the distal esophagus and comparing it with the pressure at the mouth divided by flow ($Rpulm = Ppl - Pao/\dot{V}$)

Question 2: C. Two largest values of FVC are within 0.150 L from each other

The acceptable criteria for individual spirograms consists of (1) free of artifacts; (2) good starts as defined by extrapolated volume <5% of FVC or 0.15 L, whichever is greater; and 3) satisfactory exhalation defined as ≥6 seconds, a plateau in volume time curve or patient cannot or should not continue to exhale.[1]

* *

The reproducibility criteria involves at least three individual spirograms which adhere to the acceptability criteria with the two largest FEV$_1$ and FVC within 0.150 L from each other.[1] If this is achieved, the examination can be concluded. If not, it can be repeated 8 times.

CASE 2

Question 1: A. VT and IC

During pregnancy there is a progressive decrease in expiratory reserve, residual volume, functional residual capacity, and total lung capacity secondary to the growing uterus. VT and IC increase. The VT increases up to 600 mL secondary to progesterone-mediated respiration and enhancement of hypercapnic ventilatory drive. IVC does not change.

Question 2: E. FRC

Lung volumes can be calculated by initially determining the FRC.[2] There are two approaches. One is to use gas dilution technique which works on the derivative of Boyle's law ($P_1V_1 = P_2V_2$). Nitrogen and helium dilution techniques only measure airways of communicating conducting airways.[2] With the nitrogen washout method, 100% oxygen for 3 to 7 minutes is employed or until three consecutive breaths have <1.5% nitrogen. FRC has a nitrogen concentration of 0.75 and the calculation (VFRC = [Concentration of exhaled N$_2$] [volume or (2) via body plethysmograph by measuring airway resistance (Raw = Palv − Pao/V). Raw is less than Rpulm because there is no tissue resistance.

* *

Compliance (CL = $\Delta V/\Delta Ppl$) is the change in volume secondary from a change in elastic pressure of the lung. There are two types: (1) static compliance, where there is no flow measured during total lung capacity (TLC); and (2) dynamic compliance which is Ppl measured during end inspiration and minus end expiration.[3] Normal CL is 0.150 to 0.250 L/cmH$_2$O.

* *

Hysteresis defines the major contribution of elastic recoil pressure is secondary to the surface tensions at the alveolar air–fluid interface. This elastic recoil pressure is the main determinant of maximal expiratory flow.

* *

Compliance is reduced in pulmonary fibrosis. In COPD, the static compliance is increased but the dynamic compliance maybe normal due to the heterogeneous ventilation.

* *

Choice A refers to COPD where the lung parenchyma cannot distend the airways to the extent of a nondiseased lung, Choice B is the normal range. Choice C refers to reduced ability of expiratory muscles because of reduced lung volume and increased recoil as seen in pulmonary fibrosis.

Question 2: C. III
Single breath nitrogen (SBN2) tests the distribution of ventilation. After exhaling to residual volume the patient inhales 100% of oxygen. The patient then slowly exhales through a one way valve as a nitrogen meter records the nitrogen concentration of expired air. Phase I is the anatomical dead space with no nitrogen.[3] Phase II consists of mixed concentrations of alveolar air and washing out of air from dead space.[3] Phase III consists of alveolar air, initially from dependent regions where nitrogen concentrations are lowest.[3] The slope is normally 1% to 2.5% per liter. This slope is increased in pathologic conditions where there is increased heterogeneous ventilation such as in COPD. Phase IV illustrates the end of nitrogen emptying from dependent regions and the increase reflect the abundant nitrogen concentration in the apical regions.[3] Phase IV's onset also illustrates the airway closure of the dependent areas, usually 80% to 90% of VC. Phase IV ends at the residual volume.

CASE 4

Question 1: **C. The probability of the patient having asthma is borderline due to the methacholine concentration needed to induce a 20% or greater decrease in FEV$_1$, but his lack of asthmatic symptoms give him a low pre-test probability for a diagnosis of asthma.**

* *

Methacholine challenge test maybe used to provide more evidence for an asthma diagnosis only if baseline spirometry does not show significant airway obstruction (FEV$_1$ should be ≥50% of predicted [ideally ≥60% or 70%] and ≥1 L [ideally ≥1.5 L] and there is no significant bronchodilator response).[4] The table below lists the indications and contraindications for methacholine challenge test.

Indications	Absolute Contraindications	Relative Contraindications
Assessing for a diagnosis of asthma, risk of developing asthma, response to asthma treatments Chronic cough evaluation Bronchial hyperresponsiveness assessment in patients with bronchoconstriction	FEV$_1$ <50% predicted, or <1 L CVA or MI in the last 3 months Uncontrolled HTN (SBP >200 or DBP >100) Aortic aneurysm	FEV$_1$ <60% predicted or <1.5 L or FEV$_1$ Inability to follow directions Pregnancy or location Cholinesterase inhibitor use Respiratory infection within 2 weeks Epilepsy

* *

The change in FEV_1 is primarily what is monitored during a methacholine challenge test. A fall in FEV_1 by ≥20% defines the PC20 and this is considered a significant marker of bronchial responsiveness.[4] Lowest dose of methacholine which results in a decrease in FEV_1 by ≥20% from baseline is known as the PC20. Typically, methacholine is introduced in a series of increasing concentrations until a dose of 16 mg/mL is reached or until FEV_1 decreases ≥20% from pre-test spirometry. During testing, spirometry is performed 30 and 90 seconds after each dose of diluted methacholine. If a concentration of 16 mg methacholine per mL does not result in a decrease in FEV_1 by 20% or more, then the PC20 should be reported as "greater than 16 mg/mL." If the FEV_1 is decreased by 20% or more prior to the dose reaching 16 mg methacholine per mL, then the test is terminated at that dose and the PC20 is reported as the lowest methacholine concentration which resulted in the FEV_1 falling by ≥20% from baseline. Following testing, albuterol should be administered and spirometry repeated until pre-test spirometry results are duplicated.

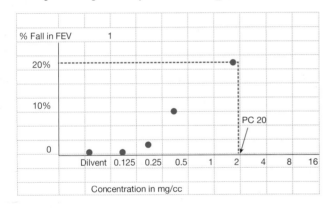

* *

The PC20 can be interpreted as below. As can be seen, in the correct clinical context, extremes in PC20 may result in more straight forward interpretation of methacholine challenge testing while intermediate dose responses become more challenging.[4]

PC20 (mg/mL)	Interpretation
Greater than 16	Normal bronchial responsiveness
4–16	Borderline bronchial hyperresponsiveness
1–4	Mild bronchial hyperresponsiveness
Less than 1	Moderate to severe bronchial hyperresponsiveness

Source: Crapo RO, Casaburi R, Coates AL, et al. Guidelines for methacholine and exercise testing-1999. This official statement of the American Thoracic Society was adopted by the ATS Board of Directors, July 1999. *Am J Respir Crit Care Med.* 2000;161:309–329.

* *

Bronchoprovocation tests, which also include histamine, mannitol, and exercise, help identify patients with asthma, exercise-induced bronchoconstriction (EIB) or other diseases with bronchial hyperresponsiveness, gauge the severity of their disease, identify triggers of their disease, and determine if there is a clinical response.[4] They can act directly (methacholine and histamine) by stimulation of airway smooth muscle receptors or indirectly (mannitol, adenosine monophosphate, and eucapnic hyperventilation) via the release of inflammatory mediators.

* *

With mannitol challenge, the subject is asked to exhale completely before taking a series of controlled deep breaths from a device containing 0 mg and then increasing doses of mannitol. The patient holds his/her breath for 5 seconds and then exhales through the mouth. At each dose level, spirometry is performed in duplicate, 60 seconds after inhalation of the dose. Consecutive doses are administered until the target is achieved, which is a 15% fall the FEV_1 or cumulative dose <635 mg. Bronchoconstriction is then reversed with albuterol.

* *

When compared to methacholine, the data is less robust for mannitol challenge. In those with symptoms of asthma, the test is 58% sensitive and a 98% specific with a positive predictive value of 91% and a negative predicted value of approximately 90%.[4] Thus a negative mannitol challenge in a patient with symptoms of asthma (and thus a high pre-test probability) makes the diagnosis of asthma unlikely but does not exclude it.

* *

Bronchoprovocation challenge test with exercise begins with pre-testing inhalation of dry air (<10 mg H_2O) from a gas cylinder with a reservoir bag and a one way valve apparatus. The exercise test should allow the patient to reach 80% to 90% of predicted maximum voluntary ventilation (MVV ≈40 × FEV_1). Spirometry is performed prior to and at 5, 10, 15, 20, and 30 minutes after the exercise test is complete. A fall in FEV_1 of 10% is suggestive but 15% is more diagnostic.

* *

Bronchoprovocation challenge test via eucapnic voluntary hypercapnia (EVH) involves inhalation of chilled hypercapnic air to a rate 80% to 85% of MVV. Two reproducible spirometries are performed at 5, 10, and

15 minutes and the test is considered positive if FEV_1 decreases by $\leq 10\%$.

Question 2: C. The patient drank a cup of regular coffee on the way to his methacholine test

Drugs which affect bronchial responsiveness should be stopped prior to the test.[5] The time frame recommended can be found in standard protocols. In addition, antihistamines need to be stopped because of the anticholinergic effect of methacholine. Note, the effect of inhaled corticosteroids on bronchial hyperresponsiveness persists for up to 3 weeks after the drug is stopped. A "negative" bronchoprovocation test while the patient is using inhaled corticosteroid and is symptomatic implies that the patient's symptoms are not due to asthma. To exclude airways hyperresponsiveness, the challenge should be performed 3 weeks after the discontinuation of inhaled corticosteroids.

* *

Methacholine, a derivative of acetylcholine, is a cholinergic agonist that causes bronchoconstriction by direct stimulation of cholinergic receptors. Before testing, a questionnaire reviewing previous asthma history, recent infection, other pertinent medical conditions, and medication is administered. Also an informed consent is obtained.

Agent	Minimum time between last exposure and testing
Short acting inhaled bronchodilators	8 hours
Medium acting inhaled bronchodilators	24 hours
Long acting inhaled bronchodilators	48 hours (Up to 1 week for tiotropium)
Oral bronchodilators	12–48 hours
Cromolyn sodium	8 hours
Hydroxyzine	3 days
Leukotriene inhibitors	24 hours
Inhaled corticosteroids	Up to 3 weeks
Caffeine containing foods	Hold on the day of study

Source: Crapo RO, Casaburi R, Coates AL, et al. Guidelines for methacholine and exercise testing-1999. This official statement of the American Thoracic Society was adopted by the ATS Board of Directors, July 1999. *Am J Respir Crit Care Med.* 2000;161:309–329.

CASE 5

Question 1: B. His COPD is severe, lung volumes are suggestive of air trapping, his DLCO is moderately decreased, and there is no evidence of hypoxemia with exertion

* *

The hallmark of obstruction is the disproportionate decrease in FEV_1 when compared to the FVC. Thus the FEV_1/FVC ratio will fall (unless the FVC also is significantly diminished, i.e., in cases of severe air trapping).[1] The low FEV_1 is a reflection of expiratory air flow slowing and results in the classic concave shape of the expiratory limb of the flow-volume loop. Abnormalities in the expiratory flow during exhalation at 75% FVC to 25% FVC (FEF 25–75) are also typically seen (as in this example) but are not specific for small airways disease.[1] However, some authorities feel that reduction in FEF 25–75 can be a sign of early obstructive physiology.

* *

As expiratory flow continues to decrease, the FVC also decreases as alluded to above. This reflects the inability of the patient to fully exhale during the forceful maneuver. The relatively high flows which occur in the FVC (forced vital capacity) maneuver can cause excessive narrowing of the intrathoracic airways, resulting in obstruction. The SVC (slow vital capacity, also referred to as VC [vital capacity]) is a slow expiratory maneuver that can eliminate some of the intrathoracic airway collapse induced during forced exhalation. The difference in SVC and FVC reflects trapped air. In severe COPD, the FVC may be significantly lower than the SVC. A significant difference in SVC and FVC is considered to be 200 mL or more.

* *

The ratio of FEV_1 to FVC (or VC [slow vital capacity, also known as SVC]) establishes the presence of obstructive disease. The best reproducible result of spirometry after several attempts and after the administration of bronchodilator should be used to classify the severity of airflow obstruction. Unfortunately, there was no postbronchodilator result reported for this patient so "the best" result is the only result listed. It therefore can be argued that this test is inadequate for classifying the severity of his COPD.

* *

As above, if FEV_1/FVC is used, severe obstruction with air trapping may result in a normal ratio ("pseudonormalization") due to the dynamic decrease in FVC along with the expected decrease in FEV_1. If FEV_1/VC is used, the ratio will be more sensitive but less specific for detecting obstructive deficits. A substantial difference between SVC and FVC (SVC − FVC >200 mL) is evidence of air trapping. As per the 1991 ATS guidelines, the FEV_1/VC should be used for detecting obstructive deficits and obstruction is considered present when the FEV_1/VC ratio is less than fifth percentile of the predicted value. However, per more recent ATS/ERS guidelines on COPD and the Global Initiative for Chronic Obstructive Lung Disease (GOLD), FEV_1/FVC should be used to screen for the presence of obstructive physiology and, per GOLD criteria, a fixed value of 0.7 or less is considered significant for obstruction.[5] The differing criteria for diagnosing obstruction can obviously lead to differing accuracy of diagnostics among interpreting physicians. Therefore, it may be wise to note the criteria used when diagnosing such issues.

**

One can see that calculated values for residual volume (RV) will differ if the FVC or VC (SVC) is used to make this calculation in patients with significant COPD. If the FVC is significantly less than the SVC and the RV is calculated by subtracting FVC from TLC (total lung capacity), the residual volume will seem higher than if the RV is calculated by subtracting SVC from TLC. Most US centers use SVC rather than FVC in calculations of static lung volumes. However, for the obstructive index in the United States, the FEV_1/FVC ratio is used whereas in Europe, the FEV_1/SVC (Tiffeneau index) is commonly used.

**

Airflow resistance is rarely used to detect obstructive deficits. However, airflow resistance may have a role in detecting extrathoracic or large central airway narrowing.

**

Classification of the severity of airflow obstruction is also important. This should be determined by the best reproducible FEV_1 (either pre- or postbronchodilator, but typically post bronchodilator) measured during the spirometry maneuvers.[1]

ATS Criteria for Severity of Any Spirometric Abnormality	FEV_1 (% Predicted)
Mild	70 or greater
Moderate	60–69
Moderately severe	50–59
Severe	35–49
Very severe	Less than 35

**

If the patient carries a clinical diagnosis of COPD, there are GOLD (Global Initiative for Chronic Obstructive Lung Disease) criteria for quantifying the severity of COPD that slightly differs from the ATS criteria classifying the degree of obstruction.[1] Please note that the best reproducible FEV_1 (Pre- or postbronchodilator) should be used in order to limit variability between tests.

GOLD Criteria for Classification of Severity of COPD[6]	FEV_1 (% Predicted. Using the best reproducible FEV_1 obtained during the testing [Pre- or Postbronchodilator])
Mild: GOLD 1	80 or greater
Moderate: GOLD 2	50–79
Severe: GOLD 3	30–49
Very severe: GOLD 4	Less than 30

**

The change in lung function over time may also be assessed if the data is available. There may be variability in testing minute to minute, day to day, week to week, etc. Therefore, it is important to determine if changes in PFTs are due to test variation or even the expected changes with age. The following displays changes felt to be significant.

Significant Changes Over Time	FVC	FEV_1	MEF (Mid Expiratory Flow) 25–75%	DLCO
Day to day				
Normal subjects	≥5	≥5	≥13	>7%
COPD patients	≥11	≥13	≥23	
Week to week				
Normal patients	≥11	≥12	≥21	>6 units
COPD patients	≥20	≥20	≥30	>4 units
Year to year	≥15	≥15		>10%

Flow-Volume Loop

The flow-volume loop must also be assessed. As below, the flow-volume loop may allude to the presence of fixed or variable obstruction, obstructive physiology, restrictive physiology, or other airways obstruction. The overall shape of the flow-volume loop must be assessed and most times is as revealing as the spirometric numbers themselves.

Normal Flow-Volume Loop

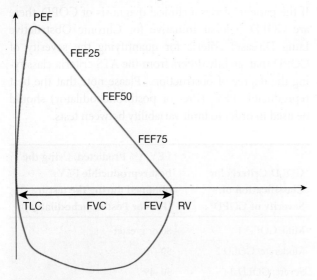

Obstructive Loops

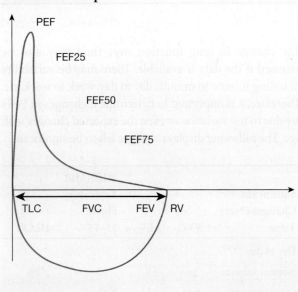

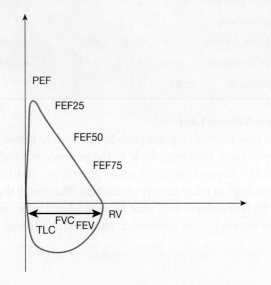

Restrictive Loops

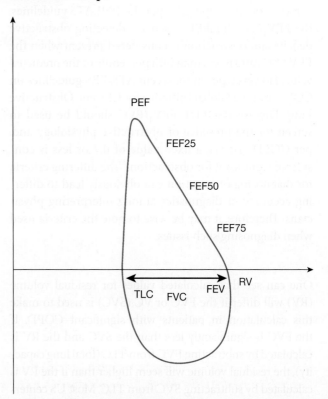

Mixed Loop

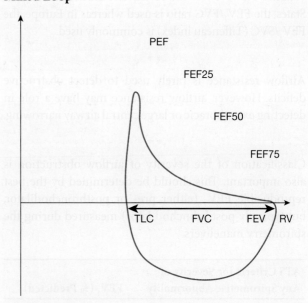

Lung Volumes

Expected (or "Normal") lung volumes are determined primarily by gender and body size (standing height being the most important size value) and ethnicity. In children and adolescents, lung growth tends to lag behind body growth during growth spurts. Thus, expected lung volumes for children and adolescents are less reliable.

Different ethnicities have slightly different proportions of thoracic size as compared to standing height. This is also true in the different sexes. The interpreter must be sure the reference values used in the study truly reflect the patient being tested.

* *

Slow vital capacity (SVC or VC) is measured along with forced vital capacity (FVC) in most US pulmonary function laboratories. In obstructive lung disease with air trapping, the FVC may be considerably smaller than the SVC due to airway collapsibility induced during the forced vital capacity maneuver. A substantial difference between SVC and FVC (SVC – FVC >200 mL) is evidence of air trapping. In obstructive lung disease with "pseudonormalization" of the FEV_1/FVC index, it may be beneficial to calculate an FEV_1/SVC index as described above.

DLCO

The diffusion capacity for carbon monoxide (DLCO) is an imperfect test but is oftentimes helpful when interpreting PFTs and attempting to make a diagnosis. The DLCO is highly dependent on the circulating hemoglobin in the lung.[7] Therefore, if the patient's hemoglobin is known the corrected DLCO (DLCOcor) should be reported and used for interpretation. If the patient's DLCO is not known, the uncorrected DLCO is often reported (DLCOunc). The convention for classifying the severity of decrease in DLCO is reported in the table below. Note, if the DLCO is above the lower level of normal (LLN), then the DLCO is considered normal.

Severity of Decrease in DLCO if Below the LLN	% of predicted DLCO
Mild	>60% but < lower limit of normal
Moderate	40–60%
Severe	<40%

* *

There can also be an increase in DLCO. This can be seen in certain conditions such as exercise, asthma, obesity, supine position, polycythemia, left to right intracardiac shunt, early pulmonary edema, and intrapulmonary hemorrhage.

* *

Adjusting DLCO for lung volume (DLCO/Va or DLCO/TLC) is controversial.[7] Conceptually, correcting the DLCO for lung volume loss (such as in pneumonectomy) seems to make sense. However, the relation of loss of lung volume and decrease in DLCO is nonlinear due to the nonuniformity of ventilation and perfusion in the lungs. Correction models have been considered but not yet validated clinically.

Six-Minute Walk Test

The 6-minute walk test (6-MWT) is a clinical tool used to objectively evaluate functional exercise capacity. As per the ATS, the 6-MWT is easy to perform, well-tolerated, and well reflects activities of daily living.[8] There is also evidence that the 6-MWT distance correlates well with formal easements of quality of life. In patients with severe COPD, reproducibility of 6-MWT distance is better than reproducibility of FEV_1. Furthermore, changes in 6-MWT distance relate well to subjective changes in dyspnea following therapeutic interventions.

* *

The primary measurement in the 6-MWT is the distance one can quickly walk on a hard, flat surface for at least 100 ft in a 6-minute time frame. Patients are permitted to slow down or stop as needed. Periods of rest are also acceptable if desired by the patient.

* *

ATS recommends the use of absolute change in 6-MWT distance until further studies are done to compare the most reliable indicator of physiologic change versus variability between attempts.[6] A normal person should be able to walk between 400 and 700 m during a 6-MWT. In previous studies of patients with pulmonary hypertension, the distance walked in 6 minutes correlated very strongly with a VO_2 as determined by cardio pulmonary exercise testing. A distance <332 m was independently associated with increased mortality. The minimally important difference (the smallest change in an outcome measures perceived as beneficial and would justify a change in medical management) was approximately 33 m.

CASE 6

Question 1: **C. True restrictive disease**
His spirometry shows restrictive physiology due to low FVC and FEV_1 with a normal FEV_1/FVC ratio. Note restrictive lung disease cannot be confirmed until lung volumes are measured and confirm a low total lung volume (TLC <fifth percentile of the predicted value or <lower limit of normal [LLN]) as is true in this case.[2] There is no significant change following the administration of bronchodilator. Lung volumes show a low total

lung capacity. This confirms the presence of restrictive lung disease. The degree of restriction is moderate based on FEV_1, though it is mild based on TLC confidence intervals (TLC predicted – TLC measured = 2.08).

Quantification of the degree of restriction:

ATS Criteria for Severity of Any Spirometric Abnormality[1]	FEV_1 (% Predicted)
Mild	70 or greater
Moderate	60–69
Moderately severe	50–59
Severe	35–49
Very severe	Less than 35

* *

Alternatively, the severity of restriction can be determined by total lung capacity confidence intervals as recommended by the Intermountain Thoracic Society. This is done by subtracting the measured total lung capacity from the predicted total lung capacity (TLC predicted – TLC measured) if the total lung capacity is below the lower limit of normal for the individual patient.

	TLC predicted – TLC measured	TLC predicted – TLC measured
Severity of Restriction Based on Confidence Intervals	Women	Men
Normal (<1 CI)	<1.08	<1.61
Mild (≥1–1.5 CI)	1.08–1.16	1.61–2.41
Moderate (≥1.5–2 CI)	1.62–2.15	2.42–3.21
Severe (≥2 CI)	>2.15	>3.21

Therefore, in this patient, his restriction is moderate per ATS criteria (best FEV_1 = 65% predicted) and is mild per confidence intervals (TLC predicted – TLC measured = 6.56 – 4.48 = 2.08).

CASE 7

Question 1: **D. Variable intrathoracic obstruction**
In this case, the pre-bronchodilator spirometry values are consistent with obstruction (FEV_1/FVC ratio <LLN) with significant response to bronchodilator (FEV_1 increases by 25% [>12%] and 0.23 L [>0.2 L]). As previously discussed, a significant response to

bronchodilator is defined as an FEV_1, FVC, or both that improve ≥12% **and** ≥200 mL following bronchodilator. This may indicate a degree of reversible bronchoconstriction.

* *

However, the flow-volume loop must not be overlooked. The flow-volume loop in this case appears to show a plateau in the expiratory limb. This is seen in both the pre- and postbronchodilator loops. The inspiratory limb of the flow-volume loop is also abnormal, but this finding is likely a manifestation of test technique rather than a physiologic condition in the patient.

* *

An irregularity in the expiratory limb may not be necessarily pathologic, but may be representative of mild small airway collapse that occurs with forced exhalation. This is especially true if the result is continually reproduced in subsequent attempts. Such a finding is commonly referred to as "Fingerprinting" or a "Signature" which aims to illustrate that the subtle shape of the flow-volume loop is unique to every patient. Fingerprinting/ Signatures do not usually change over time. If the irregularity is not reproduced in all subsequent attempts, the effect likely represents an artifact, an effort-related finding, cough during testing, etc.

* *

A plateau in the expiratory loop, such as seen here, should make one consider the possibility of a variable intrathoracic airway obstruction. Common causes of variable intrathoracic airway obstruction include tracheomalacia and tumor.

Fixed upper airway obstruction

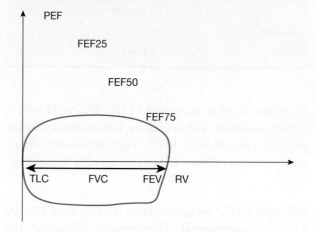

Variable extrathoracic obstruction

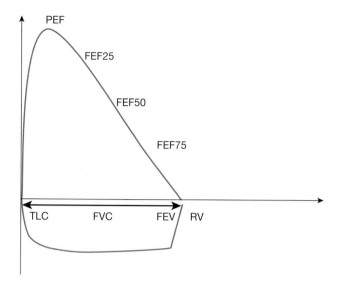

Variable intrathoracic obstruction

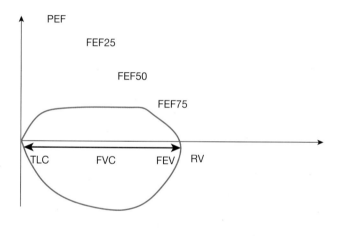

CASE 8

Question 1: A. COPD

Cardiopulmonary exercise testing (CPET) is a global assessment of the body's response to exercise. Indications include evaluation of exercise tolerance; evaluation of undiagnosed exercise intolerance and determine the extent of cardiac or pulmonary contribution; functional, prognostication of known cardiac disease and evaluation for cardiac transplantation and prescription and monitoring response for cardiac rehabilitation; functional assessment and determination of need for oxygen in patients with known pulmonary disease and pulmonary rehabilitation; and preoperative evaluation for thoracic and abdominal surgeries and lung and heart transplantation.[9,10] According to the ATS guidelines published in

2003, the absolute contraindications for CPET include: acute myocardial infarction up to 5 days, unstable angina, unstable arrhythmias, syncope, acute endocarditis or myocarditis, uncontrolled heart failure, severe aortic stenosis, pulmonary embolism, dissecting aneurysm, deep venous thrombosis, uncontrolled asthma, pulmonary edema, mental impairment, and hypoxia with O_2 sat ≤85% at rest.[9]

* *

There are two types of exercise equipment: (1) treadmill which leads to greater stress on organs but maybe difficult to determine an accurate measurement of external work rate and (2) exercise bicycle which is less expensive and smaller than the treadmill.[9] Exercise protocols include: (1) progressive incremental exercise or continuous ramp protocol; (2) multistage exercise protocol; (3) constant work rate; and (4) discontinuous protocol.

* *

The test should be terminated in the following conditions: (1) chest pain suggestive of ischemia; (2) abnormal ECG readings that suggest ischemia, ectopy, or second or third degree heart block; (3) hypotension or hypertension (SBP >220/>120); (4) desaturation <80% with symptoms; (5) symptoms such as pallor, loss of coordination, confusion, and respiratory failure.[9]

* *

Interpretation is based on correlating the patient's history, physical examination, and prior CPET studies with the current patterns noted on the physiologic measurements which include: Oxygen uptake (VO_2), CO_2 output, respiratory exchange ratio, anaerobic threshold, cardiac output, blood pressure response, and ventilation.

* *

Oxygen uptake (VO_2) is determined by the Fick equation where $VO_2 = (CO \times Ca) - (CO \times Cv)$ or $CO = VO_2/(Ca-Cv)$.[9] CO is cardiac output ($SV \times HR$) and Ca–Cv is arteriovenous difference which is approximately 75% in healthy individuals.[9] Factors that influence oxygen availability include oxygen carrying capacity, cardiac function, peripheral distribution, and tissue extraction.[2] The normal resting VO_2 is 3.5 mL/min/kg and $\Delta \dot{V}O_2/$ work rate is 8.5 to 11 mL/min/watt. In certain diseases of heart and lungs, the slope appears reduced as seen below. At a certain point, the work rate plateaus and this is the VO_2 max which is a marker of aerobic fitness. Clinically, this is not always achieved because of symptoms and

Table 2–1 SUGGESTED NORMAL GUIDELINES FOR INTERPRETATION OF CARDIOPULMONARY EXERCISE TESTING RESULTS[a]

Variables	Criteria of Normality
VO_2max or VO_2peak	>84% predicted
Anaerobic threshold	>40% $\dot{V}O_2$ max predicted; wide range of normal (40–80%)
Heart rate (HR)	HR max >90% age predicted
Heart rate reserve (HRR)	HRR <15 beats/min
Blood pressure	<220/90
O_2 pulse ($\dot{V}O_2$/HR)	>80%
Ventilatory reserve (VR)	MW − $\dot{V}O_2$ Emax:>11 L or $\dot{V}O_2$ Emax/ MW × 100: <85%
	Wide normal range: 72 ± 15%
Respiratory frequency (f_R)	<60 breaths/min
$\dot{V}E/\dot{V}CO_2$ (at AT)	<34
VD/VT	<0.28; <0.30 for age >40 years
Pa_{O_2}	>80 mm Hg
$P(A–a) O_2$	<35 mm Hg

[a]Reproduced with permission from American Thoracic Society; American College of Chest Physicians. ATS/ACCP Statement on cardiopulmonary exercise testing. Am J Respir Crit Care Med. 2003;167(2):211–277.

VO₂ peak is used as a surrogate. Main determinants are genetics and quantity of exercising muscles.

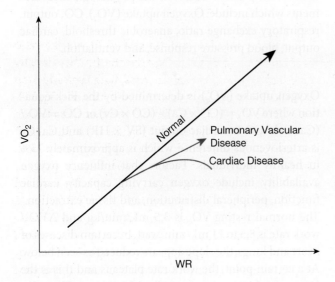

VCO_2 determinants are similar to VO_2. During the initiation of exercise, the CO_2 production is equimolar to oxygen consumption. As exercise progresses, there is more CO_2 generated due to lactic acid buffering and the slope appears steeper. The respiratory exchange ratio (RER) is equal to VCO_2/VO_2. It determines the fuels associated with that metabolic process and is a measure of gas exchange at the level of mouth. RER is also equivalent to RQ which expresses events at the tissue level. RER = 1 suggests carbohydrates while RER <1 indicates mixture of carbohydrates, fats, or protein. RER >1 can suggest hyperventilation or lactic acidosis.

* *

Anaerobic threshold (AT) marks the onset of metabolic acidosis with increased rate of lactic acid production during exercise. AT is not reached in many pathologic conditions as depicted in the graph below. However, its accuracy is in question in certain conditions such as chronic hyperventilation, exercise-induced hypoxemia, and COPD with impaired peripheral chemosensitivity and arterial blood gas might be appropriate to monitor.[2]

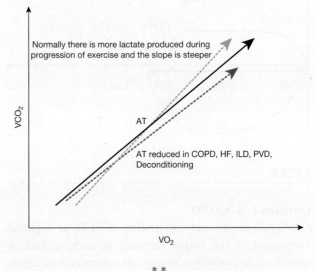

Cardiac output (SV × HR) increases with exercise. Maximal heart rate is derived from the equations 220 − age or 210 − (age × 0.65). If this is reached, patient made maximal or near maximal effort and it might suggest that exercise limitation is secondary to cardiac function. The heart rate reserve (HRR) is usually 15 beats per minute. If increased, it can suggest poor effort.

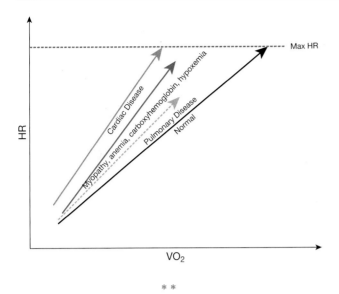

* *

The oxygen pulse (VO_2/HR) is the amount of oxygen extracted per heartbeat. Normally it increases with exercise but decrease in cardiovascular disease, decondition, early ventilator issues and symptoms.

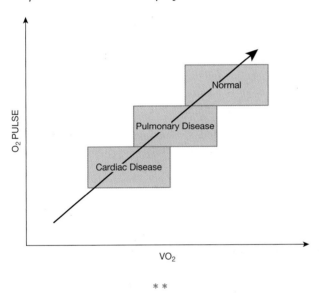

* *

Systolic blood pressure normally rises with the diastolic pressure remaining constant or slightly decline. An excessive increase could indicate hypertension and a low blood pressure response indicate cardiac limitation and the test should be aborted.

* *

Ventilation (V_E) also increases with exercise. Initially, there is an increase in frequency and tidal volume. Both will approach 80% of peak and then frequency predominates. Tidal volume (VT) is 50% to 60% of vital capacity and increases secondary to increase in end expiratory lung volume and decrease in end inspiratory lung volume. Ventilatory limitation is determined from peak exercise ventilation approaching 70% of maximal voluntary ventilation (MVV), which is determined by muscle function, genetics, aging, and disease. MVV is calculated as $FEV_1 \times 35$. Ventilatory reserve is defined as (V_E peak/ MVV $\times$ 100). VR is usually 15%. Patients with pulmonary disease such as COPD and interstitial lung disease have reduced ventilatory reserve. Ventilatory response to metabolic needs can be better assessed with V_E versus VO_2 since VO_2 is independent of V_E although this is difficult to standardize. The V_E versus VCO_2 has been contemplated and there is a strong correlation between the two. In a healthy patient, it appears linear with 23 to 25 L of V_E required to eliminate 1 L of CO_2.

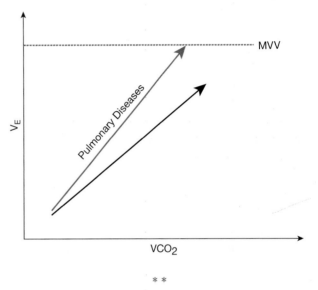

* *

Ventilatory equivalent for VO_2 and VCO_2 are the ratio of V_E to VO_2 and V_E to VCO_2, respectively. They directly correlate to V_D/V_T. During exercise, both typically drop close to its lowest level near AT and increase, V_E/VO_2 typically earlier than V_E/VCO_2 at the onset of metabolic acidosis. If there is a lack of increase, it could suggest airway resistance or increase in muscle burden. If both increase together, this could suggest anxiety, pain, or hypoxemia.[2] Increase in V_E/VCO_2 is typically followed by reduction in $PaCO_2$ and end tidal CO_2 ($PETCO_2$). End tidal O_2 ($PETO_2$) and end tidal CO_2 ($PETCO_2$) increase throughout the incremental protocol. High values when V_E/VCO_2 is at its lowest can suggest high V_D/V_T or low $PaCO_2$. A fall in $PETCO_2$ when V_E/VCO_2 is high suggest increased dead-space ventilation.[2]

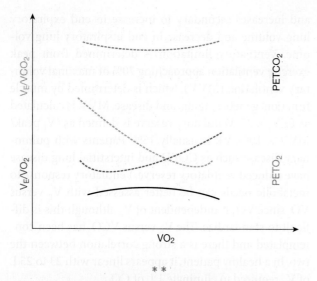

* *

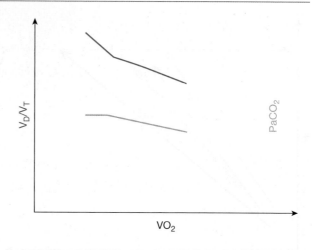

Pulmonary gas exchange indexes used in CPET include alveolar–arterial oxygen tension difference and dead space to tidal volume ratio. The alveolar–arterial (PAO_2 – PaO_2) helps determine the cause of the drop in PaO_2, where $PAO_2 = P_iO_2 – PaCO_2/R$. If both PAO_2 and PaO_2 decrease, which is suggested by a normal PAO_2 – PaO_2(usually 10 at rest and 20 with exercise), this could be secondary to inadequate ventilation or high altitude. If the PaO_2 decreases with an increased gradient (unchanged PAO_2), the potential causes include: V/Q mismatch, right to left shunt, or capillary diffusion abnormalities. PAO_2 – PaO_2 >35 gas exchange abnormality and >50 suggest underlying pulmonary disease.

* *

The dead space to tidal volume ratio (V_D/V_T) is derived from the formula $V_D/V_T = PaCO_2 – PECO_2)/PaCO_2$ and measures how much of the breath is wasted in the anatomic dead space (usually 150 mL) and physiologic dead space (underperfused alveoli). In exercise, tidal volume increases more than conducting airway; therefore the ratio falls (0.20–0.30). If it increases, it can suggest increased alveolar dead space seen in pulmonary diseases.

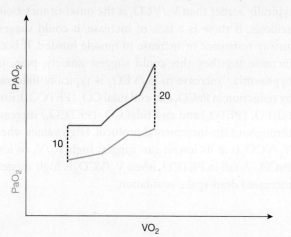

REFERENCES

1. Miller MR, Hankinson J, Brusasco, et al; "ATS/ERS Task Force. Standardisation of spirometry. *Eur Respir J.* 2005;26: 319–338.

2. Wanger J, Clausen JL, Coates A, et al; ATS/ERS Task Force. Standardisation of the measurement of lung volumes. *Eur Respir J.* 2005;26:511–522.

3. Hyatt RE, Scanlon PD, Nakamura M. *Interpretation of Pulmonary Function Tests.* 3rd ed. Wolters-Kluwer/Lippincott Williams & Wilkins; 2009.

4. Crapo RO, Casaburi R, Coates AL, et al. Guidelines for methacholine and exercise testing-1999. This official statement of the American Thoracic Society was adopted by the ATS Board of Directors, July 1999. *Am J Respir Crit Care Med.* 2000;161:309–329.

5. Miller MR, Crapo R, Hankinson J et al; ATS/ERS Task Force. General considerations of lung function testing. *Eur Respir J.* 2005;26:153–161.

6. Global Initiative for Chronic Obstructive Lung Disease. Global strategy for the diagnosis, management, and prevention of chronic obstructive pulmonary disease: GOLD executive summary. *Am J Respir Crit Care Med.* 2013;187 (4):347–365.

7. MacIntyre N, Crapo RO, Viegi G, et al. Standardisation of the single-breath determination of carbon monoxide uptake in the lung. *Eur Respir J.* 2005;26:720–735.

8. American Thoracic Society. ATS Statement: Guidelines of the six-minute walk test. *Am J Respir Crit Care Med.* 2002; 166:111–117.

9. American Thoracic Society. ATS/ACCP statement on cardiopulmonary exercise testing. *Am J Respir Crit Care Med.* 2003;167:211–277.

10. Wagner J, Clausen JL, Coates A, et al. Standardisation of the measurement of lung volumes. *Eur Respir J.* 2005;26: 511–522.

3

Chest Radiology

Mary Salvatore MD, Lea Azour MD, Adam Jacobi MD, Matthew Cham MD, Corey Eber MD, and Joseph Marchione MD

CASE 1

A 32-year-old woman presenting for pre-employment chest x-ray due to positive PPD.

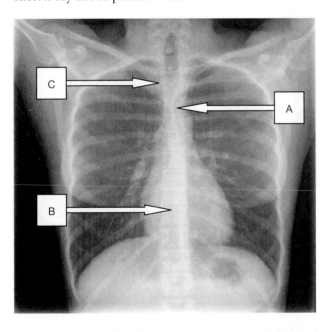

Question 1: What is the name of the structure labeled in A and what does it represent?

A. Anterior junction line: joining of pleura on right and left anteriorly

B. Posterior junction line: joining of pleura on right and left posteriorly

C. Azygos vein: returning de-oxygenated blood into right atrium

D. Superior vena cava: returning de-oxygenated blood into right atrium

E. The carina: bifurcation of right and left bronchus

Question 2: What is the name of the structure labeled in B, and its significance?

A. Coronary sinus: returning de-oxygenated blood into right atrium

B. Inferior vena cava: returning de-oxygenated blood into right atrium

C. Azygoesophageal recess: if deviated, may represent esophageal pathology

D. Para-vertebral stripe: boundary of spine on PA chest x-ray

E. Ligamentum spinosum: attachment of muscles to spinous processes

Question 3: What is the name of the structure labeled in C, and what is its significance?

A. Right paratracheal stripe: the location of the superior vena cava

B. Right superior pulmonary vein: ultimately drains into left atrium

C. Lateral wall of esophagus: becomes deviated with Zenker's diverticulum

D. Internal mammary artery: dilates with cirrhosis of the liver and shunting

E. Azygos fissure: a congenital anatomic variant

CASE 2

A 40-year-old woman presents with cough.

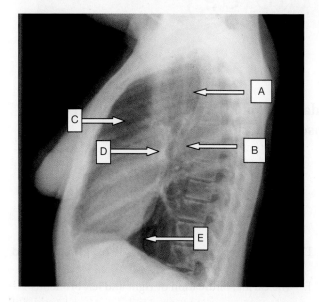

Question 1: **How do you distinguish the right hemidiaphragm from the left?**

A. Air within the stomach can identify the left hemidiaphragm

B. The heart silhouettes the right hemidiaphragm anteriorly

C. The right hemidiaphragm is usually seen in full anteroposterior dimension

D. The right hemidiaphragm is always higher because of the heart being on the left

E. The diaphragms cannot be reliably distinguished on lateral view

Question 2: **Which statement is true regarding lateral chest radiographs?**

A. In the absence of pathology, the lower thoracic spine is easier to evaluate than the upper thoracic spine

B. At least 200-mL pleural fluid is necessary to be conspicuous on a lateral film

C. Mediastinal lymphadenopathy is not appreciable on a lateral radiograph

D. The most anterior cardiac chamber is the left atrium

E. The right pulmonary artery is correctly localized posterior to the trachea

CASE 3

A 55-year-old man with history of asthma has had a persistent cough with purulent sputum. His doctor ordered a contrast CT scan of the chest. Below is the scout film and a representative axial image.

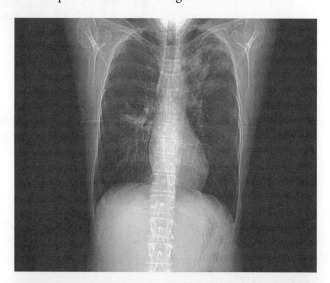

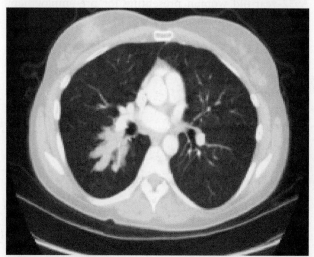

Question 1: **What is the term that best describes the radiographic pattern presented on the scout film?**

A. Batwing pattern

B. Hilar haze

C. Pulmonary vascular redistribution

D. Finger in glove

E. Tangle of vessels

Question 2: **Which form of the above disease affects immunocompromised patients?**

A. Invasive aspergillosis

B. Tuberculosis

C. Allergic bronchopulmonary aspergillosis

D. Aspergilloma

E. Cystic fibrosis

Question 3: What CT finding(s) are associated with the above images?

A. Tree in bud opacities
B. Central bronchiectasis
C. Hyperdense secretions
D. Atelectasis
E. All of the above

CASE 4

A 78-year-old woman presents with long-standing shortness of breath and wheezing. PFTs demonstrate a restrictive pattern. A contrast-enhanced CT scan of the chest is shown below.

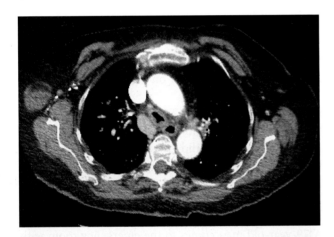

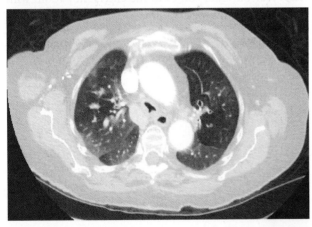

Question 1: What is the best diagnosis for the circumferential thickening of the trachea as seen on the CT scan images above?

A. Amyloidosis of the trachea
B. Relapsing polychondritis
C. Primary tracheal neoplasm
D. Iatrogenic tracheal stenosis related to intubation
E. Tracheobronchopathia osteochondroplastica

Question 2: What is the appearance of the lung parenchyma on lung window settings?

A. Mosaic attenuation
B. Crazy paving pattern
C. Hemorrhage
D. Pulmonary edema
E. Normal

Question 3: Which disease of the trachea spares the posterior wall?

A. Sarcoidosis
B. Granulomatosis polyangiitis
C. Tracheobronchitis associated with ulcerative colitis
D. Relapsing polychondritis
E. Adenoid cystic carcinoma of trachea

CASE 5

An 89-year-old woman with 50 pack-year smoking history complains of progressive shortness of breath and worsening cough.

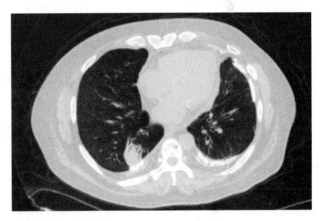

Question 1: Which disease is most likely given the imaging findings?

A. Prior empyema with residual pleural calcification
B. Adenocarcinoma of the lung with pleural involvement
C. Pulmonary infarct with Hamptons hump
D. Asbestos-related pleural disease with round atelectasis
E. Benign fibrous tumor of the pleura

Question 2: What findings are most characteristic when the above disease affects the lung parenchyma?

A. Bronchiectasis and mucoid impaction
B. Subpleural line
C. Crazy paving pattern

D. Head cheese appearance of lung parenchyma
E. Calcified granulomas

Question 3: **Which finding(s) can be seen in round atelectasis?**

A. Round opacity adjacent to pleural plaque
B. Swirling of the blood vessels
C. Normal SUV on PET scan
D. Volume loss of the involved lobe
E. All of the above

CASE 6

A 54-year-old man obtained a preadmission chest x-ray prior to elective surgery. The findings led to recommendation for a contrast-enhanced CT scan of the chest. The representative images are shown below.

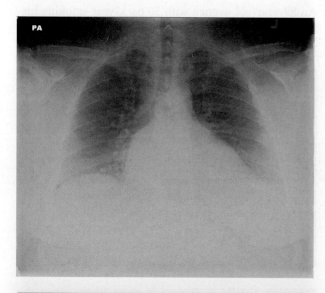

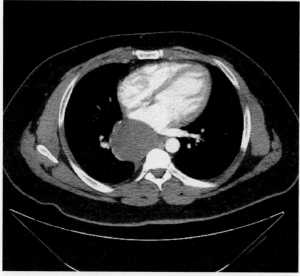

Question 1: **What is the most likely diagnosis given the imaging findings?**

A. Esophageal duplication cyst
B. Thymic cyst
C. Bronchogenic cyst
D. Lymphoma
E. Adenocarcinoma

Question 2: **What is the most common location for the above diagnosis?**

A. Intrapulmonary
B. Right paratracheal
C. Right cardiophrenic angle
D. Subcarinal
E. Chest wall

Question 3: **What would be the appearance of this entity on MRI examination?**

A. Variable signal intensity on T1, with high signal on T2
B. High signal on T1 and T2 sequences
C. Low signal on T1 and T2 sequences
D. High signal on T1 and low signal on T2
E. Low signal on T1 and low signal on T2

CASE 7

A 79-year-old man comes to the emergency room with acute onset of dyspnea.

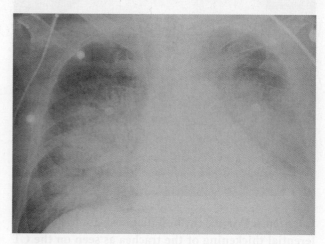

Question 1: **What is the term that best describes the radiographic pattern presented on the scout film?**

A. Batwing pattern
B. Mosaic attenuation
C. The halo sign
D. Tree in bud opacification
E. Finger in glove

Question 2: **What is the most likely diagnosis given the imaging findings?**

A. Bronchopneumonia caused by *Staphylococcus aureus*
B. Pulmonary alveolar proteinosis
C. Severe pulmonary edema
D. Organizing pneumonia
E. Allergic bronchopulmonary aspergillosis

Question 3: **What is the earliest finding on chest x-ray associated with this disease process?**

A. Pulmonary vascular redistribution
B. Centrilobular nodules
C. Interlobular septal thickening
D. Peripheral consolidation
E. Pleural effusions

CASE 8

A 57-year-old man has insidious onset of dyspnea on exertion. PFTs reveal a restrictive pattern with decreased diffusing capacity. A chest x-ray showed normal lung volumes and was followed by a CT of the chest; representative images are below.

Question 1: **What is the most likely diagnosis given the imaging features?**

A. Fibrotic NSIP
B. UIP
C. Organizing pneumonia
D. Chronic hypersensitivity pneumonitis
E. Sarcoidosis

Question 2: **Which imaging findings can help differentiate it from other diseases involving the lung interstitium?**

A. Upper lobe predominant involvement
B. Air trapping
C. Fibrosis following the bronchovascular bundles
D. Absence of extensive honeycombing
E. All of the above

Question 3: **Which term has been used to describe the lung involvement with this disease?**

A. Head cheese sign
B. Farina lung
C. Crazy paving
D. Cob web pattern
E. None of the above

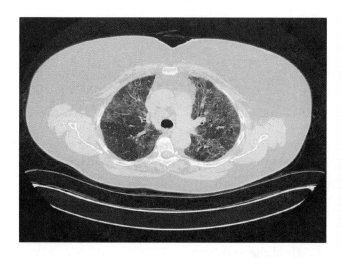
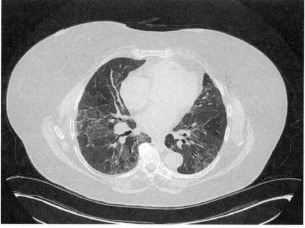

CASE 9

A 62-year-old man presents to pulmonologist with non-productive cough for several weeks.

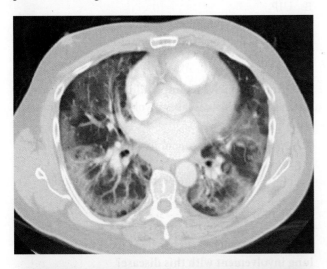

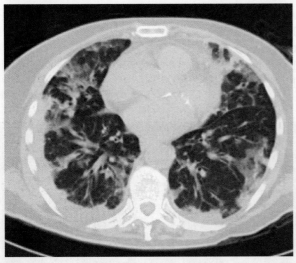

Question 1: **The distribution of the pulmonary findings is best characterized as:**

A. Centrilobular
B. Peripheral
C. Basilar
D. Perihilar
E. Random

Question 2: **The differential diagnosis for the above findings should include all of the following except:**

A. Chronic eosinophilic pneumonia
B. Sarcoidosis
C. Pulmonary lymphoma

D. Pulmonary edema
E. Bronchopneumonia

Question 3: **With which of the following is this entity associated?**

A. Pulmonary infection
B. Drug toxicity
C. Idiopathic
D. Rheumatologic disorders
E. All of the above

CASE 10

A 36-year-old man with acquired immunodeficiency syndrome presents to the emergency room with fever and cough for 5 days. A noncontrast CT scan of the chest is performed.

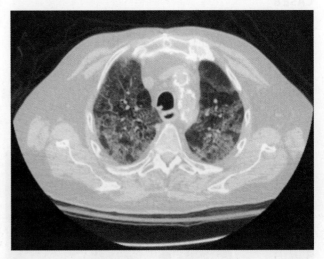

Question 1: **What is the term that best describes the radiographic pattern presented in this image?**

A. Batwing pattern
B. Miliary pattern
C. Crazy paving pattern
D. Fibrotic pattern
E. Head cheese pattern

Question 2: **Which disease(s) can have this pattern on CT of the chest?**

A. Pulmonary hemorrhage
B. Pulmonary edema
C. PCP
D. Alveolar proteinosis
E. All of the above

Question 3: **Which part of the secondary pulmonary lobule contributes to the characteristic appearance of this CT pattern of the lung?**

A. Pulmonary artery
B. Interlobular septae
C. Junctional lines
D. Terminal bronchi
E. None of the above

CASE 11

A 19-year-old man with complaint of progressive shortness of breath.

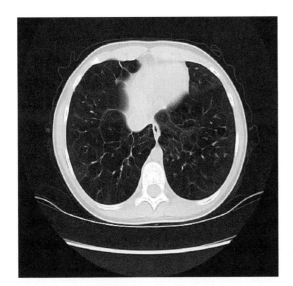

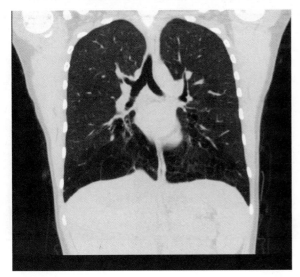

Question 1: **What is the term that best describes the radiographic pattern presented on this CT examination?**

A. Panlobular emphysema
B. Paraseptal emphysema

C. Air trapping
D. Centrilobular emphysema
E. Bullous lung disease

Question 2: **Which disease(s) may be associated with cigarette smoking?**

A. Respiratory bronchiolitis interstitial lung disease
B. Langerhans cell histiocytosis
C. Idiopathic pulmonary fibrosis
D. Centrilobular emphysema
E. All of the above

CASE 12

A 22-year-old man presents with a chronic mucopurulent productive cough and year-round nasal congestion, which has persisted since childhood. He is a nonsmoker and has no relevant environmental exposure. Physical examination reveals bibasilar crackles on auscultation. The chest CT (below) was obtained as a follow-up to an abnormal chest x-ray.

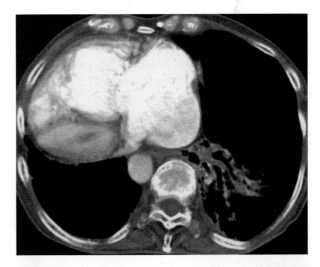

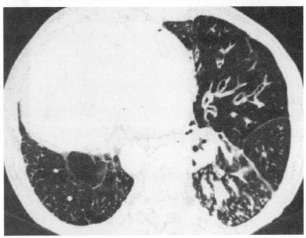

Question 1: What is the most likely diagnosis?

A. Allergic bronchopulmonary aspergillosis (ABPA)
B. Cystic fibrosis
C. Kartagener syndrome
D. Usual interstitial pneumonia (UIP)
E. Sequestration

Question 2: What other clinical manifestation is this disease likely to have?

A. Cholecystitis
B. Infertility
C. Osteoporosis
D. Renal calculi
E. Dendritic calcifications of the lung

Question 3: What is the etiology of this disease?

A. Autoimmune
B. Genetic
C. Immune deficiency
D. Maternal drug use
E. Trauma

CASE 13

A 40-year-old woman has history of 2 years of slow progressive shortness of breath and dyspnea on exertion.

Question 1: Which radiological finding(s) are present?

A. Preservation of lung volumes
B. Round cysts with uniform shape
C. Diffuse distribution with normal interspersed lung
D. Thin-walled cysts
E. All of the above

Question 2: Given the radiologic findings, what is the most likely diagnosis?

A. Centrilobular emphysema
B. Cystic fibrosis
C. Dysmotile cilia syndrome
D. Lymphangioleiomyomatosis
E. Lymphocytic interstitial pneumonia

Question 3: What additional radiographic finding is associated with this disease?

A. Renal angiomyolipoma
B. Duodenal diverticulum
C. Vertebral body hemangioma
D. Situs inversus
E. Bronchus suis

CASE 14

An 80-year-old woman presents with chief complaint of shortness of breath.

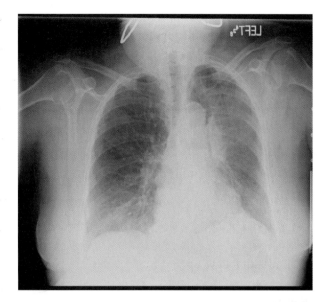

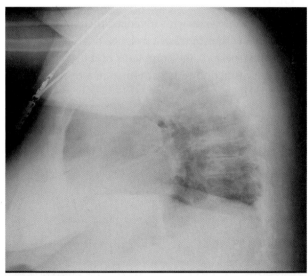

Question 1: What is the reason for the patient's shortness of breath?

A. Posterior layering pleural effusion
B. Left chest wall hematoma
C. Left upper lobe atelectasis
D. Congenital absence of the right pectoralis muscle
E. Loculated anterior left pleural effusion

Question 2: What are the findings on chest x-ray?

A. Luftsichel sign
B. Tenting of the left hemidiaphragm
C. Anterior bowing of the left major fissure
D. Veil of increased opacity over left hemithorax
E. All of the above

Question 3: What is the cause for the imaging finding?

A. Pancreatitis
B. Trauma
C. Endobronchial lesion
D. Genetic
E. Congestive heart failure

CASE 15

A 72-year-old man complains of wheezing. Inspiratory and expiratory CT scans are provided.

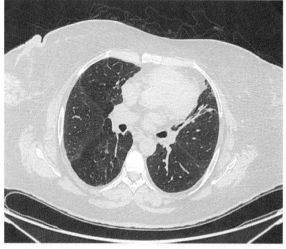

Inspiration

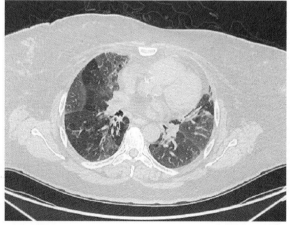

Expiration

Question 1: **What is the term used to describe the imaging findings on the inspiratory scan?**

A. Emphysema
B. Ground glass opacity
C. Pulmonary vascular redistribution
D. Mosaic attenuation
E. Halo sign

Question 2: **Why is the expiratory image useful?**

A. Worsening in appearance suggests pulmonary artery hypertension.
B. Worsening of the appearance suggests small airways disease.
C. Improvement in appearance suggests pulmonary artery hypertension.
D. Improvement in appearance suggests small airways disease.
E. It is not helpful.

Question 3: **What disease classically has the above findings?**

A. Chronic pulmonary embolism
B. Idiopathic pulmonary artery hypertension
C. Small airways disease
D. Pulmonary hemorrhage
E. Congestive heart failure

CASE 16

An 85-year-old woman with history of smoking presented for screening CT scan of the chest.

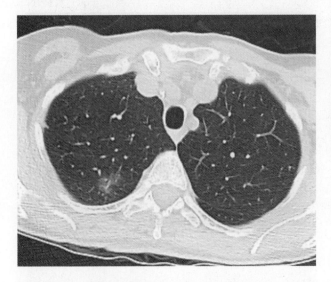

Question 1: **What is the term used to describe the imaging finding?**

A. Nonsolid pulmonary nodule
B. Part solid pulmonary nodule

C. Ground glass pulmonary nodule
D. Artifact
E. Halo

Question 2: **What is the appropriate follow-up based on Fleischner Society guidelines for this 12-mm opacity?**

A. 1-year repeat CT scan of the chest
B. 6-month repeat CT scan of the chest
C. 3-month repeat CT scan of the chest
D. No follow-up imaging required
E. 4-week follow-up after a course of antibiotics

Question 3: **What is the recommendation if the finding develops a new 6 mm solid component?**

A. PET scan
B. Biopsy
C. 3-month follow-up
D. MRI
E. 12-month follow-up

CASE 17

A 75-year-old woman with advanced rheumatoid arthritis presents with progressive dyspnea on exertion over a 1-year-time-period. She complains of a dry cough. Her pulmonary function tests demonstrate a restrictive pattern with DLCO of 35%.

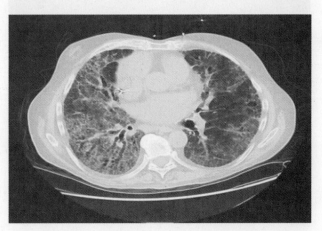

Question 1: **The CT scan of the chest demonstrates a representative image of the lung parenchyma. There is greater lower lobe involvement than upper lobe involvement. What is the main differential diagnosis given this appearance?**

A. Sarcoidosis
B. Chronic hypersensitivity pneumonitis
C. Usual interstitial pneumonia
D. Nonspecific interstitial pneumonia
E. Organizing pneumonia

Question 2: **What pathological aspect of the disease explains the radiographic manifestations?**

A. Fibroblast foci favor the lower lobes
B. Chronic inflammation causing fibrosis in various stages of evolution with temporal heterogeneity
C. Lymphocytes and plasma cells are arranged in a linear pattern
D. Presence of poorly formed granulomas in the lung interstitium
E. The presence of alveolar macrophages

Question 3: **Based on the radiographic findings, what is the most likely subtype of the disease?**

A. Acute superimposed on chronic
B. Mixed fibrotic and cellular
C. Perilymphatic
D. Mosaic type
E. Acute

CASE 18

A 55-year-old man complains of chronic shortness of breath.

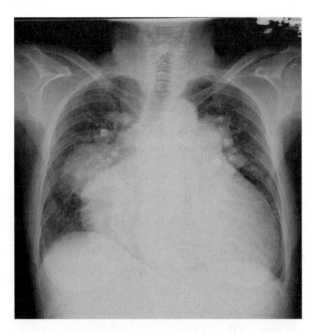

Question 1: **What is the most likely diagnosis based on the imaging findings?**

A. Primary pulmonary artery hypertension
B. Sarcoidosis
C. Lymphoma
D. Congestive heart failure
E. Metastatic disease

Question 2: **What imaging finding helps differentiate pre-capillary from post-capillary pulmonary artery hypertension?**

A. Size of pulmonary arteries
B. Cardiomegaly
C. Pulmonary edema
D. Rib notching
E. Aortic dilatation

Question 3: **Which cause(s) may result in this condition?**

A. Chronic thromboembolic disease
B. Pulmonic stenosis
C. Idiopathic
D. Pulmonary veno-occlusive disease
E. All of the above

CASE 19

A 50-year-old woman presents with acute shortness of breath following a transatlantic flight.

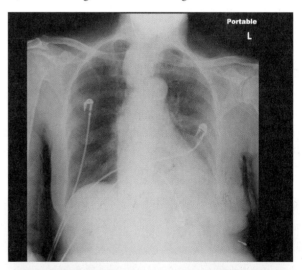

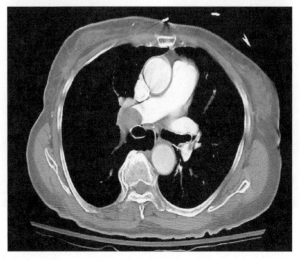

Question 1: **What is the finding on chest x-ray?**

A. Hampton hump
B. Knuckle sign
C. Westermark sign
D. Bronchial atresia
E. Visceral pleura sign

Question 2: **Based on PIOPED II, what is the best imaging study to exclude a pulmonary embolism?**

A. CTA
B. V/Q scan
C. MRA
D. Pulmonary angiogram
E. Chest x-ray

Question 3: **Which of these can cause false-positive or false-negative examinations?**

A. Insufficient contrast in pulmonary arteries
B. Respiratory motion artifact
C. Mucoid impaction of airways
D. Surgical clips in mediastinum
E. All of the above

CASE 20

A 25-year-old man presents with a history of atypical retrosternal chest pain and fever. Initial blood tests revealed leukocytosis and a mildly positive troponin. Initial chest radiograph and subsequent trans-thoracic echocardiography (TTE) images are shown below.

Question 1: **The abnormality on the frontal chest x-ray is best described as:**

A. Pulmonary edema
B. Cardiomegaly with left ventricular dilatation
C. Cardiomegaly with left atrial dilatation
D. Enlarged globular cardiac silhouette
E. No abnormality

Question 2: **How is left ventricular enlargement usually identified on chest x-ray?**

A. Displacement of the left ventricular apex inferiorly and to the left
B. Uplifting of the left ventricular apex
C. Splaying of the carina
D. "Double density" overlying right hear border
E. Obliteration of retrosternal space

Question 3: **What is the most likely cause of the above abnormality?**

A. Metastatic disease
B. Myocarditis/pericarditis
C. Myocardial infarction
D. Rheumatoid arthritis
E. Hypoalbuminemia

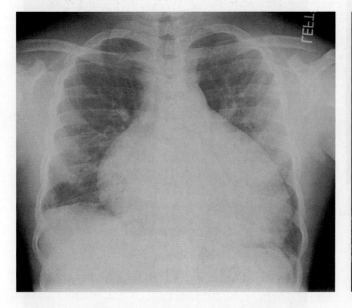

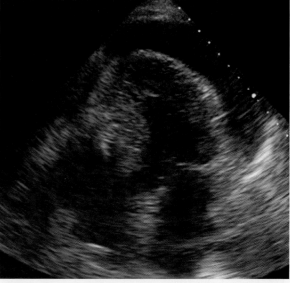

CASE 21

A 24-year-old man with history of smoking presents to the emergency room with progressive dyspnea and a chronic nonproductive cough. Initial chest x-ray reveals bilateral pneumothoraces. Chest CT was obtained after bilateral chest tube placement and is shown below.

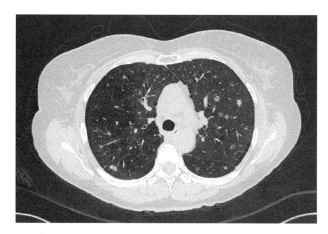

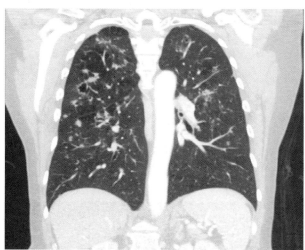

Question 1: What is the most likely diagnosis?

A. Alpha-1-antitrypsin deficiency
B. Centrilobular emphysema
C. Lymphangioleiomyomatosis
D. Pulmonary Langerhans cell histiocytosis
E. Septic emboli

Question 2: What is the most likely cause of this disease?

A. Cigarette smoking
B. Immune deficiency
C. Recurrent aspiration
D. Radiation therapy
E. IV drug abuse

Question 3: What is the initial step in treatment?

A. Anti-estrogen therapy
B. Bronchodilator
C. Enzyme replacement
D. Smoking cessation
E. Antibiotics

CASE 22

A 62-year-old man has a history of lung cancer. Two radiographs are shown; the first dated is May 20, 2012, and the second is July 2, 2014.

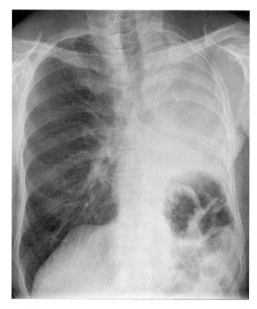

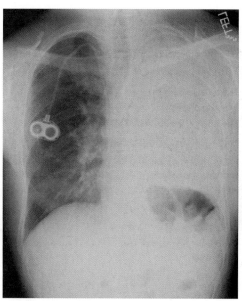

Question 1: **Which is the most likely cause of the patient's unilateral left lung "white out"?**

A. Large left pleural effusion
B. Complete collapse of the left lung
C. Pneumonectomy
D. Lung mass
E. Pneumonia

Question 2: **After undergoing pneumonectomy, how long does the thoracic cavity typically take to fill completely with fluid?**

A. 3 to 7 days
B. 3 to 7 weeks
C. 6 to 12 months
D. 1 to 2 years
E. Never

Question 3: **On the subsequent CXR, which of the following is unlikely to be the cause of the new mass effect in the left hemi-thorax?**

A. Hemothorax
B. Empyema
C. Recurrent tumor
D. Broncho-pleural fistula
E. Different techniques

Question 1: **What is the radiographic pattern?**

A. Mosaic attenuation
B. Tree-in-bud
C. Pulmonary vascular redistribution
D. Finger in glove
E. Perilymphatic nodules

Question 2: **What is the most likely diagnosis?**

A. Invasive aspergillosis
B. PCP
C. Post-primary tuberculosis
D. Neoplasm with satellite nodules
E. Septic emboli

Question 3: **Which segments of the lung are typically involved?**

A. Upper lobes posteriorly
B. Upper lobes anteriorly
C. Lower lobes inferiorly
D. No preferential distribution
E. Middle lobe and lingual

CASE 23

A 79-year-old man presents with cough productive of sputum.

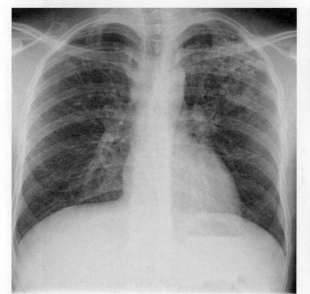
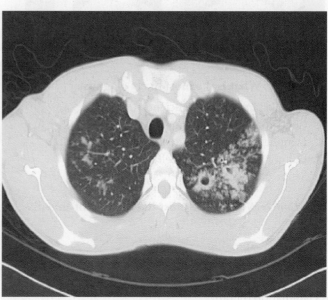

CASE 24

A 34-year-old immunocompetent woman complains of a chronic cough. No prior chest x-rays are available for comparison.

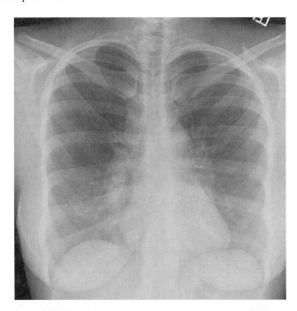

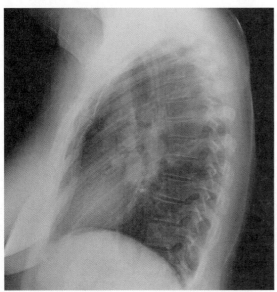

Question 1: **What is the abnormal x-ray finding?**

A. Cardiomegaly
B. Pulmonary artery hypertension
C. Lymphadenopathy
D. Lung cancer
E. Aortic dissection

Question 2: **What is the most likely diagnosis given the imaging findings?**

A. Sarcoidosis
B. Aspergillosis

C. Post-primary tuberculosis
D. Bronchogenic cyst
E. Pulmonary artery hypertension

Question 3: **What is the stage of the disease given the absence of lung nodules and fibrosis?**

A. Stage I
B. Stage II
C. Stage III
D. Stage IV
E. Stage 0

CASE 25

A 48-year-old woman presents with abnormal pre-operative chest x-ray. Initial CXR and follow-up non-contrast chest CT scan are shown below.

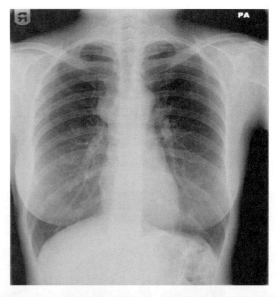

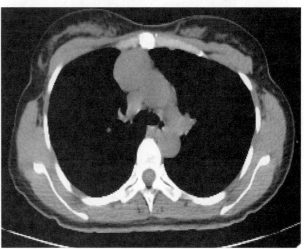

Question 1: **Which finding on this frontal chest x-ray is suggestive of an extra-pulmonary (outside the lung parenchyma) lesion?**

A. Silhouetting of the azygos arch
B. Obtuse margins with the adjacent lung
C. Absence of air bronchograms
D. Tracheal displacement
E. Splaying of ribs

Question 2: **The differential diagnosis would include all the following except:**

A. Lymphoma
B. Thymic carcinoma
C. Bronchogenic cyst
D. Thymoma
E. Teratoma

Question 3: **Which clinical manifestation is classically associated with the lesion?**

A. Palpitations
B. Gynecomastia
C. Hypoglycemia
D. Muscle weakness
E. Shortness of breath

CASE 26

A 35-year-old man complains of cough and fever.

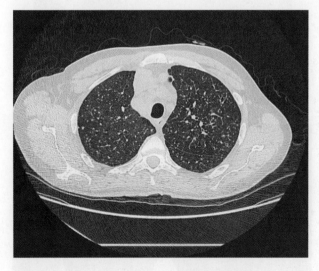

Question 1: **What is the distribution of the nodules on CT scan?**

A. Random
B. Perilymphatic
C. Centrilobular
D. Tree in bud
E. Clustered

Question 2: **What is the most likely diagnosis given the size and distribution of nodules?**

A. Sarcoid
B. Miliary TB
C. Pneumonia
D. Aspergillosis
E. Lymphangitic spread of cancer

CASE 27

A 76-year-old woman presents with nonproductive cough for past 2 months. CT images are shown.

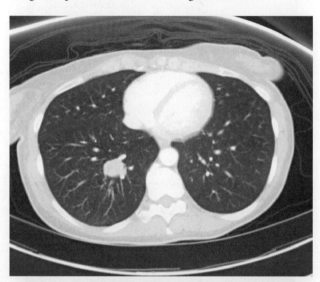

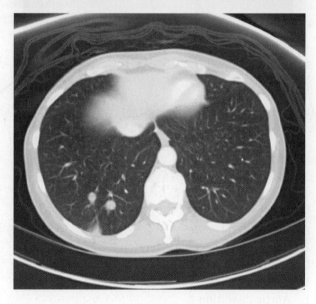

Question 1: Given that the largest right lower lobe nodule is 2 cm in size, what is the T stage for this patient based on the images shown?

A. T1b
B. T2b
C. T3
D. T4
E. T1a

Question 2: If the N and M stages are 0, is this patient a surgical candidate?

A. Yes, because they are Stage IIB
B. Yes, because the patient is Stage IIIB
C. No, because the patient is Stage IIIB
D. No, because the patient is Stage IV
E. Yes because the patient is Stage IA

Question 3: Which finding(s) would make a lesion a T3 lesion?

A. Size greater than 7 cm
B. Location within a main bronchus less than 2 cm from the carina
C. Atelectasis of the whole lung
D. Adjacent to the chest wall
E. All of the above

Question 1: What is the incidental finding?

A. Bronchus suis
B. Mounier Kuhn
C. Cylindrical bronchiectasis
D. Bilateral right-sidedness (asplenia syndrome)
E. Traction bronchiectasis

Question 2: Why is knowledge of this finding important?

A. The finding is associated with increased incidence of pneumothorax
B. Shortness of breath is often associated with this finding
C. The finding can lead to hemoptysis if not detected early
D. Intubation can cause right upper lobe atelectasis
E. Increased incidence of pneumonia

Question 3: Name additional supernumerary bronchi.

A. Subcarinal bronchus
B. Cardiac bronchus
C. Diaphragmatic bronchus
D. Pre-aortic bronchus
E. Left middle lobe bronchus

CASE 28

CT scan of the chest was performed to evaluate for metastatic disease with this incidental finding.

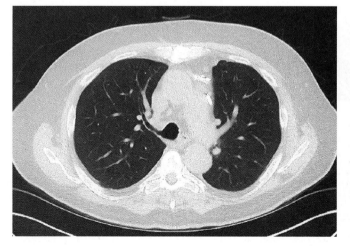
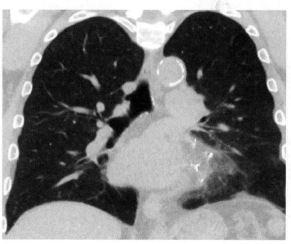

CASE 29

A 62-year-old male presents with a nonproductive cough, "Velcro" rales, and increasing dyspnea on exertion. Pulmonary function tests reveal a restrictive pattern with decreased DLCO.

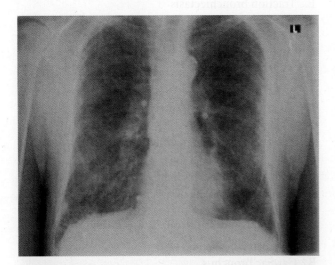

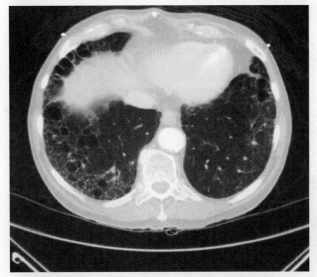

Question 1: What is the most likely diagnosis?

A. Nonspecific interstitial pneumonia (NSIP)
B. Usual Interstitial Pneumonia (UIP)
C. Asbestosis
D. Drug reaction
E. Lymphocytic interstitial pneumonia

Question 2: This disease entity may be seen with which of the following finding(s)?

A. Bronchiectasis and honeycombing
B. Pulmonary trunk and right heart enlargement
C. Rheumatoid arthritis
D. Peripheral squamous cell carcinoma
E. All of the above

Answers

Question 1: A. Anterior junction line: joining of pleura on right and left anteriorly

The anterior junction line represents the union of the parietal and visceral pleura on the right and left sides anteriorly.[1,2] This obliquely oriented lung-lung interface projects over the trachea on frontal chest radiographs and begins below the clavicles to extend to the base of the heart. In contrast, the posterior junction line represents the union of the pleura posteriorly and is a vertical line that begins above the clavicles extending to the level of the aortic arch.[1,2] The azygos vein is located along the inferior right wall of the trachea on the frontal projection, and should measure less than 1 cm in transverse dimension. Enlargement can be noted with heart failure. The superior vena cava is located to the right of the trachea, in the location of right paratracheal stripe. The carina represents the bifurcation of the trachea into left and right bronchi. A useful landmark for its level, in patients where it is difficult to localize, is the inferior aspect of the arch of the aorta.

Question 2: C. Azygoesophageal recess: if deviated, may represent esophageal pathology

The azygoesophageal recess is labeled as B and should be identified on all PA views of the chest. It is usually a straight line or bows to the left. If the recess bulges to the right, it is suggestive of disease of the esophagus or mediastinal adenopathy displacing the recess. It is true that the coronary sinus returns de-oxygenated blood into right atrium, but it cannot be identified on chest x-ray as it is inseparable from the heart. The inferior vena cava also returns de-oxygenated blood into right atrium, but it is best seen on the lateral projection where it is located posterior and inferior to the left ventricle. The para-vertebral stripe marks the boundary of spine on PA chest x-ray and is located lateral to the azygoesophageal recess.

Question 3: A. Right paratracheal stripe: the location of the superior vena cava

The right paratracheal stripe represents the interface between the right lateral tracheal wall and the radiolucent right upper lobe with interposed mediastinal fat. The right paratracheal stripe should be smooth in contour and no more than 4 mm in width. Thickening or irregularity of the paratracheal stripe may represent underlying lymphadenopathy. The right superior pulmonary vein drains into left atrium, but it is not well seen on chest x-ray. In general, veins are located laterally in the upper lobes and medially in the lower lobes. The lateral wall of the esophagus and the internal mammary artery are not routinely identified radiographically. The azygos fissure is located lateral to the paratracheal stripe with normal interspersed lung parenchyma.

Question 1: C. The right hemidiaphragm is usually seen in full anteroposterior dimension

The right hemidiaphragm is seen in its entirety on lateral chest x-ray. The left hemidiaphragm is incomplete imaged anteriorly because of the heart silhouetting it. One cannot confidently identify the left hemidiaphragm by the stomach bubble as it can be confused with a loop of bowel. Sometimes, the left hemidiaphragm is higher than the right hemidiaphragm even with the heart superior to it.

Question 2: A. In the absence of pathology, the lower thoracic spine is easier to evaluate than the upper thoracic spine

If the spine becomes more difficult to see as one looks from superior to inferior, there may be consolidation secondary to pleural effusion, pneumonia, atelectasis, or a posterior mediastinal mass. Around 150-mL pleural fluid is necessary to be seen on an upright frontal radiograph; however as little as 75 mL may be seen on a lateral chest radiograph in the posterior costophrenic angle.[3,4] Hilar lymphadenopathy is evident on the lateral chest radiograph, particularly about the trachea. In sarcoidosis, adenopathy surrounds the left bronchus on lateral projection creating the "donut sign." The anterior-most heart chamber is the right ventricle. The left atrium and ventricle are posteriorly located.

**

The following identifies the structures marked on the lateral chest radiograph:[1-4]

A. *Raider's triangle.* Created by the posterior aspect of the trachea, the superior aspect of the aortic arch and the anterior aspect of the spine. Opacification of the retrotracheal triangle may be seen secondary to etiologies including an aberrant right subclavian artery, esophageal pathology, or a posterior mediastinal mass.

B. *Left main pulmonary artery.* The left main pulmonary artery is shaped like a candy cane and drapes over the left upper lobe bronchus (hypoarterial bronchus). It should not measure more than 16 mm in transverse dimension on lateral projection.

C. *Retrosternal clear space.* Opacification of the retrosternal space is suggestive of anterior mediastinal pathology including thymoma, teratoma, and lymphoma. The right ventricle can enlarge in diseases such as pulmonic stenosis and occupy the retrosternal space. The space becomes hyperlucent and enlarged with centrilobular emphysema thus increasing the AP dimension of the chest.

D. *Right main pulmonary artery.* The right pulmonary artery cannot be measured on lateral chest radiograph as it represents a combination of structures. It can be measured on PA chest x-ray and should measure no more than 16 mm in transverse dimension.

E. *Inferior vena cava.* The IVC is seen as it enters the right atrium on lateral chest x-ray. The left ventricle is considered enlarged if it bulges far posterior (greater than 2 cm) to inferior vena cava.

CASE 3

Question 1: D. Finger in glove

The bilateral lung opacities in this patient represent the "finger in glove" pattern. This pattern is characteristic of allergic bronchopulmonary aspergillosis (ABPA) and represents mucoid impacted bronchiectasis.[5-7] This is a hypersensitivity response most often seen in asthmatics.

It characteristically affects the central bronchi. The batwing pattern refers to symmetric perihilar opacities that can be seen with pulmonary edema, PCP, and less often, pneumonia. Hilar haze has been described in Stage III sarcoidosis, parenchymal only disease, when the shrinking hilar lymph nodes cause a residual haziness around the hilum. Cephalization, also known as pulmonary vascular redistribution, is seen in the earliest stage of pulmonary vascular congestion. The upper lobe pulmonary veins become larger than their lower lobe counterparts.

Question 2: A. Invasive aspergillosis

An aspergilloma/mycetoma (saprophytic aspergillosis) is a fungus ball that occurs in a pre-existing cavity from prior infection (tuberculosis) or structural abnormality (sarcoid). It occurs in immunocompetent patients. The Monad sign describes air between the mycetoma and cavity.[5-7] Classically, the diagnosis is proven when the mucous ball moves when the patient's position is changed. This maneuver is rarely needed for a confident diagnosis on CT. Invasive aspergillosis is seen in immunocompromised patients and presents radiographically as a nodule with a ground glass halo. The halo sign is not specific to this entity. The ground glass opacity represents pulmonary hemorrhage due to vascular invasion. Tuberculosis commonly affects the upper lobes; however, it would be uncommon to see a finger in glove pattern.

Question 3: E. All of the above

Tree in bud opacities represents endobronchial mucous collections, which are most commonly associated with tuberculosis, but can occur with any infection including aspergillosis. The bronchiectasis of ABPA affects the central bronchi from the first to the fourth branching. Over the time, the secretions become hyperdense reflecting loss of water within the mucous. The presence of obstructed bronchi can be associated with atelectasis.

CASE 4

Question 1: A. Amyloidosis of the trachea

Amyloidosis causes circumferential thickening of the trachea as seen in the patient. Involvement is often diffuse and calcifications can occur.[8-10] Relapsing polychondritis and tracheobronchopathia osteochondroplastica spare the posterior portion of the trachea.[8-10] Primary tracheal neoplasms including squamous cell cancer and adenoid cystic carcinoma are more often eccentric than circumferential, as demonstrated in this case. Iatrogenic tracheal stenosis due to intubation is the incorrect answer in this patient because the location of the stenosis is too low.

Question 2: A. Mosaic attenuation

Diseases of the airways cause mosaic attenuation as demonstrated on lung window settings. The vessels in the darker areas are diminutive in size, which supports the etiology of airways disease. However, they can also be small with pulmonary artery hypertension. These two entities can be differentiated with an expiratory CT scan; if the mosaicism is accentuated, the pathology is small airways disease. If not, pulmonary artery hypertension is the diagnosis. Crazy paving is a CT pattern with ground glass opacity and interlobular septal thickening that is associated with many diseases including pulmonary alveolar proteinosis but amyloidosis. Pulmonary hemorrhage and pulmonary edema can present with ground glass opacity, which typically spares the periphery of the lung. They can demonstrate a crazy paving pattern as well.

Question 3: D. Relapsing polychondritis

Sarcoidosis, granulomatosis polyangiitis, amyloidosis, and tracheobronchitis associated with ulcerative colitis share the commonality of their involvement of the posterior wall of the trachea.[8-10] Relapsing polychondritis and traceobronchopathia osteochondroplastica (TPO) spare the posterior noncartilaginous membrane of the trachea.

CASE 5

Question 1: D. Asbestos-related pleural disease with round atelectasis

The imaging findings demonstrate bilateral calcified pleural plaque with an adjacent opacity most consistent with round atelectasis. The plaques of asbestos-related pleural disease usually begin in the posterior basilar segments and are roughly rectangular in shape.[11,12] On chest radiograph, the plaques are described as having a "holly leaf" appearance. Prior empyema or hemorrhage can cause pleural calcifications, however it is typically unilateral. Adenocarcinoma can present as a peripheral lung mass, but given its location adjacent to a pleural plaque and the swirling of the blood vessels, this is not the most likely diagnosis. Pulmonary infarct, also known as "Hamptons hump," often appears as a peripheral opacity, but the consistency is more heterogeneous. Follow-up imaging of a Hamptons hump will show decrease in size while maintaining the same configuration, which is known as the "melting ice cube sign." Benign fibrous tumor of the pleura would have obtuse margins with the chest wall because it is pleural based.

Question 2: B. Subpleural line

When asbestos affects the lung parenchyma, it most commonly demonstrates a subpleural line that runs parallel to the chest wall at approximately a 1-cm distance. A parenchymal band is also characteristic, and appears as a thick band which is perpendicular to the chest wall, usually at the lung bases. Bronchiectasis and mucoid impaction are oftentimes related to infection and inflammation such as mycobactrerium avium intracellulare (MAI). The crazy paving pattern represents thickening of the interlobular septa with ground glass opacities, and most characteristically describes alveolar proteinosis but can be seen with hemorrhage and pulmonary edema. Head cheese is a food delicacy, which is used to describe the heterogeneous appearance of chronic hypersensitivity pneumonitis with areas of fibrosis and air trapping.

Question 3: E. All of the above

Patients with asbestos exposure are at increased risk of lung cancer and mesothelioma. Therefore, it is important to differentiate benign round atelectasis from a malignancy. Round atelectasis is always adjacent to an area of abnormal pleural thickening, pleural calcification, or pleural effusion. There is swirling of the vessels, which would be expected with this atelectatic process. Because the finding is benign, the SUV uptake on PET imaging is expected to be normal; thus, differentiating round atelectasis from its malignant mimickers. Round atelectasis can increase in size despite its benign pathology.

CASE 6

Question 1: C. Bronchogenic cyst

This round unilocular subcarinal structure is most compatible with a bronchogenic cyst. There is a thin rim of calcification, which may be seen with this entity. The cyst wall may also demonstrate enhancement. An esophageal duplication cyst may also appear as a unilocular paraesophageal lesion but occurs less. Thymic cysts are most often found in the anterior mediastinum, rather than the middle mediastinum, as in this patient. Lymph nodes in lymphoma can become enlarged and may be located in the subcarinal station, but they are not typically cystic.

Question 2: D. Subcarinal

The most common location for a bronchogenic cyst is mediastinal, with 50% presenting in the subcarinal location, 20% paratracheal in location, and about 15% to 20% intrapulmonary in location.[13-16] Of the intrapulmonary bronchogenic cysts, they usually are seen in the lower lobes. Less commonly, bronchogenic cysts have been reported in the head and neck, pericardium, stomach, and retroperitoneum.

Question 3: A. Variable signal intensity on T1, with high signal on T2

When the CT appearance is hyperdense, MR imaging is particularly useful to differentiate bronchogenic cysts from other lesions. Fluid is typically high signal on T2 images and low signal on T1. The presence of protein in some cysts imparts variable signal intensity on T1 with preservation of high signal intensity on T2.

CASE 7

Question 1: A. Batwing pattern

The batwing pattern describes symmetric bilateral perihilar opacities that spare the periphery of the lung, as in this patient. Mosaic attenuation is a heterogeneous appearance of the lung parenchyma on CT, which may be seen in a variety of settings including small airway, chronic thromboembolic, or chronic veno-occlusive disease. The halo sign is classically associated with invasive aspergillosis and is a nodule surrounded by ground glass opacity representing the hemorrhage from vascular invasion. Tree in bud opacification is a cross-sectional imaging term used to describe the endobronchial spread of infection including tuberculosis.

Question 2: C. Severe pulmonary edema

The batwing pattern is most commonly associated with severe cardiogenic pulmonary edema and can occur with a large myocardial infarction or papillary muscle tear. It represents fluid within the alveoli and has high corresponding pulmonary capillary wedge pressures (>25 mm Hg).[17,18] Pulmonary hemorrhage can also spare the periphery but is usually not as extensive as pulmonary edema. Bronchopneumonia caused by *Staphylococcus aureus* manifests as bilateral patchy airspace opacities, which may cavitate. The infiltrates of *Staphylococcus aureus* do not spare the periphery of the lung. Pulmonary alveolar proteinosis (PAP) may appear similar to pulmonary edema radiographically but would lack the cardiomegaly and pleural effusions of pulmonary edema. The classic CT pattern for PAP is a "crazy paving" pattern, with prominence of the interlobular septa and ground glass opacities. Organizing pneumonia has a reverse

batwing pattern, with predominantly peripheral lung opacities. Allergic bronchopulmonary aspergillosis manifests as dilated central bronchi with mucoid impaction.

Question 3: A. Pulmonary vascular redistribution

The earliest radiographic finding of CHF is pulmonary vascular redistribution or cephalization of the vessels on an upright chest x-ray.[18] The pulmonary veins in the upper lobes become as distended as the veins in the lower lobes. In moderate CHF, there is interstitial fluid with resultant thickening of the interlobular septa creating Kerley B lines on chest x-ray. In severe CHF, there is alveolar edema, which may appear as centrilobular ground glass nodules or predominantly perihilar airspace opacity. Peripheral consolidation (reverse batwing) is seen with organizing pneumonia and chronic eosinophilic pneumonia. Pleural effusions are associated with moderate pulmonary edema.

CASE 8

Question 1: D. Chronic hypersensitivity pneumonitis

Chronic hypersensitivity pneumonitis is the best answer given the upper lung involvement with fibrosis that follows the bronchovascular bundles. Fibrotic NSIP follows the bronchovascular bundles but has lower lobe predominance and a paucity of ground glass. UIP has a peripheral and basilar predominance with sub pleural honeycombing as its hallmark finding.[22] Organizing pneumonia is predominantly peripheral, subpleural air space consolidation. Stage 4 sarcoidosis causes fibrosis of the upper lobes posteriorly, whereas chronic hypersensitivity pneumonitis affects the anterior aspect.

Question 2: E. All of the above

Chronic Hypersensitivity pneumonitis is a chronic inflammatory disease with resulting fibrosis that preferentially involves the upper lobes of the lungs. The fibrosis follows the bronchovascular bundles and is thus not a peripheral disease. There is air trapping in its advanced stage, which can be useful to distinguish it from other interstitial disease. Honeycombing is rare.

Question 3: A. Head cheese sign

The head cheese sign is typically seen in chronic hypersensitivity pneumonitis and describes the areas of fibrosis mixed with areas of air trapping and spared lung.[19-21] Farina lung is used to describe a miliary-like pattern of sarcoidosis resembling tuberculosis. Crazy paving is ground glass opacity with interlobular septal thickening, wherein the anatomy of the secondary pulmonary lobule is well defined. The crazy paving pattern is seen in alveolar proteinosis, pulmonary edema, and pulmonary hemorrhage, to name a few.

CASE 9

Question 1: B. Peripheral

The CT scan demonstrates bilateral consolidative and ground glass opacities in a peripheral or subpleural, predominant distribution. This distribution is classic for cryptogenic organizing pneumonia (COP), which can also be seen along the bronchovascular bundles, in a peribronchovascular distribution.[23,24] Centrilobular is a CT descriptor for abnormalities anatomically located centrally within the secondary pulmonary lobule. Basilar predominant ground glass opacity may be seen with nonspecific interstitial pneumonia (NSIP). Perihilar consolidation is seen in the setting of pulmonary edema or pneumocystis jiroveci pneumonia. A random distribution is associated with diseases that spread systemically such as military tuberculosis and metastatic disease.

Question 2: D. Pulmonary edema

The peripheral distribution of the pulmonary opacities is the best clue in forming the appropriate differential diagnosis. Entities that tend to have peripheral and/or peri-bronchovascular predominant distributions include chronic eosinophilic pneumonia, sarcoidosis, and pulmonary lymphoma. Chronic eosinophilic pneumonia is usually an upper lobe predominant process. Sarcoidosis typically follows the bronchovascular bundles. Pulmonary edema will classically diffuse or involve the central lung parenchyma.

Question 3: E. All of the above

Organizing pneumonia is a nonspecific inflammatory pulmonary process that may result from a number of causes. Infection is a common cause; although, other conditions such as drug reaction, radiation injury, and connective tissue disorders can also be inciting etiologies.[25] When no etiology can be elucidated, the term cryptogenic organizing pneumonia (COP) is most appropriate.

CASE 10

Question 1: C. Crazy paving pattern

"Crazy paving" consists of smooth thickened septal lines and ground glass opacities. The appearance is named after the paving stones used on an outdoor patio. A bat-wing pattern is central air space opacities that are seen with severe pulmonary edema or PCP. The miliary pattern is seen when small nodules are disseminated at the ends of the pulmonary arteries and the nodules tend to spare the periphery of the lung. There is no single pattern of fibrosis. When fibrosis is present, it is often accompanied by traction bronchiectasis, which is not seen on this image. The head cheese pattern describes chronic hypersensitivity pneumonitis with air trapping.

Question 2: E. All of the above

The crazy paving pattern has been classically described in association with pulmonary alveolar proteinosis.[26-28] However, it can be seen with many diseases of the lungs including pulmonary edema, pulmonary hemorrhage, and PCP.

Question 3: B. Interlobular septae

The characteristic appearance of the crazy paving pattern includes ground glass opacities and septal lines. The septal lines represent thickening of the interlobular septa. The pulmonary arteries and terminal bronchi are not compromised in this pattern. Junctional lines represent the union of pleura from opposite sides of the lung in the midline and are not related to the crazy paving pattern.

CASE 11

Question 1: A. Panlobular emphysema

The images show distended alveoli with lower lobe predominance, compatible with panlobular emphysema in the setting of alpha-1-antitrypsin deficiency. In panlobular emphysema, the periphery of the secondary pulmonary lobule is not preserved and the low-attenuation emphysematous lung blends in with more normal parenchyma.[29,30] There is also apparent diminution of the vessels within the emphysematous areas. Paraseptal emphysema would show distended alveoli in the periphery of the lung and would more likely be seen in an elderly person.[29,30] Air trapping is commonly associated with small airways disease and is characterized by mosaic attenuation. Centrilobular emphysema is a disease of smokers and results in destruction of the central bronchiole within the secondary pulmonary lobule. It has an upper lobe distribution.

Question 2: E. All of the above

There are multiple smoking-related interstitial lung diseases including respiratory bronchiolitis interstitial lung disease (RB-ILD), desquamative interstitial pneumonia (DIP), pulmonary Langerhans cell histiocytosis (PLCH), and idiopathic pulmonary fibrosis (IPF).[31] RB-ILD is a disease of smokers that presents on CT as small, primarily upper lobe centrilobular nodules. The nodules resolve following smoking cessation. PLCH is a disease of smokers with mid and upper lung zone bizarre-shaped cysts and nodules. The nodules frequently cavitate and the disease process characteristically spares the costophrenic angles. IPF appears as lower lobe predominant traction bronchiectasis with honeycombing.

CASE 12

Question 1: C. Kartagener syndrome
Chest CT demonstrates bronchiectasis and situs inversus. These two findings, coupled with the provided history of sinusitis, complete the triad of Kartagener syndrome. The bronchiectasis in Kartagener syndrome has a middle and lower lobe propensity. All other options may also present with bronchiectasis but are not associated with situs inversus. Allergic bronchopulmonary aspergillosis is a hypersensitivity reaction with mucoid impacted bronchiectasis. Cystic fibrosis is an autosomal recessive disorder with upper lobe predominant bronchiectasis. Usual interstitial pneumonia demonstrates peripheral and basal bronchiectasis with honeycombing. Sequestrations show opacification of a segment of the lung with an aberrant arterial supply.

Question 2: B. Infertility
The vast majority of men with Kartagener syndrome have immotile spermatozoa and are therefore infertile.[33-36] Up to 50% of women with this disease are also infertile.[33-36] All other options are not associated with Kartagener syndrome.

Question 3: B. Genetic
Kartagener syndrome is an autosomal recessive disease; although, genetic testing is not part of the initial evaluation. Screening tests for Kartagener syndrome typically include nasal nitric oxide and mucociliary clearance measurement followed by ciliary function testing and microscopy.[33-36] Kartagener syndrome is a subset of primary ciliary dyskinesia, which includes all genetic disorders with impaired ciliary function.

CASE 13

Question 1: E. All of the above
The chest x-ray demonstrates normal lung volumes, which would be uncommon for UIP and NSIP. Scattered

throughout, the lungs are cysts of variable sizes with thin walls. The distribution of the cysts is in both upper and lower lobes, and there are areas of interspersed normal lung parenchyma.

Question 2: D. Lymphangioleiomyomatosis
The combination of cysts throughout the lung with normal interspersed lung and maintained lung volumes in 40-year-old women is most compatible with lymphangioleiomyomatosis (LAM).[37-41] Centrilobular emphysema is characterized by hypoattenuation within the center of the secondary pulmonary lobule, without a well-defined wall. The lung volumes with emphysema are preserved or increased. However, the cystic change has upper lobe predominance. Cystic fibrosis does not have the homogeneity of this disease entity and has upper lung predominance. Dysmotile cilia syndrome typically affects the middle and lower lobes, and the main finding is bronchiectasis, which is not the main finding in our current patient. Lymphocytic interstitial pneumonia is an interstitial lung disease with cysts that is associated with Sjogren's disease and HIV.

Question 3: A. Renal angiomyolipoma
Renal angiomyolipomas are frequently seen in patients with LAM. Extrathoracic findings can also include lymphagioleiomyomas in the abdomen and pelvis and uterine fibroids. Within the thorax, pneumothorax and chylous pleural effusions may occur. Doudenal diverticuli and vertebral body hemangiomas are not associated with the disease. Situs inversus can be seen with dysmotile cilia syndrome, and known as Kartagner's syndrome.

CASE 14

Question 1: C. Left upper lobe atelectasis
There is increased veil-like density over the left lung with signs of volume loss, including leftward mediastinal shift and elevation of the left hemidiaphragm. All findings are compatible with left upper lobe atelectasis. A left chest wall hematoma might cause increased opacity over the left hemithorax. However, it would not be associated with volume loss. Posterior layering pleural effusions show increased opacity; they are usually most prominent at the lung bases. No basilar opacity is appreciated on the lateral film in this patient. Furthermore, pleural effusions are not associated with ipsilateral volume loss and mediastinal shift. Absence of a pectoralis muscle, known as Poland syndrome, may cause the contralateral lung to appear relatively dense, but there would be no

associated volume loss. Congenital loss of the pectoralis muscle, Poland's syndrome, causes relative hyperlucency of the lung on the involved side.

Question 2: E. All of the above

Left upper lobe atelectasis on chest x-ray demonstrates a veil of increased density over the left hemithorax, which is most conspicuous on the lateral radiograph. On the frontal radiograph, a crescentic lucency is seen between the mediastinum and collapsed left upper lobe with the lucency representing the Luftsichel sign ("air sickle" in German). The Luftsichel sign signifies air from the hyper-aerated superior segment of the left lower lobe insinuating itself between the aorta and pulmonary artery on frontal radiograph.[42] In addition, left upper lobe atelectasis will result in left-sided volume loss with ipsilateral mediastinal shift, elevation (or tenting) of the left hemidiaphragm also known as the juxtaphrenic peak sign, and anterior bowing of the left major fissure.[43]

Question 3: C. Endobronchial lesion

Left upper lobe atelectasis can be caused by an endobronchial nodule, mucous plug or foreign body. Pancreatitis can be associated with an isolated left pleural effusion, which is not the case in the current examination.

CASE 15

Question 1: D. Mosaic attenuation

Mosaic attenuation refers to heterogeneity of the lungs reminiscent of mosaic tiles. It may be seen in large and small airways diseases (e.g., cystic fibrosis, asthma, and bronchiolitis), as well as pulmonary vascular diseases (primary pulmonary hypertension, chronic pulmonary embolism, or pulmonary veno-occlusive disease).[44-46] In emphysema, a pattern of centrilobular, panlobular, or paraseptal lucency would be seen. Ground glass opacity is characterized by areas of increased attenuation which do not obscure underlying vessels. Pulmonary vascular redistribution refers to the initial stage of pulmonary vascular congestion. There is redistribution of pulmonary blood flow from the lower lobes to the upper lobes.

Question 2: B. Worsening of the appearance suggests small airways disease

Mosaic attenuation can be secondary to airways disease or vascular disease. Worsening or exaggeration of the mosaic attenuation pattern on expiratory imaging is known as air trapping and is suggestive of small airways disease. At end-expiration, one would expect the lung parenchyma to increase in attenuation. In small airways disease, such as asthma, prominent areas of hyperlucency and maintained volume are seen at end-expiration, representing "trapped" air. Pulmonary artery hypertension is characterized by the central redistribution of blood flow, which may lead to a heterogeneous attenuation pattern. However, this pattern would not be expected to change on expiratory scanning. Associated findings are central pulmonary arterial enlargement with peripheral vessel pruning and possible bowing of the interventricular septum would be expected.

Question 3: C. Small airways disease

Small airways disease demonstrates mosaic attenuation that worsens on expiratory images as demonstrated in this case. Chronic pulmonary embolism and pulmonary artery hypertension for any reason can have mosaic attenuation, but it does not worsen with expiration. Pulmonary hemorrhage and congestive heart failure can have mosaic attenuation but the vessels in the more lucent area are normal in caliber.

CASE 16

Question 1: A. Nonsolid pulmonary nodule

The finding is a nonsolid pulmonary nodule with visualization of vessels through the nodule without any solid component. The previously used term was "ground glass nodule." We cannot assume that this nonsolid nodule is an artifact based on its imaging appearance. In smaller nonsolid nodules, 1-mm thin slices may be obtained to confirm a true nonsolid nodule. A halo typically refers to ground glass opacity surrounding a nodule in the case of invasive aspergillosis.

Question 2: C. 3-month repeat CT scan of the chest

Fleischer Society Guidelines recommend 3-month follow-up for nonsolid nodules that are greater than 5 mm in size, and if stable, yearly follow-up thereafter for a minimum of 3 years.[47,48] Smaller nodules require no CT scan follow-up.

Question 3: B. Biopsy

If the nonsolid nodule develops a solid component ≥5 mm, the recommendation would be for further evaluation to exclude neoplasm with either biopsy or surgical resection.[47,48] Three-month follow-up is recommended if the solid component is <5 mm with yearly surveillance thereafter.[47,48] PET may be considered for part-solid nodules that are >10 mm; however, given findings that part-solid nodules with solid component >5 mm are likely to be malignant, biopsy/resection is a better answer choice.

CASE 17

Question 1: D. Nonspecific interstitial pneumonia

Nonspecific interstitial pneumonia is a lower lobe predominant disease with ground glass opacity, traction bronchiectasis and little, if any, honeycombing. The disease follows the bronchovascular bundles. UIP occurs in a peripheral and basal distribution with the hallmark of honeycombing. Organizing pneumonia is a predominantly peripheral lung disease. Sarcoidosis and chronic hypersensitivity pneumonitis are both upper lobe predominant diseases.

Question 2: C. Lymphocytes and plasma cells arranged in a linear pattern

NSIP is characterized pathologically by lymphocytes and plasma cells arranged in a linear pattern with collagen deposition and/or inflammation causing interstitial thickening.[49-51] It may be seen in the setting of collagen vascular diseases such as scleroderma, rheumatoid arthritis, or polymyositis. Fibroblastic foci are the hallmark of UIP. NSIP is temporally homogeneous rather than temporally heterogeneous like UIP. Poorly formed granulomas are characteristic of chronic hypersensitivity pneumonitis.

Question 3: B. Mixed fibrotic and cellular

The imaging demonstrates prominent reticular markings and ground glass opacities likely representing mixed fibrotic and cellular disease. In the cellular type, inflammatory cells predominate; whereas in the fibrotic pattern, there is interstitial collagen deposition. A greater degree of fibrosis portends a worse prognosis.

CASE 18

Question 1: A. Primary pulmonary artery hypertension

There is cardiomegaly with marked enlargement of the right atrium and right ventricle, as well as dilated main pulmonary arteries. These findings are compatible with pulmonary artery hypertension. There is also "pruning" of the peripheral vessels.[52-54] Sarcoidosis and lymphoma may cause enlargement of the pulmonary hila secondary to lymphadenopathy. However, they are not usually associated with the additional finding of cardiomegaly. There is

no evidence of pulmonary vascular redistribution, pleural effusion, or airspace opacity to suggest pulmonary edema. Metastatic pulmonary nodules are not identified on this film.

Question 2: C. Pulmonary edema

Pulmonary edema is a finding that may be encountered in post-capillary pulmonary hypertension. Pre- and post-capillary pulmonary hypertension refers to abnormalities in the arterial and venous pulmonary circulations, respectively. Pre-capillary pulmonary hypertension may be due to pulmonary arterial thromboembolic disease or chronic interstitial lung disease, among other etiologies. Post-capillary pulmonary hypertension affects the pulmonary veins distal to the capillaries and may be caused by anything that affects pulmonary venous drainage: atrial myxoma or mitral stenosis, peripheral veno-occlusive disease, left ventricular dysfunction, or mediastinal fibrosis with mass effect on the pulmonary veins. As such, engorgement of the pulmonary veins, pulmonary edema, and pleural effusions may be seen. Both pre-and post-capillary pulmonary hypertensions have enlarged pulmonary arteries and right-sided heart dysfunction with resultant cardiomegaly. Neither is associated with rib notching, which is seen in coarctation of the aorta due to dilated intercostal collateral arteries.

Question 3: E. All of the above

Pulmonary hypertension has many causes including idiopathic, interstitial lung disease, chronic pulmonary emboli, collagen vascular disease, medications (particularly diet medications), and infections such as HIV or schistosomiasis. It may also occur with post stenotic dilatation of the pulmonary artery in the setting of pulmonic stenosis.

CASE 19

Question 1: C. Westermark sign

The chest x-ray demonstrates right lung oligemia or the Westermark sign. In this case, the right-sided oligemia or paucity of vessels is secondary to the large right main pulmonary artery filling defect seen on the CT image. Pulmonary emboli can lead to pulmonary arterial enlargement giving the appearance of a hilar knuckle, which is not the case in this examination. A Hampton hump is a wedge-shaped peripheral opacity representing lung infarct, which occurs in fewer than 10% of cases of embolic disease. As pulmonary infarcts resolve, they maintain their wedge shape as they "melt;" this is known as the "melting ice cube" sign. Bronchial atresia can have surrounding hyper-lucent lung with a bronchial filling defect.

Question 2: A. CTA

Prospective investigation of pulmonary embolism diagnosis (PIOPED) II compared CTA and V/Q scan for the diagnosis of PE and found CTA to be the preferred examination.[56] PIOPED I compared V/Q scan and pulmonary angiogram for the diagnosis of pulmonary embolus (PE).[55] PIOPED III compared MRA and CTA for the evaluation of PE and found that MRA was more difficult to adequately obtain; it should only be performed at institutions with experience in performing the test.[57]

Question 3: E. All of the above

False positive and false negative CTAs for evaluation of pulmonary embolism occur.[56] If there is insufficient contrast in the pulmonary circulation, small emboli can go undetected. If there is respiratory motion artifact, the examination should not be considered negative because small emboli can be missed. In addition, because bronchi parallel the course of the pulmonary arteries, mucoid impaction can mimic arterial filling defects.

CASE 20

Question 1: D. Enlarged globular cardiac silhouette

The patient's chest x-ray demonstrates a featureless, globular, enlarged cardiac silhouette. In combination with a narrow vascular pedicle, this gives the cardiac silhouette a symmetric "water bottle configuration." The subsequent trans-thoracic echocardiography (TTE) reveals anechoic fluid within the pericardium anterior to the left ventricle compatible with a pericardial effusion. Though cardiomegaly is often seen with pulmonary edema, patchy airspace opacities would be the main finding. Isolated left ventricular or left atrial dilatation would not result in the "water bottle" configuration.

Question 2: A. Displacement of the left ventricular apex inferiorly and to the left

In contrast to pericardial effusion, which is characterized by uniform globular enlargement, cardiac chamber enlargement appears as a contour irregularity. With left ventricular enlargement, the LV apex will be displaced inferiorly, posteriorly (on the lateral film), and more leftward than expected. One of the most common signs of right ventricular dilatation and hypertrophy on the frontal CXR is uplifting of the left ventricular apex producing

the "boot-shaped" appearance of the heart, classically found in patients with Tetralogy of Fallot.[58–60] Splaying of the carina, a "double density" sign over the right heart border, and posterior displacement of the superior heart border on the lateral CXR are all findings typically found with left atrial dilatation. Obliteration of the retrosternal space is seen with right ventricular enlargement.

Question 3: B. Myocarditis/pericarditis

Myocarditis or pericarditis is the most likely etiology of pericardial effusion. Echocardiography is the method of choice to confirm the diagnosis of pericardial effusion, estimate the volume of fluid, and most importantly, assess the hemodynamic impact of the pericardial effusion. Given the patient's young age, clinical complaints, and findings of a pericardial effusion, the most likely diagnosis is myocarditis/pericarditis. Metastatic disease to the heart and pericardium is uncommon, but the presenting sign is often malignant pericardial effusion. Post myocardial infarction syndrome, also known as Dressler's syndrome, is autoimmune pericarditis after cardiac insult, often manifested by pericardial effusion. Rheumatoid arthritis is a rare cause of pericarditis, which can subsequently cause pericardial effusion.

CASE 21

Question 1: D. Pulmonary Langerhans cell histiocytosis

Pulmonary Langerhans cell histiocytosis (PLCH) is characterized by thick-walled, bizarre irregular-shaped cysts with upper lobe predominance. Nodules may also be present and are up to 5 mm in size.[61–64] They may be difficult to detect with increasing disease severity.[61–64] Alpha-1 antitrypsin deficiency is characterized by cysts with barely perceptible walls with diffuse upper and lower lobe involvement. This patient is likely too young to have smoking-related centrilobular emphysema, which would appear as areas of low attenuation at the center of the secondary pulmonary lobule without appreciable wall. Lymphangioleiomyomatosis (LAM) is characterized by diffuse thin-walled cysts and occurs almost exclusively in women.

Question 2: A. Cigarette smoking

PLCH is caused by cigarette smoking in patients with an underlying immune system abnormality. Essentially, all affected patients are smokers or former smokers. An abnormally increased immunoglobulin G may be found during bronchoalveolar lavage.

***Question 3*: D. Smoking cessation**

The initial step in management is smoking cessation, which results in disease remission for most patients. In uncontrolled disease, the major cause of death is respiratory failure.

CASE 22

***Question 1*: C. Pneumonectomy**

The initial CXR demonstrates complete opacification of the left hemithorax ("white out"). The best indicator of the etiology is the left sided volume loss as evidenced by the ipsilateral mediastinal and tracheal shift as well as elevation of the left hemidiaphragm. These findings are unlikely to be the result of a large pleural effusion or mass because these processes would tend to push the mediastinum to the contralateral side. Complete atelectasis of the left lung does cause volume loss; however, given the surgical clips within the left chest and abrupt cut-off of the left main stem bronchus, the patient has likely undergone prior pneumonectomy.

***Question 2*: B. 3 to 7 weeks**

Predictable anatomic changes occur following pneumonectomy. Typically after pneumonectomy, the empty thoracic cavity is filled with air.[65–67] The rate of accumulation of fluid in the post-pneumonectomy space is extremely variable. In most cases, within the first 4 to 5 postoperative days, approximately half of the space is filled with fluid. After the first week, the air-fluid level gradually rises, filling the entire cavity within several weeks to months.[65,66]

***Question 3*: D. Broncho-pleural fistula**

On the subsequent chest x-ray 2 years later, there is new rightward mediastinal shift and inferior displacement of the left hemi-diaphragm from a space occupying process other than typical fluid. As there is no air or air-fluid level within the left chest, a broncho-pleural fistula is unlikely to contribute to the findings. Although post-pneumonectomy empyema is usually diagnosed in the peri-operative period, some cases are not detected until months or even several years later.[67] The pathogenesis of late-onset empyema is sometimes difficult to establish because of the many possible sources of infection in the post-pneumonectomy space. In two-thirds of all patients who undergo pneumonectomy, the post-pneumonectomy space remains fluid-filled and marginated by thickened pleura. In the remaining one-third of patients, the space is obliterated by fibrous tissue or

normal mediastinal structures. The persistence of fluid in the postoperative space exposes patients to the risk of late-occurring empyema as was the case in this patient.

CASE 23

***Question 1*: B. Tree-in-bud**

The finding in the left upper lobe is primarily tree-in-bud opacity with small nodules that follow the course of the bronchovascular bundles. There is also a cavitary lesion in the left upper lobe. Mosaic attenuation refers to heterogeneity of the lung parenchyma with areas of increased attenuation and hyperlucency. Pulmonary vascular redistribution is distension of the upper lobe pulmonary veins or cephalization on an upright chest x-ray. The finger in glove pattern represents mucoid impaction in allergic bronchopulmonary aspergillosis (ABPA).

***Question 2*: C. Post-primary tuberculosis**

Tree-in-bud opacity represents the endobronchial spread of infection and is most characteristic of tuberculosis, but it can be seen with any infection. Tuberculomas seen in post-primary tuberculosis may cavitate with satellite lesions about the tuberculoma. Nodules with surrounding ground glass halos characterize invasive aspergillosis. PCP appears as ground glass opacity with pneumatoceles.

***Question 3*: A. Upper lobes posteriorly**

Post-primary tuberculosis typically affects the posterior segments of the upper lobes and the superior segments of the lower lobes.[68,69] Manifestations of post-primary tuberculosis include patchy upper lobe consolidation, cavitating tuberculomas, and tree-in-bud opacity. Primary tuberculosis presents with lymphadenopathy, airspace opacity with a lower-zone predilection, and pleural effusion. The miliary pattern of small randomly distributed nodules may be seen in both primary and postprimary tuberculosis.

CASE 24

***Question 1*: C. Lymphadenopathy**

The radiograph demonstrates symmetric paratracheal and bilateral hilar adenopathy. On the lateral view, the lymphadenopathy forms what looks like a donut, which is a classic sign differentiating this finding from enlarged pulmonary arteries. The heart size is less than half the transverse diameter of the thorax, so the patient does not have cardiomegaly. No lung cancer is identified, and adenopathy associated with lung cancer is more often unilateral.

Question 2: A. Sarcoidosis

The appearance of the lymphadenopathy is classic for sarcoidosis, wherein the hilar lymph nodes appear potato-like with a gap between them and the heart.[70–73] The lateral view demonstrates the classic donut sign caused by hilar lymphadenopathy. Aspergillosis is not typically associated with bulky lymphadenopathy. Primary tuberculosis or tuberculosis in an immunocompromised patient may present with lymphadenopathy; however, it is not the case in this immunocompetent patient. A bronchogenic cyst can cause bulging of the right paratracheal stripe but would not affect the pulmonary hila.

Question 3: A. Stage I

Stage I sarcoidosis is comprised of hilar and mediastinal lymphadenopathy with the so-called garland sign or 1–2–3 sign as seen in this patient.[70–73] Stage II sarcoidosis represents a combination of lymphadenopathy and pulmonary nodules, which the patient does not demonstrate. The pulmonary nodules in stage II sarcoidosis may include perilymphatic nodules along the bronchovascular bundles and subpleural regions. In stage III sarcoidosis, the lymph nodes shrink in size while the pulmonary parenchymal findings persist; this may result in a "hilar haze."[73] In stage IV, there is fibrosis of the upper lobes that extends laterally on chest x-ray, creating the appearance of a swag curtain.

CASE 25

Question 1: B. Obtuse margins with the adjacent lung

In the provided radiograph, there is a right paratracheal mass. The main radiographic finding that supports the lesion's extra-pulmonary (outside the lung parenchyma) location is the obtuse margins it creates with adjacent lung most likely placing it in the mediastinum. In contrast, a lung mass would abut the mediastinal and/or pleural surface, creating acute angles with the adjacent lung. In this patient, the mass can be placed within the anterior mediastinum on the accompanying chest CT because it is located anterior to the great vessels (prevascular space).

Question 2: C. Bronchogenic cyst

The differential diagnosis for an anterior mediastinal mass includes the four T's: thymus, teratoma, thyroid (and parathyroid), and (terrible) lymphoma.[74–79] Thymic masses include thymoma, thymic carcinoma, and thymic cysts. Thymomas are the most common anterior mediastinal mass and are usually unilateral. They may occur at any level in the anterior mediastinum from the thoracic inlet to the cardiophrenic angle. Masses in the upper anterior mediastinum may obscure the retrosternal clear space or displace the anterior junction line. At the level of the hila, an anterior mediastinal mass will not obscure the hilum, a middle mediastinal structure; this is known as the hilum overlay sign. A mass in the inferior anterior mediastinum may obscure the cardiophrenic angle. Bronchogenic cysts are typically located in the middle mediastinum; they are most commonly subcarinal in location.

Question 3: D. Muscle weakness

While 10% to 15% of patients with myasthenia gravis have a thymoma, up to 50% of patients with thymoma may have myasthenia gravis. The main symptom of myasthenia gravis is muscle weakness.

CASE 26

Question 1: A. Random

Multiple tiny nodules appear randomly distributed. There are three main distributions seen in the setting of multiple nodules: centrilobular, perilymphatic, and random. When multiple nodules are seen, the first step is to determine the presence or absence of subpleural nodules. A predominance of pleural nodules is not seen in the centrilobular pattern or random pattern. To distinguish between centrilobular and random patterns, determine whether the nodules are well defined. If the nodules are well defined, they are random; if not they are centrilobular.

Question 2: B. Miliary TB

Given the tiny nodule size seen in a random distribution, miliary TB is most likely.[80,81] Hematogenous metastases and fungal infections may also follow the miliary pattern. Sarcoid follows the bronchovascular bundles and subpleural regions and is perilymphatic in distribution. Lymphangitic carcinomatosis and silicosis also demonstrate this pattern. Infections can often appear as centrilobular nodules, particularly hypersensitivity pneumonitis.

CASE 27

Question 1: C. T3

The International Association for the Study of Lung Cancer provides recommendations for lung cancer staging revisions. The 7th edition of the TNM staging system for lung cancer incorporates knowledge acquired from a world database.[82] The CT of the chest shows a dominant right lower lobe pulmonary nodule measuring 2 cm in size, which in isolation would be a T1 a lesion. T1 a lesions are ≤2 cm with T1b lesions >2 but ≤3 cm. However, the presence of two additional nodules in the same lobe makes this a T3 lesion. If the additional nodules had been in a different lobe of the ipsilateral lung, this would be a T4 lesion. If the nodules had been in the contralateral lung, then they would be considered metastases (M1 a).

Question 2: B. Yes, because the patient is Stage IIIB

The 7th edition TNM staging of the lung states that a T3N0M0 lesion is Stage IIB. Lesions less than STAGE IIIB are considered for surgical resection. N3 lymph nodes or additional M1a or M1b disease would preclude this patient from having surgery.

Question 3: E. All of the above

T3 lesions are greater than 7 cm in size. They invade the chest wall, mediastinal pleura, diaphragm, or pericardial pleura. They can be located in major airways closer than 2 cm from the carina. They can have additional nodules in the same lobe or can cause atelectasis of a whole lung. T2 lesions are less than or equal to 7 cm in size, may cause lobar atelectasis, and are ≥2 cm from the carina. A tumor in the carina is T4 as in invasion of the heart, great vessels, trachea, esophagus, or spine.

CASE 28

Question 1: A. Bronchus suis

The CT images demonstrate an accessory tracheal bronchus, which is also known as a bronchus suis. Tracheal bronchi are nearly always right-sided.[83-85] They may be supernumerary, coexisting with normal bronchi or correspond to an aberrant bronchus. Mounier Kuhn is tracheobronchomegaly with tracheal diameters greater than 3 cm. Cylindrical bronchiectasis is an acquired disease of the airway rather than congenital abnormality. In bilateral right sidedness, the patient has two right lungs, which is associated with asplenia, the absence of the left-sided spleen. That is not the case in our patient.

Question 2: D. Intubation can cause right upper lobe atelectasis

Tracheal bronchus can lead to right upper lobe atelectasis if the patient is intubated. There is no significant

increased incidence of pneumothorax, pneumonia, shortness of breath, or hemoptysis.

Question 3: B. Cardiac bronchus

There are many variants of bronchial branching. The most common supernumerary bronchi are the tracheal bronchus and the cardiac bronchus, which originates from the bronchus intermedius and travels medially toward the heart.

CASE 29

Question 1: B. Usual Interstitial Pneumonia (UIP)

The radiograph demonstrates increased peripheral and basilar reticular markings with intermixed cystic lucencies. The companion chest CT reveals subpleural and basilar predominant honeycombing. Honeycombing represents clustered cysts with well-defined walls stacked upon one another. Usual interstitial pneumonia (UIP) refers to the histologic pattern of IPF, which is temporally heterogeneous.[86] NSIP has basilar predominant ground glass opacity. Asbestosis usually has concomitant pleural plaque. Drug toxicity may lead to fibrotic lung disease, among other patterns of lung disease; however, it is not the most specific answer for the images presented. Exclusion of other known causes of interstitial lung disease such as drug toxicity is among the criteria required for the diagnosis of IPF in the absence of biopsy.

Question 2: E. All of the above

Bronchiectasis and honeycombing are predominant features in IPF. Fibrotic lung disease may lead to secondary pulmonary artery hypertension. Collagen vascular disease is associated with pulmonary findings with rheumatoid arthritis, which is most commonly associated with the IPF pattern (scleroderma is more commonly associated with NSIP).[87,88]

REFERENCES

1. William EB, Clyde AH. *Fundamentals of Diagnostic Radiology*. 4th ed. Philadelphia, PA: Wolters Kluwer/Lippincott Williams & Wilkins; 2012.
2. Gibbs JM, Chandrasekhar CA, Ferguson EC, et al. Lines and stripes: where did they go?—From conventional radiography to CT. *Radiographics*. 2007;27(1):33–48.
3. Raoof S, Feigin D, Sung A, et al. Interpretation of plain chest roentgenogram. *Chest*. 2012;141(2):545–558.
4. Webb WR, Charles BH. *Thoracic Imaging: Pulmonary and Cardiovascular Radiology*. 2nd ed. Philadelphia, PA: Wolters Kluwer/Lippincott Williams & Wilkins Health; 2011.

5. Franquet T, Müller NL, Giménez A, et al. Spectrum of pulmonary aspergillosis: Histologic, clinical, and radiologic findings. *Radiographics.* 2001;21(4):825–837.

6. Gotway MB, Dawn SK, Caoili EM, et al. Pictorial Essay: The Radiologic Spectrum of Pulmonary Aspergillus Infections. *J Comput Assist Tomogr.* 2002;26(2):159–173.

7. Thompson BH, Stanford W, Galvin JR, et al. Varied radiologic appearances of pulmonary aspergillosis. *Radiographics.* 1995;15(6):1273–1284.

8. Kwong JS, Muller NL, Miller RR. Diseases of the trachea and main-stem bronchi: Correlation of CT with pathologic findings. *Radiographics.* 1992;12(4):645–657.

9. Grenier PA, Beigelman-Aubry C, Brillet PY. Nonneoplastic tracheal and bronchial stenoses. *Radiol Clin North Am.* 2009;47(2):243–260.

10. Prince JS, Duhamel DR, Levin DL, et al. Nonneoplastic lesions of the tracheobronchial wall: Radiologic findings with bronchoscopic correlation. *Radiographics.* 2002;22:S215–S230.

11. Chong S, Lee KS, Chung MJ, et al. Pneumoconiosis: Comparison of imaging and pathologic findings. *Radiographics.* 2006;26(1):59–77.

12. Roach HD, Davies GJ, Attanoos R, et al. Asbestos: When the dust settles an imaging review of asbestos-related disease. *Radiographics.* 2002;22:S167–S184.

13. Odev K, Guler I, Altinok T, et al. Cystic and cavitary lung lesions in children: Radiologic findings with pathologic correlation. *J Clin Imaging Sci.* 2013;3:60.607514.124087. eCollection 2013.

14. Berrocal T, Madrid C, Novo S, et al. Congenital anomalies of the tracheobronchial tree, lung, and mediastinum: Embryology, radiology, and pathology. *Radiographics.* 2004;24(1):e17.

15. Jeung MY, Gasser B, Gangi A, et al. Imaging of cystic masses of the mediastinum. *Radiographics.* 2002;22:S79–S93.

16. Pradeep KE. Cutaneous bronchogenic cyst: An under-recognised clinicopathological entity. *J Clin Pathol.* 2009;62(4):384.

17. Ware LB, Matthay MA. Clinical practice. Acute pulmonary edema. *N Engl J Med.* 2005;353(26):2788–2796.

18. Mueller-Lenke N, Rudez J, Staub D, et al. Use of chest radiography in the emergency diagnosis of acute congestive heart failure. *Heart.* 2006;92(5):695–696.

19. Hirschmann JV, Pipavath SN, Godwin JD. Hypersensitivity pneumonitis: A historical, clinical, and radiologic review. *Radiographics.* 2009;29(7):1921–1938.

20. Silva CI, Churg A, Muller NL. Hypersensitivity pneumonitis: Spectrum of high-resolution CT and pathologic findings. *AJR Am J Roentgenol.* 2007;188(2):334–344.

21. Glazer CS, Rose CS, Lynch DA. Clinical and radiologic manifestations of hypersensitivity pneumonitis. *J Thorac Imaging.* 2002;17(4):261–272.

22. Lynch DA, Travis WD, Muller NL, et al. Idiopathic interstitial pneumonias: CT features. *Radiology.* 2005;236(1):10–21.

23. Cordier JF. Cryptogenic organizing pneumonia. *Clin Chest Med.* 2004;25(4):727–738, vi-vii.

24. Kim SJ, Lee KS, Ryu YH, et al. Reversed halo sign on high-resolution CT of cryptogenic organizing pneumonia: Diagnostic implications. *AJR Am J Roentgenol.* 2003;180(5):1251–1254.

25. Ujita M, Renzoni EA, Veeraraghavan S, et al. Organizing pneumonia: Perilobular pattern at thin-section CT. *Radiology.* 2004;232(3):757–761.

26. Ishii H, Trapnell BC, Tazawa R, et al. Comparative study of high-resolution CT findings between autoimmune and secondary pulmonary alveolar proteinosis. *Chest.* 2009;136(5):1348–1355.

27. Frazier AA, Franks TJ, Cooke EO, et al. From the archives of the AFIP: Pulmonary alveolar proteinosis. *Radiographics.* 2008;28(3):883–899; quiz 915.

28. Rossi SE, Erasmus JJ, Volpacchio M, et al. "Crazy-paving" pattern at thin-section CT of the lungs: Radiologic-pathologic overview. *Radiographics.* 2003;23(6):1509–1519.

29. Stern EJ, Frank MS. CT of the lung in patients with pulmonary emphysema: Diagnosis, quantification, and correlation with pathologic and physiologic findings. *AJR Am J Roentgenol.* 1994;162(4):791–798.

30. Webb WR. Radiology of obstructive pulmonary disease. *AJR Am J Roentgenol.* 1997 ;169(3):637–647.

31. Hidalgo A, Franquet T, Gimenez A, et al. Smoking-related interstitial lung diseases: Radiologic-pathologic correlation. *Eur Radiol.* 2006;16(11):2463–2470.

32. National Lung Screening Trial Research Team, Church TR, Black WC, Aberle DR, et al. Results of initial low-dose computed tomographic screening for lung cancer. *N Engl J Med.* 2013;368(21):1980–1991.

33. Jain K, Padley SP, Goldstraw EJ, et al. Primary ciliary dyskinesia in the paediatric population: Range and severity of radiological findings in a cohort of patients receiving tertiary care. *Clin Radiol.* 2007;62(10):986–993.

34. Kennedy MP, Noone PG, Leigh MW, et al. High-resolution CT of patients with primary ciliary dyskinesia. *AJR Am J Roentgenol.* 2007;188(5):1232–1238.

35. Rossman CM, Forrest JB, Lee RM, et al. The dyskinetic cilia syndrome. Ciliary motility in immotile cilia syndrome. *Chest.* 1980;78(4):580–582.

36. Barbato A, Frischer T, Kuehni CE, et al. Primary ciliary dyskinesia: A consensus statement on diagnostic and treatment approaches in children. *Eur Respir J.* 2009;34(6):1264–1276.

37. Abbott GF, Rosado-de-Christenson ML, Frazier AA, et al. From the archives of the AFIP: Lymphangioleiomyomatosis: Radiologic-pathologic correlation. *Radiographics.* 2005;25(3):803–828.

38. Avila NA, Dwyer AJ, Moss J. Imaging features of lymphangioleiomyomatosis: Diagnostic pitfalls. *AJR Am J Roentgenol.* 2011;196(4):982–986.

39. Pallisa E, Sanz P, Roman A, et al. Lymphangioleiomyomatosis: Pulmonary and abdominal findings with pathologic correlation. *Radiographics.* 2002;22:S185–S198.

40. McCormack FX. Lymphangioleiomyomatosis: A clinical update. *Chest.* 2008;133(2):507–516.

41. Rappaport DC, Weisbrod GL, Herman SJ, et al. Pulmonary lymphangioleiomyomatosis: High-resolution CT findings in four cases. *AJR Am J Roentgenol.* 1989;152(5):961–964.

42. Blankenbaker DG. The luftsichel sign. *Radiology.* 1998;208(2):319–320.

43. Mullett R, Jain A, Kotugodella S, et al. Lobar collapse demystified: The chest radiograph with CT correlation. *Postgrad Med J*. 2012;88(1040):335–347.

44. Ridge CA, Bankier AA, Eisenberg RL. Mosaic attenuation. *AJR Am J Roentgenol*. 2011;197(6):W970–W977.

45. Abbott GF, Rosado-de-Christenson ML, Rossi SE, et al. Imaging of small airways disease. *J Thorac Imaging*. 2009;24(4):285–298.

46. Agrawal A, Agrawal A, Bansal V, et al. A systematic approach to interpretation of heterogeneous lung attenuation on computed tomography of the chest. *Lung India*. 2013;30(4):327–334.

47. Naidich DP, Bankier AA, MacMahon H, et al. Recommendations for the management of subsolid pulmonary nodules detected at CT: A statement from the fleischner society. *Radiology*. 2013;266(1):304–317.

48. Henschke CI, Yankelevitz DF, Mirtcheva R, et al. CT screening for lung cancer: Frequency and significance of part-solid and nonsolid nodules. *AJR Am J Roentgenol*. 2002;178(5):1053–1057.

49. Akira M, Inoue Y, Kitaichi M, et al. Usual interstitial pneumonia and nonspecific interstitial pneumonia with and without concurrent emphysema: Thin-section CT findings. *Radiology*. 2009;251(1):271–279.

50. Kligerman SJ, Groshong S, Brown KK, et al. Nonspecific interstitial pneumonia: Radiologic, clinical, and pathologic considerations. *Radiographics*. 2009;29(1):73–87.

51. Silva CI, Muller NL, Hansell DM, et al. Nonspecific interstitial pneumonia and idiopathic pulmonary fibrosis: Changes in pattern and distribution of disease over time. *Radiology*. 2008;247(1):251–259.

52. Frazier AA, Galvin JR, Franks TJ, et al. From the archives of the AFIP: Pulmonary vasculature: Hypertension and infarction. *Radiographics*. 2000;20(2):491–524; quiz 530–1, 532.

53. Pena E, Dennie C, Veinot J, et al. Pulmonary hypertension: How the radiologist can help. *Radiographics*. 2012;32(1):9–32.

54. Galie N, Torbicki A, Barst R, et al. Guidelines on diagnosis and treatment of pulmonary arterial hypertension. The task force on diagnosis and treatment of pulmonary arterial hypertension of the European Society of cardiology. *Eur Heart J*. 2004;25(24):2243–2278.

55. PIOPED Investigators. Value of the ventilation/perfusion scan in acute pulmonary embolism. results of the prospective investigation of pulmonary embolism diagnosis (PIOPED). *JAMA*. 1990;263(20):2753–2759.

56. Stein PD, Fowler SE, Goodman LR, et al. Multidetector computed tomography for acute pulmonary embolism. *N Engl J Med*. 2006;354(22):2317–2327.

57. Stein PD, Chenevert TL, Fowler SE, et al. Gadolinium-enhanced magnetic resonance angiography for pulmonary embolism: A multicenter prospective study (PIOPED III). *Ann Intern Med*. 2010;152(7):434–443, W142–W143.

58. Zamorano JL. *The ESC Textbook of Cardiovascular Imaging*. New York, NY: Springer; 2010.

59. Chiles C, Woodard PK, Gutierrez FR, et al. Metastatic involvement of the heart and pericardium: CT and MR imaging. *Radiographics*. 2001;21(2):439–449.

60. Parker MS, Chasen MH, Paul N. Radiologic signs in thoracic imaging: Case-based review and self-assessment module. *AJR Am J Roentgenol*. 2009;192(3 Suppl):S34–S48.

61. Mendez JL, Nadrous HF, Vassallo R, et al. Pneumothorax in pulmonary Langerhans cell histiocytosis. *Chest*. 2004; 125(3):1028–1032.

62. Schonfeld N, Dirks K, Costabel U, et al; Wissenschaftliche Arbeitsgemeinschaft fur die Therapie von Lungenkrankheiten. A prospective clinical multicentre study on adult pulmonary langerhans' cell histiocytosis. *Sarcoidosis Vasc Diffuse Lung Dis*. 2012;29(2):132–138.

63. Kim HJ, Lee KS, Johkoh T, et al. Pulmonary langerhans cell histiocytosis in adults: High-resolution CT-pathology comparisons and evolutional changes at CT. *Eur Radiol*. 2011;21(7):1406–1415.

64. Mogulkoc N, Veral A, Bishop PW, et al. Pulmonary langerhans' cell histiocytosis: Radiologic resolution following smoking cessation. *Chest*. 1999;115(5):1452–1455.

65. Goodman LR. Postoperative chest radiograph: II. alterations after major intrathoracic surgery. *AJR Am J Roentgenol*. 1980;134(4):803–813.

66. Wechsler RJ, Goodman LR. Mediastinal position and airfluid height after pneumonectomy: The effect of the respiratory cycle. *AJR Am J Roentgenol*. 1985;145(6):1173–1176.

67. Kerr WF. Late-onset post-pneumonectomy empyema. *Thorax*. 1977;32(2):149–154.

68. Jeong YJ, Lee KS. Pulmonary tuberculosis: Up-to-date imaging and management. *AJR Am J Roentgenol*. 2008; 191(3):834–844.

69. Burrill J, Williams CJ, Bain G, et al. Tuberculosis: A radiologic review. *Radiographics*. 2007;27(5):1255–1273.

70. Criado E, Sanchez M, Ramirez J, et al. Pulmonary sarcoidosis: Typical and atypical manifestations at high-resolution CT with pathologic correlation. *Radiographics*. 2010;30(6):1567–1586.

71. Prabhakar HB, Rabinowitz CB, Gibbons FK, et al. Imaging features of sarcoidosis on MDCT, FDG PET, and PET/CT. *AJR Am J Roentgenol*. 2008;190(3 Suppl):S1–S6.

72. Lynch JP,3rd, Ma YL, Koss MN, et al. Pulmonary sarcoidosis. *Semin Respir Crit Care Med*. 2007;28(1):53–74.

73. Rabinowitz JG, Ulreich S, Soriano C. The usual unusual manifestations of sarcoidosis and the "hilar haze"–a new diagnostic aid. *Am J Roentgenol Radium Ther Nucl Med*. 1974;120(4):821–831.

74. Webb WR, Charles BH.. "*The Mediastinum: Mediastinal Masses*." *Thoracic Imaging: Pulmonary and Cardiovascular Radiology*. Philadelphia, PA: Wolters Kluwer/Lippincott Williams & Wilkins Health; 2011.

75. Nasseri F, Eftekhari F. Clinical and radiologic review of the normal and abnormal thymus: Pearls and pitfalls. *Radiographics*. 2010;30(2):413–428.

76. Tecce PM, Fishman EK, Kuhlman JE. CT evaluation of the anterior mediastinum: Spectrum of disease. *Radiographics*. 1994;14(5):973–990.

77. Takahashi K, Al-Janabi NJ. Computed tomography and magnetic resonance imaging of mediastinal tumors. *J Magn Reson Imaging*. 2010;32(6):1325–1339.

78. Brown LR, Aughenbaugh GL. Masses of the anterior mediastinum: CT and MR imaging. *AJR Am J Roentgenol*. 1991; 157(6):1171–1180.

79. Raoof S, Amchentsev A, Vlahos I, et al. Pictorial essay: Multinodular disease: A high-resolution CT scan diagnostic algorithm. *Chest*. 2006;129(3):805–815.

80. Hong SH, Im JG, Lee JS, et al. High resolution CT findings of miliary tuberculosis. *J Comput Assist Tomogr*. 1998; 22(2):220–224.

81. Oh YW, Kim YH, Lee NJ, et al. High-resolution CT appearance of miliary tuberculosis. *J Comput Assist Tomogr*. 1994; 18(6):862–866.

82. UyBico SJ, Wu CC, Suh RD, et al. Lung cancer staging essentials: The new TNM staging system and potential imaging pitfalls. *Radiographics*. 2010;30(5): 1163–1181.

83. Doolittle AM, Mair EA. Tracheal bronchus: Classification, endoscopic analysis, and airway management. *Otolaryngol Head Neck Surg*. 2002;126(3):240–243.

84. Ghaye B, Szapiro D, Fanchamps JM, et al. Congenital bronchial abnormalities revisited. *Radiographics*. 2001;21(1):105–119.

85. Wu JW, White CS, Meyer CA, et al. Variant bronchial anatomy: CT appearance and classification. *AJR Am J Roentgenol*. 1999;172(3):741–744.

86. Raghu G, Collard HR, Egan JJ, et al; ATS/ERS/JRS/ALAT Committee on Idiopathic Pulmonary Fibrosis. An official ATS/ERS/JRS/ALAT statement: idiopathic pulmonary fibrosis: evidence-based guidelines for diagnosis and management. *Am J Respir Crit Care Med*. 2011;183(6):788–824.

87. Lynch DA. Lung disease related to collagen vascular disease. *J Thorac imaging*. 2009;24(4):299–309.

88. Gutsche M, Rosen GD, Swigris JJ. Connective tissue disease-associated intersitial lung disease: A review. *Curr Respir Care Rep*. 2012;1:224–232.

4

Chronic Obstructive Pulmonary Disease

Jason Filopei MD, Lisa Bajpayee MD, and Ronaldo Collo Go MD

CASE 1

A 62-year-old man has been complaining of progressive shortness of breath, worsening cough, and increased sputum production for several days. He is an active smoker with a history of chronic obstructive pulmonary disease (COPD) on fluticasone/salmeterol and albuterol. His exercise tolerance is now limited to getting out of bed, significantly worse than his baseline of two city blocks. His physical examination is remarkable for a respiratory rate of 42 breaths per minute, oxygen saturation of 79% on room air, diffuse bilateral wheezing, and a prolonged expiratory phase.

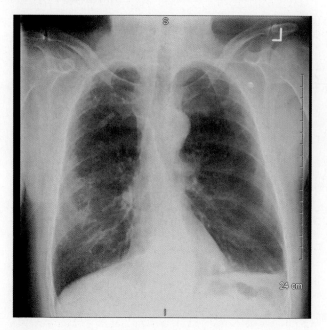

* *

A venous blood gas shows pH 7.08 and pCO_2 of 116. Recent pulmonary function test (PFT) from his outpatient pulmonologist show:

PFT	Result
FVC	3.52 L
FEV_1	1.41 L
FEV_1/FVC	40%
TLC	6.3L (150%)
DLCO	23.1%
Bronchodilator response	(–)

* *

The patient is intubated and treated with intravenous corticosteroids and inhaled bronchodilators. He is extubated on day 3.

Question 1: **Which of the following medications would decrease his likelihood for hospital readmission?**

A. Increase the dose of fluticasone/salmeterol.
B. Start theophylline 300 mg daily.
C. Start inhaled tiotropium 18 μg/cap daily.
D. Add inhaled ipratropium bromide every 6 hours.
E. Continue with current medications.

Question 2: **Based on the 2014 Global Initiative for Chronic Obstructive Lung Disease (GOLD) guidelines, what is considered to be the most appropriate treatment dose and duration of steroids for a COPD exacerbation?**

A. Five-day course of oral prednisone
B. Fourteen-day course of oral prednisone
C. Seven-day course of intravenous solumedrol
D. Fourteen-day course of intravenous hydrocortisone
E. Five-day course of intravenous solumedrol

Question 3: **What about this patient's pulmonary function test is most suggestive of chronic obstructive pulmonary disease?**

A. A decreased diffusion capacity
B. A decreased FEV_1/FVC ratio
C. A positive bronchodilator response
D. A decreased total lung volume
E. Both A and B.

CASE 2

A 59-year-old man with COPD and 60 pack-year smoking history comes to your office for a follow-up visit. Despite continued smoking, his COPD has been stable over the past year on tiotropium and albuterol. The patient has tried to quit multiple times, but has never gone more than 4 days without a cigarette. His brother, who is also a smoker, recently is diagnosed with advanced small cell lung cancer. Your patient is concerned for his health and wants to know what he can do to increase his life span and reduce his chances of developing lung cancer.

Question 1: **What could be done to reduce the patient's mortality risk from chronic obstructive pulmonary disease?**

A. Start the patient on daily systemic steroid therapy.
B. Refer the patient for a pulmonary rehabilitation.
C. Start a low dose inhaled corticosteroid.
D. Start smoking cessation counseling and subsequent pharmacological therapy.
E. Start inhaled tiotropium daily.

Question 2: **The patient is interested in pharmacological therapy to help in his efforts to quit smoking. After he scores 0 points on the PHQ-2 questionnaire and he states he has no history of a seizure disorder, what would be the most appropriate medication to provide the patient?**

A. Bupropion
B. Bupropion and nicotine replacement patch
C. Varenicline
D. Combination nicotine replacement therapy using both patch and gum
E. Varenicline and nicotine replacement therapy

CASE 3

A 55-year-old woman with COPD and a 30- pack-year history is being discharged from the hospital for COPD exacerbation. She still smokes one to two cigarettes daily. Upon discharge, she is asked to continue her inhaler therapy and a short course of oral prednisone. It has been recommended that she follows up for enrollment in pulmonary rehabilitation.

Question 1: **When is the appropriate time to refer this patient to pulmonary rehabilitation?**

A. After she finishes her course of prednisone
B. As soon as she is discharged from the hospital
C. One month after she is discharged
D. She is not a candidate for pulmonary rehabilitation
E. After she quits smoking

Question 2: **During follow-up at the pulmonary clinic, discussion regarding lung volume reduction surgery (LVRS) is entertained. Which of the below answer choices is an indication for performing lung volume reduction surgery?**

A. Age >75 years
B. Five months of smoking cessation
C. Pre-rehabilitation of 140 m achieved during 6-minute walk test but low maximal achieved cycle ergometry
D. Post-rehabilitation of 140 m achieved during 6-minute walk test with low maximal achieved cycle ergometry
E. Patients with both an FEV_1 <20% and DLCO <20% predicted

Question 3: **Which patient group is associated with the highest mortality risk after lung volume reduction surgery?**

A. Patients with FEV_1 <20% predicted and homogeneous emphysema
B. Patients with upper lobe emphysema and low-exercise capacity
C. Patients with upper lobe emphysema and high-exercise capacity
D. Patients with FEV_1 <20%%predicted and upper-lobe emphysema
E. None of the above

CASE 4

A 35-year-old man with a 5 pack-year smoking history who quit 2 years ago has been complaining of shortness of breath with exertion. He denies any sick contacts. Chest radiograph reveals hyper lucencies in the lower lobes and computed tomography of his chest shows panacinar emphysema of the lower lobes. His family history is significant for his grandfather who suffered from unexplained liver disease and bronchiectasis. Blood work performed is remarkable for slightly abnormal liver enzymes.

Question 1: What could be one of the initial screening tests for this patient's clinical presentation?

A. Alpha-1 antitrypsin level (AAT)
B. ANCA
C. ANA
D. Alpha-1 antitrypsin phenotyping
E. Functional assay of AAT antiprotease

Question 2: Patient is found to have a positive C-ANCA. He is also noted to have an AAT level of 7 umol/L. Pulmonary function test reveals reduced FEV/FVC with FEV_1 40% predicted. Which phenotype is most closely associated with lung disease?

A. MM
B. PI*ZZ
C. PI*M
D. PI*MZ
E. None of the above

Question 3: What is the appropriate treatment?

A. Aerosolized human pooled AAT
B. Weekly intravenous administration of AAT
C. Gene therapy
D. Lung volume reduction surgery
E. None of the above

Question 4: What should be checked prior to the initiation of augmentation therapy?

A. Pulmonary function test
B. IgA level
C. TMPT deficiency
D. IgE level
E. None of the above

CASE 5

A 75-year-old man presents to outpatient clinic for a preoperative evaluation prior to a right total knee replacement. He has been oxygen dependent for the past 2 years and continues to smoke one pack of cigarettes daily, with a 55 pack-year history. He reports that at baseline he has significant shortness of breath when walking and has to stop every few minutes to "catch breath." His other

medical problems include diabetes mellitus type 2 with neuropathy, atrial fibrillation, gastric ulcer disease, irritable bowel syndrome, and anxiety disorder. His medications are albuterol as needed, tiotropium, fluticasone/salmeterol, metformin, diltiazem, coumadin, omeprazole, and wellbutrin. His temperature is 98°F, blood pressure 120/76 mm Hg, pulse 80 per minute, respirations at 16 per minute and unlabored, and oxygen saturation is 95% on 2 L oxygen. His general physical examination shows an obese gentleman, BMI 30, expiratory wheezing on lung examination, and the remainder of his examination is unremarkable. A 6-minute walk test is performed and the patient is able to walk 230 m.

* *

His laboratory results are as follows:

WBC	7.0/uL
Hemoglobin	12.6 g/dL
Platelets	200,000/uL
Sodium	142 mEq/L
Potassium	4.0 mEq/L
Chloride	108 mEq/L
Bicarbonate	26 mEq/L
BUN	14 mg/dL
Creatinine	0.8 mg/dL
Albumin	4.0 g/dL

* *

A chest radiograph performed 2 months ago shows hyperinflation but no other abnormalities. Results of his pulmonary function studies are shown below. After inhaling a short-acting beta-agonist, the FEV_1 has shown a 5% improvement.

PFT	Result
FVC	3.1 L (73%)
FEV_1	0.7 L (23%)
FEV_1/FVC ratio	23%
TLC	9.7 (150%)
DLCO	0.9 (19%)

Question 1: As his pulmonologist, you are asked to perform a preoperative pulmonary risk assessment.

In addition to a complete history and physical examination, what else are you required to order as part of his preoperative evaluation?

A. Repeat pulmonary function test
B. Arterial blood gas
C. Chest radiograph
D. Arterial blood gas and chest radiograph
E. No further testing is indicated

Question 2: Which of the following is not a statistically significant risk factor for the development of postoperative pulmonary complications?

A. Cigarette smoking
B. General health status (ASA class >II)
C. Age >50 years
D. Upper respiratory infection 2 weeks ago
E. Chronic obstructive pulmonary disease (COPD)

Question 3: The patient's upcoming surgery and need for preoperative pulmonary evaluation has raised his concern regarding his long-term prognosis. Which of the following is the best way to predict his long-term prognosis?

A. FEV_1, DLCO, and current smoking status
B. FEV_1, exercise capacity, patient's perceived dyspnea, and BMI
C. FEV_1, exercise capacity, presence of hypercapnia during acute COPD exacerbations
D. Current smoking status, presence of chronic hypercapnia, gender
E. Currently, there is no good way to predict long-term prognosis

Question 4: You counsel your patient regarding his long-term prognosis for COPD. Your patient expresses understanding of his risk factors. He then proceeds to ask, "Do any of my other medical problems worsen my chance of survival in COPD?" Which of the following is the MOST accurate response?

A. No. There is no evidence that coexisting medical problems affect mortality in COPD.
B. No. There are medical problems that affect mortality in COPD, but you do not have any medical problems that should affect your mortality.
C. Yes. Based on the COTE index, your diabetes, irritable bowel syndrome, and anxiety increase your mortality risk in COPD.
D. Yes. Based on the COTE index, your diabetes with neuropathy, atrial fibrillation, and gastric ulcer disease increase your mortality risk in COPD.

E. Yes. Based on the BODE index, your diabetes with neuropathy, atrial fibrillation, and gastric ulcer disease increase your mortality risk in COPD.

CASE 6

A 69-year-old man with severe COPD is referred to you for management of his condition. He recently has stopped smoking 6 months ago but prior to this, has had a 50- pack-year smoking history. He has a minimal exercise tolerance and usually stops multiple times when walking short distances. He correlates his subjective dyspnea as "Grade 3" on the breathlessness questionnaire, Modified British Medical Research Council (mMRC). He is on 3 L oxygen continuously and is on multiple lung medications including long-acting theophylline. His last COPD exacerbation has been 2 years ago, for which he was treated with a short steroid course and antibiotics. The possibility of lung transplant is raised, but the patient refuses. He has no other medical conditions. Physical examination reveals a SaO_2 of 95% on 3 L/min nasal cannula; his other vital signs are normal.

* *

His pulmonary function studies are shown below.

PFT	Result
FVC	1.82 L (55%)
FEV_1	0.39 L (15%)
FEV_1/FVC ratio	0.21

Question 1: You congratulate the patient on his tobacco cessation and counsel him on how his lung function will be affected. Which of the following is the most accurate statement?

A. Your lung function (FEV_1) will decline at a slower rate.
B. Your lung function (FEV_1) will decline at a faster rate.
C. Your lung function (FEV_1) will no longer decline, but stay the same for the rest of your life.
D. Your lung function (FEV_1) will improve to the level of a nonsmoker at a similar age.
E. Your lung function (FEV_1) will supersede that of a nonsmoker at a similar age.

Question 2: You perform an assessment of the patient's COPD severity. Which of the following is not a criterion used in the combined COPD assessment?

A. Patient's subjective symptom assessment, including breathlessness

B. The degree of airflow limitation based on spirometry

C. The risk of COPD exacerbations

D. The use of supplemental oxygen

E. Both A and D

Question 3: Based on the combined assessment of COPD, which of the following is an appropriate initial pharmacologic regimen for this patient?

A. Fluticasone and salmeterol

B. Levoalbuterol and ipratropium bromide

C. Fluticasone/salmeterol and po prednisone

D. Budesonide, tiotropium, and beclomethasone

E. The patient does not need medication at this time

Question 4: Upon review of the patient's medications, you notice that the patient is taking theophylline, which was started by his previous healthcare provider. Which of the following is not a potential metabolic complication of theophylline toxicity?

A. Hyperglycemia

B. Metabolic acidosis

C. Hypokalemia

D. Hyperkalemia

E. Hypophosphatemia

Question 5: You review the patient's current vaccination history. Which of the following is most accurate concerning vaccines in COPD patients?

A. Vaccines are contraindicated in severe COPD patients.

B. Flu vaccines are recommended yearly in COPD patients.

C. The flu vaccine and pneumococcal polysaccharide vaccine should be administered only in COPD patients 65 years and older.

D. The flu vaccine should be administered yearly in COPD patients. The pneumococcal polysaccharide vaccine should be administered once in patients younger than 50 years who have COPD with an FEV_1 <40% or with significant comorbid conditions and then readministered in patients greater than 50 years.

E. The flu vaccine should be administered yearly in COPD patients. The pneumococcal polysaccharide vaccine should be administered once in patients <65 years who have COPD with an FEV_1 <40% or with significant comorbid conditions and then readministered in patients >65 years of age.

CASE 7

A 50-year old-man, nonsmoker, has been complaining of productive cough for the last three years. He denies any smoking history or sick contacts. He tries to exercise but is limited by his cough. His family history is significant for his father having COPD and mother having asthma. He has had chest radiography and pulmonary function test last year, both of which were essentially unremarkable. He has been recently admitted to the hospital for progressive shortness of breath and cough, and has been discharged on bronchodilators and short course of steroids. The repeat pulmonary function test 1 month later has shown the following:

PFT	Result
FEV_1	50%
FEV_1/FVC	60%
Bronchodilator Response	(–)

Question 1: What is your diagnosis?

A. Asthma

B. COPD—emphysema

C. COPD—chronic bronchitis

D. Asthma—COPD overlap syndrome

E. Diffuse panbronchiolitis

Question 2: Which of the following agents has been shown to reduce COPD exacerbations in this type of patient?

A. Oxygen

B. Roflumilast

C. Theophylline

D. Oral corticosteroids

E. None of the above

Answers

CASE 1

Question 1: C. Start inhaled tiotropium daily.

Adding tiotropium, a long-acting anti-muscarinic antagonist (LAMA), is the correct choice in a patient who is GOLD Stage III to IV already on an inhaled corticosteroid (ICS) and long-acting beta-agonist (LABA). Tiotropium is a LAMA that selectively blocks the M1 and M3 receptors found on airway smooth muscle cells that normally cause bronchoconstriction. Large randomized clinical trials have shown tiotropium to reduce COPD exacerbations with ranges of 14% to 25%, improvement, overall health status, and outcomes on pulmonary rehabilitation. The Understanding potential long-term improvements in function with tiotropium (UPLIFT) trial is the landmark trial examining the effects of tiotropium.[1] It is a 4-year randomized placebo-controlled clinical trial examining 5,922 patients with moderate-to-severe COPD permitted to be on ICS, LABA, or both that evaluated the decline in FEV_1. Secondary end points includes lung function, quality of life measures, rate of exacerbations, exacerbation-related hospitalizations, and overall mortality. While the results fail to show an effect of tiotropium on the rate of decline of FEV_1, it has shown improvements in lung function and health-related quality of life that are sustained and a reduction in the risk of exacerbations. Although increasing the dose of the combination inhaler fluticasone/salmeterol might be an appropriate adjustment in therapy for this patient, it is not the best choice of those listed. Salmeterol is a LABA with roughly an 8- to 12-hour half-life. Alone, salmeterol has been shown in both the TORCH and TRISTAN trials to significantly reduce the rate of COPD exacerbations (not mortality). Fluticasone is an inhaled corticosteroid very effective in the treatment of asthma; however, as single therapy for COPD has mixed and controversial data (however in TORCH it is shown to have small improvements in respiratory health status and reductions in exacerbation rates). The combination of these two inhaled therapies as for COPD has also been studied in another arm of both the TORCH[2] and TRISTAN[3] trials. These has demonstrated improvements in FEV_1, QOL, and decreased exacerbation rates by as much as 25% as compared to monotherapy in patients with moderate obstruction (FEV_1 50–79%). Although the difference was modest and the exacerbation rate was low in both the study groups, a number needed to treat analysis demonstrated that treating four patients for 1-year time prevented one exacerbation versus each therapy separately. The POET-COPD investigators have demonstrated in a head to head analysis that in patients with moderate to very severe COPD, tiotropium is more effective than salmeterol in reducing exacerbations (0.85, [95% CI, 0.80–0.90]) versus (1.13 [95% CI 1.07–1.20]).[4] When combination salmeterol and fluticasone versus tiotropium is studied in the INSPIRE trial, both drugs have been found to prevent COPD exacerbations equally as well.[5] Finally, the use of "triple therapy" for patients with COPD is studied in a randomized controlled trial from the Annals of Internal Medicine and showed similar reductions in COPD exacerbations to the TRISTAN and TORCH trials while showing a 50% reduction in hospitalization rates along with greater rates of improved symptoms and spirometric lung function.[6]

* *

Theophylline, a methylxanthine derivative, functions as a nonselective competitive phophodiesterase inhibitor and inhibits the degradation of cyclic adenosine monophosphate. Mechanisms include a bronchodilator effect that has been to shown to improve FEV_1 and vital capacity and reduction in the systemic inflammatory response inherent to COPD. Mixed data from the past has shown theophylline to improve disease sequeale of COPD including dyspnea, exercise capacity, and respiratory mechanics via surrogate markers such as FEV_1 and vital capacity. The current GOLD guidelines recommend its use only as third-line therapy or when inhaled bronchodilators are not available. This is due to its narrow therapeutic window and significant degree of intolerance by patients' secondary to gastrointestinal side effects.

**

According to the most recent GOLD guidelines, treatment with an inhaled corticosteroid and long-acting beta-agonist could represent an appropriate treatment option; however, more recent data has suggested there are modest benefits to triple therapy in patients with Gold 3–4 classification who still have uncontrolled symptoms. Therefore, making no changes to this patient's medication regiment would be incorrect.

Question 2: A. Five-day course of oral prednisone

Five days of oral prednisone is the most current GOLD recommendation for treatment of COPD exacerbation. Previously, a 10- to 14-day course of systemic steroids has been recommended. This is primarily based on data from a New England Journal of Medicine study from 1999 examining treatment of patients at a Veterans Affair hospital.[7] Currently, there remains insufficient data concerning the optimal duration, appropriate route of administration, and dose of corticosteroid therapy creating a wide spectrum steroid therapy in real world practice. Most recently, the REDUCE trial shows that 5 days of oral prednisone is noninferior to 14 days of oral prednisone. This trial has examined 314 patients mostly with severe COPD (an average FEV_1 of 40%) and randomized these patients to receive 5 versus 14 days of 40 mg of prednisone.[8] Prior to this, shorter courses have never studied against a longer 10- to 14-day course. These patients also have received broad-spectrum antibiotics for 7 days, inhaled triple therapy, and as needed nebulizer bronchodilators. Besides the shorter course being shown to be noninferior to the traditional longer course, the decreased cumulative exposure of 65% to corticosteroids has decreased the degree of steroid induced side effects a patient might experience.

**

In the previous GOLD 2013 guidelines,[9] a grade D recommendation has existed for a 10- to 14-day course of systemic corticosteroid treatment; however, there still remains insufficient data to continue to recommend this course in the light of new data suggesting that shorter courses are noninferior.

**

In the last 10 years, it has been shown that oral steroids are noninferior to intravenous steroids in the treatment

of COPD exacerbations that require hospitalization. De Jong and colleagues have shown this in detail in 2007 with a double blinded randomized trial of 435 patients comparing the two forms of administration.[10] It has also been shown by Lindenauer and colleagues in an epidemiological cohort study that administration of oral steroids did not have worse outcomes than the use of intravenous steroids.[11]

Question 3: E. Both A and B

Diffusion capacity (DLCO) measures the ability of the lung to transfer gas from inspired air to the red blood cells in the pulmonary capillaries. Although it is not required for the diagnosis of COPD, a decreased DLCO can be indicative of the degree of emphysema that exists on the alveolar level. Traditionally, this value was always considered to be decreased in patients with COPD; however, it is now known that patients with chronic obstructive disease can have a normal DLCO secondary to their airway limitation from chronic bronchitis. Beyond this, DLCO remains a strong predictor for desaturation with exertion and need for oxygen therapy. The patient described in the vignette has a very low diffusion capacity secondary to the large component of emphysematous disease.

**

The patient has an FEV_1/FVC ratio of 29%. According to the GOLD criteria, it is required to have the presence of post-bronchodilator FEV_1/FVC <0.70 to confirm the diagnosis of COPD. The FEV_1 represents the area under the curve of the FVC that a patient is able to complete within 1 second of beginning expiration. Values below 80% predicted for the FEV_1 are used to define airflow obstruction. The FVC represents the volume of air forcibly exhaled from the point of maximal inspiration. It is a simple diagnostic criterion that unlike other spirometric values is independent of reference values. The use of a single value allows for both simplicity and consistency for clinicians when evaluating a patient with suspected COPD.

**

COPD is traditionally characterized by airflow limitation not fully normalized after an inhaled bronchodilator. The traditional mechanism of progressive lung destruction in patients with emphysema starts in small airways that are generally devoid of smooth muscle fibers progressing often to the medium-sized airways where beta-agonist receptors exist. These smooth muscle fibers found in medium airways are the target of beta-agonist therapies. The presence of a post-bronchodilator FEV_1/FVC <0.70 confirms the presence of airflow limitation. This differs from the other traditional obstructive disease which sees nearly full reversibility of airflow limitation with therapy; however, there exists a well-described cohort of patients with COPD phenotype that exhibits a >12% increase in FEV_1 after bronchodilator administration.

* *

The most common lung volume measurements include total lung capacity, functional residual capacity, and residual volume. Lung volume measurements are not needed for all patients that are suspected to have COPD. However, it can provide insight into a decreased FVC value whether it is secondary to air trapping, hyperinflation, or other restrictive ventilator defects.

CASE 2

Question 1: D. Start smoking cessation counseling and subsequent pharmacological therapy.

Smoking cessation counseling combined with pharmacological interventions has been shown to increase patients' quit rates, improve long-term mortality, and slow the decline of FEV_1.[12] FEV_1 declines normally with aging by approximately 30 mL each year, but in some smokers the decline exhibited can be as much as double this.[13,14] According to the United States Public Health Service, brief smoking cessation should be addressed at every single office visit, whether performed by the physician or other healthcare provider. The "Five A's" approach is often recommended as the framework for brief counseling and includes ask, advise, assess, assist, and arrange. In addition to brief counseling, providers in addition should offer pharmacological interventions when appropriate as this has been shown to be more effective than either medication or counseling alone. On average, it takes seven attempts for a smoker to successfully quit. Patients who attempt smoking cessation should be warned about withdrawal symptoms including headache, irritability, and weight gain, and avoid high-risk smoking situations.

* *

There is limited evidence to suggest that placing a patient with COPD on chronic systemic corticosteroids improves outcomes including hospitalization rates and mortality. A study published in 2003 by Aaron et al.

suggested that there is a decrease in relapse rate of COPD exacerbation if patients were treated with an additional 10 days of oral prednisone upon discharge from the hospital; however, this endpoint did not reach statistical significance.[15] There has been no other convincing evidence for chronic steroid use.

* *

Pulmonary rehabilitation has shown improvements across many different parameters measured for patients with chronic obstructive pulmonary disease including symptoms such as dyspnea, exercise tolerance in the form of improved 6-minute walk tests, measurements in forced expiratory volume over 1 second, and various questionnaires targeted at quality of life measures; however, it has not been shown to have a significant impact on overall survival. Recently published data suggests that pulmonary rehabilitation can have a significant improvement on mortality if a patient enrolls within 10 days of an exacerbation.

* *

As discussed earlier, neither inhaled corticosteroid nor inhaled tiotropium have been shown to reduce long-term mortality in patients suffering from COPD. Both randomized controlled clinical trials and Cochrane reviews of all existing evidence have failed to show a mortality benefit for either of these agents, especially in those who are active smokers.

Question 2: C. Varenicline

Varenicline is a weak nicotine receptor partial agonist to reduce cravings and decrease the pleasurable effects of tobacco products. In a recent Cochrane review of all the literature on smoking cessation therapy, a pooled odds ratio for sustained smoking cessation at 12 months versus placebo has been found to be 3.22 (95% CI, 2.43–4.27) while the pooled odds ratio for varenicline versus bupropion has been 1.66 (95% CI, 1.28–2.16).[16] At 1-year follow-up of the varenicline group, the sustained quit rate was found to be 27% versus placebo.[16] In terms of the black box warning of increased suicide risk and connection to increased cardiac risk, subgroup analysis performed from these Cochrane reviews found limited incidence of either neuropsychiatric or cardiac events in patients on therapy.[16]

* *

Bupropion is a realistic choice of medication for this patient but not the best answer choice listed (as stated above). Its mechanistic role in smoking cessation is unclear, but is believed to play a role in mitigating withdrawal symptoms that stem from nicotine. As sole therapy, it nearly doubles the odds of smoking cessation versus placebo therapy.[17] Bupropion can be appropriate if the patient does not have a predilection for seizures since it is a rare, but major side effect (1 in 1,000). Bupropion in combination with a form of nicotine replacement therapy (gum, patch, inhaler, tablets, lozenges) has not been shown to increase the odds of smoking cessation as compared to monotherapy with bupropion alone.

* *

Combination nicotine replacement therapy has been shown to outperform single formulations of NRT in clinical trials and meta-analysis performed; however, it does not have a greater efficacy than either varenicline or bupropion as monotherapy.[18]

* *

Varenicline combined with NRT has become an increasingly more studied treatment modality for smoking cessation; however, the results are mixed. Within the last year (2014), two well-designed randomized controlled clinical trials have been resulted with conflicting data. Ramon et al. in a randomized controlled trial published results in BMC Medicine that the combination of varenicline and nicotine patch did not improve abstinence rates at 12 and 24 weeks compared with varenicline used as monotherapy when all smokers were analyzed as a whole, independent of consumption level.[19] On the other hand, Koegelenberg et al. has studied this same intervention with their data showing >10% abstinence rates at 12 weeks and 24 weeks respectively, combination varenicline and a nicotine patch versus varenicline alone.[20] More large-scale clinical trials are needed along with meta-analysis data to ensure there is in fact an increased abstinence rate with combination therapy.

CASE 3

Question 1: B. As soon as she is discharged
The Joint Committee of American Thoracic Society and the European Respiratory Society defines "pulmonary rehabilitation is a comprehensive intervention based on a thorough patient assessment followed by patient tailored therapies that include, but are not limited to, exercise training, education, and behavior change, designed to improve the physical and psychological condition of people with chronic respiratory disease and to promote the long-term adherence to health-enhancing behaviors."[21]

* *

A Cochrane review published by Puhan et al. in 2011 that examined nine trials of moderate methodological quality involving 432 patients with recent COPD exacerbations suggests that pulmonary rehabilitation is a highly effective and safe intervention immediately post-discharge to reduce the rate of hospital readmissions (Number Needed to Treat = 4) as well as improve health-related quality of life in COPD patients.[22]

* *

There is no data to suggest that performing pulmonary rehabilitation immediately following discharge leads to worsening outcomes or increased readmissions; rather the data supports early intervention. One reason for this may be that pulmonary rehabilitations are often tailored to individual patients, and although most of the data exists for patients with an FEV_1 <50%, pulmonary rehabilitation can be offered to all patients with an FEV_1 <80%. Although it has not been definitively shown to reduce mortality in patients suffering from COPD, pulmonary rehabilitation is a cornerstone of COPD management with a large supporting body of evidence. For example, a Cochrane review published in 2006 shows statistically and clinically significant improvements in dyspnea, fatigue, and emotional status. Beyond this, a large meta-analysis performed by Cambach and colleagues shows improvements in exercise capacity, walking distance, and scores in the chronic respiratory disease questionnaire.[23]

* *

There are no specific inclusion or exclusion criteria for pulmonary rehabilitation enrollment. Active smoking is not a contraindication to joining pulmonary rehabilitation and these patients most likely benefit the same advantages as nonsmokers as well as the added benefit of smoking cessation counseling that would be incorporated into their pulmonary rehabilitation program.

Question 2: D. Post-rehabilitation of 140 m during 6-minute walk test with low maximal achieved cycle ergometry
Much of the existing data on LVRS including indications for surgery, patient selection, and long-term outcomes are based on data from the National Emphysema Treatment Trial Research Group. This is a randomized controlled trial of 1,218 patients with severe emphysema who underwent

pulmonary rehabilitation and randomly assigned to undergo lung volume reduction surgery or to receive standard medical treatment. It has found that overall in the entire population studied, LVRS did not provide a survival benefit, but did improve exercise capacity in certain populations.[24] Within a subgroup analysis of patients with predominantly upper- lobe emphysema and low base–line exercise capacity, there exists a significant mortality benefit.[24] The patient population that dictates what the eventual indications for surgery are to this day.

* *

The indications for surgery are as follows:[24]

1. Age <75 years
2. Former smoker, ideally having quit for more than 6 months
3. Continued dyspnea despite maximal inhaler therapy and completion of pulmonary rehabilitation
4. FEV_1 <45% of predicted after administration of a bronchodilator.
5. Hyperinflation on lung volume measurements on spirometry including
   a. TLC >100% predicted
   b. RV >150%
6. As highlighted in answer choice D, a post-rehabilitation 6-minute walk distance >140 m
7. A low post-rehabilitation maximal achieved cycle ergometry watts, based on sex-specific standards
8. Chest radiograph showing hyperinflation
9. High resolution CT (HRCT) confirming severe emphysema, ideally with upper- lobe predominance

With these in mind, there also exists several relative contraindications to the procedure that are derived from the exclusion criteria from the NETT trial and include the following:

1. Age >75 years
2. Active cigarette smoking, defined as smoking with the last 6 months
3. A comorbid illness such as clinically significant coronary artery disease or systolic heart failure with a decreased ejection fraction less than 40%.
4. HRCT findings consistent with homogeneous emphysema, pulmonary nodules of unknown significance, interstitial lung disease, or giant bullae
5. An FEV_1 <20% of predicted
6. Severe derangements on blood gas analysis including Pa02 <45 mm Hg or $PaCO_2$ >60 mm Hg
7. A diffusion capacity <20% of predicted
8. History of severe alpha-1 antitrypsin deficiency

Question 3: A. Patients with FEV_1 <20% predicted and homogeneous emphysema

The NETT trial identifies patients with FEV_1 <20% of the predicted and a carbon monoxide diffusion capacity <20% of the predicted or homogeneous distribution of emphysema as high risk of mortality and minimal functional gains postoperatively.

* *

Patients with upper- lobe predominant emphysema and relative sparing of other portions of the lung have experienced improved outcomes compared to patients with homogeneous emphysema. The physiological thought process behind these results stems from speculation that removal of focal portions of dysfunctional lung will result in the following: (1) allow other healthy portions of the lung to expand appropriately (increase elastic recoil) thereby improving expiratory airflow; (2) decrease hyperinflation allows diaphragmatic and chest wall mechanics to improve thereby decreasing the overall work of breathing; and (3) decrease intra-throracic pressures would improve left-ventricular filling and cardiac index. Patients with homogeneous emphysema do not have clear areas of diseased lung but rather diffuse emphysematous disease that removing portions would not benefit other portions of the lung with a similar disease load.

CASE 4

Question 1: A. Alpha-1 antitrypsin

Alpha-1 antitrypsin deficiency (AAT) is an under-recognized genetic disease involving the lung, liver, and skin. There are three million cases worldwide with 80,000 to 100,000 cases in the US. Onset of emphysema in the fourth decade of life should clue the clinician to the possible presence of AAT. AAT is a protease inhibitor mainly produced in the liver and functions to protect the lung against proteolytic damage. A serum AAT level of 11 micromoles/L represents the protective threshold. A serum level <11 with phenotype testing is used to diagnose AAT. The testing of ANCA or ANA does not have any role in the diagnosis of alpa-1 antitrypsin.

* *

In very rare or unclear circumstances, an additional third test may be considered in patients with clinical features highly consistent with that of AAT deficiency but whose serum levels are within the normal range. This serum test must be sent to a specialized laboratory that can perform a functional assay of alpha-1 antiprotease that essentially measures the ability of the patient's serum to inhibit human leukocyte elastase in vitro. Such a defect is extremely rare and costly.

Question 2: B. PI*ZZ

AAT deficiency is inherited in an autosomal codominant pattern with numerous alleles having been identified on the long arm of chromosome 14. The classification pattern of PI is chosen since alpha-1 antitrypsin represents a protease inhibitor by function. The MM refers to the normal pattern of the gene resulting in a normal phenotype while the Z designation refers to the most common genetic mutation that leads to clinically significant emphysema.

Question 3: B. Weekly intravenous administration of AAT

Currently, the only FDA approved treatment is weekly infusion of AAT-purified protein. The American Thoracic Society has treatment recommendations based on research data derived mainly from a prospective cohort study conducted by the National Registry of Patients with severe deficiency of alpha-1 antitrypsin.[25] This study has shown both a mortality reduction as well as reduction in rate of decline in FEV_1 for those patients receiving weekly augmentation therapy. The patients in particular that are studied are carriers of the highest risk phenotype PI*ZZ, have had serum plasma levels of AAT less than 11 umol/L, and have established airflow obstruction with an $FEV_1 < 80\%$ predicted.

* *

Aerosolized delivery of AAT to the lung via inhalation remains an experimental therapy with no existing clinical studies to support its use. Due to the short half-life of intravenous AAT, direct delivery was investigated as a way to achieve higher more steady levels in the lung epithelial. Although animal studies show success in achieving higher concentrations with minimal side effects, there are no clinical trials in humans to justify its use.

* *

Similar to aerosolized AAT therapy, gene therapy is also an experimental treatment for AAT. The concept behind this therapy would be to "transplant" the DNA needed to code for AAT in deficient patients so that it could code for endogenous generation of the protein. Although there

is some initial promising data, it remains too scarce of therapy.

* *

Lung volume reduction surgery outcomes are studied during the NETT with a small patient population enrolled in this study suffering from AAT deficiency. Of the 1,218 patients in this study, 16 have suffered from severe AAT deficiency and 10 have had LVRS showing a 20% increase in mortality in this group compared to medical therapy.[24] Beyond this, the FEV_1 increase is shown to be of lower magnitude and shorter duration. Although the data set is small, clinicians should proceed with caution when offering this procedure to patients with AAT deficiency.

Question 4: B. IgA level

Some of the side effects of augmentation therapy include flu-like symptoms and low-grade fevers; however, a more serious anaphylaxis reaction can occur. Pooled human plasma alpha-1 antiprotease is known to contain small amount of IgA and individuals with IgA-deficiency who have developed anti-IgA antibodies represent a markedly increased risk of anaphylaxis. Prior to initiating intravenous AAT therapy, it is recommended to check for IgA deficiency or anti-IgA antibodies even though these reactions are exceedingly rare. Pulmonary function test would most likely already be known in a patient that is undergoing a work-up for AAT deficiency. Although there are some documented cases of anaphylaxis via an IgE-mediated pathway, it represents an extremely rare reaction to infusion.

CASE 5

Question 1: E. No further testing is indicated

The American College of Physicians (ACP) has developed guidelines for preoperative risk assessment for the development of postoperative pulmonary complications.[26] These guidelines are developed to guide physicians on the clinical and laboratory workup needed before a non-cardiothoracic surgery and reduce the risk of postoperative pulmonary complications. In general, for patients undergoing a low risk or intermediate risk surgery, a complete history and physical examination are the most important factors of a preoperative risk assessment for pulmonary complications. If someone has undiagnosed lung disease and symptoms of dyspnea, exercise intolerance, or cough, further workup and investigation is required. In this example, the patient has known COPD and underwent a complete history and physical examination for a low-risk surgery. No further testing is indicated.

* *

Obtaining a repeat pulmonary function test is not indicated in this patient. This patient already has a well-established diagnosis of COPD with prior PFTs. Repeating a pulmonary function test would only reconfirm a known diagnosis and add very little to the clinical estimation of risk. In addition, studies have failed to consistently show that obtaining PFTs prior to surgery is superior to history and physical examination in predicting postoperative pulmonary complications.[27–30] There is no spirometric threshold value that prohibits a patient from being a candidate for surgery. In this case, the patient already had PFTs performed in the past and thus, no further PFT testing is indicated. It is important to note that there are specific situations in which repeat PFT testing should be done prior to surgery: (1) before lung resection surgery, (2) in determining candidacy for coronary artery bypass, and (3) in patients with undiagnosed suspected lung disease.

* *

Presently, the data does not support the routine use of preoperative arterial blood gas (ABG) in risk assessment of postoperative pulmonary complications. Several small case studies suggest that preoperative hypercarbia or hypoxemia is associated with increased postoperative pulmonary complications, however this is yet to be proven in a large scale study, and further investigation will need to be done regarding the utility of ABGs prior to surgery.[31–32] For now, preoperative ABG is not recommended.

* *

There is much controversy over the obtainment of a routine CXR for preoperative pulmonary risk assessment. According to the ACP guidelines, a routine CXR is not indicated for preoperative evaluation.[26] This is largely because current literature has failed to show that finding an abnormal imaging study actually changes perioperative management.[33] One specific study showed that preoperative CXRs were abnormal 23.1% of the time, but only 3% had findings clinically important enough to change management.[34] Some experts believe that patients over the age of 50 years who are undergoing a

high-risk surgery, or who have known cardiopulmonary disease, should have a CXR within the past 6 months.[35] In this question, the patient is undergoing a low-risk surgery and has a recent CXR that was performed 2 months ago.

***Question 2*: D. Upper respiratory infection 2 weeks ago**
As of now, there is no statistically significant risk factor between a current or recent upper respiratory infection and the development of postoperative pulmonary complications. This is largely secondary to the limited trials performed in adults with respiratory infections. Most of the data regarding the impact of URIs on perioperative morbidity are for children undergoing surgery, which have shown minor postoperative complications including oxygen desaturation but failed to demonstrate an increase in morbidity.[36] Despite this, it would be reasonable to defer elective surgery if he had an acute upper respiratory infection. In this case, the patient's URI was 2 weeks ago and poses less of a threat. The most common postoperative pulmonary complications include: atelectasis, bronchospasm, exacerbation of underlying chronic lung disease, infection, prolonged mechanical ventilation, and respiratory failure. In this patient, his cigarette smoking, general health status, and chronic lung conditions are all known risk factors for the development of postoperative pulmonary complications.

* *

Smoking cessation at least four weeks prior to surgery reduces the risk of postoperative complications; some studies indicate that longer periods of smoking cessation, greater than 8 weeks, is even more effective.[37] In addition, smokers with a greater than 20- pack-year smoking history have a higher incidence of postoperative complications than those with a lesser pack-year history.[38]

* *

Poor general health status is a strong predictor of complications. The widely used American Society of Anesthesiologists (ASA) classification is highly predictive of postoperative pulmonary complications.[39] The ASA classification system is based on the presence or absence of systemic disturbances: absent (class 1), mild (class 2), moderate (class 3), severe (class 4), or almost certain death (class 5). Patients with an ASA class >2 confer a 4.87-fold increase in risk.

Age >50 years old is an important independent risk factor for developing postoperative pulmonary complications. Compared to patients <50 years old, patients aged 50 to 59 years, 60 to 69 years, 70 to 79 years, and >80 years have an odds ratio of 1.50 (CI 1.31–1.71), 2.28 (CI 1.86–2.80), 3.90 (CI 2.70–5.65), and 5.63 (CI 4.63–6.85), respectively for developing pulmonary complications.[35] In this case, the patient is 75-year-old and based on age alone, carries a significant risk for pulmonary complications.

**

Known chronic lung disease such as COPD is an important risk factor for postoperative pulmonary complications. Unadjusted relative risk of postoperative pulmonary complications range from 2.7 to 6.0.[40] Studies have shown that patients with severe COPD (FEV$_1$ <50% predicted) increase the mortality and severity of postoperative pulmonary complications.[41] Despite this, there is no prohibitive FEV$_1$ level for which surgery is absolutely contraindicated. The benefit of surgery must be weighed against the known risks.

Question 3: B. FEV$_1$, exercise capacity, patient's perceived dyspnea, and BMI

The BODE index is currently the best way to predict mortality in stable COPD patients. The BODE index utilizes four factors, including BMI (B), FEV$_1$—which quantifies the degree of airway obstruction (O), patient's perceived level of dyspnea (D), and patient's exercise capacity—using a 6-minute walk test (E).

**

Calculating the BODE index: The index is broken down into the four subgroups mentioned above and for each subgroup, a point value is assigned. The calculated total value is used to predict 4 year survival.

MMRC DYSPNEA SCALE[a]	
Points	**Patient's Perceived Level of Dyspnea**
0	Dyspnea on strenuous exercise
1	Dyspnea on walking a slight hill
2	Dyspnea on walking level ground; must stop occasionally due to breathlessness
3	Must stop for breathlessness after walking 100 yards or after a few minutes
4	Cannot leave house; breathless on dressing/undressing

[a]MMRC is the Modified Medical Research Council Scale for Dyspnea.

BODE INDEX Approximate 4-Year Survival	
Points	**Percent Survival (%)**
0–2	80
3–4	67
5–6	57
7–10	18

In this case, the patient has a total score of seven which correlates to an 18% survival in 4 years.

**

Although forced expiratory volume in 1 second (FEV$_1$) can be used to predict mortality, studies have shown that the multidimensional BODE index is superior to the unidimensional FEV$_1$ in predicting mortality.[42] In addition, FEV$_1$ by itself has been inconsistent in accurately predicting mortality.[43-44] FEV$_1$ is more commonly used to characterize the disease severity of COPD and aid in pharmacologic management. More specifically, FEV$_1$ is the backbone of the Global Initiative for Chronic Obstructive Lung Disease (GOLD) Classification.[9] Diffusion capacity of the lung for carbon monoxide

	POINTS				
BODE PARAMETERS	**1**	**2**	**3**	**4**	**SCORE**
BMI	<21	≥21			
FEV$_1$ % predicted	>65%	54–64%	36–49%	≤35%	
Dyspnea questionnaire	0–1	2	3	4	
Six-minute walk test	≥350 m	250–349 m	150–249 m	≤149 m	
					TOTAL:___

(DLCO) is a good index for disease progression. However it is inconsistent as a predictor of mortality. Finally, although active cigarette smoking increases the risk for progression of lung disease and cancer, there is no clear predictive model for tobacco use and prognosis for COPD.

* *

The development of hypercapnia during COPD exacerbations has not been shown to increase mortality compared to eucapnic individuals.[45] It is important to note that although acute hypercapnia does not affect long-term prognosis, chronic hypercapnia is a known prognostic factor for COPD.

* *

As mentioned above, active tobacco use is not a good predictor for COPD mortality. Unlike acute hypercapnia, several studies have demonstrated that patients with chronic hypercapnia have an increased mortality compared to patients who are eucapnic.[45,46] Finally, gender also affects mortality in COPD patients. In general, the male gender is associated with a higher all-cause and respiratory mortality compared to their female counterparts, 40 versus 18% and 24 versus 10%, respectively.[47] Interestingly however, the female gender reports more anxiety and depression, worse symptoms, lower exercise tolerance, more airway hyperresponsiveness, and worse health-related quality of life than males with COPD.[48–52] Despite chronic hypercapnia and gender being prognostic factors for COPD, the BODE index remains the best way to predict long-term mortality.

Question 4: D. Yes. Based on the COTE index, your diabetes with neuropathy, atrial fibrillation, and gastric ulcer disease increase your risk of mortality in COPD.

The risk for death in COPD has long been calculated by multidimensional indices such as the BODE (body mass index, FEV_1, dyspnea scale, and exercise capacity) index. However, this index and related COPD mortality indices do not account for the contribution of comorbid conditions. COPD patients frequently have multiple comorbidities and until recently, there was limited prospective data that evaluated which specific comorbid condition contributed the greatest to COPD mortality risk. The COPD specific comorbidity test (COTE) index evaluated 79 comorbid conditions in COPD patients and found 12 statistically significant conditions that independently increased the risk of death in COPD. These 12 comorbid conditions include cancers of the lung, pancreas, esophagus, and breast, followed by pulmonary fibrosis, atrial fibrillation/flutter, congestive heart failure, coronary artery disease, gastric/duodenal ulcers, liver cirrhosis, diabetes with neuropathy, and anxiety.[53] It is important to note that anxiety is only a risk factor for women, not men. Even though this index is the first of its kind, it has not come without criticism. Despite some limitations of the COTE index,[54] this comorbidity scale has been generally well-accepted and a necessary consideration when assessing a patient's mortality risk. Finally, one prospective study has demonstrated that COPD and BODE are complimentary and improved mortality prediction.[55]

* *

In the question above, the patient has diabetes mellitus type 2 with neuropathy, atrial fibrillation, gastric ulcer disease, irritable bowel syndrome, and anxiety disorder. According to the COTE index, choice D is the best answer as he has an increased risk of mortality for COPD based on his comorbid conditions of diabetes with neuropathy, atrial fibrillation, and gastric ulcer disease. It is important to note that even though diabetes with neuropathy has been proven to increase mortality in COPD patients, diabetes without neuropathy has not been. In addition, anxiety is a known risk factor in female COPD patients, however given this patient is a male, anxiety does not play a role. Irritable Bowel Syndrome is not a known risk factor in the COTE index. The BODE index does not account for comorbid conditions in COPD. The BODE index utilizes four factors, including BMI (B), FEV_1—which quantifies the degree of airway obstruction (O), patient's perceived level of dyspnea (D), and patient's exercise capacity—using a 6-minute walk test (E).

CASE 6

Question 1: A. Your lung function (FEV_1) will decline at a slower rate.

Lung function in a nonsmoker normally increases in childhood and adolescence as the lungs grows. In your mid-20s, lung function plateaus and then begins to gradually decline with age. This decline with age is normal. Smokers who develop COPD, have an accelerated rate of lung function decline (contributing to their development of COPD). Most frequently, when smokers with COPD stop smoking, their rate of lung function decline decreases compared to that of who continue to smoke.[13,56–59] There is no data to suggest that COPD patients accelerate their lung function decline after smoking cessation. Although COPD patients who stop smoking may experience an initial slight improvement in FEV_1/FVC, the lung function of a COPD patient does not normalize to that of a non-COPD of similar age. COPD patients may have a slight improvement in their FEV_1/FVC, but it does not normalize or supersede the lung function of a non-COPD patient of a similar age.

Question 2: D. The use of supplemental oxygen

The Global Initiative for Chronic Obstructive Lung Disease (GOLD) has revised its criteria for the determination of disease severity in COPD in December 2011.[60] The old GOLD criteria for COPD staging has been based solely on spirometry data, namely FEV_1. Based on a patient's FEV_1, the patient is placed into a disease severity category, and this guides their therapeutic regimen. This revised criteria takes into account that not all COPD patients with similar FEV_1, will behave similarly. For example, it is often the case that one patient with moderate COPD has severe breathlessness while another patient with mild-COPD is more prone to acute exacerbations. This new assessment tool is called the Combined COPD assessment and is based on patient's subjective symptoms, spirometry classification, and risk of exacerbations. Among the answer choices above, the use of supplemental oxygen is not a factor of the combined COPD assessment tool.

**

The patient's subjective symptom assessment is a component of the combined COPD assessment tool. The patient's symptoms should be assessed using either the COPD Assessment Test (CAT) or the Modified British Medical Research Council (mMRC). Both of these questionnaires measure the health status and symptom severity of the patient. If a patient has a score of mMRC 0 to 1 or CAT <10, then he is in the "less symptoms" group versus a score of mMRC ≥2 or CAT ≥10, places a patient in the "more symptoms" group.

**

The degree of airflow limitation based on spirometry data is also a component of the combined assessment scale. This classification has not changed from prior GOLD classifications. GOLD 1 is characterized as mild disease if an FEV_1 ≥80% predicted. GOLD 2 is characterized as moderate disease if the spirometry shows 50% ≤FEV_1 <80% predicted. GOLD 3 is characterized as severe disease if spirometry shows 30% ≤FEV_1 <50% predicted. Finally, GOLD 4 is characterized as very severe disease if spirometry shows FEV_1 <30% predicted.

**

Finally, the risk of COPD exacerbations is the final factor in the combined assessment tool. A COPD exacerbation is defined as an acute worsening of any symptoms—cough, sputum production, or dyspnea. If a patient has two or more exacerbations within the last year or an FEV_1 <50% of predicted value, they are classified as "high-risk" exacerbations. If a patient has less than two exacerbations per year or an FEV_1 >50% of predicted value, they are classified as "low-risk" exacerbations.

**

Shown below is the table used to assess a patient's severity score in the Combined Assessment of COPD.

COMBINED ASSESSMENT OF COPD					
When assessing risk, choose the highest risk according the GOLD grade or exacerbation history					
GOLD Classification: FEV₁	3–4	**C** High risk, low symptoms	**D** High risk, more symptoms	≥2	**Exacerbation History**
	1–2	**A** Low risk, less symptoms	**B** Low risk, more symptoms	0–1	
		mMRC 0–1 or CAT <10	mMRC ≥2 or CAT ≥10		

* *

In this clinical case, the patient falls in category D. Let's go through the assessment. First, assess the patient's symptoms. The patient has a score of three on the mMRC scale, which according to the chart above, places the patient into category "D" or "B." In regards to spirometry, he has an FEV_1 of 15% predicted, which translates to GOLD stage 4, placing him in the "C" or "D" category. In regards to his exacerbation history, he has not had an exacerbation in greater than 2 years, but has an FEV_1 <50% predicted, which places the patient into a high risk exacerbation category, "C" or "D." Putting it all together, the patient has more symptoms and is high risk, thus falling into category "D." Once the patient category has been determined—A, B, C, or D—steps are taken to reduce his symptoms, decrease his risk factors, and determine his appropriate pharmacotherapy based on the patient's ABCD category. This will be explained in more detail in the subsequent questions.

Question 3: A. Fluticasone and salmeterol

This patient falls into patient category D of the GOLD criteria, based on his symptoms, FEV_1, and risk for exacerbations. The GOLD criteria suggest that an initial treatment regimen for a patient in category D is an inhaled corticosteroid + long-acting beta$_2$-agonist or a long-acting anticholinergic.[60] Fluticasone is an inhaled corticosteroid and salmeterol is a long-acting beta$_2$-agonist, making this the best answer choice. If a patient's symptoms are not well controlled with this initial regimen, it would be reasonable to add on additional pharmacologic class until the symptoms are well controlled. A table with the updated pharmacologic recommendations is included below.

* *

Levoalbuterol and ipratropium bromide are not the best pharmacologic regimen for a patient with GOLD patient category D. Levoalbuterol is a short-acting beta$_2$-agonist and ipratropium bromide is a short-acting anticholinergic. Both of these medications would be appropriate for a patient with GOLD patient category A, but longer-acting agents should be used in severe COPD. Tiotropium is a long-acting anticholinergic, which would be an appropriate treatment regimen for a patient with category D COPD. Budesonide and beclomethasone are both inhaled corticosteroids and it would not be appropriate to give a patient two agents from the same pharmacologic class.

* *

Below is an updated list of GOLD's recommended therapy in stable COPD patients.

GOLD's Recommended Pharmacologic Therapy for Stable COPD		
Patient Group	**First Choice**	**Second Choice**
A	SA anticholinergic prn or SA beta$_2$-agonist prn	LA anticholinergic or LA beta$_2$-agonist or SA anticholinergic and SA beta$_2$-agonist
B	LA anticholinergic or LA beta$_2$-agonist	LA anticholinergic and LA beta$_2$-agonist
C	ICS + LA beta$_2$-agonist or LA anticholinergic	LA anticholinergic and LA beta$_2$-agonist
D	ICS + LA beta$_2$-agonist or LA anticholinergic	ICS + LA anticholinergic or ICS + LA anticholinergic and LA beta$_2$-agonist or ICS + LA beta$_2$-agonist and PDE-4 inhibitor or LA anticholinergic and LA beta$_2$-agonist or LA anticholinergic + PDE-4 inhibitor

SA, short acting; LA, long acting, ICS, inhaled corticosteroid; PDE-4, phosphodiesterase 4.

Question 4: D. Hyperkalemia

Theophylline is used as a last line pharmacologic agent for uncontrolled COPD. It is used as a last line agent because of its narrow therapeutic index, which can sometimes cause life-threatening toxicities.[61-63] In general, theophylline toxicity affects five major categories: (1) cardiovascular, (2) neurologic, (3) metabolic, (4) gastrointestinal, and (5) musculoskeletal. The most common metabolic derangements observed are hypokalemia and hyperglycemia. Other metabolic complications include metabolic acidosis, hypercalcemia, and hypophosphatemia. Of the above answer choices, HYPERkalemia is incorrect as theophylline toxicity usually presents with HYPOkalemia.

* *

The most common cardiovascular manifestations are arrhythmias—sinus tachycardia, ventricular arrhythmias, and supraventricular tachycardia. The most common neurologic manifestations include tremors, agitation, restlessness, hallucinations, and seizures. The most common GI manifestations include nausea/vomiting and abdominal pain. The most feared musculoskeletal complication is rhabdomyolysis.

***Question 5:* E. The flu vaccine should be administered yearly in COPD patients. The pneumococcal polysaccharide vaccine should be administered once in patients <65 years who have COPD with an FEV$_1$ <40% or with significant comorbid conditions and then readministered in patients >65 years of age**
The Global Initiative for Chronic Obstructive Lung disease (GOLD) recommends yearly influenza vaccines for all COPD patients. In addition, the pneumococcal polysaccharide vaccine should be given to COPD patients >65 years and once in patients <65 years if they have a FEV$_1$ <40% or have significant comorbidities.[9] These vaccinations have been shown to reduce serious respiratory illness in COPD patients.

CASE 7

***Question 1:* C. COPD—chronic bronchitis**
COPD has several different subtypes including emphysema, chronic bronchitis, and asthma-COPD overlap syndrome. Even though the distinction between these various subtypes in not necessary, identifying a patient's COPD phenotype may help guide epidemiologic and therapeutic purposes.

* *

COPD—Chronic Bronchitis is defined as a chronic productive cough for at least 3 months in a 2-year time frame, in which other causes of chronic cough have been ruled out. Chronic bronchitis can precede air flow limitation and can persist after air flow limitation has been established. In this clinical case, the patient has been experiencing a chronic productive cough for the last three years, making chronic bronchitis the best answer choice.

* *

Asthma is a chronic inflammatory disorder that is associated with airway hyperresponsiveness. This in turn leads to recurrent episodes of wheezing, breathlessness, chest tightness, and coughing, most pronounced at night. PFTs may show an obstructive airflow pattern but the key to distinguishing asthma from COPD is that asthma is reversible—either spontaneously and with treatment—whereas COPD is irreversible. In this clinical case, the patient has a negative bronchodilator response during his PFT test, suggesting an irreversible obstructive lung disease.

* *

COPD—Emphysema is defined as permanent dilated airways distal to the terminal bronchioles and is secondary to the destruction of the airspace walls. Emphysema is not associated with excess mucus production, making this answer choice less likely.

* *

Asthma-COPD Overlap syndrome (ACOS) is recognized by the Global Initiative for Chronic Obstructive Lung disease (GOLD) as a separate entity from asthma or COPD.[60] Patients with this syndrome have persistent airway obstruction with several features associated with asthma and several features associated with COPD. Patients with ACOS usually have more pronounced symptoms after the age of 40 years but may have had some symptoms in childhood and are frequently diagnosed by doctors as having childhood asthma. Airflow limitation is not fully reversible in this population but symptoms are significantly reduced with treatment.

* *

Diffuse Panbronchiolitis is a rare syndrome, most frequently seen in the Japanese descent, which is characterized by bronchiolitis and chronic sinusitis. Diffuse lesions appearing throughout both lungs that represent inflammation of the respiratory bronchioles. Patients with this rare syndrome typically present with intense coughing and large amounts of sputum production.

Question 2: B. Roflumilast
Roflmilast is a phosphodiesterase 4 inhibitor that is a once a day oral medication that has no direct bronchodilator activity but works to reduce inflammation by inhibiting the breakdown of intracellular cyclicAMP. It has been shown to improve FEV$_1$ in patients treated with salmeterol or tiotropium. In addition, Roflumilast has been shown to reduce moderate to severe exacerbations in patients with chronic bronchitis, severe to very severe

COPD, and a history of exacerbations (Evidence A).[60] Oxygen has been shown to improve mortality in patients with COPD that are hypoxic, but it does not reduce the frequency of COPD exacerbations. Theophylline is a controversial medication that has a narrow therapeutic index and is less effective and less well tolerated than long-acting bronchodilators. The regular use of theophylline is not currently recommended and should only be used if long-acting bronchodilators are not available or as a last line COPD agent. Theophylline has not been shown to reduce COPD exacerbations. Long-term monotherapy with oral corticosteroids is not recommended in the management of COPD.

REFERENCES

1. Tashkin DP, Cellie B, Senn S, et al. A 4 year trial of tiotropium in chronic obstructive pulmonary disease. *N Engl J Med.* 2008;359;1543–1554.
2. Vestbo J. The TORCH (towards a revolution in COPD health) survival study protocol. *Eur Respir J.* 2004;24(2): 206–210.
3. Calverley P, Pauwels R, Vertbo J, et al. Combined salmeterol and fluticasone in the treatment of chronic obstructive pulmonary disease; a randomized controlled trial. *Lancet.* 2003;361:449–456.
4. Hoogendoorn M, Al MJ, Beeh KM et al. Cost-Effectiveness of Tiotropium Versus Salmeterol: the POET-COPD trial. *Eur Respir J* 2013;41:556–564.
5. Wedzicha JA, Calverley PM, Seemungal TA et al. The prevention of chronic obstructive pulmonary disease exacerbations by salmeterol/fluticason propionate or tiotropium bromide. *Am J Respir Crit Care Med.* 2008;177:19–26.
6. Aaron SD, Vandemheen KL, Fergusson D, et al. Tiotrpium in combination with placebo, salmterol or fluticasone-salmterol for treatment of chronic obstructive pulmonary disease: A Randomized Trial. *Ann Intern Med.* 2007;146(8): 545–555.
7. Niewoehner DE, Erbland ML, Deupree RH, et al. Effect of systemic glucocorticoids on exacerbations of COPD. *N Engl J Med.* 1999;340:1941–1947.
8. Leuppi JD, Schuetz P, Bingisser R, et al. Short-Term vs conventional glucocorticoid therapy in acute exacerbation of chronic obstructive pulmonary disease: the REDUCE randomized clinical trial. *JAMA.* 2013;309:2223–2231.
9. Global Initiative for Chronic Obstructive Lung Disease (GOLD). Global strategy for the diagnosis, management and prevention of chronic pulmonary disease, 2013. http://www.goldcopd.org/Guidelines/guidelines-resources.html.
10. De Jong YP, Uil SM, Grotjohan HP, et al. Oral or IV Prednisolone in the treatment of COPD exacerbations: a randomized, controlled, double-blind study. *Chest.* 2007;132 (6):1741–1747.
11. Lindenauer PK, Pekow PS, Lathi MC, et al. Association of corticosteroids dose and route of administration with risk of treatment failure in acute exacerbation of chronic obstruct pulmonary disease. *JAMA.* 2010:303(23);2359–2367.
12. Anthonisen NR, Skeans MA, Wise RA, et al. Lung Health Study Research Group. The effects of a smoking cessation intervention on 14.5 year mortality: a Randomized Clinical Trial. *Ann Intern Med.* 2005;142(4):233–239.
13. Anthonisen NR, Connett JE, Kiley JP, et al. Effects of smoking intervention and the use of an inhaled anticholinergic bronchodilator on the rate of decline of FEV1. The Lung Health Study. *JAMA.* 1994;272:1497–1505.
14. Lee PN, Fry JS. Systematic Review of the evidence relating FEV1 decline to giving up smoking. *BMC Med.* 2010; 8:84.
15. Aaron S, Vandemheen KL, Hebert P, et al. Outpatient oral prednisone after emergency treatment of chronic obstructive pulmonary disease. *N Engl J Med.* 2003;348: 2618–2625.
16. Cahill K, Stead LF, Lancaster T. Nicotine receptor partial agonists for smoking cessation. *Cochrane Database Syst Rev.* 2007;(1):CD006103.
17. Cahill K, Stevens S, Perera R, Lancaster T. Phamacological interventions for smoking cessation: an overview and network meta-analysis. *Cochrane Database Syst Rev.* 2013:5: CD009329.
18. Cahill K, Stevens S, Lancaster T. Pharmacological treatments for smoking cessation. *JAMA.* 2014;311(2):193–194.
19. Ramon JM, Morchon S, Baena A, et al. Combining varenicline and nicotine patches: a randomized controlled trial study in smoking cessation. *BMC Med.* 2014;12(1):172.
20. Koegelenberg CF, Noor F, Bateman ED, et al. Efficacy of varenicline combined with nicotine replacement therapy vs. varenicline alone for smoking cessation: a randomized clinical trial. *JAMA.* 2014;213(2):155–161.
21. Spruit MA, Singh SJ, Garvey C, et al; ATS/ERS Task Force on Pulmonary Rehabilitation. An Official American Thoracic Society/European Respiratory Society Statement: Key concepts and advances in pulmonary rehabilitation. *Am J Respir Crit Care Med.* 2013;188(8):e13–e64.
22. Puhan MA, Gimeno-Santos E, Scharplatz M, et al. Pulmonary rehabilitation following exacerbations of chronic obstructive pulmonary disease. *Cochrance Database Syst Rev.* 2011;:(10):CD005305.
23. Cambach W, Wagenaar RC, Koelman TW, et al. The long-term effects of pulmonary rehabilitation in patients with asthma and chronic obstructive pulmonary disease; a research synthesis. *Arch Phys Med Rehabil.* 1999;80(1): 103–111.
24. National Emphysema Treatment Trial Research Group. A randomized trial comparing lung reduction surgery versus medical therapy for severe emphysema. *NEJM.* 2003;348:2059–2073.
25. American Thoracic Society/European Respiratory Society Statement: Standards for the Diagnosis and Management of Individuals with Alpha-1 Antitrpysin Deficiency, 2002.
26. Qaseem A, Snow V, Fitterman N, et al. Risk assessment for and strategies to reduce perioperative pulmonary

complications for patients undergoing noncardiothoracic surgery: a guideline from the American College of Physicians. *Ann Intern Med.* 2006;144:575–580.

27. Lawrence VA, Dhanda R, Hilsenbeck SG, et al. Risk of pulmonary complications after elective abdominal surgery. *Chest* 1996;110:744–750.

28. Brooks-Brunn JA. Predictors of postoperative pulmonary complications following abdominal surgery. *Chest.* 1997; 111:564–571.

29. De Nino LA, Lawrence VA, Averyt EC, et al. Preoperative spirometry and laparotomy: blowing away dollars. *Chest.* 1997;111:1536–1541.

30. Lawrence VA, Page CP, Harris GD. Preoperative spirometry before abdominal operations. A critical appraisal of its predictive value. *Arch Intern Med.* 1989;149:280–285.

31. Tisi GM. Preoperative evaluation of pulmonary function. Validity, indications, and benefits. *Am Rev Respir Dis.* 1979;119:293–310.

32. Milledge JS, Nunn JF. Criteria of fitness for anaesthesia in patients with chronic obstructive lung disease. *Br Med J.* 1975;3:670–673.

33. Hamoui N, Kim K, Anthone G, et al. The significance of elevated levels of parathyroid hormone in patients with morbid obesity before and after bariatric surgery. *Arch Surg.* 2003;138:891–897.

34. Archer C, Levy AR, McGregor M. Value of routine preoperative chest x-rays: a meta-analysis. *Can J Anaesth.* 1993;40:1022–1027.

35. Smetana GW, Lawrence VA, Cornell JE, et al; American College of Physicians. Preoperative pulmonary risk stratification for noncardiothoracic surgery: systematic review for the American College of Physicians. *Ann Intern Med.* 2006;144:581–595.

36. Tait AR, Malviya S. Anesthesia for the child with an upper respiratory tract infection: still a dilemma? *Anesth Analg.* 2005;100:59–65.

37. Mills E, Eyawo O, Lockhart I, et al. Smoking cessation reduces postoperative complications: a systematic review and meta-analysis. *Am J Med.* 2011;124:144–154.e8.

38. Wong J, Lam DP, Abrishami A, et al. Short-term preoperative smoking cessation and postoperative complications: a systematic review and meta-analysis. *Can J Anaesth.* 2012; 59:268–279.

39. Wolters U, Wolf T, Stützer H, et al. ASA classification and perioperative variables as predictors of postoperative outcome. *Br J Anaesth.* 1996;77:217–222.

40. Smetana GW. Preoperative pulmonary evaluation. *N Engl J Med.* 1999;340:937–944.

41. Kroenke K, Lawrence VA, Theroux JF, et al. Operative risk in patients with severe obstructive pulmonary disease. *Arch Intern Med.* 1992;152:967–971.

42. Ong KC, Earnest A, Lu SJ. A multidimensional grading system (BODE index) as predictor of hospitalization for COPD. *Chest.* 2005;128:3810–3816.

43. Vestbo J, Edwards LD, Scanlon PD, et al. Changes in forced expiratory volume in 1 second over time in COPD. *N Engl J Med.* 2011;365:1184–1192.

44. Celli BR, Cote CG, Marin JM, et al. The body-mass index, airflow obstruction, dyspnea, and exercise capacity index in chronic obstructive pulmonary disease. *N Engl J Med.* 2004;350:1005–1012.

45. Costello R, Deegan P, Fitzpatrick M, et al. Reversible hypercapnia in chronic obstructive pulmonary disease: a distinct pattern of respiratory failure with a favorable prognosis. *Am J Med.* 1997;102:239–244.

46. Ahmadi Z, Bornefalk-Hermansson A, Franklin A, et al. Hypo- and hypercapnia predict mortality in oxygen-dependent chronic obstructive pulmonary disease: a population-based prospective study. *Respir Res.* 2014;15:30.

47. de Torres JP, Cote CG, López MV, et al. Sex differences in mortality in patients with COPD. *Eur Respir J.* 2009;33:528–535.

48. Laurin C, Lavoie KL, Bacon SL, et al. Sex differences in the prevalence of psychiatric disorders and psychological distress in patients with COPD. *Chest.* 2007;132:148–155.

49. Martinez F, Curtis J, Sciurba F, et al. Gender differences in severe pulmonary emphysema. *Am J Respir Crit Care Med.* 2007;176(3):243–252.

50. Tashkin DP, Altose MD, Bleecker ER, et al. The Lung Health Study: airway responsiveness to inhaled methacholine in smokers with mild to moderate airflow limitation. The Lung Health Study research Group. *Am Rev Respir Dis.* 1992;145:301–310.

51. Ferrer M, Villasante C, Alonso J, et al. Interpretation of quality of life scores from the St George's Respiratory Questionnaire. *Eur Respir J.* 2002;19:405–413.

52. de Torres JP, Casanova C, Hernandez C, et al. Gender associated differences in determinants of quality of life in patients with COPD: a case series study. *Health Qual Life Outcomes.* 2006;4:72.

53. Divo M, Cote C, de Torres JP, et al. Comorbidites and risk of mortality in patients with chronic obstructive pulmonary disease. *Am J Respir Crit Care Med.* 2012;186:155–161.

54. Dodd J, Jones P. Potential limitation of the COTE index in assessing the impact of comorbidities on mortality in chronic obstructive pulmonary disease. *Am J Respir Crit Care Med.* 2012;186:804–805.

55. de Torres JP, Casanova C, Marin JM, et al. Prognostic evaluation of COPD patients: GOLD 2011 versus BODE and the COPD comorbidity index COTE. *Thorax.* 2014;69:799–804.

56. Xu X, Weiss ST, Rijcken B, et al. Smoking, changes in smoking habits, and rate of decline in FEV1: new insight into gender differences. *Eur Respir J.* 1994;7:1056–1061.

57. Løkke A, Lange P, Scharling H, et al. Developing COPD: a 25 year follow up study of the general population. *Thorax.* 2006;61:935–939.

58. Postma DS, Burema J, Gimeno F, et al. Prognosis in severe chronic obstructive pulmonary disease. *Am Rev Respir Dis.* 1979;119:357–367.

59. Weiss S. (2014, June 10). Chronic obstructive pulmonary disease: Risk factors and risk reduction. Retrieved from http://www.uptodate.com/contents/chronic-obstructive-

pulmonary-disease-risk-factors-and-risk-reduction, accessed on August 31, 2014.

60. Global Initiative for Asthma. Global strategy for the diagnosis, management and prevention of Asthma, COPD, and Asthma-COPD Overlap Syndrome, 2014. http://www.goldcopd.org/Guidelines/guidelines-resources.html, accessed on November 2014.

61. McKay SE, Howie CA, Thomson AH, et al. Value of theophylline treatment in patients handicapped by chronic obstructive lung disease. *Thorax*. 1993;48(3):227–232.

62. Ram FS, Jardin JR, Atallan A, et al. Efficacy of theophylline in people with stable chronic obstructive pulmonary disease: a systematic review and meta-analysis. *Respir Med*. 2005;99(2):135–144.

63. Ram FS, Jones PW, Castro AA et al. Oral theophylline for chronic obstructive pulmonary disease. *Cochrane Database Syst Review*. 2002;(4):CD003902.

5

Asthma

Sarun Thomas DO and Alfred Astua MD

CASE 1

A 42-year-old man with history of asthma since childhood, well controlled on inhaled steroid/long-acting beta agonist and albuterol PRN, hypertension on lisinopril for 3 years, and alcohol abuse was recently admitted to the hospital for new onset atrial fibrillation. In the hospital, he was placed on an amiodarone drip and has since been on amiodarone 200 mg PO daily. His HbA1C was found to be 9 and he was started on sitagliptin. One month later, he complained of a rhinorrhea and a new cough. Hematologic studies, chest radiograph and high resolution computed tomography of his chest were performed and essentially unremarkable.

Question 1: **Which statement is true regarding the patient's cough?**

A. Patient will benefit from the addition of montelukast
B. Patient has cough from amiodarone 200 mg PO daily
C. The cough is likely related to lisinopril
D. The cough is likely related to sitagliptin
E. The cough is GERD related secondary to alcohol intake

Question 2: **All the statements are true regarding the cough reflex except:**

A. Rapidly acting receptors are the predominant receptor beyond the respiratory bronchioles
B. During the mechanism of cough, the diaphragm and the intercostal muscles contract creating a negative pressure
C. The afferent neural pathway of cough travels to the vagus nerve into the medulla
D. Stimulation of auricular nerve in ear can also trigger a cough

E. Afferent and efferent pathways involve the superior and inferior laryngeal nerves, respectively

CASE 2

A 22-year-old morbidly obese man complains of nocturnal cough for the past 3 months. He denies any sore throat or dyspnea on exertion. He occasionally smokes but has stopped recently. His complete blood cell count reveals no leukocytosis but with eosinophils 5%. His chest radiograph is essentially unremarkable. He has a pulmonary function test with spirometry performed and the results are below:

Spirometry	Actual	% Predicted	Post bronchodilator	% Change
FVC (liters)	2.81	85	3.31	5.7%
FEV1 (liters)	2.49	82	3.00	20%
FEV1/FVC	88.6%		90%	
Quality	Good			

Question 1: **What is your diagnosis?**

A. Asthma
B. COPD
C. Chronic bronchitis
D. Exercise-induced bronchospasm
E. Restrictive lung disease

CASE 3

A 19-year-old woman who lives in Colorado has been experiencing shortness of breath and dry cough. She is a member of her college snowboarding team and notices symptoms 30 minutes into her training. Her symptoms are bothersome up to 30 to 90 minutes after she stops exercising. She is a nonsmoker and denies any pets or sick contacts.

Question 1: **What is the next step most reasonable for this patient?**

A. Avoid exercise

B. Albuterol before her work out routine

C. Azithromycin

D. Benzodiazepines

E. Acetazolamide administration

CASE 4

A 32-year-old woman is evaluated at a follow-up visit for uncontrolled asthma. She is started on low-dose inhaled fluticasone for mild persistent asthma and returns after 4 weeks stating that her asthma keeps her from getting her work done only a little of the time. She has shortness of breath about three times a week that require her to use her short-acting beta2 agonist. Her symptoms have not woken her up at night. She fills out her asthma control test form prior to seeing you and rates her asthma as well controlled.

Question 1: **What is her Asthma control test (ACT) score?**

A. 16

B. 17

C. 18

D. 19

E. 20

Question 2: **All of the following are reasonable adjustments to make to her medications except:**

A. Increase her inhaled fluticasone to medium dose

B. Add a long-acting beta2 agonist to her current therapy

C. Add montelukast to her current therapy

D. Increase her inhaled fluticasone to medium dose and add a long-acting beta2 agonist to her current therapy

E. Add theophylline to her current therapy

Question 3: **The patient loses her insurance for a period of time and will be unable to afford her medication indefinitely and has improving asthma symptoms which currently require an inhaled corticosteroid and long-acting beta2 agonist. She is determined to have good control of her asthma and wants to know**

when she can be on less medication and which medication should be stopped first.

A. After 2 weeks of controlled asthma, her inhaled corticosteroid can be stopped

B. After 6 weeks of controlled asthma, her long-acting beta2 agonist can be stopped

C. After 3 months of controlled asthma, her long-acting beta2 agonist can be stopped

D. After 6 months of controlled asthma, her inhaled corticosteroid can be stopped

E. After 6 months of controlled asthma, her long-acting beta2 agonist can be stopped as long as the FEV1 is well above 80%

CASE 5

A 38-year-old woman with a history of asthma is referred for persistence of her shortness of breath. She has recurrent bouts of colds and uses over-the-counter cold medications. After use of her over-the-counter medications, she claims her chest tightens and she notices audible wheezes. She previously saw an ENT specialist who stated she has sinusitis and even surgically has removed a nasal polyp which has decreased her symptoms for 3 years.

Question 1: **All of the following medications are helpful in her condition except:**

A. Zafirlukast

B. Montelukast

C. Zileuton

D. Roflumilast

E. Intranasal steroids

Question 2: **You place her on a leukotriene receptor inhibitor and she shows some improvement until her cardiologist placed her on a medication for her atrial fibrillation (patient has a CHADS score of 1). What is a reasonable next option for this patient?**

A. CT sinuses to rule out sinusitis

B. Antibiotics to treat an upper respiratory infection

C. Aspirin desensitization

D. Pulmonary rehabilitation

E. Cardiopulmonary exercise testing

Question 3: **Your patient is curious regarding aspirin desensitization and wants to know what is done if she becomes symptomatic prior to the maximum dose of aspirin.**

A. Desensitization is always aborted

B. Aspirin dose will be increased

C. The same dose is kept until no reaction is seen
D. This is considered the maximum dose the patient can ever receive
E. Aspirin dose can be increased as long as oral steroids are added.

CASE 6

An 18-year-old pregnant woman, 14 weeks age of gestation, is referred to you by her obstetrician as she states she has a history of wheezing and shortness of breath as a child and currently gets woken up by her symptoms once a week. Her pulmonary function tests show reversible airflow obstruction characteristic of asthma. She is afraid of taking any medications as she thinks it will harm her baby.

Question 1: **You give her a script for a rescue albuterol inhaler. What additional medication would you start her on after an explanation of risks and benefits?**

A. Inhaled low-dose budesonide
B. Oral prednisone
C. Omalizumab
D. Inhaled high-dose budesonide with a long-acting bronchodilator
E. Beclomethasone inhaler

CASE 7

A 50-year-old man, nonsmoker presents with the complaint of 4-month history of wheezing and shortness of breath. Symptoms began after cleaning a chemical spill at a pool supply store. Chest radiography is unremarkable and pulmonary function tests show airflow obstruction and with a positive bronchodilator response.

Question 1: **What is the most likely diagnosis?**

A. COPD
B. Reactive airway dysfunction syndrome
C. Allergic rhinobronchitis
D. Refractory asthma
E. Irritant-induced asthma

Question 2: **How would you treat this individual besides limiting further exposure to toxic fumes?**

A. Inhaled long-acting beta2 agonist
B. Inhaled nasal fluticasone
C. Montelukast
D. Inhaled corticosteroids
E. Inhaled cromolyn

CASE 8

A 30-year-old woman is referred to you after her recent hospitalization for asthma exacerbation. Specifically she has two hospitalizations in the last 6 months. She has been on high doses of inhaled corticosteroid with long-acting beta2 agonist, montelukast, and oral prednisone. Despite this she claims she has needed albuterol four to six times every day. She is recently started on a proton-pump inhibitor by her primary care physician. She demonstrates good technique with her inhalers. Besides obesity, her physical examination is unremarkable. Her laboratory tests were unremarkable except for a serum eosinophils level of 500/μL and her chest radiography shows no acute pulmonary disease.

Question 1: **Which of the following tests can test for control and compliance in this patient?**

A. Repeat sputum eosinophil count
B. Amount of medications left over at each visit
C. Exhaled nitric oxide
D. Peripheral eosinophil count
E. Repeated pulmonary function testing

CASE 9

A 50-year-old man with a history of glaucoma is brought into the emergency room by his family after falling and hitting his head at home. His family states that he is getting over a "head cold" and has been using his albuterol inhaler every single hour without any relief of symptoms and thinks he may have passed out. His peak flow volume is normally around 400 mL. He is currently in the emergency room and has received intravenous corticosteroids, continuous nebulizers, intravenous magnesium, and subcutaneous epinephrine without any improvement in his dyspnea. His peak flow is 125 mL. He appears fatigued and using accessory muscles. ABG shows a pH of 7.35, a CO_2 of 50, and O_2 of 60 receiving oxygenation through a nonrebreather mask.

Question 1: **Which of the following interventions is the most reasonable next step at this time?**

A. High-flow nasal cannula titrating to O_2 saturation >92%
B. Intubation with ventilator settings of 400/20/80/15
C. Intubation with ventilator settings of 400/12/80/5
D. Intravenous ketamine
E. Subcutaneous terbutaline

Question 2: **The patient becomes intubated. A few minutes later, the nurse states the patient continues to struggle to breathe and the ventilator continues to alarm. Which of the following ventilator changes can you make to help alleviate this problem?**

A. Check an end expiratory pressure and increase the extrinsic positive end expiratory accordingly
B. Increase the tidal volume and respiratory rate
C. Decrease the respiratory rate
D. Decrease level of sedation
E. Decrease the inspiratory flow

Question 3: **In asthmatics, during exacerbations—what affect does hypoxia have on a patient's respiratory drive?**

A. Hypoxia heightens symptom perception
B. Hypoxia depresses symptom perception
C. Hypoxia minimally affects respiratory drive in asthma
D. Hypoxia affects all asthmatics differently
E. Hypoxia does not play a role in asthmatics respiratory failure

CASE 10

A 60-year-old woman has been seeing an asthma specialist for 1 year and despite treatment with high-dose inhaled glucocorticoids often in combination with long-acting beta agonists, multiple types of leukotriene receptor antagonists, and very frequently oral glucocorticoids. She has symptoms daily requiring short-acting beta agonists and requires hospitalization once every other month. She frequently runs out of her medications. Her exacerbations appear "random" and are not associated with any triggers which you confirm with her asthma symptom diary which she is very meticulous about keeping.

Question 1: **What type of asthma does she have?**

A. Atopic asthma
B. Refractory asthma
C. Exercise-induced bronchoconstriction
D. Occupational-induced asthma
E. No asthma is present, likely has tracheal stenosis

Question 2: **Which of the following therapies has not shown any benefit in difficult to control asthmatics?**

A. Bronchial thermoplasty
B. Tiotropium

C. Azithromycin
D. Theophylline
E. Doubling dose of inhaled corticosteroid

CASE 11

A 36-year-old woman comes to your office for ongoing evaluation and treatment of hard to treat asthma. She is compliant with all her medications, has no pets, and is a secretary. She is also being treated for GERD, rhinitis and tells you that she plans to join a gym to lose weight (BMI 36).

Question 1: **Which of the following is false regarding asthma and sleep disorders?**

A. Obstructive sleep apnea–induced GERD can be a trigger for asthma
B. Hypoxemia can act as a trigger for the carotid body leading to bronchoconstriction and worsening of asthma symptoms. This has been shown to decrease in sheep after carotid denervation
C. Most experts recommend looking for OSA in patients with hard to treat asthma
D. The decreased vagal tone of patients with OSA stimulate the muscarinic receptors in the central airways leading to nocturnal asthma symptoms
E. Hard to control asthma is not a cause of central sleep apnea

CASE 12

A 38-year-old man with known GERD, obesity, allergic rhinitis, and asthma is seen at your office. He is taking a proton-pump inhibitor, intranasal steroid, statin, beta blocker, and daily aspirin. His hard to control asthma has remained a problem no matter what combination or doses of medications for asthma he has tried. Imaging, blood work, ENT evaluation, and allergy testing have proven unfruitful for symptoms improvement. He has no pets, no significant exposures, and besides being a lifelong nonsmoker he takes medications as prescribed. He is aware of the interaction regarding obstructive sleep apnea and asthma.

Question 1: **Which of the following statements regarding inflammatory theories/associations of OSA and asthma are correct?**

A. Increased intrathoracic pressure secondary to repeated Mueller's maneuvers is associated with decreased tracheal collapsibility in mild as compared to severe OSA patients with asthma (tracheal tug theory)

B. Airway epithelial cells produce adipocyte-derived factors such as leptin which have been found to be elevated in obese males with OSA and associated with increased levels of airway hyper reactivity (leptin theory)

C. Sleep fragmentation is likely beneficial in OSA patients with asthma by causing less hypoventilation opportunity during the night (sleep architecture theory)

D. Lower levels of vascular endothelial growth factor noted in asthma and OSA are protective against hypoxemia present in more severe cases (vascular theory)

E. The inflammatory response in OSA patients can be blunted in lower BMI patients (blunted response theory)

Question 2: The patient was diagnosed with OSA by a split night in laboratory sleep study. His AHI is 42 and was optimally treated on testing night with a CPAP of 11 cm of water. He asks about the associated impact that the CPAP will have on his OSA, asthma, and gout. Your best answer to his question is:

A. The CPAP treatment will treat his OSA, help in his asthma but not his gout

B. The CPAP treatment will treat his OSA, but not help his asthma or gout

C. It is not clear whether the CPAP will help, he needs to first have a full night sleep study

D. An auto servo ventilator will best serve him for treatment of the OSA and asthma but not the gout

E. The CPAP will help his asthma only if his blood pressure is also controlled

Answers

CASE 1

Question 1: D. The cough is likely related to sitagliptin

An acute cough is defined as being present for less than 3 weeks, while subacute would be between 3 and 8 weeks and chronic would be for more than 8 weeks.[1,2]

* *

With well-controlled asthma since childhood, it is doubtful montelukast will be helpful unless you suspect aspirin-induced asthma. Drug-induced lung disease (DILD) is a consideration in patients with cough and review of medications and duration of use is important. There have been numerous case reports regarding cough secondary to sitagliptin. The mechanism of cough is thought to be secondary to increased nasal engorgement, mucosal thickening, and increased substance P-induced vasodilation. Topical and nasal corticosteroid treatment can generally control symptoms. ACE inhibitor (ACEI) such as lisinopril can cause cough and should be considered as the cause in all patients with cough, however in our case, the lisinopril has been a chronic medication for 3 years. ACEIs usually cause cough within the first four

4 weeks and sometimes can be delayed up to 6 months. Although it is possible for an ACEI to cause symptoms at any point while taking it, it becomes less likely. If an ACEI is used, a period of discontinuation should be attempted to determine whether symptom relief occur if that is suspected to be the cause of cough. Amiodarone can also induce cough but the mechanism is not direct as with ACEI. Amiodarone causes interstitial changes but with normal high-resolution CT scan imaging it is unlikely secondary to amiodarone. It should also be noted that interstitial changes caused by amiodarone are often dose related. People who receive 400 mg or more daily for greater than 2 months are at higher risk. Those that take 200 mg daily usually need to be on the drug for over 2 years prior to any symptoms of pulmonary toxicity.

* *

GERD typically is a cause of chronic cough and the patient mentioned has a cough with duration of only 30 days. Furthermore, no other accompanying GERD like symptoms such as chest pain or acid taste in the mouth is mentioned.

Acute	Subacute	Chronic Cough
• Infectious etiology (usually viral) • Sinusitis • Exacerbation of obstructive lung disease • Allergic rhinitis • Environmental irritants • Medications	• Postinfectious cough • Bacterial sinusitis • Cough variant asthma • Upper airway cough syndrome • Medications	• Upper airway cough syndrome • Cough variant asthma • GERD • Nonasthmatic eosinophilic bronchitis • Chronic bronchitis secondary to cigarette smoking • Bronchogenic carcinoma • Carcinomatosis • Sarcoidosis • Chronic infections: Tuberculosis, cystic fibrosis • Left ventricular heart failure • Aspiration due to pharyngeal dysfunction • Medications • Psychogenic

Question 2: **A. Rapidly acting receptors are the predominant receptor beyond the respiratory bronchioles**

Sensory nerve receptors responding to stimuli that cause cough are defined by conductive properties. They are identified as rapidly acting receptors, slowly acting receptors, or c-fiber receptors. In the lungs these receptors are absent beyond the respiratory bronchioles. Afferent fibers from the cough receptors travel through the vagus nerve to the nucleus tractus solitarius in the medulla where the cough response is generated. A cough has three phases: (1) an inspiratory phase (diaphragm and internal intercostal muscle create negative pressure); (2) forced expiration against a closed glottis; and (3) opening of the glottis with rapid expiration (diaphragm relaxes and abdominal and expiratory muscles contract). Stimulation of the auricular branch of the vagus nerve, which can be done by irritating the external auditory meatus can also stimulate cough through what is known as Arnold's reflex. Both the afferent and efferent pathways involve the superior laryngeal nerve stemming from the vagus nerve.

CASE 2

Question 1: **A. Asthma**

Reversible airflow obstruction is characteristic of asthma, and this is demonstrated during spirometric testing by an increase in 200 mL of FEV1 along with >12% increase in FEV1 after receiving a short-acting inhaled beta2 agonist. This patient's changes in pulmonary function tests are not normal due to the bronchodilator response and fits with asthma. COPD has obstructive changes (FEV1/FVC ratio <70%) and usually does not show reversibility. Chronic bronchitis will also not have significant improvement in FEV1 in response to bronchodilators. Exercise-induced asthma occurs when several minutes of vigorous exercise stimulate bronchoconstriction. It is theorized that the addition of mouth breathing to nasal breathing which occurs during exercise allows colder air that has not had time to be humidified by the upper airway and the resulting dehydration irritates the bronchial lining causing edema. Exercise-induced asthma is usually treated with a short-acting beta2 agonist 15 minutes prior to exercise. People with exercise-induced asthma should have normal pulmonary function tests during rest and normal breathing which eliminates it as a choice in this question. Features of restrictive lung disease might include decreased FVC and lung volumes, none of which are represented by the offered spirometric values.

CASE 3

Question 1: **B. Albuterol before her work out routine**

This young woman has symptoms typical of exercise-induced bronchoconstriction (EIB). The mechanism is increased blood flow to nasal passages from cold, unhumidified air causing edema, and subsequently bronchoconstriction.[3] Two catalysts are the nature of inspired air (water content and temperature) and intensity of the exercise. Treatment is a short-acting beta2 agonist 15 minutes prior to exercise, although frequent use may cause tolerance. Additional pharmacological treatments can include an inhaled corticosteroid (which can take 4 weeks to have an effect), a leukotriene receptor agonist and a mast cell stabilizing agent. Inhaled corticosteroids immediately prior to exercise are not recommended and use of an inhaled anticholinergic agent is a weak recommendation. Nonpharmacologic treatment should also be used, consisting of increased warm up times and methods to humidify air if exercising in a cold environment, such as breathing through a face mask or scarf. Better overall conditioning and optimization of asthma in general has also been found to help decrease symptoms.

CASE 4

Question 1: D. 19

Asthma control test (ACT) is for >12 years of age to assess asthma control in the last 4 weeks.[4,5] An ACT score of 19 or less provided a sensitivity (71%) and specificity (71%) for detecting uncontrolled asthma.[4,5] It consists of a scale of five questions which range from 1 to 5 points.

**

The questions are listed below:

1. How much of the time did your asthma keep you from getting as much done at work, school, or at home? (1: all of the time, 2: most of the time, 3: some of the time, 4: a little of the time, 5: none of the time)

2. How often have you had shortness of breath? (1: >1 day, 2: once daily, 3: 3–6 × a week, 4: once or twice a week, 5: not at all)

3. How often did your asthma symptoms (wheezing, coughing, shortness of breath, chest tightness, or pain) wake you up at night or earlier than usual in the morning? (1: 4 or more nights a week, 2: 2 or 3 nights a week, 3: once a week, 4: once or twice, 5: not at all)
4. How often have you used your rescue inhaler or nebulizer medication (such as albuterol)? (1: 3 or more times per day, 2: 1 or 2 times per day, 3: 2 or 3 times per week, 4: once a week or less, 5: not at all)
5. How would you rate your asthma control during the past 4 weeks? (1: not controlled at all, 2: poorly controlled, 3: somewhat controlled, 4: well controlled, 5: completely controlled)

***Question 2:* D. Increase her inhaled fluticasone to medium dose and add a long-acting beta2 agonist to her current therapy**
Guidelines from the National Asthma Education and Prevention program publish a stepwise approach for managing asthma along with a classification of asthma severity guideline and assessment of asthma control. Different guidelines are present and updated dependent on age, below are the NHLBI guidelines (revise September 2012) for ages 12 and above.[6]

* *

INITIAL VISIT: CLASSIFYING ASTHMA SEVERITY AND INITIATING THERAPY FOR AGES ≥12.[6]

Components of Severity	Intermittent	Mild Persistent	Moderate Persistent	Severe Persistent
Symptoms	≤2 days/week	>2 days/week but not daily	Daily	Throughout the day
Nighttime awakenings	≤2 ×/month	3–4 ×/month	>1 ×/week but not nightly	Often 7 ×/week
SABA use for symptom control	≤2 days/week	>2 days/week but not daily or more than once daily	Daily	Several times per day
Interference with normal activity	None	Minor	Some limitation	Extremely limited
Lung function FEV1 (% pred) FEV1/FVC	>80% Normal	>80% Normal	60–80% Reduced 5%	<60% Reduced >5%
Recommended step	STEP 1	STEP 2	STEP 3	STEP 4 or 5

FOLLOW-UP VISIT: ASSESSING ASTHMA CONTROL AND ADJUSTING THERAPY FOR AGES ≥12.[6]

Components of Control	Well Controlled	Not Well Controlled	Very Poorly Controlled
Symptoms	≤2 days/week	>2 days/week but not daily	Throughout the day
Nighttime awakenings	≤2 ×/month	1–3 ×/month	≥4×/week
Interference with normal activity	None	Some Limitation	Extremely limited
SABA use for control	≤2 days/week	>2 days/week	Several times per day
Lung function FEV1 FEV1/FVC	>80% Not applicable	60–80% Not applicable	<60% Not applicable
Questionnaires ACT	≥20	16–19	≤15
Action for treatment	Maintain current Step, reevaluate every 1–6 months	Step up 1 Step, reevaluate in 2–3 weeks	Step up 1–2 steps and consider short course of oral systemic steroids, reevaluate in 2 weeks

STEP-WISE TREATMENT[6]

	Step 1	Step 2	Step 3	Step 4	Step 5	Step 6
	Intermittent Asthma	**Persistent Asthma (A specialist is recommended at Step 4 and higher)**				
Preferred treatment	SABA as needed	Low-dose ICS	Low-dose ICS + LABA or medium-dose ICS	Medium-dose ICS + LABA	High-dose ICS + LABA and consider omalizumab for patients who have allergies	High-dose ICS + LABA + Oral corticosteroid and consider omalizumab for patients who have allergies
Alternative treatment		Cromolyn, LTRA, or theophylline	Low-dose ICS + either LTRA, theophylline, or zileuton	Medium-dose ICS either LTRA, theophylline, or zileuton		

SABA, short-acting beta2 agonist; ICS, inhaled corticosteroid; LABA, long-acting beta2 agonist; LTRA, leukotriene receptor agonist.

In persistent allergic asthma, subcutaneous allergen immunotherapy should be considered.

* *

There are some differences that can be noted between the initial assessment and follow-up visits such as nighttime awakenings. Also it should be noted that under questionnaires, the Asthma control Questionnaire (ACQ) and the Asthma Therapy Assessment Questionnaire (ATAQ) are also validated tools that can be used.

* *

Our patient is using her SABA three times a week with an ACT score of 19 which places her in the not well-controlled category and recommended action for treatment would be to move up one step. She is already on a low-dose inhaled corticosteroid and the next step would be a low-dose ICS + LABA or a medium-dose ICS. Alternative treatment can also be attempted which would be low-dose ICS + LTRA, theophylline, or zileuton.

Question 3: C. After 3 months of controlled asthma, her long-acting beta2 agonist can be stopped

Stepping down therapy is also important in asthmatics and is generally done in patients after at least 3 months of controlled asthma. Long-acting beta2 agonist should never be used alone to control asthma symptoms. A blackbox warning exist that states that LABA treatment without concurrent long-term asthma control such as an inhaled corticosteroid is contraindicated and treatment

mitigates increased risk of asthma related death from a long-acting beta2 agonist. In this answer, only choice C is a reasonable option. Symptomatic control and control evaluation using the ACT do not take spirometric values into account.

CASE 5

Question 1: D. Roflumilast

This 38-year-old woman has aspirin-induced asthma. Other names include aspirin exacerbation respiratory disease (AERD), aspirin sensitivity, or aspirin intolerant asthma. A typical patient will have the triad first described by Samter and Beers and consists of nasal polyps, asthma, and aspirin sensitivity.[7] The pathophysiology is secondary to an aberrant metabolism of arachidonic acid, leading to suppression of COX-1 and overexpression of COX-2, which leads to overexpression of inflammatory prostanoids. This syndrome is not restricted to aspirin and can be catalyzed by NSAIDs, particularly COX-1 inhibitors such as Ibuprofen and naproxen while drugs such as meloxicam acetaminophen, celecoxib are considered safer but still have risk of inducing symptoms.[7] Asthma may be subclinical therefore in doubtful cases, nasal provocation with lysine asthma can be used to as a test as it is relativity safe and very specific for aspirin-induced asthma but our scenario is very typical. Nasal polyps are first generally treated with intranasal steroids often with success but in some scenarios where resolution is unsatisfactory, endoscopic polyp surgery has also shown success. Leukotriene inhibitors should be used in aspirin-induced asthma. Leukotriene inhibitors affect two pathways—either they inhibit 5-lipooxygenase pathway such as zileuton (liver monitoring is required) or they antagonize specific cysteinyl LT receptors as in the case of zafirlukast or montelukast. Roflumilast is a medication for COPD and does not have any proven benefits in aspirin-induced asthma. Roflumilast and its metabolites acting inhibit PDE4 (phosphodiesterase 4) which causes an accumulation of cAMP (cyclic adenosine monophosphate) and is thought to decrease anti-inflammatory effects through cytokine release suppression, it has no role in AERD.

Question 2: C. Aspirin desensitization

The cause in aspirin sensitivity is an increase in proinflammatory leukotrienes via the 5-lipooxygenase pathways and via increased synthesis of cysteinyl leukotrienes (LTS). Aspirin inhibits cyclooxygenase which decreases PGE2 which normally inhibits leukotriene synthesis. When these leukotrienes are uninhibited, it leads to mast cell degranulation. Desensitization lowers Il-4 and cys-LT receptors. The preferred treatment for our patient would be aspirin desensitization. Small incremental doses of oral aspirin are given in a monitored setting generally over 48 hours. After completion, they are kept on a maintenance dose. Benefits include fewer hospitalizations from asthma, fewer number of sinus infections, decreased use of corticosteroids, and an improved sense of smell.[8] Considering the overall safety of this therapy, it is should be considered a viable therapeutic adjunct in patients with aspirin-induced asthma. There are currently no indications for CT sinuses and our vignette does not describe any signs of an active infection. There is currently no role for pulmonary rehabilitation in aspirin-induced asthma. Cardiopulmonary exercise testing is a test that may be elected to be performed in patients with dyspnea of unclear etiology.

Question 3: C. The same dose is kept until no reaction is seen

It is almost universal among all aspirin desensitization protocols that if a mild reaction is seen to the dose of asthma throughout the desensitization protocol it is repeated until the patient no longer mounts a reaction. A mild reaction is not necessarily a reason to abort desensitization unless a systemic hypersensitivity reaction or anaphylaxis is seen. A mild reaction to aspirin would be a rash, hives, or itching. A moderate reaction to aspirin would be abdominal cramps and/or swelling of the eyelids. A severe reaction to aspirin is wheezing, shortness of breath, or tongue swelling. Anaphylaxis would be multisystem dysfunction inclusive of hypotension. Addition of oral steroids plays no role in aspirin desensitization.

CASE 6

Question 1: A. Inhaled low-dose budesonide

Our patient's asthma is not well controlled and falls into the category of mild persistent asthma as she has three to four nighttime awakenings per month, a normal FEV1/FVC ratio and an FEV1 of >80% which would place her into the category of step 2 in the treatment algorithm. The recommended treatment of step 2 is a low-dose inhaled corticosteroid, of which budesonide would be preferred in pregnant patients.

**

Counseling by their physician is required to make sure pregnant women have an understanding of their condition. Asthma exacerbations that require medical attention occur in about 20% of women and they primarily occur in the late second trimester after viral illnesses and nonadherence to therapy. Women with uncontrolled asthma with exacerbations during pregnancy are at higher risk for babies with lower birth weight and inhaled corticosteroids may reduce exacerbation rates. Budesonide is the ICS that was used in the majority of the studies of pregnant women with asthma making it the drug of choice although other inhaled corticosteroids have not been shown to be unsafe.[9-11] Inhaled beclomethasone may not be wrong but because of the amount of evidence supporting budesonide, it becomes the best option. The use of inhaled corticosteroids in appropriate doses has not been shown to have adverse effects to the fetus and this should be conveyed to the patient. An asthma action plan should also be developed and given to the patient.

**

Prednisone is pregnancy category D but should be used during severe exacerbations as the maternal and fetal benefits generally outweigh fetal risk during severe exacerbations. Omalizumab is pregnancy category B; first-trimester studies do not exist in humans but animal studies have shown no adverse fetal effects. Our patient is not at the point where she requires a medication such as omalizumab. Our patient does not need a high-dose ICS at this point but this may be required in the future. The amount of trials done studying long-acting beta2 agonists are limited, but epidemiological studies done with salmeterol have not shown any adverse effects in pregnant women.

CASE 7

Question 1: **B. Reactive airway dysfunction syndrome**
Reactive airway dysfunction syndrome is defined as onset of symptoms after a single specific high-dose exposure to a respiratory irritant to a nonatopic patient. Symptoms, which include cough, wheezing, and dyspnea, begin 24 hours after exposure and persist for at least 3 months to years in some patients. Pulmonary function tests will show airflow obstruction but unlike COPD, reversibility is seen with bronchodilators. Patients generally also have no respiratory complaints prior to the episode. Toluene, chlorine, sulfuric acid, hydrochloric acid, and smoke inhalation are common inciting agents. It is proposed that inhalation injury produces significant epithelial injury with release of proinflammatory and toxic mediators. In general, improvement is seen with healing of the epithelium but a selected group of people with chronic symptoms are thought to have a lower threshold of receptor reactivity resulting in chronic symptoms. COPD is usually a persistent and progressive disease of airflow obstruction caused by chronic inflammation. This patient has obstructive findings but our scenario fits best with reactive airways disease. Allergic rhinitis is an allergic inflammation of the airways with rhinorrhea, congestion, and is sometimes associated with asthma. Our patient does not have an atopic presentation. Refractory asthma is asthma with persistent symptoms despite being on medications such as prednisone and frequent reevaluations with a specialist for over 6 months. Our patient has never been on medications previously and his clinical picture points toward reactive airways disease.

Question 2: **D. Inhaled corticosteroids**
Reactive airways disease is treated similarly to acute asthma. Sequential biopsies done in patients with reactive airways disease show a decrease in inflammation with inhaled corticosteroid use often requiring very high doses. Reactive airways disease seems to be less responsive to beta agonists although patients with the disease should be given a short-acting beta2 agonist in emergencies. Montelukast is used for atopic or aspirin-induced asthma and has not shown benefit in reactive airways disease. Inhaled nasal fluticasone would be the treatment for allergic rhinitis not for reactive airways disease. The best answer in this scenario would be an inhaled corticosteroid. Inhaled cromolyn works by stabilizing mast cells.

CASE 8

Question 1: **C. Exhaled nitric oxide**
This patient has eosinophilic airway disease which is a subphenotype of asthma classified by the pattern of inflammatory cells in the airway. It is associated with thickening of the basement membrane and often (not always) responsiveness to corticosteroids.[12] The ability to induce sputum has helped management of this disease as sputum eosinophil counts decrease with better control and normalization of sputum eosinophils has been shown to prevent exacerbations. Peripheral blood eosinophilia does not always correlate with sputum eosinophil levels but elevated levels generally point toward asthma severity. Blood eosinophil levels >300/μL has a positive predictive value of 50%. Inducing sputum eosinophils may not be an option in someone who found it difficult to do especially on a long-term basis. Exhaled nitric oxide is a simple, noninvasive, and safe method of measuring airway inflammation. Nitric oxide is present in the exhaled breath of all humans and is elevated in airway inflammation. The official American Thoracic Society guidelines (2011) recognizes exhaled nitric oxide as a test to diagnose eosinophilic airway disease, determine likelihood of responsiveness to steroids, unmasking noncompliance, and quantifying level of airway inflammation.[13] Strong evidence supports using greater than 25 ppb as indication that eosinophilic inflammation and steroid responsiveness.[12] In our patient—this is the safest, simplest, and best next test to use. It is important to see how often medications are filled but inhaler use can be difficult to measure in terms of how much and when medication was used. Repeated pulmonary function testing although frequently ordered do not give any information about compliance and seldom correlate to asthma control.

CASE 9

Question 1: C. Intubation with ventilator settings of 400/12/80/5

This patient's peak flow decline >50% is indicative of a severe asthma exacerbation, severe acute asthma, or asthmatic flare. It is not always possible to perform peak flow during an asthmatic exacerbation and the need for mechanical ventilation is a clinical decision. Signs and symptoms include inability to talk in full sentences, need for the tripod position, use of accessory muscles, diaphoresis, and inability to lie supine. Risk factors include history of near fatal asthma requiring mechanical ventilation, asthma-related hospitalizations within the last year, oral corticosteroid use, overuse of SABA, psychiatric or psychosocial problems, poor adherence to medications, and food allergies. Intubation is appropriate as our patient has not shown improvement after many therapies and his ABG is worrisome as well. Intravenous corticosteroids, continuous nebulizers, intravenous magnesium, and subcutaneous epinephrine have all shown some level of benefit in patients with severe asthma exacerbations. Our patient has not improved with these modalities and our ABG shows CO_2 retention which is indicative of our patient's impending and worsening respiratory failure. A normal ABG is generally a marker of fatigue as a patient in respiratory distress should have a respiratory alkalosis from an increased respiratory rate and exhaling CO_2. In asthmatics and patients with obstructive lung disease, setting high respiratory rates can often lead to elevated end expiratory pressures (also known as intrinsic peep or auto-peep) due to longer expiratory times needed in patients with asthma exacerbations and this can be dangerous hemodynamically. Lower extrinsic peep is what is generally used in intubated asthmatics to prevent excess hyperinflation and to reduce already elevated airways pressures. Intravenous ketamine is a modality that can be used in asthma, especially during intubation due to its bronchodilatory properties while preserving respiratory drive. However, contraindications include elevated ICP after hitting his head and elevated intraocular pressures (history of glaucoma). High-flow nasal cannula does not have an indication in acute asthma exacerbations as ventilation rather than oxygenation is the primary issue. Terbutaline at times can be used in the setting of acute asthma as an adjunct treatment. Its dose is 0.25 mg by subcutaneous injection every 20 minutes for total of three doses. Epinephrine or terbutaline can be used as parenteral beta agonist but not simultaneously. Our patient already has failed epinephrine administration. Below is a table listing common medications to treat asthma exacerbation.

* *

COMMON MEDICATIONS USED TO TREAT ASTHMA IN ADULTS IN THE URGENT CARE SETTING

Medication	Dose	Comment
Short-acting inhaled beta2 agonist (albuterol)	2.5–5 mg every 20 minutes by nebulizer Or 10–15 mg over 1 hour as a continuous nebulizer	Levoalbuterol can be used at half the dose of albuterol but has not been studied as a continuous nebulizer in critical ill patients
Anticholinergics (ipratropium)	0.5 mg every 20 minutes by nebulization or 8 puffs every 20 minutes × 3 hours by MDI	Can be mixed in nebulizer with albuterol.
Corticosteroids (prednisone or methylprednisone)	40–80 mg qdaily (in 1 or 2 doses)	Given normal absorption is present, IV and PO have equal efficacy, it should be noted that corticosteroids may not show effect until 6 hours after administration
Magnesium sulfate	2 g IV over 20 minutes, can be repeated once more after 20 minutes	Magnesium is considered an adjunctive therapy, it has not been shown to help in routine use but has shown benefit when used in the acute setting
Epinephrine	0.3–0.5 every 20 minutes × 3 doses subcutaneously	Recommended for people who are poorly responding to above therapies first

Question 2: **C. Decrease the respiratory rate**

Positive end expiratory pressure (PEEP) is the pressure present in the alveoli after the end of expiration. In severe asthma, hyperinflation is present due to the inability to exhale secondary to heterogeneous airflow obstruction. Unlike COPD, during a severe asthma exacerbation, the predominant site of airflow obstruction happens in the central noncollapsible airways and the pressures in the alveoli are usually positive even during expiration. In COPD, the alveolar attachments that keep small airways open are lost and airway can collapse during expiration and increasing extrinsic peep can create a pneumatic stent to aid in ventilation. Methods to decrease autoPEEP include increasing the expiratory time which can be accomplished by decreasing the respiratory rate (even allowing permissive hypercapnia) and decreasing tidal volumes. It is also important to make sure the patient is not anxious and well sedated; paralytics are sometimes required where ventilator synchrony is difficult to maintain. Increasing not decreasing the inspiratory flow speed can be helpful in obstructive disease patients that are intubated and ventilated. By increasing the speed of the delivered breath will ultimately allow more expiratory time during the respiration cycle.

Question 3: **B. Hypoxia depresses symptom perception**

Hypoxia acts a central nervous system depressant and impairs cognitive function during severe asthma exacerbations.[14] It is therefore very important to treat hypoxia in asthma and it could take up to an hour to regain a normal perception of the magnitude of airway obstruction. Hypercapnia normally acts as a strong respiratory stimulant but in asthmatics this may also impair cognitive function and blunt a patient ability to recognize the severity of their obstruction although there are conflicting reports on this. The effects of hypoxia are very likely a major part of why severe asthmatics do not seek help early and have a delay in treatment.

CASE 10

Question 1: **B. Refractory Asthma**

Since 1999 refractory asthma has been defined as difficult to control asthma despite on nebulizers and corticosteroids by the European Respiratory Society, American Thoracic Society, World Health Organization, and Innovative Medicine Initiative.[14-16] As with all pulmonary medicine a thorough social history is necessary. Atopic asthma specifies that an allergic component is present.

During history taking, assessing symptoms during their vacations away from their homes and symptoms when they are not around their pets can be helpful. Exercise-induced bronchoconstriction usually has a clear inciting agent whether it is just inhalation of cold dry air or increased respiratory rate from exertion. Occupational asthma generally has an environmental trigger and a thorough symptom diary can often narrow down that symptoms specifically occur only at work or in certain areas. Measuring peak expiratory flow rates is a relatively easy test that the patient who suspects occupational asthma can perform when they are around the suspected environmental trigger or begin to have symptoms. Our particular patient is seeing a specialist and has difficult to manage symptoms making refractory asthma the best answer. Tracheal stenosis is the least likely diagnosis since patients with tracheal have a history of previous intubation unlike our patient. Taking a history that includes previous intubations should raise suspicion to asthma mimickers such as tracheal stenosis but not on this particular case.

Question 2: **C. Azithromycin**

Chronic infections can contribute to asthma. Infections with *Chlamydia pneumonia and mycoplasma pneumonia* have been associated with reduced FEV1 however trials with azithromycin have not shown statistical improvement in asthma outcomes or reduced infection rate.[17] Bronchial thermoplasty may benefit in severe refractory asthmatics although long-term follow-up and objective measurements of asthma control are needed.[18-20] It targets the smooth muscle of the large- to medium-sized airways with the idea that thermal energy generated results in long-term reduction of airway smooth muscle mass. With less airway smooth muscle, airway obstruction that occurs during exacerbations would be decreased because of less smooth muscle present to augment bronchoconstriction. Tiotropium is another option for a patient with poorly controlled asthma despite use of a long-acting beta2 agonist and inhaled corticosteroids. This may be due to an overlap syndrome that spans across COPD and asthma.[21] Benefits include increased length of time to the next seen asthma exacerbation and bronchodilatory effects. Theophylline has anti-inflammatory properties and is an effective brochodilator and can be used in asthma. Toxicity is more often seen in the elderly population and requires monitoring of blood levels with goal ranges between 8 and 15. Cardiac arrhythmias, seizures, nausea, vomiting, and diarrhea are unlikely to occur unless supratherapeutic levels are present. Doubling the dose on inhaled corticosteroids as a treatment algorithm plays no role in the management of acute or chronic asthma including hard to control asthma.

CASE 11

Question 1: D. The decreased vagal tone of patients with OSA stimulate the muscarinic receptors in the central airways leading to nocturnal asthma symptoms

Despite multiple tests and compliance to medications, the patient still has resistant asthma. It is thought that OSA and asthma may have many components in common that may make one augment the other. OSA has many inflammatory markers associated with it that may cause unwanted systemic inflammation such as leptin, tumor necrosis factor alpha, and interleukin 6 to name a few. It has been seen that treatment of OSA has improved the GERD and asthma symptoms in patients with OSA. It is thought that the OSA/asthma relationship can turn into a cycle of inflammation. Nocturnal hypoxemia that can be seen with OSA has also been implicated in the inflammatory pathway that may make asthma hard to control as is this patient. The vagal tone in OSA patients is increased not decreased. This increase is vagal tone can in fact trigger the muscarinic receptors in the central airways and cause nocturnal asthma symptoms. It is known that OSA-induced GERD as well as hypoxemia can lead to increased asthma symptoms. Even before the 2007 National Asthma Education and Prevention Program Expert Panel Report 3 (EPR3) which recommended that clinicians evaluate symptoms that suggest OSAS in unstable, poorly controlled asthmatic patients, particularly those who are overweight or obese many experts would agree to the above. It is known that hypoxemia can cause and be a trigger for bronchconstriction via carotid body signaling as seen in sheep. The most common causes of central sleep apnea include post stroke/BTI patients, patients with heart failure and those with high doses of medications such as methadone. Most experts to recommend looking for OSA in appropriately treated hard to control asthmatics.

CASE 12

Question 1: B. Airway epithelial cells produce adipocyte-derived factors such as leptin which have been found to be elevated in obese males with OSA and

associated with increased levels of airway hyper reactivity (leptin theory)

It is known that leptin is produced by epithelial cell in inflammatory response to antigens. Patients that are obese and have OSA have up to 50% more leptin than patients that are obese with no OSA. The tracheal tug theory has to do with asthma patients having typically lower lung volumes during sleep (e.g., FRC), which may attenuate the tracheal tug (stiffening) on the pharyngeal segment leading to more easily, increased collapsibility. The vascular theory deals with increased levels of VEGF for both asthma and OSA patients. This increased VEGF stems from hypoxemia leading to increased AHR. The sleep architecture theory deals with sleep fragmentation leading to increased resistance and obstruction along with blunted response to bronchoconstriction. There exists no blunted response theory of OSA and asthma.

Question 2: A. The CPAP treatment will treat his OSA, help in his asthma but not his gout

It should be pointed out that during a recent study of asthmatics that underwent a sleep study evaluation, there was a stronger prevalence of OSA in asthmatics. Using CPAP as a treatment for OSA has shown a positive impact on asthma symptoms. It has also shown to have a positive influence on levels of inflammatory cytokines. Of special interest is this older patient with asthma, in a recent study it was found that among the older patients, OSA was strongly associated with severe asthma (nearly 7 times more likely to have severe asthma) making undiagnosed OSA a possible existing reason in older patients with severe asthma. It is not necessary to have another sleep test if he has already been diagnosed and titrated appropriately. Auto servo ventilator has no role at this time in simple OSA with or without asthma. It is known that OSA treatment has a role in the improved care in asthma patients as well as in the care of patients with high blood pressure (especially those with resistant hypertension). What is not recorded is that the blood pressure must be controlled in such asthmatics patients in order to gain benefit.

REFERENCES

1. Chung KF, Pavord ID. Prevalence, pathogenesis, and causes of chronic cough. *Lancet.* 2008;371(9621):1364–1374.
2. Dicpinigaitis PV. Chronic cough due to asthma: ACCP evidence-based clinical practice guidelines. *Chest.* 2006; 129(1 suppl):75S–79S.
3. Parsons JP, Hallstrand TS. An official American Thoracic Society Clinical Practice Guideline: Exercise-induced bronchoconstriction. *Am J Respir Cril Care Med.* 2013;187 (9):1016–1027.

4. ASTHMA CONTROL TEST™ *Test Your Asthma Control.* GlaxoSmithKline, n.d. Web. 8 June 2014.

5. Schatz M, Sorkness CA, Li JT, et al. Asthma control test: Reliability, validity, and responsiveness in patients not previously followed by asthma specialists. *J Allergy Clin Immunol.* 2006;117(3):549–556.

6. National Asthma Education and Prevention Program. Expert Panel Report 3 (EPR-3): Guidelines For The Diagnosis And Management Of Asthma Summary Report 2007. *J Allergy Clin Immunol.* 2007;120(5):S94–S138.

7. Babu KS. Aspirin and asthma. *Chest.* 2000;118(5):1470–1476.

8. Xu J, Sowerby L, Rotenberg BW. Aspirin desensitization for aspirin-exacerbated respiratory disease (Samter's Triad): A systematic review of the literature. *Int Forum of Allergy Rhinol.* 2013;3(11):915–920.

9. Murphy VE. Asthma exacerbations during pregnancy: Incidence and association with adverse pregnancy outcomes. *Thorax.* 2006;61(2):169–176.

10. Murphy VE, Gibson P. Asthma in pregnancy. *Clin Chest Med.* 2011;32(1):93–110.

11. Namazy JA, Murphy VE, Powell H, et al. Effects of asthma severity, exacerbations and oral corticosteroids on perinatal outcomes. *Euro Respir J.* 2013;41(5):1082–1090.

12. Walford H, Doherty T. Diagnosis and management of eosinophilic asthma: A US perspective. *J Asthma Allergy.* 2014;7:54–65.

13. Dweik, RA, Boggs PB, Erzurum SC, et al. An official ATS clinical practice guideline: Interpretation of exhaled nitric oxide levels (FENO) for clinical applications. *Am J Respir Crit Care Med.* 2011;184(5):602–615.

14. Eckert DJ. Hypoxia suppresses symptom perception in asthma. *Am J Respir Crit Care Med.* 2004;169(11):1224–1230.

15. Leatherman, JW, Mcarthur C, Shapiro RS. Effect of prolongation of expiratory time on dynamic hyperinflation in mechanically ventilated patients with severe asthma. *Crit Care Med.* 2004;32(7):1542–1545.

16. Brasier AR, Sundar V, Boetticher G, et al. Molecular phenotyping of severe asthma using pattern recognition of bronchoalveolar lavage derived cytokines. *J Allergy Clin Immunol.* 121(1):30–37.e6.

17. Cheney S. Azithromycin for prevention of exacerbations in severe asthma: A multicentre randomized double blind placebo-controlled trial. *J Emerg Med.* 2013;45(3):480.

18. Castro M, Rubin AS, Cox G, et al. Two-year persistence of effect of bronchial thermoplasty (BT) in patients with severe asthma: AIR2 trial. *Chest.* 2010;138(4):768A–768A.

19. Castro M, Cox G. Asthma outcomes from bronchial thermoplasty in the AIR2 trial. *Am J Respir Crit Care Med.* 2011; 184(6):743–744.

20. Wechsler ME, Hanania NA, Leeds WM et al. Bronchial thermoplasty: Long-term safety and effectiveness in patients with severe persistent asthma. *J Allergy Clin Immunol.* 2013;132(6):1295–1302.e3.

21. Gibson PG, Simpson JL. The overlap syndrome of asthma and COPD: What are its features and how important is it? *Thorax.* 2009;64(8):728–735.

6

Bronchiectasis

Daniel Greenblatt Fein MD, Stacy Verzosa MD, and Patricia Walker MD

CASE 1

An 18-year-old woman with a history of asthma is referred to your clinic for follow-up after a recent visit to the ER for an episode of chest pain and cough. A computed tomography with angiogram is performed to rule out pulmonary embolism. She has not had any pain since the day of her ER visit and denies exertional dyspnea. Vital signs including temperature, heart rate, and oxygen saturation are all within normal limits. Lungs are clear to auscultation bilaterally. Serum IgE level is 320 kU/L. Serum precipitins to Aspergillus fumigatus are also negative.

Question 1: **What is this patient's abnormality?**

A. Bronchogenic cyst
B. Congenital bronchial atresia
C. Intrapulmonary sequestration
D. Allergic bronchopulmonary aspergillosis
E. Foreign-body aspiration

Question 2: **What would be the most appropriate next step in the management of this patient?**

A. Thoracic surgery referral for lobectomy or segmentectomy
B. Bronchoscopy with BAL for microbiologic studies

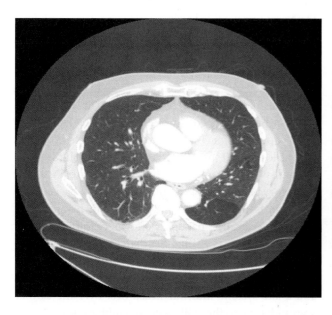
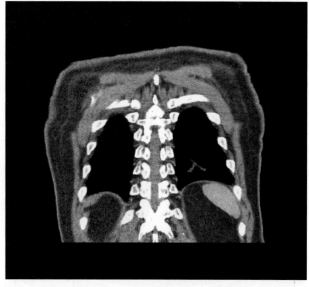

C. Four-week course of amoxicillin clavulanate followed by repeat CT of the chest

D. Observation and follow-up

E. Extended course of oral corticosteroids

CASE 2

A 35-year-old woman is referred to your clinic with recurrent upper respiratory infections. She complains of longstanding sinus congestion and a daily wet cough that does not vary seasonally. She denies dry eyes, dry mouth or parotid gland enlargement. Physical examination is notable for coarse crackles at the left lung base. Neurologic examination is unremarkable. Laboratory studies are notable for normal white blood cell count without eosinophilia. Urine analysis is within normal limits. Serum IgE is 22 kU/L. Serologic testing for anti-Ro, anti-La, rheumatoid factor is negative. Sweat chloride testing is performed and noted to be 30 mmol/L. Rapid HIV testing is negative. Urinalysis is negative for hematuria and is otherwise unremarkable.

Pulmonary function testing:

- FEV_1: 55% of predicted
- FVC: 68% of predicted
- FEV_1/FVC: 56%
- TLC: 87% of predicted
- FRC: 110% of predicted
- DLCO: 63% of predicted

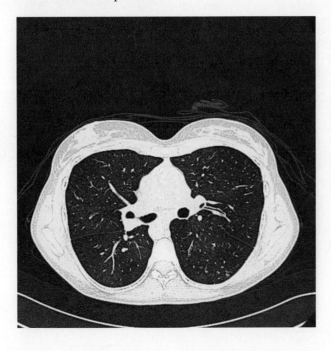

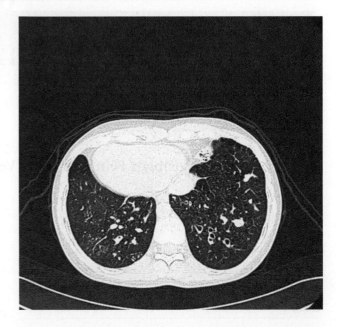

Question 1: **What is the patient's most likely diagnosis?**

A. Cystic fibrosis

B. Granulomatosis with polyangiitis

C. Primary ciliary dyskinesia

D. Eosinophilic granulomatosis with polyangiitis

E. Lymphoid interstitial pneumonia

Question 2: **What is the best test to confirm the diagnosis in this patient?**

A. Measurement of mucociliary clearance

B. Electron microscopy of ciliary structure

C. CFTR gene sequencing

D. Nasal nitric oxide levels

E. Antineutrophil cytoplasmic antibody (ANCA) testing

CASE 3

A 68-year-old woman is referred to your clinic complaining of a productive cough of 6 months. Review of systems is positive for 3 months of night sweats as well as weight loss of 10 lbs in the last 3 months. She is given 4 months of azithromycin by her primary care doctor for refractory bronchitis. She denies history of tobacco abuse but reports that her husband smoked in her presence for many years. The patient is a former clothing factory worker and reports visiting her daughter in New Mexico 7 months prior to presentation. Physical examination is notable for kyphoscoliosis, coarse rales in all lung fields and a late systolic murmur heard best over the cardiac apex radiating to the axilla with an audible click.

Pulmonary Function Testing

- FEV$_1$: 65% of predicted
- FVC: 56% of predicted
- FEV$_1$/FVC: 86%
- TLC: 70% of predicted
- FRC: 86% of predicted
- DLCO: 48% of predicted

Imaging studies are shown below.

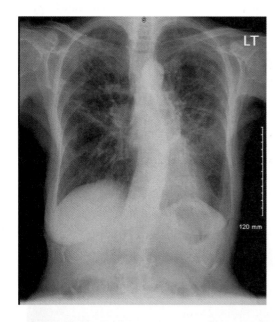

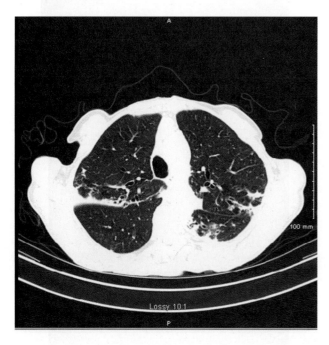

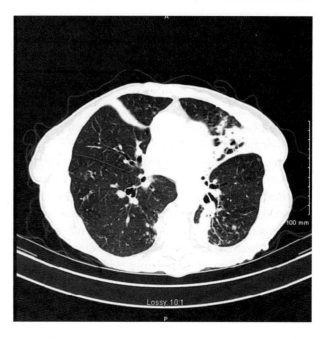

Question 1: **What would be the next appropriate diagnostic test?**

A. Three sputum collections with AFB smear and culture
B. Sweat chloride testing
C. Placement of tuberculin skin test
D. Bronchoscopy with BAL for Langerhans cells
E. Modified barium swallow

Question 2: **What would be the appropriate initial treatment plan for this patient?**

A. Azithromycin daily
B. Watchful waiting with frequent follow-up
C. Ethambutol, rifampin, and azithromycin daily
D. Rifampin, ethambutol, and clarithromycin or azithromycin three times per week
E. Omeprazole

Question 3: **Therapy is initiated and your patient tolerates the medications well. She returns to clinic after 1 year of therapy complaining of continued night sweats and productive cough which she feels limits her daily routine. Follow-up sputum reveals macrolide resistance. How should this patient be managed further?**

A. Daily azithromycin therapy
B. Daily levofloxacin + azithromycin
C. Surgical resection plus streptomycin for initial 3 to 6 months with subsequent daily isoniazid, rifampin, and ethambutol

D. Rifampin, ethambutol, and clarithromycin or azithromycin three times a week

E. Observation

CASE 4

A 58-year-old man presents to your clinic with dyspnea after walking five blocks. He reports vague episodic chest discomfort and daily cough productive of thick sputum. Vital signs are notable for oxygen saturation of 96% while breathing ambient air, blood pressure 140/84, pulse 88, and temperature 97°F. On examination, mild wheeze is found in all lung fields with diffused inspiratory and expiratory crackles. There is no clubbing or edema. Pulmonary function testing and imaging are shown below.

Pulmonary Function Testing
- FEV$_1$: 78% of predicted
- FVC: 82% of predicted
- FEV$_1$/FVC: 69%
- TLC: 94% of predicted
- FRC: 97% of predicted
- DLCO: 67% of predicted

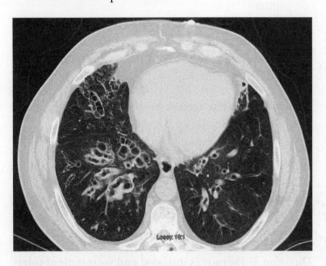

Question 1: **Initial workup for this patient's lung disease should include which of the following?**

A. Fiberoptic bronchoscopy

B. Measurement of rheumatoid factor

C. Measurement of serum immunoglobulins (IgG, IgA, and IgM)

D. Tuberculin skin testing

E. Measurement of nasal nitric oxide levels

Question 2: The same patient presents to the emergency room with chief complaint of worsening dyspnea on exertion. Review of systems is also positive for worsening cough productive of blood-tinged sputum. Vital signs are unremarkable with the exception of saturation 95% on room air. He is breathing comfortably and lung auscultation is notable for diffuse wheezing and inspiratory crackles. Prior sputum cultures obtained in clinic were not indicative of *Pseudomonas aeruginosa* or beta-lactamase positive *Haemophilus influenzae*. Chest x-ray is shown below.

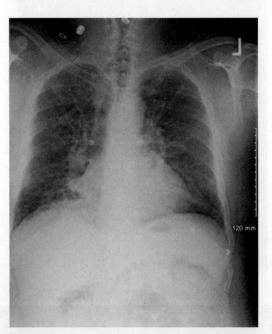

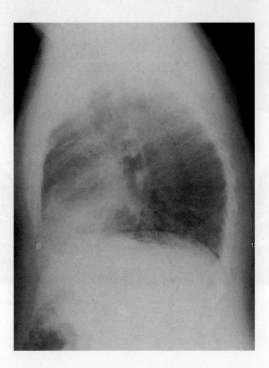

What organism is most likely responsible for this patient's exacerbation?

A. *H. influenzae*
B. *P. aeruginosa*
C. *Staphylococcus aureus*
D. Nontuberculous mycobacteria
E. *Streptococcus pneumoniae*

Question 3: **What antibiotics should be administered?**

A. Oseltamavir 150 mg two times a day
B. Amoxicillin 500 mg three times daily for 14 days
C. Ciprofloxacin 750 mg two times daily
D. Amoxicillin 500 mg three times a day for 7 days
E. Vancomycin 15 mg/kg every 12 hours

Question 4: **Your patient improves dramatically in the ER and is discharged home. Six months later he presents again to the emergency department with dyspnea and cough productive of dark sputum. Vital signs are temperature 100.7°F, blood pressure 130/82, pulse 105, respiratory rate 33, oxygen saturation 88% while breathing ambient air. Recent outpatient sputum culture is as follows:**

Gram stain moderate (3+) polymorphonuclear leukocytes
Rare (1+) gram-negative bacilli
Culture, moderate (3+) *P. aeruginosa*
Amikacin susceptible
Aztreonam susceptible
Cefepime susceptible
Ceftazidime susceptible
Gentamicin resistant
Imipenem resistant
Levofloxacin resistant
Piperacillin resistant
Tobramycin resistant

What antibiotics should be administered?

A. Nebulized tobramycin 300 mg two times a day plus oral ciprofloxacin 750 mg two times a day
B. Ciprofloxacin 750 mg by mouth two times a day
C. Tobramycin IV 5 mg/kg daily
D. Cefepime 2 g IV every 8 hours plus Amikacin 20 mg/kg IV daily
E. Amoxicillin 500 mg three times a day for 10 days

Question 5: **Which of the following therapies have been shown to reduce the frequency of exacerbations in patients with non-CF bronchiectasis?**

A. Azithromycin 500 mg three times a week
B. Noninvasive ventilation at night
C. Nebulized hypertonic saline two times per day
D. Nebulized mannitol two times per day
E. Aerosolized recombinant human DNase two times daily

CASE 5

A 46-year-old woman is referred to your pulmonary clinic with chief complaint of intermittently coughing up blood. She reports of shortness of breath after walking one block and chronic productive cough of many years duration. Past medical history is notable for diabetes and small bowel obstruction requiring surgical resection at age 17. Social history is notable for active smoking with 30-pack years and she was a bus driver. Vital signs are unremarkable with the exception of oxygen saturation of 94% on room air. Physical examination is unremarkable. The patient has a sputum culture that grows *H. influenzae, S. aureus,* and normal respiratory flora.

Pulmonary Function Testing

- FEV_1: 54% of predicted
- FVC: 77% of predicted
- FEV_1/FVC: 70% of predicted
- TLC: 84% of predicted
- FRC: 91% of predicted
- DLCO: 59% of predicted

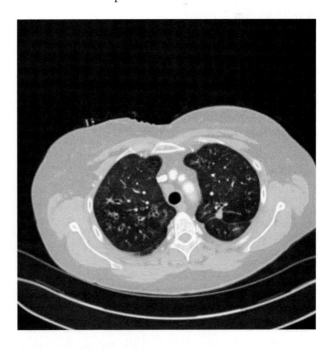

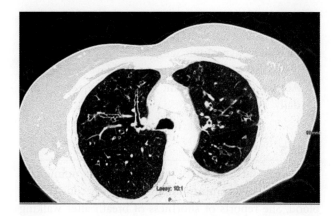

Question 1: **What is the next diagnostic test that you can perform on this patient to confirm diagnosis?**

A. Skin prick test for aspergillus
B. Rheumatoid factor measurement
C. Sweat chloride testing
D. Nasal brushing with subsequent examination with high speed microscopy
E. Flexible bronchoscopy with bronchoalveolar lavage for microbiologic testing

Question 2: **Sweat chloride testing was performed on this patient and found to be 113 mmol/L. Genotype sequencing found mutations to delta F508 on exon 10 and a mutation to G551D on exon 24 of the CFTR gene. Based on this finding, this patient can be classified as which of the following?**

A. Nonclassic cystic fibrosis
B. CFTR-related disease
C. Classic cystic fibrosis
D. Idiopathic bronchiectasis
E. Tracheobronchomegaly

Question 3: **Which of the following chronic therapies would most likely improve FEV1 and decrease rate of exacerbation in this patient?**

A. Daily albuterol therapy
B. Daily high-dose ibuprofen
C. Ivacaftor 150 mg two times a day
D. Aerosolized aztreonam 75 mg three times a day
E. Inhaled budesonide two times daily

CASE 6

A 21-year-old woman with longstanding asthma presents to your clinic with chief complaint of dyspnea on exertion. She tells you that she has had several months of cough productive of dark, thick mucus. Review of systems is positive for chest pain and subjective fever. She does not smoke and works as a waitress. Family history is notable for asthma in her sister and children. Vital signs are normal. Diffuse wheezing is noted in all lung fields on examination. There is no clubbing or peripheral edema.

Pulmonary Function Testing

- FEV_1: 51% of predicted
- FVC: 74% of predicted
- FEV_1/FVC: 52%
- TLC: 88% of predicted
- FRC: 85% of predicted
- DLCO: 58% of predicted

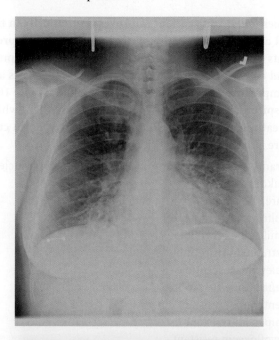

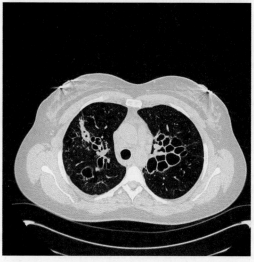

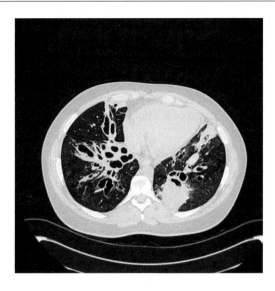

the upper extremity digits without cyanosis or edema. Laboratory studies are as follows:

WBC: 7.9 k/UL normal (4.5–10.8)

Sweat chloride testing: 28 mmol/L

CD4 count: 413 normal (393–1,771)

IgG level: 243 mg/dL (normal 768–1,728 mg/dL)

IgA level: 31 mg/dL (normal 99–396 mg/dL)

IgM level: 35 mg/dL (normal 38–266 mg/dL)

Pulmonary Function Testing

- FEV_1: 51% of predicted
- FVC: 74% of predicted
- FEV_1/FVC: 52%
- TLC: 88% of predicted
- FRC: 85% of predicted
- DLCO: 58% of predicted

Question 1: **Which of the following would be the next appropriate diagnostic test?**

A. Sputum culture

B. Skin prick test for aspergillus

C. Flexible bronchoscopy with transbronchial biopsy

D. CFTR gene sequencing

E. Alpha-1 antitrypsin level

Question 2: **This patient's skin prick test and serum Aspergillus-specific IgE and IgG were found to be positive. Serum IgE was 5305 mg/dL. What medical therapy should be initiated on this patient?**

A. Prednisone 40 mg daily

B. Omalizumab 300 mg intravenous every 4 weeks

C. Immunotherapy with fungal allergens

D. Prednisone 40 mg daily and oral itraconazole 200 mg two times daily

E. Nebulized amphotericin B and nebulized budesonide once daily

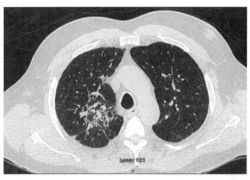

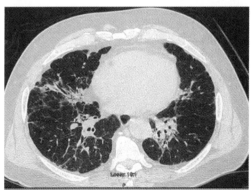

CASE 7

A 33-year-old man presents to your clinic complaining of cough. He reports a history of multiple respiratory infections requiring treatment with antibiotics as well as chronic rhinosinusitis and multiple episodes of gastroenteritis for as long as he can remember. Vital signs are all within normal limits. The patient appears chronically ill. He has nasal discharge and coarse crackles in multiple lung fields on pulmonary auscultation. The abdomen is soft with significant splenomegaly. Cardiac examination is within normal limits. There is noted clubbing of

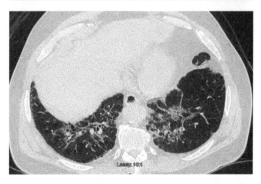

Question 1: **What would be the next appropriate diagnostic test?**

A. Sputum culture and smear for bacteria, mycobacteria, and fungi
B. Assessment of patient's response to protein and polysaccharide-based vaccines
C. Flow cytometry
D. Molecular analysis with genetic sequencing
E. CFTR gene sequencing

Question 2: **What would be the most appropriate treatment for this patient's condition?**

A. Trimethoprim—sulfamethoxazole 800 mg/160 mg three times weekly
B. Immune globulin 500 mg/kg every month
C. Allogenic stem cell transplantation
D. Splenectomy
E. Interleukin-2 therapy

Answers

CASE 1

Question 1: B. Congenital bronchial atresia

The first image in this question shows focal air trapping and a central nodule. The soft tissue window displays a low-density central nodule with branching consistent with a mucocele. These findings are consistent with congenital bronchial atresia. It is a congenital interruption of a segmental or subsegmental bronchus resulting in a distal bronchial segment without associated proximal airway.[1,2] It is secondary to fetal trauma or ischemia during the intrauterine process of lung formation.[1-3] Congenital bronchial atresia is often discovered around the age of 17 and may be asymptomatic or with recurrent pulmonary infection, wheezing, or dyspnea.

* *

Radiographs of patients with congenital bronchial atresia may show a branching, tubular, or nodular area of opacification surrounded by hyperlucent lung parenchyma which correlates clinically with mucous impaction and resultant hyperinflation.[3] As was seen in this case, CT scan findings of congenital bronchial atresia are usually significant for a mucocele with distal air trapping. The hyperinflation is from collateral ventilation of adjacent airways. Focal oligemia may be seen and is thought to be due to intrapulmonary vascular compression and hypoxic vasoconstriction. The most common affected segment is the apicoposterior segment of the left upper lobe followed by the right upper lobe, right middle lobe, and less commonly the right lower lobe. On gross inspection the affected lung unit is often suggestive of focal infection or mucocele with associated hyperinflation.

* *

Bronchogenic cysts occur due to anomalous budding of the foregut during development. Patients generally present during the second decade of life with cough, wheeze, or infection. On chest radiograph, it appears as a mass with water density and an air fluid level. On chest CT, it shows a sharply marginated cystic mediastinal or intrapulmonary mass.[3] Pathologic examination will demonstrate a unilocular cyst filled with thick fluid that does not communicate with the tracheobronchial tree. Persistence of symptoms warrants surgical intervention. Given the location and characteristics of this patient's pulmonary finding, it is unlikely to be a bronchogenic cyst.

* *

Bronchopulmonary sequestration is a nonfunctioning mass of lung tissue that does not communicate with the tracheobronchial tree and receives its blood supply from the systemic circulation. On chest radiograph and CT, it may appear as an opacification or mass with or without an air-fluid level.[3] These findings were not consistent with this patient's imaging. Bronchopulmonary sequestration is thought to be caused by an anomaly of tracheobronchial branching with retention of the embryonic systemic arterial supply. This condition may be found incidentally or when a patient presents with either infectious complaints or less commonly hemoptysis. Management may be dictated by whether the patient has an intralobar or extralobar pathology. Intralobar abnormalities are generally resected whether the patient has symptoms or not in order to prevent future infections. If the patient has extralobar disease, they may be followed clinically if asymptomatic.

* *

Allergic bronchopulmonary aspergillosis is a hypersensitivity reaction to aspergillus antigens that typically occurs in patients with asthma or cystic fibrosis. Patients may present with wheezing, productive cough, chest pain or fever. Chest x-ray may be normal in the early stages of disease but may also manifest as fleeting infiltrates and mucoid impaction. Later manifestations include band-like opacities emanating from the hilum with rounded distal margins (gloved finger), central bronchiectasis, or fibrosis. In patients without central bronchiectasis, criteria for diagnosis include asthma, immediate skin reactivity to aspergillus, serum IgE level greater than 1000 ng/mL, pulmonary infiltrates, and elevated Aspergillus IgE and IgG antibodies. Although this patient has a prior diagnosis of asthma and a pulmonary infiltrate, the absence of central bronchiectasis with normal IgE and negative serum precipitins to *Aspergillus fumigates* makes ABPA unlikely. This patient displayed an impacted airway but the above clinical criteria are not met for the diagnosis of ABPA.

* *

While a foreign-body aspiration may exhibit indication of air trapping as seen in this case, the appearance and density of the abnormality is more suggestive of mucocele and thus congenital bronchial atresia.

Question 2: D. Observation and follow-up

Congenital bronchial atresia generally has an indolent and nonprogressive course. For this reason, often no treatment or intervention is necessary.[1,2] At the time of evaluation, this patient is asymptomatic and so observation would be appropriate. Surgical intervention for congenital bronchial atresia with either lobectomy or segmentectomy may be indicated if there is significant infection or damage to the adjacent lung parenchyma. There is no role for bronchoscopy with BAL in the evaluation of bronchial atresia in an asymptomatic patient. A trial of antibiotics in a patient with congenital bronchial atresia could be considered if there was indication of pulmonary infection. In this case antibiotics would be inappropriate. Corticosteroids would be indicated if this patient presented with an exacerbation of her asthma or a new diagnosis of ABPA. However, the presentation, laboratory results, and imaging findings are more consistent with congenital bronchial atresia. Steroids have no role in the management of congenial bronchial atresia.

CASE 2

Question 1: C. Primary ciliary dyskinesia

This patient has the triad of sinusitis, bronchiectasis and situs inversus known as Kartangener syndrome and therefore most likely has primary ciliary dyskinesia (PCD). It is a recessive disorder of ciliary function that results in neonatal respiratory distress, chronic oto-sinus disease, male infertility, organ laterality defects, and pulmonary disease.[4]

* *

PCD in infancy and childhood results in recurrent/chronic bacterial infections of the lower airways which lead to the development of bronchiectasis in nearly all patients. Patients are frequently colonized with *H. influenzae, S. aureus, S. pneumoniae,* and *P. aeruginosa.* In up to 15% of adult patients nontuberculous mycobacteria is also discovered.

* *

Bronchiectasis may be visualized on imaging in nearly all adult patients with PCD. Mucous plugging, peribronchial thickening, subsegmental atelectasis and evidence of air trapping or ground glass are also common. The right middle lobe, lingula, and basal segments are most frequently affected. This patient's CT findings are indicative of situs inversus, bronchiectasis, mucoid impaction, scattered regions of nodular, linear densities, and a small area of atelectasis.

* *

Laterality defects, as seen in this patient, may be found in up to 60% of pediatric patients and 50% of adults and reflect defective cilia function during embryogenesis (patients radiograph shown below).[4] Infertility is almost universal in men with PCD due to dysmotile sperm. Women may also have reproductive difficulties due to impaired ciliary function of the fallopian tubes. Pectus excavatum is also a common finding in patients with PCD as compared to the general population and may be seen in up to 10% of affected patients.[4]

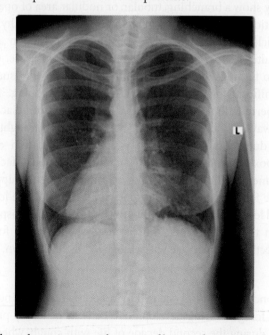

Although patients with cystic fibrosis frequently have bronchiectasis and sinus disease, this patient's negative sweat chloride testing and the presence of situs inversus makes PCD more likely.

* *

Granulomatosis with polyangiitis (GPA) is an ANCA associated vasculitis that may manifest with sinus disease and pulmonary infiltrates. Radiographic findings generally include nodules, fixed infiltrates or cavities rather than bronchiectasis. There is often abnormal urine sediment consisting of microscopic hematuria with or without red cell casts. Given the absence of cavities and hematuria as well as findings consistent with PCD, GPA in this patient is less likely.

* *

Eosinophilic granulomatosis with polyangiitis (formerly called Churg–Strauss syndrome) is a vasculitis of the small- and medium-sized arteries that frequently presents with asthma, migratory pulmonary infiltrates, peripheral eosinophilia, mononeuropathy, and sinus disease. Biopsy may show blood vessels with accumulation of eosinophils in extravascular areas. The above patient has asthma and sinus disease but presence of bronchiectasis and absence of neuropathy and elevated peripheral eosinophils make this disease unlikely.

* *

Lymphoid interstitial pneumonia is an uncommon interstitial lung disease characterized by infiltration of the pulmonary interstitium and alveolar spaces by lymphocytes, plasma, cells, and other lymphoreticular elements. When it does occur, it is most frequently found in patients with either HIV or autoimmune disease such as Sjögren's syndrome. Absence of indication of these conditions as well as the presence of sinusitis and situs inversus makes primary ciliary dyskinesia more likely.

Question 2: D. Nasal nitric oxide levels
Nasal nitric oxide levels in patients with PCD are generally low and accurate measurement by aspiration of nasal air is thought to be a reliable test for PCD.[4] However, nasal nitric oxide may be falsely low in the setting of acute infection or in the presence of cystic fibrosis. Therefore it is performed after CF has been ruled out with CFTR genetic studies and should be compared to the patient's baseline.

* *

Direct measurement of mucociliary clearance has also been used in the past to evaluate for PCD but may be confounded by cough or pre-existing bronchiectasis of other etiologies. Electron microscopy of ciliary structure has traditionally thought to be the gold standard for diagnosis of this condition. Unfortunately, as many as

30% of the patients with PCD may have normal ciliary ultrastructure and so this test is no longer considered the gold standard for ruling out PCD.[4] Assessment of ciliary motility from fresh biopsies of the airway is another traditional approach to diagnosing PCD but it requires an experienced investigator and many confounders exist to collect an effective sample.

* *

In most patients, a normal sweat chloride test is sufficient to rule out cystic fibrosis. CFTR gene sequencing may be considered for patients in whom sweat chloride testing is intermediate (40–59 mmol/L in adults). This patient's normal sweat testing and clinical picture make cystic fibrosis less likely.

* *

If there were suspicion for an ANCA associated pulmonary disease, consideration may be made for checking antineutrophil cytoplasmic antibodies. The triad of sinusitis, bronchiectasis and situs inversus makes primary ciliary dyskinesia more likely in this case.

CASE 3

Question 1: A. Three sputum collections with AFB smear and culture
This patient likely has mycobacterium avium complex (MAC) infection with associated fibronodular bronchiectasis. Up to 12% of the patients with MAC may demonstrate a reticular, fibrotic pattern rather than cavitary disease. In contrast to patients with MAC and cavitary disease, patients with fibronodular bronchiectasis from MAC are predominantly Caucasian postmenopausal women without a history of smoking or pre-existing lung disease. This syndrome is frequently referred to as Lady Windermere Syndrome.

* *

The most frequent associated symptoms are cough and sputum production. Fatigue, dyspnea, fever, chest pain, weight loss, and hemoptysis are also common with constitutional symptoms seen more frequently in advanced disease. Though MAC is the most commonly associated pathogen in fibronodular bronchiectasis, *M. abscessus*, and *M. kansasii* may also be implicated. Patients frequently have respiratory cultures positive for *P. aeruginosa*. It is unknown if bronchiectasis is the result of mycobacterial infection or due to some alternative process that then predisposes the patient to mycobacterial infection. Typical CT findings include small peripheral nodules centered on a bronchovascular tree with cylindrical bronchiectasis also known as "tree in bud."

* *

According to the official ATS/IDSA statement regarding nontuberculous mycobacteria (NTM), the minimum evaluation of a patient suspected of having NTM lung disease should include at least three sputum specimens for AFB, a chest radiograph or high-resolution CT scan (if there is no cavitation on chest radiograph), and exclusion of alternative disease processes such as tuberculosis.[5] The minimum requirement for microbiologic diagnosis includes either:

1. Positive culture results from at least two separate expectorated sputum samples.
2. Positive culture results from at least one bronchial washing or lavage.
3. Transbronchial biopsy with mycobacterial features and positive culture for NTM or biopsy with mycobacterial features and one or more culture positive sputum or bronchial washings.

* *

There are currently no consensus guidelines regarding routine testing for cystic fibrosis or alpha one antitrypsin deficiency (A1AT) in patients suspected of having nodular bronchiectatic MAC. Generally in the case of cystic fibrosis the central airways are more involved. The absence of bulla and lower lobe predominance makes A1AT less likely.

* *

NTM-specific skin antigen testing has been developed but is not currently commercially available. Available tuberculin skin tests do not distinguish between NTM and latent or prior *Mycobacterium tuberculosis*. For this reason these tests are not recommended for screening of NTM disease.

* *

Langerhans cells may be present in the lungs of normal individuals and quantities less than 5% are not considered pathogenic. The presence of elevated Langerhans cells is not associated with the development of NTM pulmonary disease.

* *

Though chronic aspiration may be considered for this patient, a thorough history and physical examination indicative of a swallowing disorder should be obtained prior to further diagnostic testing for gastrointestinal pathology. A modified barium swallow study may be utilized if there is high suspicion of esophageal, stomach, or duodenal pathology.

Question 2: D. Rifampin, ethambutol, and clarithromycin or azithromycin three times per week

Clarithromycin testing is recommended for previously untreated MAC disease.[5] For macrolide susceptible, nodular/bronchiectatic MAC, clarithromycin 1,000 mg or azithromycin 500 mg with ethambutol 25 mg/kg and rifampin 600 mg three times a weekly is generally suggested.

* *

The goals of therapy for NTM disease include symptomatic, radiographic and microbiologic improvement including negative sputum cultures.[5] The patient should be followed clinically on a monthly basis for symptom resolution and culture conversion. Patients should exhibit clinical improvement within 3 to 6 months and sputum conversion within 12 months of treatment initiation. Treatment failure could be secondary to medication noncompliance due to drug intolerance, drug resistance, or anatomic limitations such as cystic or cavitary disease should be investigated. Patients who have 12 months of culture negative sputum may be considered cured of their disease. If cultures are positive after 12 months, reinfection rather than recurrence is likely.

* *

A macrolide with a single companion drug such as ethambutol may be considered for nodular/bronchiectatic disease, but macrolide monotherapy should be avoided out of risk for the development of resistance.

* *

Given the substantial side effects of therapy for NTM disease, in the absence of systemic symptoms or in the presence of significant comorbidity, it may be reasonable to observe a patient over time. This would involve monitoring for symptomatic and radiographic worsening as well as regular sputum collection. Given this patient's symptoms and lack of substantial comorbid complaints, pharmacologic treatment may be more reasonable.

* *

In patients with cavitary or severe nodular/bronchiectatic MAC-related disease, treatment may include a daily regime of ethambutol, rifampin, and a macrolide.

Given the absence of cavitary disease in this patient, it is reasonable to start with rifampin, ethambutol, and clarithromycin or azithromycin three times weekly instead.

* *

Although proton pump inhibitors such as omeprazole may be utilized to minimize the complications of gastroesophageal reflux disease, there is no evidence that they improve swallowing function in the setting of chronic aspiration.

Question 3: C. Surgical resection plus streptomycin for initial 3 to 6 months with subsequent daily isoniazid, rifampin, and ethambutol

A drug regimen using a parenteral aminoglycoside (streptomycin or amikacin) and surgical debulking most likely leads to treatment success in patients with clarithromycin resistant MAC. Risk factors for initial drug resistance in this population included macrolide monotherapy or a combination of a macrolide and quinolone only. Macrolide resistance developed in only 4% of patients whose initial regimen was consistent with American Thoracic Society guidelines for the treatment of MAC.[5-7] Although rifampin, ethambutol, and clarithromycin or azithromycin three times a week may be a good choice for the initial treatment of NTM disease, in a patient with macrolide resistance an alternative course should be considered. Although observation is generally a reasonable alternative in the management of patients with NTM disease, this patient's distressing symptoms, consistent organism isolation, and prior tolerance to medical therapy make observation less of an appropriate strategy.

CASE 4

Question 1: C. Measurement of serum immunoglobulins (IgG, IgA, and IgM)

This patient exhibits a clinical picture and imaging consistent with a new diagnosis of bronchiectasis. Bronchiectasis is the anatomic distortion of conduction airways resulting in chronic cough, sputum production, and recurrent infections. It is the result from inflammatory or infectious damage to bronchial and bronchiolar walls that leads to a viscous cycle of airway injury with further infection and inflammation.[8,9] The signet ring sign, an internal bronchial diameter greater than the bronchial artery, and/or lack of bronchial tapering defines bronchiectasis on CT scan. Traditional radiographic descriptions

of bronchiectasis include cylindrical, varicose or cystic/saccular but patients may have all three. Cystic bronchiectasis is associated with *Pseudomonas* colonization and worse prognosis.

* *

The differential diagnosis for the etiology of underlying bronchiectasis includes post-infectious, genetic disease such as cystic fibrosis, primary ciliary dyskinesia or Alpha-1 antitrypsin deficiency, chronic aspiration, immune deficiency, rheumatoid arthritis, inflammatory bowel disease, ABPA, asthma, or idiopathic.

* *

The British Thoracic Society suggests measuring serum immunoglobulins (IgG, IgA, and IgM), serum electrophoresis and antibody titers to pneumococcal serotypes before and 4 weeks after vaccination.[9] In all patients the possibility of underlying cystic fibrosis should be considered with low threshold for screening with sweat chloride testing and CFTR genetic mutation analysis should be undertaken. Adult patients should be ruled out for asthma if no other cause of bronchiectasis is identified. Evaluation for ABPA with serum IgE, *Aspergillus fumigatus* RAST/CAP and aspergillus precipitins may be investigated when clinically appropriate in all patients found to have a new diagnosis of bronchiectasis of unclear etiology.

* *

Bronchoscopy may be indicated when bronchiectasis is focal in nature and local obstruction is suspected but is not part of a standard workup. There is a recognized association between rheumatoid arthritis and other connective tissue diseases however in the absence of appropriate clinical presentation, screening for rheumatic diseases is not necessary in the initial work up for bronchiectasis. A tuberculin skin test is not a sensitive marker of active *Mycobacterium tuberculosis* infection and not part of the initial work up for bronchiectatic disease. Measurement of nasal nitric oxide levels may be performed if there is high suspicion for primary ciliary dyskinesia. In the absence of sinusitis and situs inversus, primary ciliary dyskinesia is less likely.

Question 2: A. H. influenzae

A bronchiectasis exacerbation is characterized by an acute clinical deterioration with increased cough, dyspnea, hemoptysis, sputum volume, change in viscosity, purulence or increased wheezing. Mucopurulent sputum or colonization with atypical airway pathogens is alone not reason for antibiotic therapy in patients with bronchiectasis.

* *

The initial management of a bronchiectasis exacerbation should include sending a sputum sample prior to empiric antibiotic administration. In most studies of adult patients with bronchiectasis the most common organism cultured is *H. influenzae.* Although *P. aeruginosa* is much more common in adults with noncystic fibrosis-related bronchiectasis than it is in children, *H. influenzae* is still cultured more frequently. *S. aureus,* atypical mycobacteria, and *S. pneumoniae* may also be found in the respiratory tracts of patients with bronchiectasis but less common.

Question 3: B. Amoxicillin 500 mg three times daily for 14 days

There are no randomized placebo-controlled trials to evaluate antibiotic choice in bronchiectasis exacerbations. Antibiotic choice is generally empiric and may be guided first by prior sputum cultures and then by local microbial patterns and cost. Patients may be treated with oral antibiotics unless a patient is particularly unwell or there is treatment failure. Because the most commonly cultured organism is *H. influenzae,* it is appropriate to initiate treatment with amoxicillin 500 mg three times a day for 14 days. In patients who fail to respond, the dose can be escalated to 1 g three times a day or 3 g two times a day.

* *

Although exacerbations may be triggered by viral infections, there are no studies to evaluate the role of antiviral agents in bronchiectasis exacerbations. If there are prior sputum cultures positive of *Pseudomonas* or high clinical suspicion of this organism, an oral fluoroquinolones are indicated. Fluoroquinolones are associated with high rates of antibiotic resistance and *Clostridium difficile* colitis. Therefore, they should be used judiciously.

* *

There are a number of studies that suggest that inflammation may be improved after 7 days of therapy but takes 10 to 14 days of therapy for symptomatic relief. For this reason expert consensus dictates that all patients with bronchiectasis exacerbation should be treated for 14 days.

* *

Vancomycin may be considered if methicillin-resistant *S. aureus* were to have grown on prior sputum culture in the setting of bronchiectasis exacerbation but would not be indicated in this case.

Question 4: D. Cefepime 2 g IV every 8 hours plus Amikacin 20 mg/kg IV daily

British Thoracic Society guidelines recommend that intravenous antibiotics be considered for bronchiectasis exacerbation in patients who are particularly ill, have resistant organisms, or have failed to respond to oral therapy.[9] This patient's clinical status requires hospital admission and IV antimicrobial therapy with agents that match his most recent sputum sensitivities. Combination antibiotics are recommended when there are strains of *Pseudomonas* resistant to one or more antipseudomonal antibiotics. Antibiotics should be further modified and repeat sputum culture should be performed if there is no clinical improvement.

* *

In patients colonized with *P. aeruginosa* the addition of nebulized tobramycin to ciprofloxacin has been shown to decrease microbial load without overt clinical benefit.[11] Due to lack of data and this patient's spectrum of drug resistance this combination would be inappropriate. Further studies are thought to be needed before inhaled aminoglycosides added to oral fluoroquinolones can be adopted as an accepted treatment strategy.

* *

Patients who have cultured *P. aeruginosa* and exhibit clinical stability may be considered for an oral fluoroquinolone but this patient's progression of symptoms and hypoxemia warrants hospital admission for IV therapy. Additionally this patient has exhibited resistance to fluoroquinolones. These drugs would therefore be inappropriate.

* *

Intravenous aminoglycosides require careful dosing and monitoring systems with the goal of avoiding renal and ototoxicities. This patient has displayed resistance to tobramycin and this drug would therefore be inappropriate.

* *

Amoxicillin therapy may be considered for a bronchiectasis exacerbation in patients who do not have microbiologic evidence of pseudomonas or beta-lactamase positive *H. influenza.* This patient has microbiologic culture indicating pseudomonas with extensive drug resistance. Amoxicillin would therefore be an inappropriate choice in this case

Question 5: A. Azithromycin 500 mg three times a week
A multicenter, randomized, double-blind placebo controlled trial found that azithromycin reduced the frequency of exacerbations in patients with non-CF bronchiectasis.[10] The patients were given 500 mg of azithromycin three times per week or placebo over 6 months. During the study period, the rate of exacerbations was .59 per patient in the treatment group and 1.57 in the placebo arm.[10] Of note, administration of azithromycin was not shown to significantly affect lung function or health-related quality of life. Prior to administration of a macrolide antibiotic, all patients should have sputum culture to rule out the presence of nontuberculous mycobacterial disease.

* *

Inhaled antibiotics have also been found to be helpful to decrease rates of bronchiectasis exacerbations. In a double-blind placebo-controlled trial involving 30 patients with non-CF bronchiectasis, 6 months of 300 mg inhaled tobramycin was shown to reduce the number of hospital admissions and density of pseudomonas.[11] Inhaled tobramycin was associated with bronchospasm but not with ototoxicity or nephrotoxicity. The British Thoracic Society guidelines therefore suggest that patients with non-CF bronchiectasis who have more than three exacerbations per year requiring antibiotic therapy be given a trial of nebulized antibiotics.[9] This treatment therapy should especially be considered for patients colonized with *P. aeruginosa*.

* *

Though it has been shown in small patient groups that noninvasive ventilation may improve quality of life in some patients with bronchiectasis, there has been no indication that this mode of therapy may decrease rate of exacerbations. Nebulized hypertonic saline is often used in patients with bronchiectasis to augment mucous expectoration. A randomized study of 40 patients with noncystic fibrosis bronchiectasis found no difference in rates of exacerbations between patients that used nebulized hypertonic saline or isotonic saline.[13] Mannitol is a hyperosmolar agent that is thought to promote mucous clearance. There is no quality data to suggest that the use of nebulized mannitol decreases rates of bronchiectasis exacerbations. Although use of aerosolized recombinant human DNase has been shown to improve pulmonary function and reduce hospitalizations in patients with cystic fibrosis, it has not been found to be effective in patients with noncystic fibrosis-related bronchiectasis and may in fact lead to more exacerbations and greater decline of FEV_1.[12,13]

CASE 5

Question 1: C. Sweat chloride testing
This patient's CT scan is indicative of bronchiectasis and her clinical history is strongly suggestive of cystic fibrosis (CF). Criteria for the diagnosis of cystic fibrosis includes at least one organ system known to be involved with CF and the demonstration of cystic fibrosis trans-membrane conductance regulator (CFTR) dysfunction.[13-16] Typical clinical manifestations of CF include sino-pulmonary disease, gastrointestinal or nutritional abnormalities, and salt wasting or male urogenital pathology resulting in azospermia. CFTR dysfunction may be demonstrated by a sweat chloride level greater than 60 mmol/L, the presence of two CFTR mutations known to be associated with CFTR dysfunction or evidence of CFTR ion transport abnormalities by measurement of nasal potential difference.[13-17] Measurement of nasal potential difference may be particularly useful in the case of inconclusive sweat chloride values.

* *

Cystic fibrosis is a genetic disorder resulting from mutations of the cystic fibrosis transmembrane conductance regulator gene.[13-16] The CFTR gene is a cAMP-activated anion channel expressed in the epithelial cells and sub-mucosal glands of the airway. Mutations in CFTR result in abnormal airway ion movements with subsequent depletion of airway surface liquid, decreased pH and impaired mucociliary clearance. Bronchiectasis from cystic fibrosis results from a vicious cycle of airway infection, inflammation, and mucous obstruction.

* *

Performance of a skin prick test for aspergillosis is the first step to make the diagnosis of allergic bronchopulmonary aspergillosis. Although it is reasonable to investigate ABPA in all patients with a new diagnosis of bronchiectasis and elevated clinical suspicion, this patient's history is strongly suggestive of cystic fibrosis. In addition, when bronchiectasis is found in the setting of ABPA it is classically central in location.

* *

Although connective tissue disease, particularly rheumatoid arthritis may predispose patients to bronchiectasis, in the absence of strong clinical indication and presence of high clinical suspicion for cystic fibrosis, it is not necessary to perform further work up for rheumatic disease.

* *

Patients in whom there is suspicion for primary ciliary dyskinesia, nasal brushing with a bronchoscopy brush may be used to obtain ciliate epithelium for examination with high speed video microscopy. This technique is technically difficult therefore nasal nitric oxide measurement is suggested. Because this patient's history is more consistent with cystic fibrosis, evidence of CFTR dysfunction should be investigated first.

* *

Although respiratory tract culture for cystic fibrosis associated pathogens is part of the initial workup of a patient with newly diagnosed disease, bronchoscopy is generally not needed for this purpose.

Question 2: C. Classic cystic fibrosis
Using clinical features, patients with CFTR dysfunction may be classified as classic cystic fibrosis, nonclassic cystic fibrosis, or CFTR-related disease. This patient meets criteria for classic CF. Classic CF is defined as demonstration of clinical disease in one or more organ system along with an elevated sweat chloride test above 60 mmol/L. As is the case with this patient, most patients with classic CF have multiorgan system disease.

* *

Nonclassic CF may be defined as those individuals demonstrating manifestation of CF in at least one organ system but with sweat chloride that is normal (less than 40 mmol/L) or borderline (between 40 and 60 mmol/L). Only 2% of the patients who fulfill criteria for a diagnosis of CF fall into the nonclassic CF category.[14] In general patients with nonclassic CF tend to have less incidence of pancreatic insufficiency and often have milder lung disease. Males may demonstrate fertility. Although patient with nonclassic CF are often diagnosed beyond childhood this patient has an abnormally elevated sweat chloride test and so meets criteria for classic CF.

* *

Cystic fibrosis transmembrane conductance regulator-related diseases are conditions that have been associated with mutations of the CFTR gene that do not fit the criteria for cystic fibrosis or follow a Mendelian inheritance pattern. Allergic bronchopulmonary aspergillosis, chronic sinusitis, and idiopathic bronchiectasis have been found to coexist with CFTR mutations and are thus termed CFTR-related disease. This patient meets criteria for classic CF and therefore is not categorized as having cystic fibrosis transmembrane conductance regulator-related disease.

* *

Idiopathic bronchiectasis is generally defined as bronchiectasis of unknown etiology despite extensive evaluation. This patient meets criteria for cystic fibrosis and therefore does not have idiopathic bronchiectasis.

* *

Idiopathic giant trachea (IGT) is a rare condition that presents during adulthood and is thought to be secondary to atrophy of elastic fibers and thinning of the muscularis mucosa of the trachea. When this defect extends to the central bronchi it may be termed tracheobronchomegaly or Mounier–Kuhn syndrome. Tracheobronchomegaly may be diagnosed when the diameter of the trachea exceeds 3 cm, the right mainstem bronchus exceeds 2.4 cm, and the left mainstem bronchus is greater than 2.3 cm. This patient meets criteria for classic CF and does not meet the above criteria for tracheobronchomegaly.

Question 3: C. Ivacaftor 150 mg two times a day
A recent randomized, double-blind, placebo-controlled trial evaluated the CFTR potentiator ivacaftor in cystic fibrosis patients with at least one G551D-CFTR mutation.[13-15] It was found that ivacaftor was associated with significant improvements in FEV_1 after 2 weeks and that these improvements were sustained throughout the 48 week study period. Subjects receiving ivacaftor were 55% less likely to have a pulmonary exacerbation and the drug was also associated with improved respiratory symptoms and weight gain. Interestingly, the concentration of sweat chloride, viewed as a surrogate for CFTR activity, was substantially lower in the patients who had received ivacaftor. For this reason, recent guidelines suggest initiating ivacaftor in patients older than 6 years who have at least one G551D CFTR mutation in order to improve lung function, quality of life and reduce exacerbations.[15] This patient has a mutation of the G551D gene and ivacaftor should therefore be initiated.

* *

Additional grade A recommendations regarding chronic medications for cystic fibrosis include administration of daily nebulized dornase alpha for moderate to severe disease.[12,13] For patients who grow persistent *P. aeruginosa* with moderate to severe disease either standing inhaled tobramycin or inhaled aztreonam are suggested. Grade B recommendations for any CF patient include regular inhaled hypertonic saline and chronic ibuprofen for patients younger than 18.[13] In any patient growing *pseudomonas*, azithromycin is suggested. For patients with mild disease and *pseudomonas* colonization inhaled tobramycin, aztreonam or dornase alpha are suggested.

* *

Earlier guidelines had recommended the use of beta-2 adrenergic receptor agonists for chronic, standing use in cystic fibrosis patients. On subsequent review of the literature it was determined that there is insufficient evidence to recommend chronic daily use of inhaled bronchodilators in patients for the purpose of improvement of quality of life or prevention of exacerbations. Because of bronchospasm inducing alternative CF therapies these agents may still be considered in patients with documented airway hyper-reactivity.

* *

High-dose ibuprofen can slow the progression of lung disease in cystic fibrosis patients but it is thought that this effect is mostly seen in children aged 6 to 17 years. It is thought that ibuprofen at doses sufficient to maintain a level of 50 to 100 mg/mL are effective at inhibiting neutrophil migration and thus progression of loss of lung function. Despite this, there is little data to suggest that high-dose ibuprofen has benefits in patients over the age of 18.

* *

The CF foundation strongly recommends the chronic use of inhaled aztreonam for patients who persistently grow *P. aeruginosa* on sputum culture with strong evidence for this therapies ability to improve lung function and improve quality of life.[13] This patient did not grow Pseudomonas on culture and should therefore not be initiated on standing inhaled aztreonam.

* *

Inhaled glucocorticoids have not been proven to be beneficial to patients with cystic fibrosis in the absence of asthma or allergic bronchopulmonary aspergillosis and are therefore not indicated in this case.

CASE 6

Question 1: B. Skin prick test for aspergillus

Allergic bronchopulmonary aspergillosis (ABPA) is a syndrome of asthma, eosinophilia, and bronchiectasis caused by a complex hypersensitivity reaction to Aspergillus colonization of the airways. ABPA more commonly occurs in patients with cystic fibrosis or steroid dependent asthma than in the general population. Patients frequently present with a history of asthma, cough productive of brown mucous plugs, chest pain, fever, and wheezing. Chest x-ray often shows findings suggestive of bronchiectasis and hyperinflation. As is the case in this patient, CT scan may show central predominant bronchiectasis and mucoid impaction. Often mucoid impaction may be seen as band-like opacities emanating from the hilum with rounded distal margins also known as gloved finger appearance. Although this patient does not show finger in glove, her radiographic findings are otherwise characteristic.

* *

The diagnosis of ABPA requires strong clinical suspicion followed by skin prick reactivity to the aspergillus antigen. If the skin prick test is negative, the patient is unlikely to have ABPA. If skin prick is positive, total serum IgE should be measured along with aspergillus-specific IgE and IgG levels.[18,19] If serum IgE is above 1,000 ng/mL and aspergillus-specific IgE and IgG levels are positive than the patient likely has ABPA.[18,19] If both are negative the patient is unlikely to have ABPA and if only one is positive then the patient should be followed with repeat testing as clinically indicated.[18,19]

* *

Because of the presence of central bronchiectasis, this patient's diagnosis can be confirmed with only a history of asthma, a positive immediate skin test reactivity to Aspergillus antigens, precipitating serum antibodies to A fumigatus and serum total IgE concentration greater than 1,000 ng/mL. This patient would be classified as ABPA-CB where the absence of bronchiectasis in a patient meeting the remainder of the clinical criteria would be termed ABPA-S (seropositive).[18,19]

* *

Positive sputum culture for Aspergillosis may be present in up to two thirds of patient with ABPA and is supportive but not required to make this diagnosis. Aspergillosis is a ubiquitous fungal organism, found as an airway colonizer of both healthy and diseased patients.

* *

On pathologic examination the Aspergillus organism may be visualized in the airway lumen without invasion into bronchial mucosa. Mucoid impaction, eosinophilic infiltration, granuloma formation and findings consistent with the histologic presentations of asthma may also be visualized. Although supportive of the diagnosis, transbronchial or open lung biopsy is not part of the criteria for diagnosis of ABPA.

* *

Although CFTR gene mutations are associated with increased frequency in patients with a diagnosis of ABPA, CFTR gene investigation is not currently part of the diagnostic workup for ABPA.

* *

Although measurement of alpha-1 antitrypsin (A1AT) level may be indicated in many young patients without history of smoking who present with persistent airflow obstruction and emphysema, this patients history and imaging findings are more consistent with ABPA. Measurement of A1AT level is not indicated before workup for ABPA is complete.

Question 2: D. Prednisone 40 mg daily and oral itraconazole 200 mg two times daily

Because of the presumed pathophysiologic nature of ABPA as a disease of hypersensitivity, corticosteroids have been a longstanding mainstay of therapy. Steroids have been shown to improve pulmonary function and result in fewer episodes of pulmonary consolidation. More recently studies have looked at the use of the antifungal itraconazole to decrease the burden of Aspergillus in airways. Two separate randomized, double-blind, placebo-controlled trials demonstrated that the addition of itraconazole two times daily resulted in decreased use of corticosteroids, improved pulmonary function and exercise tolerance as well as decreased sputum eosinophilia and IgE concentration.[18–20] Given the above data the current clinical practice guidelines of the Infectious Diseases Society of America for treatment of Aspergillosis recommend combination of corticosteroids and itraconazole for treatment of ABPA.[18–20]

* *

The literature to support the use of corticosteroids as monotherapy is limited to small, low-quality trials. In addition, chronic administration of these drugs is associated with substantial side effects. For these reasons, itraconazole therapy has become a useful adjunct to steroid therapy in patients with ABPA.

* *

Omalizumab is a monoclonal antibody directed against IgE that has been shown to be effective in treating patients with asthma who posses a strong allergic component. There are case reports of effective treatment of steroid dependent patients with cystic fibrosis and ABPA who experienced clinical improvement with Omalizumab.[21] Unfortunately, these were small observational studies that did not include noncystic fibrosis patients. Omalizumab is therefore not part of standard therapy for ABPA at this time.

* *

Therapeutic reagents for fungal immunotherapy are difficult to standardize and so high-quality trials of to suggest that immunotherapy improves outcomes in patients who suffer from ABPA are not available. For this reason, immunotherapy is not recommended for patients with ABPA

* *

Case reports exist of clinical improvement of ABPA using a combination of nebulized corticosteroids and amphotericin B but current guidelines do not advocate for the use of this treatment combination.

CASE 7

Question 1: B. Assessment of patient's response to protein and polysaccharide-based vaccines

This patient has history suggestive of common variable immunodeficiency (CVID) and imaging studies indicative of resultant bronchiectasis. CVID is a genetic syndrome characterized by significant decrease of immunoglobulin G, immunoglobulin A and/or immunoglobulin M levels with poor or absent antibody production and exclusion of alternative causes for hypogammaglobulinemia.

* *

Along with respiratory tract infections and resultant bronchiectasis, there is generally an increased incidence of rhinosinusitis, hepatic dysfunction, and gastrointestinal malabsorption along with an increased incidence of autoimmune disease, lymphoid proliferation and malignancy. Although often thought to be a disease of childhood, 95% of patients will present after the age of 6 with an average age of diagnosis of 26.6. Because of the heterogeneous manifestations of the disease, patients may present to a variety of medical specialties with an average 8.9 years delay in the diagnosis being made.[22-24] This delayed diagnosis may contribute to early mortality, commonly from respiratory failure of age 55.4 in females and age 28.8 in males.[22-24] The most common presenting complaint, as was the case with this patient, is recurrent chest infection followed by productive cough.

* *

The initial evaluation of any patient with suspected CVID should include measurement of immunoglobulin levels, measurement of response to vaccinations, and exclusion of other disease processes. Measurement of response to protein-based vaccines is performed by testing for IgG levels to tetanus and diphtheria and measurement of response to polysaccharide vaccines is performed by testing for IgG antibodies to serotypes in the pneumococcal vaccine. Imaging findings of CVID are nonspecific but include nodules, air trapping or ground glass and bronchiectasis as seen in this patient.

* *

Sputum culture is a standard test in the evaluation of a patient with a new diagnosis of bronchiectasis but is not needed to make the diagnosis of CVID.

* *

Flow cytometry of leukocytes is not required for the diagnosis of CVID but may reveal reduced numbers of certain subclasses of B cells.

* *

Molecular analysis for genetic defects is not necessary to diagnose CVID. This testing may be considered if there are other affected family members and a specific defect needs to be investigated.

* *

Although this patient's history of sinus and gastrointestinal along with bronchiectasis on imaging may raise suspicion for cystic fibrosis, the normal sweat chloride test and abnormal immunoglobulin levels are more concerning for CVID.

Question 2: B. Immune globulin 500 mg/kg every month.

The primary treatment for CVID is the replacement of immune globulin antibody via the infusion of 400 to 600 mg/kg monthly. Immune globulin replacement has been found in retrospective reviews to reduce the number of infections, decrease antibiotic usage, number of hospitalizations and slow the progression of lung disease as measured by pulmonary function testing and CT scan

findings.[25] Immune globulin therapy has not been found to affect the course of systemic granulomatous disease, autoimmune dysfunction, lymphoid hyperplasia, gastrointestinal complications or the development of cancer in patients with CVID.

* *

In addition to immune globulin therapy it is suggested that all patients with CVID have yearly evaluations including basic laboratory studies, serum IgG, chest radiograph, and pulmonary function testing. CT scan should be performed every 3 to 4 years or in the case of change in therapy or clinical status. Patients should have age appropriate cancer screening and further directed investigation should concerning symptoms or signs of malignancy arise.

* *

The utility of prophylactic antibiotics for patients with CVID has not been studied and is therefore not routinely recommended.

* *

There have been isolated cases of allogeneic stem cell transplant in patients who either have severe CVID or associated hematologic malignancy with variable outcomes. This therapy may be considered in select cases but is not standard management for patient with CVID.

* *

Lymphoid hyperplasia and enlarged spleen are found in 20% of patients with CVID.[26] As in this case, splenomegaly can be massive but often does not cause symptoms. Splenectomy is generally not recommended unless there is uncontrolled autoimmunity or concern for lymphoma.

* *

In small investigations interleukin-2 (IL-2) has been shown to modulate T-cell function in CVID patients but has failed to improve clinical outcomes in a meaningful manner and therefore should only be considered in refractory disease.[27]

REFERENCES

1. Jederlinic PJ, Sicilian LS, Baigelman W, et al. Congenital bronchial atresia. A report of 4 cases and a review of the literature. *Medicine (Baltimore).* 1987;66(1):73–83.
2. Gipson MG, Cummings KW, Hurth KM. Bronchial Atresia. *Radiographics.* 2009;29(5):1531–1535.
3. Zylak CJ, Eyler WR, Spizarny DL, et al. Developmental lung anomalies in the adult: Radiologic-pathologic correlation. *Radiographics.* 2002;22:S25–S43.

4. Knowles MR, Daniels LA, Davis SD, et al. Primary ciliary dyskinesia. Recent advances in diagnostics, genetics, and characterization of clinical disease. *AJRCCM*. 2013;188(8): 913–922.

5. Griffith DE, Aksamit T, Brown-Elliott BA, et al. An official ATS/IDSA statement: diagnosis, treatment, and prevention of nontuberculous mycobacterial diseases. *AJRCCM*. 2007;175(4):367–416.

6. Griffith DE, Brown-Elliott BA, Langsjoen B, et al. Clinical and molecular analysis of macrolide resistance in Mycobacterium avium complex lung disease. *AJRCCM*. 2006;174(8):928–934.

7. Field SK, Cowie RL. Lung disease due to the more common nontuberculous mycobacteria. *Chest*. 2006;129(6): 1653–1672.

8. O'Donnell AE. Bronchiectasis. *Chest*. 2008;134(4):815.

9. Pasteur MC, Bilton D, Hill AT; British Thoracic Society Bronchiectasis (non-CF) Guideline Group. British Thoracic Society guideline for non-CF bronchiectasis. *Thorax*. 2010;65(Suppl 1):i1–i58

10. Wong C, Jayaram L, Karalus N, et al. Azithromycin for prevention of exacerbations in non-cystic fibrosis bronchiectasis (EMBRACE): a randomised, double-blind, placebo-controlled trial. *Lancet*. 2012;380(9842):660–667.

11. Drobnic ME, Suñé P, Montoro JB, et al. Inhaled tobramycin in non-cystic fibrosis patients with bronchiectasis and chronic bronchial infection with Pseudomonas aeruginosa. *Ann Pharmacother*. 2005;39(1):39–44.

12. O'Donnell AE, Barker AF, Ilowite JS, et al. Treatment of idiopathic bronchiectasis with aerosolized recombinant human DNase I. rhDNase Study Group. *Chest*. 1998;113(5): 1329–1334.

13. Mogayzel PJ, Naureckas ET, Robinson KA, et al. Cystic fibrosis pulmonary guidelines: Chronic medications for maintenance of lung health. *AJRCCM*. 2013;187(7): 680–689.

14. Boyle MP. Nonclassic cystic fibrosis and CFTR-related diseases. *Curr Opin Pulm Med*. 2003;9(6):498–503.

15. Jain M, Goss CH. Update in cystic fibrosis. 2013. *AJRCCM*. 2014;189(10):1181–1186.

16. Farrell PM, Rosenstein BJ, White TB, et al. Guidelines for diagnosis of cystic fibrosis in newborns through older adults: Cystic fibrosis foundation consensus report. *J Pediatr*. 2008;153(2):S4–S14.

17. Ramsey BW, Davies J, McElvaney NG, et al. A CFTR Potentiator in Patients with Cystic Fibrosis and the *G551D* Mutation. *NEJM*. 2011;365(18):1663–1672.

18. Agarwal R. Allergic bronchopulmonary aspergillosis. *Chest*. 2009;135(3):805.

19. Walsh TJ, Anaissie EJ, Denning DW, et al. Treatment of aspergillosis: Clinical practice guidelines of the infectious diseases society of America. *Clin Infect Dis*. 2008;46(3): 327–360.

20. Wark PA, Hensley MJ, Saltos N, et al. Anti-inflammatory effect of itraconazole in stable allergic bronchopulmonary aspergillosis: a randomized controlled trial. *J Allergy Clin Immunol*. 2003;111(5):952–957.

21. Zirbes JM, Milla CE. Steroid-sparing effect of omalizumab for allergic bronchopulmonary aspergillosis and cystic fibrosis. *Pediatr Pulmonol*. 2008;43(6):607–610.

22. Cunningham-Rundles C. How I treat common variable immune deficiency. *Blood*. 2010;116(1):7–15.

23. De Gracia J, Vendrell M, Alvarez A, et al. Immunoglobulin therapy to control lung damage in patients with common variable immunodeficiency. *Int Immunopharmacol*. 2004; 4(6):745–753.

24. Thickett KM, Kumararatne DS, Banerjee AK, et al. Common variable immune deficiency: respiratory manifestations, pulmonary function and high-resolution CT scan findings. *QJM*. 2002;95(10):655–662.

25. Busse PJ, Razvi S, Cunningham-Rundles C. Efficacy of intravenous immunoglobulin in the prevention of pneumonia in patients with common variable immunodeficiency. *J Allergy Clin Immunol*. 2002;109(6):1001–1004.

26. Quinti I, Soresina A, Spadaro G, et al. Long-term follow-up and outcome of a large cohort of patients with common variable immunodeficiency. *J Clin Immunol*. 2007;27(3): 308–316.

27. Rump JA, Jahreis A, Schlesier M, et al. A double-blind, placebo-controlled, crossover therapy study with natural human IL-2 (nhuIL-2) in combination with regular intravenous gammaglobulin (IVIG) infusions in 10 patients with common variable immunodeficiency (CVID). *Clin Exp Immunol*. 1997;110(2):167–173.

7

Diffuse Parenchymal Lung Diseases

Ronaldo Collo Go MD

CASE 1

A 64-year-old man complains of progressive dyspnea on exertion. In the emergency department, he is noted to have chest pain and atrial fibrillation. He has electrocardioversion and is started on an amiodarone drip. He is a construction worker and has a 30 pack-year history. His physical examination was otherwise unremarkable except for crackles at the bases on auscultation and irregularly irregular heart rate. His laboratory tests including complete blood count, electrolytes, BNP, and echocardiogram are otherwise unremarkable. Coronal view of his chest computed tomography is shown below.

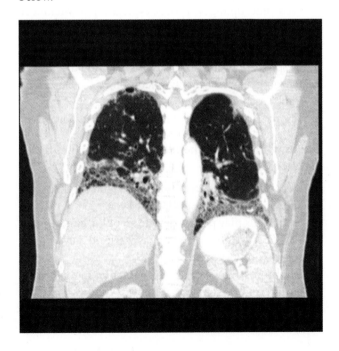

Question 1: **What is the least invasive approach to obtain the histologic diagnosis of his pulmonary disease?**

A. Surgical lung biopsy
B. Bronchioalveolar lavage
C. Transbronchial biopsy
D. Connective tissue disease serologies
E. None of the above

Question 2: **What treatment would you prescribe for curative intent?**

A. Pirfenidone 2,403 mg PO daily
B. Nintedanib 150 mg PO BID
C. Lung transplantation
D. Acetylcysteine PO 600 mg PO BID
E. Prednisone 40 mg PO daily

Question 3: **Patient is evaluated in pulmonary clinic. What objective parameters would you use to determine progression of his disease?**

A. 6 MWT, DLCO, FVC, HRCT
B. Serial high-resolution CT scan of his chest
C. DLCO
D. FEV/FVC, FEV_1
E. Serial CXR

Question 4: **His daughter is concerned that she might have inherited his pulmonary disease. What genetic abnormalities are responsible for familial interstitial pneumonia?**

A. TERT
B. TERC

C. MUC5B

D. Surfactant protein A1

E. All of the above

Question 5: After 2 months, the patient is sent to the emergency department for worsening shortness of breath, fevers, and chills for a week. He was desaturating to 80% on room air and requires nonrebreather. His WBC is found to be elevated and CXR shows new bilateral opacities. What would be the appropriate management?

A. Solumedrol 1 g IV daily for 3 days

B. Panculture and obtain BNP

C. Mechanical ventilation

D. Anticoagulation

E. Bronchoscopy

CASE 2

A 70-year-old woman with history of dermatomyositis complains of shortness of breath. She was never a smoker and has worked as a secretary in the past. Her husband is a construction worker and they have parakeets at home. She has a family history of rheumatoid arthritis, diabetes mellitus, and hypertension.

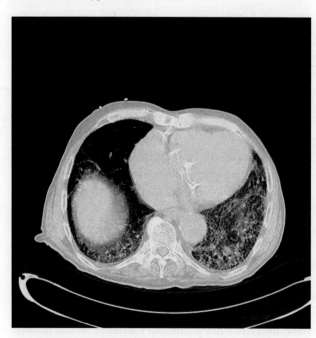

Question 1: Based on her HRCT above, what is your likely diagnosis?

A. Usual interstitial pneumonia

B. Cellular nonspecific interstitial pneumonia

C. Fibrotic nonspecific interstitial pneumonia

D. Chronic hypersensitivity pneumonitis

E. Idiopathic pleuroparenchymal fibroelastosis

Question 2: Patient had a surgical lung biopsy which showed temporal homogeneity of interstitial fibrosis with no fibrotic foci, eosinophils, or granulomas. Her pulmonary function test showed moderate restriction with mild gas transfer. During the 6-minute walk test, she had to stop after the third minute for shortness of breath. There was no desaturation during the test. Which medication would you prescribe?

A. Prednisone 1 mg/kg PO daily

B. Cellcept 1,000 mg PO BID

C. Imuran 100 mg PO daily

D. Methotrexate 5 to 15 mg PO daily

E. Cyclophosphamide 100 mg/kg PO daily

CASE 3

A 55-year-old man, 30 pack-years and current smoker has complained of worsening dyspnea on exertion and nonproductive cough for the past 6 months. He is not hypoxic on room air, bilateral crackles on auscultation, and no JVD or lower extremity edema. HRCT scan shows bilateral patchy ground glass opacities and centrilobular ill-defined nodules. PFT shows restriction with mild gas transfer defect.

Question 1: Surgical lung biopsy shows brownish pigmented macrophages in the respiratory bronchioles. What is the diagnosis?

A. Respiratory bronchiolitis

B. Respiratory bronchiolitis interstitial lung disease

C. Chronic hypersensitivity pneumonitis

D. Panbronchiolitis

E. Idiopathic pulmonary neuroendocrine hyperplasia

Question 2: What is the likely clinical course of this disease?

A. Complete resolution of symptoms with smoking cessation

B. Symptoms may persist despite smoking cessation.

C. Early corticosteroid therapy is warranted even prior to smoking cessation.

D. Symptoms may worsen despite smoking cessation and steroid therapy.

E. None of the above

CASE 4

A 30-year-old-man has been complaining of fever, shortness of breath, cough, and pleuritic chest pain for 2 weeks. He has recently traveled to South America and claims to have started smoking cigarettes. He denies any recreational drug use. He is noted to have an oxygen saturation of 80% on room air. On nonrebreather his oxygenation improves to 89%. He appears more tachypneic and is subsequently intubated. The patient is started on piperacillin-tazobactam and vancomycin.

Laboratory results:

WBC 10K
Neutrophils 80%
Eosinophils 3%

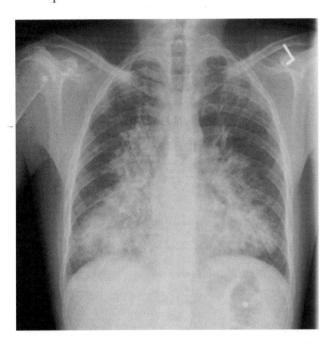

Question 1: **BNP 100 and echocardiogram show normal LVEF RVSP 25. ECG shows right bundle branch block. Cell count from bronchial alveolar lavage shows eosinophils 40%. Serum galactomannan is positive.**

What is your diagnosis?

A. Acute interstitial pneumonia
B. Acute eosinophilic pneumonia
C. Desquamative interstitial pneumonia
D. Airway enlargement with fibrosis
E. Lipoid pneumonia

Question 2: **The patient is given solumedrol 125 mg IV every 6 hours and improves.**

What would you advise the patient?

A. Stop smoking
B. Relapse is possible and should be given year long course of oral corticosteroids
C. He should be ruled out for asthma since this is a risk factor for AEP
D. Serial CT is warranted to determine progression of underlying ILD
E. None of the above

CASE 5

A 50-year-old man, current smoker and HIV with CD4 500, has been complaining of shortness of breath and nonproductive cough for 5 months. He is previously treated with antibiotics but his symptoms have failed to improve. In the emergency department, he is noted to be hypoxic on room air and crackles on auscultation of his lungs.

* *

His WBC 16,000; Hgb 14; Plt 300; LDH 500.
He had a chest CT which is shown below:

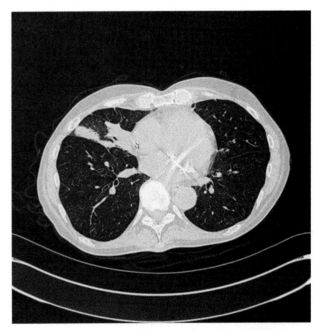

Question 1: **The cell count from the bronchial alveolar lavage reveals eosinophils 5%, lymphocytes 15%, neutrophils 15%. The transbronchial biopsy shows inflammatory intraluminal plugs consisting of granulation**

tissue with fibroblasts and myofibroblasts in connective matrix, in small airway, ducts and alveoli with mild interstitial inflammation. There is preservation of architecture and uniform appearance. What is your presumptive diagnosis?

A. Chronic eosinophilic pneumonia
B. Cryptogenic organizing pneumonia
C. Desquamative interstitial pneumonia
D. Acute fibrinous and organizing pneumonia
E. Acute eosinophilic pneumonia

Question 2: The patient has been discharged on prednisone 20 mg PO daily for 4 weeks. However, he returns, complaining of fatigue and shortness of breath. He is noted to have oxygen saturation of 95% on room air and afebrile. Repeat radiographs show new central sparing infiltrates on the left lung. Cultures are obtained which are negative. What would be the next appropriate step?

A. Prednisone 20 mg PO daily
B. Solumedrol 1 g IV daily for 3 days
C. Piperacillin–Tazobactam 3.375 mg IV every 6 hours with vancomycin 1 g IV every 12 hours
D. Cellcept 1,000 mg PO every 12 hours
E. Amphotericin B

CASE 6

A 62-year-old woman comes into the emergency department from her PCP complaining of shortness of breath and cough. She has a past medical history of multi-site, low-grade monoclonal B-cell lymphoma and has been on multiple chemotherapies. She has suffered multiple chemo-related complications such as an allergic reaction to rituxan and thrombocytopenia from CVP. She is found to have an oxygen saturation of 83% on room air which improved with oxygen supplementation via nasal cannula. She has a temperature of 38.8°C and she is hemodynamically stable. She has a known allergy to sulfa.

BNP 25
WBC 0.4 (3.9–10.7 10^3/μL)
Hemoglobin 8.9 (12.0–14.7 g/dL)
Hematocrit 27.5 (37.1–45.4%)
Final Platelets 150 (126–373 10^3/μL)
PCP–DFA negative
Sputum culture AFB +

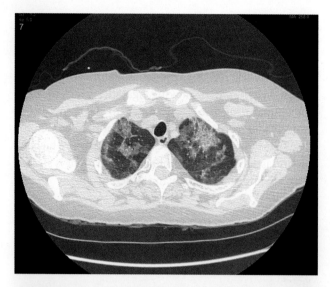

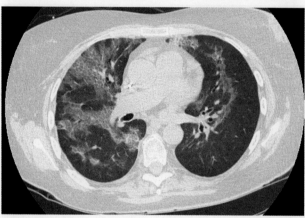

* *

Neupogen is subsequently started. Her leukocytes continue to improve but her oxygenation requirements increase. There is no worsening infiltrates on subsequent radiographs. She has defervesce and is discharged on the treatment above. However, she continues to have dyspnea on exertion and requires oxygen supplementation. Bronchoscopy reveals milky lavage with lymphocytosis.

Question 1: What is your diagnosis?

A. Lymphoproliferative disorders
B. Pulmonary alveolar proteinosis
C. Immune reconstitution syndrome
D. Chronic hypersensitivity pneumonitis
E. Malignancy-associated sarcoidosis

Question 2: What would be the appropriate treatment?

A. Rituximab
B. High-volume bronchial lavage

C. GM-CSF supplementation

D. Plasmapheresis

E. Steroids

CASE 7

A 40-year-old African-American woman with progressive shortness of breath is noted to have an abnormal chest radiograph which prompted the chest computed tomography below. She denies any recent travel or sick contacts. She works in an office and her husband is a social worker. Family history is unremarkable.

* *

The biopsy of the lesion below shows noncaseating granulomas. Cultures were negative.

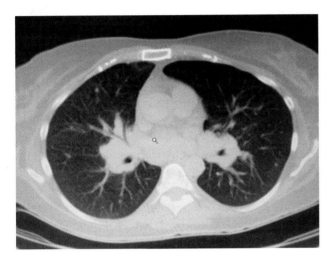

Question 1: **What is the likely mechanism of the diagnosis?**

A. An overexaggerated immune response

B. T1 helper cell response leads to production of IFN-gamma and IL-2

C. Increased clonal proliferation of the lymphatics

D. Proliferation of neuroendocrine cells

E. Two hit mechanism involving a genetic or prior environmental exposure prompting the progression to the disease with antigen exposure

Question 2: **What is the genetic basis of this disease?**

A. HLA-DRB1*03

B. BTNL2

C. 5p

D. 5q

E. All of the above

Question 3: **Her chest radiograph shows bilateral hilar adenopathy with scattered pulmonary nodules. Based on this, which of the following is true?**

A. The severity of the radiographic finding correlates with the pulmonary function test.

B. The severity of the radiographic finding correlates with degree of dyspnea.

C. It has been implied that severity of radiographic findings has prognostic significance although interpretation has high inter-observer variability.

D. It has been used to measure response with treatment.

E. Severity of radiographic findings has prognostic significance.

Question 4: **She claims her exercise tolerance has decreased from walking 15 city blocks to 5 city blocks. She cannot walk two flights of stairs. What treatment do you recommend?**

A. Prednisone 40 mg PO daily for 3 months

B. Motrin 400 mg PO daily

C. Solumedrol 1 g IV daily × 3 days

D. Cellcept 1,000 mg PO twice a day for 2 months

E. Methotrexate 5 mg weekly

Question 5: **Another patient is found to have hilar adenopathy, rash on anterior surface of legs, fever, and arthritis. How would you diagnose this patient?**

A. Biopsy of rash

B. Kveim test

C. Bronchoscopy with bronchoalveolar lavage

D. Biopsy of hilar adenopathy

E. None of the above

CASE 8

A 59-year-old housewife is referred to you from her primary physician for an abnormal chest CT. She has a dry cough, malaise, weight loss, and progressive dyspnea on exertion for the past year. Her cough has worsened after cleaning her house with chlorine and when washing her husband's clothes. She is a nonsmoker but her husband is a smoker. She denied any recent travels and claims she doesn't own any pets. Her current husband works in an animal store specializing in birds. Physical examination is remarkable for oxygen saturation of 85% on room air and crackles on auscultation of her lungs. Pulmonary function test shows no obstruction or bronchodilator response. There is restriction with moderate gas transfer defect.

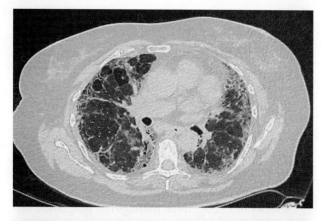

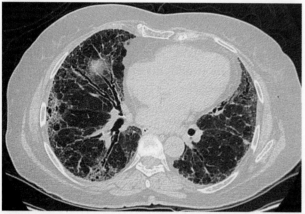

Question 1: **A bronchoscopy was performed and the BAL showed lymphocytosis with a low CD4/CD8 ratio. The transbronchial biopsy was not diagnostic. Therefore, she had a surgical lung biopsy which revealed architectural distortion, interstitial bronchiolocentric pneumonitis with lymphocytes, plasma**

cells and occasional eosinophils and neutrophils. With cathepsin K, poorly formed granulomas were seen. Which of the following best describes the diagnosis?

A. Exaggerated immune response to a repeated exposure to an inhaled antigen involving Th1 and Th17 T cells

B. Exaggerated immune response to repeated exposures to an inhaled antigen involving immune complexes

C. T cell–mediated disease with major histocompatibility complex mismatch and enhanced stimulation of toll-like receptors

D. Nonimmunologic response to repeated exposure to low-dose inhaled irritant

E. Nonimmunologic response to single large dose exposure to inhaled irritant

CASE 9

A 30-year-old woman with a history of asthma had been on high dose of inhaled corticosteroids and long-acting beta-agonist. Because she ran out of these medications, she decided to use montelukast when she went on a trip to South America for 1 month. When she returned home, she complained of progressive abdominal pain radiating to her back for the past 3 weeks and tingling sensation in the soles of her feet. Physical examination is significant for crackles and wheezes on the right upper and left lung field. Significant laboratory findings include WBC 17 with 90% eosinophils, IgE 750, ANCA negative, RF negative, ANA negative DS DNA. Helminth serologies, and stool ova and parasites are negative. Sequential chest radiographs, 2 days apart, are shown below:

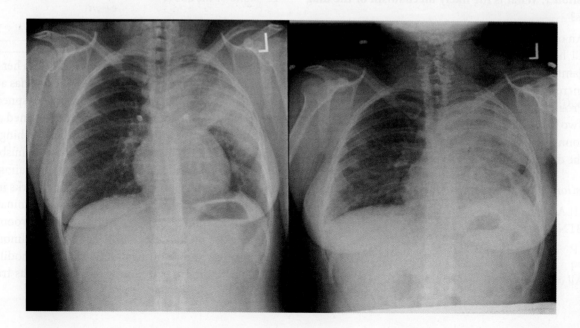

* *

Cell count from bronchoalveolar lavage showed 90% eosinophils and transbronchial biopsy is below:

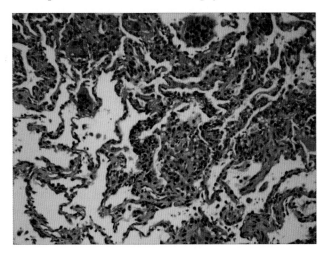

Question 1: What is the diagnosis?

A. Eosinophilic granulomatosis with polyangiitis
B. Chronic eosinophilic pneumonia
C. Loeffler's syndrome
D. Acute eosinophilic pneumonia
E. None of the above

Question 2: What is the most common cause of mortality in this disease?

A. Myocardial infarction
B. Acute renal failure
C. Status asthmaticus
D. Cerebral hemorrhage
E. Gastrointestinal bleeding

CASE 10

A 58-year-old man with hyperthyroid on PTU from a recent trip to South America is complaining of fevers, chills, and shortness of breath. He denies any sick contacts and is a nonsmoker. On physical examination he is noted to have an oxygen saturation of 95% on room air. He appears to have a saddle nose with epistaxis, diffuse rales on auscultation, and further inquiry reveals he has hematuria.

WBC 13.1 K/uL
Hemoglobin 10.1 g/dL
Hematocrit 37.7%
Platelet 194 K/uL
Sodium 138 mmol/L
Potassium 4.3 mmol/L
Chloride 102 mmol/L
CO_2 31 mmol/L

Urea nitrogen 31 mg/dL
Creatinine 4 mg/dL
INR 1

* *

Computed tomography of the chest shows bilateral cavitary nodules with areas of ground glass and intralobular septal thickening. A bronchoscopy is perfomed with sequential bronchoalveolar lavage. Three aliquots of 60 mL of sterile saline show progressive, nonresolving hemorrhage. Echocardiogram is unremarkable.

IgG and IgM anticardiolipid antibodies (anti–B2-glycoprotein I) negative
Lupus anticoagulant negative
Antistreptolysin O antibodies negative
Hyaluronidase negative
ANA negative
Anti-glomerular basement antibodies negative
PR3-ANCA positive
MPO-ANCA negative
Urine drug screen negative
Nasal swab positive for MRSA
Blood cultures negative

Question 1: What is the next step to confirm the diagnosis?

A. No additional testing is warranted
B. Transbronchial biopsy
C. Renal biopsy
D. Nasal biopsy
E. Serial ANCA

Question 2: What is your treatment?

A. Plasmapheresis + IV cyclophosphamide + IV corticosteroids
B. IV cyclophosphamide + IV corticosteroids
C. Oral cyclophosphamide + oral corticosteroids
D. Methotrexate
E. Azathioprine

Question 3: The patient's symptoms have improved and slowly transitioned to remission medications. He is started on trimethoprim–sulfamethoxazole. What purpose does that serve?

A. PCP prophylaxis
B. PCP prophylaxis and to eradicate Staphylococcus aureus colonization
C. Treat concomitant pneumonia
D. PCP prophylaxis and improve renal function
E. None of the above

CASE 11

A 28-year-old man who worked at a textiles factory in Rhode Island had been complaining of shortness of breath and dry cough for the last 2 months. He had a chest radiograph which was unremarkable. He was prescribed albuterol by his primary physician. Spirometry was normal. He had started working at the textiles factory 3 months prior, and he claimed his symptoms would subside a couple of hours after leaving work. He was a nonsmoker and his brother had history of asthma. Referral to a pulmonologist was followed by high-resolution computed tomography which showed subtle dependent ground glass opacities and a reduced DLCO. He subsequently had a bronchoscopy which revealed 15% neutrophils and 20% lymphocytes. Rheumatologic workup was negative. Transbronchial biopsy showed lymphocytic inflammation.

Question 1: **What is the main treatment of this disease?**

A. Avoidance of antigen
B. Avoidance of antigen and early initiation of steroids, prednisone 40 mg PO daily for 4–6 weeks and re-evaluate with a pulmonary function test
C. Avoidance of antigen and long-acting albuterol and inhaled steroid
D. Early referral for lung transplantation
E. None of the above

CASE 12

A 72-year-old Korean woman with hypertension, Hepatitis C, hepatocellular carcinoma, and orthotropic liver transplant 3 months prior, complained of 3 days of abdominal pain with nonbloody, nonbilous vomiting.

* *

An endoscopy showed gastritis. Because of shortness of breath, pulmonary consult was called. The patient migrated from Korea to the United States in 1981. She denied any sick contacts. She had no pets, no travel history, and lived with her family.

* *

Home medications included prednisone 10 mg daily, tacrolimus 3 mg BID, and mycophenolate 1,000 mg BID. On consultation, patient's vital signs were normal except her oxygen saturation was 85% on room air. She had bilateral crackles and decreased breath sounds on the right. She had nonblanching maculopapular rash on her abdomen and lower extremities. Admission laboratory values showed WBC count 1,500/uL, eosinophil 6.2%, neutrophil

57%, BNP 183, creatinine 0.6 mg/dL, albumin 2.6 g/dL, total bilirubin 0.7 mg/dL, ALT 20 U/L, AST 25 U/L, and INR 1. Serum viral studies, including CMV and HIV, were negative. Chest radiograph showed bilateral patchy opacities and right-sided pleural effusion as seen below. Pleural fluid was transudative and glucose 131 mg/dL. Pleural cytology and culture, serum galactomannan, and echocardiography were unremarkable. Broad spectrum antibiotics and diuretics offered no improvement. She was intubated for bronchoscopy.

* *

Coagulated blood was seen in all airways. Serial alloquots of BAL had bloody return that did not clear. Transbronchial biopsy showed nonspecific chronic inflammation with reactive pneumocyte hyperplasia. Cultures from bronchoalveolar lavage were positive for enterococcus and klebsiella. RUL clot was removed and sent for pathologic examination which is seen below.

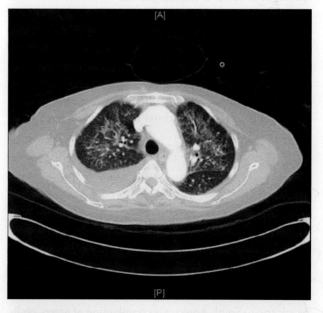

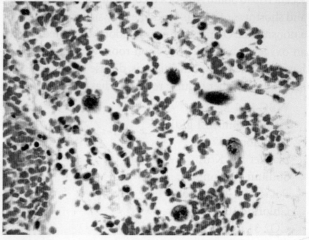

***Question 1:* What is the primary treatment for this disease?**

A. Corticosteroids 1 g IV × 3 days

B. Corticosteroids 1 g IV × 3 days followed by rituximab

C. Plasmapheresis

D. Amphotericin B

E. Ivermectin and abendazole

CASE 13

A 50-year-old man who recently migrated from Turkey is complaining of progressive shortness of breath and dry cough. He claims he is a nonsmoker and has been an office worker in his native country. He denies any sick contacts, pets, or significant family history. On physical examination he is noted to have scattered crackles. Laboratory studies are unremarkable. Chest radiograph shows bilateral sand-like densities concentrated in the lower two-thirds obliterating the diaphragm, mediastinum, and cardiac borders. The mediastinal windows of a high-resolution computed tomography show polyglonal densities along the bronchovascular bundles, subpleural regions, and perilobular densities. The patient has a surgical lung biopsy which shows intra-alveolar calcospherites. There are no granulomas or bone formation. Cultures are negative.

***Question 1:* What is your diagnosis?**

A. Tuberculosis

B. Sarcoidosis

C. Pulmonary alveolar microlithiasis

D. Idiopathic pulmonary ossification

E. Sequelae of varicella pneumonia

***Question 2:* What is the least invasive approach in confirming the diagnosis?**

A. Induced sputum

B. Bronchoalveolar lavage

C. Transbronchial biopsy

D. Chest radiography

E. High-resolution computed tomography

***Question 3:* What is your treatment?**

A. Corticosteroids

B. Chelating agents

C. Repeated bronchoalveolar lavage

D. Bisphosphonates

E. Lung transplantation

CASE 14

A 40-year-old woman is complaining of shortness of breath, dry cough, and fever 39.4°C for the last 2 weeks. She is a social smoker and has recently starting using the hot tub daily. She used her hot tub last year without any symptoms. Her husband and friends would join her in the hot tub, and they claim to have no symptoms. She also owns some birds and works as a chemist.

* *

Physical examination is unremarkable except for some fine crackles in both lung fields. Chest radiograph is normal and high-resolution computerized tomography shows patchy ground glass opacities with ill-defined nodules. Pulmonary function tests show mild restriction with mild gas transfer defect.

***Question 1:* Based on the current information, what is your diagnosis?**

A. Organic dust syndrome

B. Acute hypersensitivity pneumonitis

C. Community-acquired pneumonia

D. Vanishing lung syndrome

E. Shrinking lung syndrome

CASE 15

A 60-year-old man, who has recently migrated from China, has been complaining of shortness of breath and cough for the last 6 months. He can barely walk two blocks. He has a distant history of tuberculosis. He is a former smoker and quit 30 years ago and socially drinks. He has worked in an office in the past and denies any fever, chills, or sick contacts. His oxygen saturation is 95% at rest but he quickly is noted to desaturate to 85% after walking a few steps.

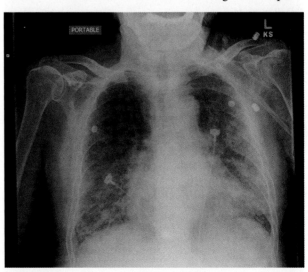

Question 1: **He had connective tissue serologies:**

Anti–ThRNP negative
Anti–PM-SCL negative
Topoisomerase I negative
Fibrillin negative
RNP negative
RF positive
ACCP positive
ANA positive
Anti-SSA negative
CK negative
Aldolase negative
Anti–Jo-1 negative
SSA/Ro negative
SSA/La negative

What is your diagnosis?

A. Scleroderma
B. Rheumatoid arthritis
C. Sjögren's syndrome
D. SLE
E. Dermatomyositis

Question 2: **After further inquiry, he complains of symmetrical joint pain that is worse when he wakes up. He is started on prednisone and later switches to methotrexate. His symptoms persist and he is started on leflunomide 1 month ago. He also claims he has been taking naproxen intermittently for his joint pain. Six months later, he returns to your clinic and a pulmonary function test shows a decreased in DLCO and VC by 15%. His oxygen saturation is 90% on room air. HRCT shows the following:**

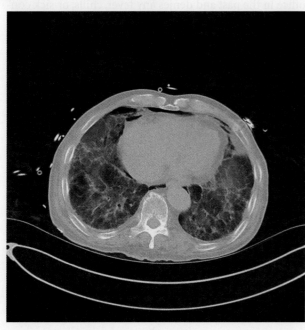

What will aide in your diagnosis?

A. Echocardiogram
B. Bronchoscopy
C. Serial CTD serologies
D. Chest tube
E. Blood cultures

Question 3: **Echocardiogram shows preserved EF with RVSP 15. Blood cultures are negative. Serial CTD serologies have lower values compared to prior. Transbronchial biopsy shows fibrosis with lymphocytes. Bronchioalveolar lavage shows eosinophils 1% and lymphocytes 15%. What is the etiology of his decompensation?**

A. Drug-induced pneumonitis
B. Naproxen
C. Infection
D. RA-ILD exacerbation
E. None of the above

CASE 16

A 55-year-old man who recently quit smoking after 20 years is noted to have progressive shortness of breath on exertion. He is given albuterol by his primary care physician and is referred to you after no resolution of his symptoms. He claims he had discoloration of his hand upon exposure to cold weather and has noted difficulty swallowing.

* *

Chest computed tomography is done, which prompts connective tissue disease workup below.

Anti–ThRNP negative
Anti–PM-SCL negative
Topoisomerase I positive
Fibrillin negative
RNP negative
RF negative
ACCP negative
ANA positive
Anti-SSA negative
CK negative
Anticentromere negative
Aldolase negative
Anti–Jo-1 negative
SSA/Ro negative
SSA/La negative
Anti-endothelial positive

Question 1: **Which of the antibodies is associated with formation of interstitial lung disease?**

A. Topoisomerase I and anti-endothelial
B. Fibrillin and RNP
C. Anticentromere
D. RF and ACCP
E. SSA/Ro and SSA/La

Question 2: **What is the treatment?**

A. Prednisone
B. Cyclophosphamide
C. Mycophenolate mofetil
D. Stem cell transplantation
E. Solumedrol 1 g IV × 3 days

CASE 17

A 50-year-old man, RSV negative, CMV negative, with history of acute leukemia is a recipient of allogeneic hematopoietic stem cell transplantation from RSV negative CMV positive donor. Forty-five days after transplantation, he develops fever 38.8°C, shortness of breath on minimal exertion, diaphoresis, and dry cough. High-resolution computed tomography of his chest shows thickening of interlobular and intralobular septa with superimposed ground glass opacities. Cultures from his urine, blood and sputum are negative. Bronchoscopy with bronchoalveolar lavage and transbronchial biopsy is unremarkable for microorganisms. BNP is 100 and serum galactomannan is negative. Continued evaluation shows that patient is comfortable on 50% venturi mask with a respiratory rate of 22 although he quickly desaturates to 80% on room air. He denies any chest pain.

Question 1: **What is the diagnosis?**

A. CMV pneumonitis
B. Pulmonary veno-occlusive disease
C. Idiopathic pneumonia syndrome
D. Pulmonary cytologic thrombi
E. None of the above

Question 2: **What is the appropriate treatment for this patient?**

A. Mechanical ventilation
B. Solumedrol >4 mg/kg/day
C. Solumedrol 2 mg/kg/day
D. Adding antifungal to antibiotics
E. Lasix 40 mg IV daily

CASE 18

A 60-year-old Caucasian man, former smoker 1 PPD for 30 years went for a routine physical. He complained of decreased exercise tolerance. He complained of some subjective fevers and chills and on physical examination noted wheeze on the lower lobes. His chest radiograph showed multiple nodules on the lower lobes. He subsequently went for surgical lung biopsy which showed some bone tissue with marrow elements in a branching pattern located within the alveolar spaces.

Question 1: **This disease is associated with all of the following EXCEPT:**

A. Idiopathic pulmonary fibrosis
B. Asthma
C. Busulfan
D. Pyloric stenosis
E. Mitral valve disease

Answers

CASE 1

Question 1: E. None of the above

According to ATS guidelines, high-resolution chest computed tomography (HRCT) is diagnostic for usual interstitial pneumonia (UIP) histology, with positive and negative predictive value of 90% and 100%, respectively if all four of the UIP characteristics are present.[1,2] If less than four of the features are present, a surgical lung biopsy is necessary for histologic diagnosis. Except in certain diffuse parenchymal lung diseases such as sarcoidosis, hypersensitivity pneumonitis, and Langerhan's histiocytosis, transbronchial biopsies are often inadequate for histologic diagnosis.

* *

The presence of honeycombing is suggestive but not pathognomonic for UIP. Honeycombing associated with UIP are generally macrocystic (>4 mm) and appear in a stacking pattern. Microcysts (<4 mm) can be seen in NSIP, chronic HP with NSIP features, and DIP. Paracicatricial emphysema are emphysematous changes associated with scarring from pulmonary infarction, granulomatous disease such as tuberculous or silicosis, or prior infections. They can be confused as honeycombing.

* *

UIP is a histologic pattern associated with connective tissue diseases such as rheumatoid arthritis and scleroderma, drug-induced lung diseases such as methotrexate, occupational lung diseases such as silicosis, or the end spectrum of other interstitial lung diseases such as chronic hypersensitivity pneumonitis. Therefore, review of the patient's medications, occupational history or environmental exposure, connective tissue disease serologies, hypersensitivity panel, and bronchoscopy for alveolar lavage may be necessary. Investigation of an underlying disease is warranted before classifying UIP as idiopathic pulmonary fibrosis (IPF) because pulmonary manifestations may precede rheumatologic manifestations and identifying risk exposure history or treatment of underlying disease may delay progression of the pulmonary disease.

* *

Connective tissue disease (CTD) or rheumatologic disease serologies are listed below. Caveats to CTD testing include: (1) elevated levels of ANA and RF are seen in IPF; and (2) pulmonary disease may manifest before rheumatologic manifestations and therefore repeat serologies and clinical evaluation is warranted to monitor for development of the CTD.[3]

* *

Even though the evidence is weak, bronchial alveolar lavage (BAL) can be used to provide adjunct evidence of an underlying lung disease such as chronic hypersensitivity pneumonitis or sarcoidosis. To perform an adequate sample of BAL, at least 100 mL of normal saline should be instilled with >30% return to obtain a good sample study. At least 5 mL is required for cell count with differential. If there is <5% return from the BAL, the procedure should be aborted at the risk of further tissue

UIP Pattern (All Four)	Possible Features	Inconsistent Features
Subpleural basal predominance	Subpleural base predominance	Upper or middle
Reticular	Reticular	Peribronchovascular
Honeycombing	Absence of inconsistent features	Extensive ground glass (greater than reticular)
Absence of inconsistent features		Profuse micronodular
		Discrete cysts away from honeycombing
		Diffuse mosaicism and air trapping (≥3 lobes)
		Consolidation

Rheumatologic Disease	Manifestations	Serologies
Systemic Sclerosis (SSc)—heterogeneous disorder of excessive collagen deposition	Both groups have esophageal reflux with esophageal dilatation in up to 80% of patients in the absence of symptoms plus: Below the elbows and knees (distal extremities) and above clavicles Proximal extremities and torso	Anticentromere antibodies Anti-ThRNP Anti–PM-SCL Topoisomerase I antibodies (Scl-70) Fibrillin and ribonucleoprotein (RNP) antibodies anti-RNP polymerase I and III (high frequency of renal cell crisis)
Limited SSc—more commonly associated with pulmonary HTN from fibrosis and hypoxia-induced vascular remodeling		
Diffuse Ssc—more commonly associated with ILD although Scleroderma Lung Study showed similar frequency of ILD in both limited and diffuse SSc		
Rheumatoid arthritis is a chronic inflammation of the small joints		Rheumatoid factor, anticyclic citrullinated peptide
Dermatomyositis and polymyositis involving inflammation of skeletal muscle and lung. It is more common with black women. CD8+ cells are mediators in polymyositis and CD4+ in dermatomyositis and ILD Variants: Amyopathic dermatomyositis—no muscle involvement Antisynthetase antibody syndrome	Violaceous erythematous rash over interphalangeal joints, knuckles, elbows or knees (gottron sign), eyelids (heliotrope rash) or nape of neck and upper chest or back Myositis, ILD, fever, Raynaud phenomenon or erythema, hyperkeratosis, and mechanic's hands	ANA, anti-Ro antibody (anti-SSA), creatine kinase, aldolase Anti–CADM-140 (MDA-5) antibodies Antiaminoacyl tRNA synthetase antibodies such as Jo-1 If ANA and anti–Jo-1 negative, anti–PL-12
Sjögren's syndrome is an autoimmune disease involving lymphocytic infiltration of exocrine glands.		SSA/Ro and SSA/La
Mixed connective tissue disease		Normal anti-RNP antibody excludes this disease

rupture and release of inflammatory mediators due to overdistention. It has been suggested that BAL should be performed within 6 weeks of HRCT. With nutrient poor media (saline), the analysis should be performed within 1 hour or stored at 4°C.

* *

Other abnormalities include: nonresolving or increasing heme with serial aliquots suggestive of diffuse alveolar hemorrhage, milky fluid with positive periodic acid, Schiff staining that settles with gravity within 15 to 20 minutes that is suggestive of pulmonary alveolar proteinosis, and lymphocyte proliferative response to beryllium antigen suggestive of chronic beryllium disease.[4] CD4/CD8 ratio >4 is suggestive of sarcoidosis.[4] CD4/CD8 ratio

<1 suggests acute HP, with a predominance of CD8+. A predominance of CD4+ might suggest chronic HP.

Question 2: C. Lung transplantation

There are few medications available to delay the progression of IPF. Acetylcysteine is a precursor to glutathione which can be depleted in IPF. Two large studies have suggested that acetylcysteine at 600 mg PO twice a day in adjunct to azathioprine and prednisone, was shown to have decreased rate of decline of vital capacity and DLCO in 12 months.[5,6] However, a recent randomized study did not show any benefit when acetylcysteine is administered as monotherapy.[7] A recent phase three trial of an oral antifibriotic, pirfenidone (2,403 mg PO daily) administered randomly to patients

CELL COUNT IN BRONCHOALVEOLAR LAVAGE

Alveolar macrophages	Normal (nonsmokers) >85%	Predominance of macrophages with smoking related inclusion bodies suggestive of RB, RBILD, DIP or pulmonary Langerhan's cell histiocytosis Predominance of hemosiderin-laden macrophages is suggested of hemosiderosis or alveolar hemorrhage.
Lymphocytes	10–15%	>15% sarcoidosis, NSIP, drug-induced pneumonitis, radiation pneumonitis, COP, lymphoproliferative disorder >25% granulomatous disease (sarcoidosis, HP, berryllium disease), cellular NSIP, drug reaction, LP, COP, lymphoma >50% cellular NSIP or HP
Neutrophils	≤3%	>3% collagen-vascular disease, IPF, aspiration pneumonia, infection, bacterial, fungal, asbestosis, ARDS, DAD, bronchitis >50% acute lung injury, aspiration pneumonia, suppurative infection
Eosinophils	≤1%	>1% drug-induced pneumonitis, BMT, asthma, bronchitis, ABPA, helminitic, PCP, bacterial, fungal, Hodgkin's >25% eosinophilic lung disease
Squamous epithelial/ ciliated columnar epithelial cells	≤5%	>5% epithelial cells suggest suboptimal study Presence of squamous cells suggest upper airway secretion contamination
Langerhan's cells	≤4%	>5% Langerhan's histiocytosis

or placebo for 52 weeks showed a relative reduction by 47.9% of patients with >10% in the percentage of predicted FVC; relative increase by 132.5% of patients with no decline in FVC (P <0.001); decreased decline in 6-minute walk test (P = 0.04) and increased progression-free survival (P <0.001).[8] In pooled analysis, the between group difference of pirfenidone was significant for death from any other causes (P = 0.01) and from idiopathic pulmonary fibrosis (P = 0.006).[8] Nintedanib 150 mg PO BID, an intracellular inhibitor of tyrosine kinases such as VEGF, FGF, and PDGF, was studied in a randomized double blinded placebo-controlled parallel group trial and was shown to have decreased annual decline in FVC compared to placebo (−114.7 mL vs. −239.9 mL 95% CI 77.7–172.8 INPULSIS-1 and −113.6 mL vs. −207.3 mL 95% CI 44.8–142.7 P <0.001 in INPULSIS-2).[9]

* *

The decision between pirfenidone or nintedanib can be dependent on adverse effects. Pirfenidone was found to have increased risk of headaches, rash, nausea, vomiting, dyspepsia, and diarrhea. Nintedanib has a higher risk for diarrhea.

* *

Other discharge planning considerations for this patient include referral to pulmonary rehabilitation to alleviate symptoms, increase exercise tolerance and functional ability and pantoprazole since the high association of GERD with interstitial lung diseases. Nocturnal hypoxemia is common and associated with fatigue and impaired daytime functioning and best predictor is daytime oxygen saturation. Currently this patient is not hypoxic.

* *

Indications for lung transplantation referral for IPF symptomatic patients <65 years of age with a DLCO <39% predicted and/or evidence of FVC decline of >10% over 6 months. Lung transplantation has been the treatment of choice for advance IPF; with 50% to 60% survival. Without it, mean survival for patients is 2.5 to 3.5 years. Prednisone has not been shown to be of benefit in IPF without exacerbations and amiodarone causes lung toxicity at a dose of 400 mg PO daily for at least 2 months or 200 mg PO daily for 2 years.

Question 3: A. 6 MWT, DLCO, FVC, HRCT

The clinical course of idiopathic pulmonary fibrosis can follow three patterns: (1) stable for years, (2) slow progression, or (3) rapid progression.[1] Sequential physiologic studies every 3 to 4 months to monitor FVC and DLCO. Improvement is defined as >10% increase in FVC or TLC, >15% increase in DLCO or >4% mm increase in PaO_2 during exercise.[10] HRCT may be used to monitor radiographic progression of disease and also to monitor for the development of exacerbations and/or occurrence of infections or malignancy.

Question 4: E. All of the above

Familial interstitial pneumonitis (FIP) is defined as two or more probable or definite interstitial lung disease in individuals related within at least three degrees. Radiographic and histologic presentations usually have a UIP, NSIP, or organizing pneumonia pattern. Evidence for genetic susceptibility includes (1) familial clusters of pulmonary fibrosis in monozygotic twins raised in different environments, consecutive generations in the same family, and in families separated at an early age; (2) pulmonary fibrosis in genetic disorders such as IgG4 sclerosing disease, hermansky-pudlak syndrome, neurofibromatosis, tuberous sclerosis, niemann-pick disease, gaucher disease, famlial hypocalciuric hypercalcemia, and familial surfactant protein C mutation; (3) variability in workers exposed to fibrogenic antigens; and (4) variability of susceptibility to fibrogenic agents in inbred mice.[11] Gene mutations associated with this disease include telomerase gene mutation, which consists of TERT, TERC, DKC, TIN2, MUC5B, surfactant proteins A1 (SP2-A2) and C (SFTPC).[12,13]

* *

Telomerase is a polymerase, with hTERT, catalytic telomerase reverse transcriptase, and RNA component, hTR, that adds telomere sequence, TTAGG, to the ends of chromosomes to counter shortening during DNA replication. Eventually telomeres shorten and lead to DNA damage response and apoptosis. Mutations in either hTERT or hTR have been implicated in familial IPF.[14]

* *

hTERT is commonly found in germ cells, cells with high turnover such as the bronchial epithelium, and cancer cells and loss of function mutations are found in 18% of kindreds with familial pulmonary fibrosis and 3% sporadic. In one prospective study, it has been found that extrapulmonary manifestations (hepatic and hematologic) are found in carriers who are <40 years of age. They are found to have low RBC and platelets, and high MCV and MCHC and early graying of hair. However, it is difficult to discern the sole impact of this mutation on the development of IPF since 90% were smokers.

* *

One theory emphasized peripheral distribution of pulmonary fibrosis as a consequence of mechanical stress and premature aging as highlighted by decreased levels of dehydroeiandrosterone (DHEA) and sulfated form DHEA. These are believed to decrease fibroblast proliferation and differentiation to myofibroblast, collagen proliferation from TGF- beta1, and fibroblast migration from platelet-derived growth factor. Polymorphism of MUC5B gene leads to increased risk of IPF through interference with normal repair process of the epithelium, direct toxic effect, and as a stimulus for fibroproliferative response. Humoral immunity and innate immunity with activation of toll-like receptor (TLR) 9 and TLR 3 have also been implicated in the pathogenesis.

Question 5: B. Panculture and obtain BNP

Acute exacerbations occur mostly in IPF but can occur in other forms of interstitial lung diseases. It is a diagnosis of exclusion. It is suggested by worsening dyspnea within 30 days, new ground glass opacities or consolidation via HRCT, worsening hypoxemia from baseline ABG, no evidence of infection and exclusion of congestive heart failure exacerbation, pulmonary embolism or other causes of acute lung injury.[15] Pathologically, it would have diffuse alveolar damage superimposed on UIP. Initiation of treatment such as high-dose steroids or anticoagulation without further workup would be incorrect. Mechanical ventilation has been shown to have worse survival in patients with ILD. Patient is requiring high amounts of oxygen and bronchoscopy might not be performed without mechanical ventilation.

CASE 2

Question 1: C. Fibrotic nonspecific interstitial pneumonia

Nonspecific interstitial pneumonia (NSIP) is commonly associated with connective tissue disease, except for rheumatoid arthritis. Other causes include hypersensitivity pneumonitis, drugs, postinfectious and idiopathic. Smoking is not a risk factor. NSIP consists of temporal homogeneity on histology. Radiographically, there is bilateral, lower lobe predominance with ground glass opacities (GGO), traction bronchiectasis, and rarely microcystic honeycombing. Subpleural sparing may be noted. There are three subtypes: Cellular NSIP, mixed, and fibrotic NSIP. Cellular NSIP consists of predominant GGO and histologically there is lymphocytes and plasma cells with chronic interstitial inflammation, uniform but patchy lung involvement, with absent eosinophils, granulomas, and lung injury pattern. Recently the mixed and fibrotic NSIP have been grouped together because of their similar prognostic implications. Fibrotic NSIP consists of predominantly reticulation, traction bronchiectasis and rarely microcystic honeycombing. Histologically, there is temporal homogeneity with collagen deposition, interstitial fibrosis with rare fibroblastic foci, and absent acute lung injury and eosinophils and granulomas. Data for diagnosing NSIP based on radiographic findings is not as robust as UIP and usually surgical lung biopsy is needed for confirmation.

* *

As stated in Case 1, UIP can be diagnosed via HRCT if it has the four typical features. Histologically, there is mild chronic interstitial inflammation, temporal heterogeneity, fibroblastic foci and absent acute lung injury, eosinophils and granulomas.

* *

Idiopathic pleuroparenchymal fibroelastosis (PPFE) consists of upper-lobe fibrosis suggested by traction bronchiectasis with associated architectural distortion and volume loss and/or irregular pleural-based reticular opacities. Histologic studies show elastotic intra-alveolar fibrosis and sometimes UIP.[1] A typical patient

has an age >50 years with recurrent infections or pneumothorax.

* *

Chronic hypersensitivity pneumonitis (CHP) is a parenchymal lung disease from an inhalation exposure, with occasional positive serum precipitations and compatible clinical, radiographic, and physiologic findings. Radiographically, it might be difficult to distinguish CHP from fibrotic NSIP and UIP; although the presence of centrilobular nodules, lobular areas with decreased attenuation and vascularity, and lack of lower lobe predominance might favor its diagnosis. CHP may also have similar histologic patterns as fibrotic NSIP or UIP.[16] Distinction may be possible if there are areas on acute HP or subacute HP, poorly formed granulomas, Schaumann bodies, or peribronchiolar fibrosis.

Question 2: A. Prednisone 1 mg/kg PO daily

Definitive diagnosis in patients with ILD is necessary for therapeutic and prognostic implications. Given that she is not in acute exacerbation, cyclophosphamide and rituximab might not be necessary. Cellcept, imuran, and methotrexate might take weeks to achieve therapeutic benefits.

MEDICATIONS FOR INTERSTITIAL LUNG DISEASE

Medications	Dose		Side Effects
Prednisone	1 mg/kg/day to start then taper (max 60 mg/day)	Avoid or lower dose with scleroderma since might precipitate renal crisis	Osteoporosis Psychosis Gastric ulcers Diabetes
Cyclophosphamide	100 mg/kg/day oral 200 mg max or 750 mg/m^2 body surface area		Pancytopenia
Hematuria			
Azathioprine (Imuran)	1.5 mg/kg/day (maximum daily dose 150 mg/day)	Myelotoxic in TMPT deficiency, therefore check this enzyme prior to use	Pancytopenia Lymphoma
Mycophenolate moteil (cellcept)	1,000–3,000 mg/day in divided doses and usually takes 2 months to reach therapeutic levels		Bleeding, rash, diarrhea, GI upset, deep venous thrombosis
Rituximab	Initial infusion: 50 mg/h IV and increase by 50 mg/h every 30 minutes up to 400 mg/h Subsequent infusion: 100 m/h IV and increase by 100 mg every hour up 400 mg/h		Hypotension, bronchospasm, angioedema
Methotrexate	5–15 mg PO weekly		ILD, pleural effusions, pulmonary nodules

CASE 3

Question 1: **B. Respiratory bronchiolitis interstitial lung disease**

Respiratory bronchiolitis interstitial lung disease (RBILD) is part of the smoking-related interstitial lung diseases which include respiratory bronchiolitis (RB), acute eosinophilic pneumonia, desquamative interstitial lung disease (DIP), airspace enlargement with fibrosis, and Langerhan's cell histiocytosis.[17,18] Respiratory bronchiolitis is a physiologic response to smoking and consists of brown and granular pigmented macrophages within respiratory bronchioles and adjacent alveoli. Radiographs may be normal. HRCT findings typically include ground glass opacities thought to be secondary to macrophage accumulation in alveoli and alveolar ducts, either upper lobe predominant or diffuse, ill-defined 2 to 3 mm centrilobular nodules thought to represent bronchiolectasis with peribronchiolar fibrosis, and areas of hypoattenuation on inspiratory more so on expiratory HRCT. RB may not be clinically relevant, and is difficult to distinguish between RB and RBILD based on histology and HRCT. RBILD is diagnosed via clinical severity, pulmonary function impairment, HRCT and histology. Pulmonary function tests in RBILD would show predominant restrictive with mild–moderate obstructive pattern and mild to moderate decrease in DLCO. Diagnosis can be suggested by bronchoalveolar lavage with macrophages in the absence of lymphocytosis. Surgical lung biopsy is used more to rule out other diagnosis.

Pan Asian

Panbronchiolitis is an obstructive disease and was once restricted to Japan but has now been found in Western countries such as Italy, France, UK, Germany, Norway, and the United States.[19] It is an inflammatory disease of the respiratory bronchioles, coexisting sinusitis, and isolate of *Haemophilus influenzae*, *Streptococcus pneumoniae*, and if advanced *Pseudomonas aurginosa*. Etiology is unknown although certain HLA types such as HLA-A11 and HLA-Bw54, bare lymphocyte syndrome (BLS), and HTLV-1 associated bronchiolitis are suspected.[19] Pathology shows respiratory bronchioles infiltrated by plasma cells, histiocytes, and occasional centrilobular granulation tissue tufts. There is marked mucous production secondary to aberrant expression of MUC5B, goblet cell metaplasia, and expression of EGFR.[19] Patients generally present between the second and the fifth decade with productive cough followed by exertional dyspnea. Sputum volume exceeds 50 mL/day.

HRCT grading system has been proposed: Stage 1, small nodules <5 mm in diameter at the end of bronchovascular branching structures; stage 2 tree in bud; stage 3 cystic dilation of nodules; and stage 4 large cysts connected to dilated proximal bronchi. ESR, RF, CRP, and IgA may be elevated. BAL and serum sialyl stage-specific embryonic antigen and sialyl lewis (a) is increased. Nasal nitric oxide is low. Pulmonary function test may show airflow limitation with occasional restrictive defect. Diagnosis is based on this criteria: (1) persistent cough, sputum, and exertional dyspnea, (2) chronic paranasal sinusitis; (3) radiographic findings; (4) coarse crackles; (5) FEV_1/FVC <70% and PaO_2 <80 mm Hg; and (6) cold haemagluttin >64.[19] Definitive diagnosis is fulfilling 1 to 3 of the criteria and at least 2 from 4 to 6. Ten-year survival is >90% with treatment. Treatment would consist of erythromycin 400 or 600 mg daily or clarithromycin 200 or 400 mg PO daily for at least 6 months even if there is clinical improvement. Treatment should be continued for 2 years and prolong if symptoms reoccur.

* *

Neuroendocrine cells are part of normal cell maturation and diminish with age; but persist in diffuse idiopathic pulmonary neuroendocrine cell hyperplasia (DIPNECH).[20,21] Given the female predominance, there might be a genetic or hormonal component involved. The proliferation is confined to the airway mucosa of small bronchi and bronchioles. Tumorlets (<0.5 cm) is the term for extraluminal proliferation. If tumorlets >0.5 cm, it is considered as carcinoid tumors which appear to be more peripheral. DIPNECH can cause luminal narrowing and mural scarring, causing constrictive bronchiolitis. Radiographically, there are nodules, ground glass attenuation/mosaic pattern, air trapping, and sometimes bronchiectasis. Patients with reversible airflow obstruction might benefit from corticosteroids, inhaled or systemic, or bronchodilators. If symptoms are severe, surgical intervention is warranted via resection or transplantation.

* *

Smoking was once been thought to be protective from chronic hypersensitivity pneumonitis. HP can occur in smokers, a more treatment-resistant form.

Question 2: **B. Symptoms may persist despite smoking cessation**

Serial bronchoalveolar lavage shows macrophages return to nonsmoker levels within 3 years although clinically symptoms can persist for years. This can be attributed to peribronchiolar fibrosis or concomitant centrilobular emphysema.

CASE 4

Question 1: B. Acute eosinophilic pneumonia

Acute eosinophilic pneumonia (AEP) is a primary eosinophilic syndrome, characterized by rapid onset of cough and dyspnea within 1 to 4 weeks with associated fever 38°C, pleuritic chest pain, and myalgias. The pathogenesis involves increased production of IL-5 and IL-18, suggestive of antigenic stimulation of TH2 lymphocytes and macrophages.[22–24] Eosinophilic granules are released into the interstitium and damage the lung. It usually has no peripheral eosinophilia although on occasion it can occur between 7 and 30 days of onset, with mean counts 1,700 cells/mm³. Other inflammatory markers such as erythrocyte sedimentation rate, C-reactive protein, and IgE are elevated although nonspecific. Radiographically, it manifests as diffuse bilateral ground glass opacities with occasional pleural effusions with marked eosinophilia. Cell count from bronchoalveolar lavage shows eosinophilia >25%. The patient had a risk factor, initiation of smoking, and the BAL showed elevated eosinophils. The galactomannan was positive, but it was probably secondary to the piperacillin-tazobactam.

* *

Acute interstitial pneumonia (AIP) is idiopathic and characterized by 7 to 14 prodromal illness with fever, cough, and progressive shortness of breath in a previously healthy individual, usually >40 years of age, and leads hypoxic respiratory failure with diffuse alveolar opacities.[25] Histologic appearance of AIP consists of diffuse alveolar damage (DAD) with temporal uniformity. Diagnostic workup is to determine other potential causes and treatment is largely supportive, with some benefit with high-dose corticosteroids (up to 2 g per day). Mortality remains high (>50%), although those that recover can have a near baseline quality of life. Relapse is possible.

* *

Desquamative interstitial pneumonia (DIP) is found in smokers, nonsmokers with surfactant protein gene mutations and CTD. High-resolution CT scan findings include bilateral lower-lobe ground glass opacities and some basal irregular linear opacities, traction bronchiectasis, and peripheral cystic lesions. Diagnosis is made via CT scan findings and surgical lung biopsy. Pathologic findings of DIP include diffuse infiltration of macrophages. Pulmonary function test in DIP shows restrictive pattern with reduced DLCO.

* *

Airway enlargement with fibrosis is not a distinct interstitial lung disease and is an incidental finding of interstitial fibrosis, and emphysema.

* *

Lipoid pneumonia is the accumulation of fats via endogenous means, from the release of cholesterol esters from destroyed alveolar walls, or exogenous, via aspiration of oil-based material such as milk, poppy seed oils, petroleum jelly or from occupational exposure to paraffin or oil blasting.[26] Clinical presentation is nonspecific and radiographically can manifest as nodules, masses, crazy paving pattern, or consolidation. Negative attenuation values (−150 and −30 HU) in a densely consolidated area free of aerated parenchyma or air bronchograms on chest computed tomography is highly suggestive. Broncholveolar lavage of whitish or turbid fluid with fat on the surface is also suggestive. Biopsy, via transbronchial or surgical, might be necessary if diagnosis is still in question despite clinical history and other studies. Specimens are limited to frozen section given the lipids will dissolve if placed into paraffin and the dyes must be specific for lipids. Treatment is largely supportive and elimination of exposure. There is anecdotal evidence for whole lung lavage although treatment might not be beneficial in the event of lipid phagocytosis by macrophages.[26] Complications include superinfections such as *nocardia* or nontuberculous mycobacteria, pulmonary fibrosis, and hypercalcemia.

Question 2: A. Stop smoking

Initiation of cigarette smoking is a risk factor for this disease. Although usually idiopathic, AEP can be associated with BCG vaccination, minocycline, fludrabine, progesterone IM, sertraline, firework smoke, WTC demolition dust, cave exploration, woodpile moving, and plant repotting. Chronic eosinophilic pneumonia (CEP) is associated with asthma. AEP responds quickly with corticosteroids and there is a low degree of relapse. There is a higher degree of relapse with CEP. Steroid course varies from 2 to 12 weeks.

CASE 5

Question 1: B. Cryptogenic organizing pneumonia

Cryptogenic organizing pneumonia (COP) is a histologic diagnosis comprised of intra-alveolar buds of granulation tissue consisting of intermixed myofibroblasts and connective tissue with no known precipitating disease. It has many multiple radiographic manifestations which include: central sparing, bilateral migratory infiltrates; upper lobe sometimes cavitary focal opacity; infiltrative pattern; bronchocentric pattern; linear or band-like pattern; or reverse halo sign.[1,27] Diagnosis depends on histological examination via transbronchial biopsy, and if tissues are insufficient, surgical lung biopsy. Bronchial alveolar lavage may have elevated levels of lymphocytes and to a lesser degree, neutrophils and eosinophils.

* *

The search for the cause of the organizing pneumonia should be elicited. Often, an infectious etiology is contemplated and the organizing pneumonia can persist despite eradication of the microbe. Drugs and underlying diseases, such as connective tissue disease, common variable hypogammaglobulinemia, ulcerative colitis, thyroid disease, and sarcoidosis, should also be investigated.

INFECTIONS AND DRUGS THAT CAN CAUSE ORGANIZING PNEUMONIA

Infections	*Burkholderia, chlamydia, coxiella, legionella, mycoplasma, nocardia, pseudomonas, serratie, Staphylococcus aureus, streptococcus,* adenovirus, CMV, herpes, HIV, *influenza, parainfluenza,* RSV, *plasmodium, dirofilaria, Cryptococcus, penicillium,* and PCP
Drugs	5-Aminosalicyclic acid, acebutolol, amiodarone, amphoterin B, Bleomycin, Busulfan, Cyclophosphamide with Busulfan, Carbamazepine, Cephalosporin, Chlorambucil, Doxorubicin, Fluvastatin, Gold salts, Hexamethonium, Interferon-a, Intereron-a2b, Interferon-a + cytosine, Interferon_ribavarin, Interferon-B1a, L-tryptophan, mesalzaine, methotrexate, minocycline, nilutamide, nitrofuranitoin, phenytoin, siolimus, sotalol, sulfasaazline, tacrolimus, ticopidine, trastuzumb, vinbarbital-aprobarbital

* *

Chronic eosinophilic pneumonia (CEP) is an important differential for COP; although not necessarily mutually exclusive. There are cases with both COP and CEP in the same patient at the same time. It is suggestive by cough and dyspnea for 2 weeks with peripheral eosinophilia ($>1,000/mm^3$) and BAL eosinophilia $>25\%$.

* *

Acute fibrinous and organizing pneumonia is a patchy histologic pattern of fibrinous intraalveolar deposition with organizing pneumonia and no hyaline membranes.[1] It can be idiopathic or associated with other diseases such as hypersensitivity pneumonitis, eosinophilic pneumonia, rheumatoid arthritis, infectious or drugs.

* *

For a discussion on AEP and DIP, refer to the answer portion of Case 4.

Question 2: A. Prednisone 20 mg PO daily

The patient appears to had a relapse, which manifests as worsening symptoms with reoccurrence of prior or new infiltrates. They are common during steroid taper. Predictors of relapse include delayed treatment and mild increases with alkaline phosphatase and gammaglutamyltransferase. Proposed taper of medications include prednisone 0.75 mg/kg/day for 4 weeks; followed by 0.5 mg/kg/day for 4 weeks, and then 20 mg daily for 4 weeks, 10 mg for 6 weeks, and 5 mg daily for 6 weeks. If relapse occurs while dose <20 mg daily, increase dose to 20 mg daily and slowly taper accordingly.[27] Treatment of COP includes steroids from 0.75 to 1.5 mg/kg/day with usual duration of up to 1 year.

CASE 6

Question 1: B. Pulmonary alveolar proteinosis

Pulmonary alveolar proteinosis (PAP) has abnormal accumulation of surfactant, which is a mixture of proteins (SP-A, SP-B, SP-C, and SP-D) and lipids (phosphatidylcholine). Surfactant lowers surface tension, preventing alveolar collapse, and is involved in defense against infections. Surfactant is produced by pneumocytes type II and cleared by alveolar macrophages and pneumocytes type II. GMCSF, a cytokine and growth factor for monocytes and granulocytes, has been hypothesized to have a role based on clinical PAP in two populations: (1) animal models who lack this cytokine and (2) patients with absent or mutated GM-CSF receptors but elevated serum and alveolar GM-CSF.[28]

* *

In this patient, it is secondary to alveolar macrophages unable to clear the surfactant secondary to functional or quantitative impairment of alveolar macrophages secondary to defect of expression of GM-CSF receptor. Clinically, patients present with acute respiratory insufficiency, neutropenia, and fever. Prognosis is generally poor with median survival of 16 months. Treatment of the underlying malignancy can improve this form of secondary PAP.

* *

PAP from hematologic disorders and inhalation of toxins, such as silica, talc, cement, aluminium, titanium, indium, and cellulose, are classified as secondary PAP. Anti–GM-CSF antibodies have been isolated in patients with secondary PAP due to toxic inhalation, suggesting an autoimmune trigger.

* *

There are two other variants called autoimmune (previously called primary or idiopathic) PAP, which accounts for 90% of PAP, and genetic PAP. In autoimmune PAP, there are neutralizing anti–GM-CSF immunoglobulin antibodies that bind to GM-CSF and block the clearance of surfactant. This also modifies neutrophils and lymphocytes and allows presence of opportunistic infections. Five percent of autoimmune PAP is present with opportunistic infections such as *Nocardia*, *Aspergillus*, or Mycobacterium. Prevalence varies per country but generally 4 to 40 cases per million and incidence is 0.2 cases per million.[28] Autoimmune PAP is rarely associated with other autoimmune diseases.

* *

Genetic PAP may be secondary to mutations of surfactant proteins such as SFTPB or SFTPC, ATP-binding cassette 3(ABCA3), NK2 homeobox 1 (NKX2-1), GM-CSF receptor alpha or beta subunit, or lysurinic protein intolerance.

* *

Diagnosis can be suggested by "crazy-paving" pattern of ground glass opacities with superimposed septal thickening or reticulation in a geographic pattern of normal and abnormal zones. Bronchoalveolar lavage of milky fluid with foamy macrophages with eosinophilic granules with hyaline material and positive periodic acid-Schiff (PAS) is suggestive of PAP. If diagnosis is still not obtained, surgical lung biopsy might be considered.

Anti–GM-CSF antibodies are specific for auto-immune PAP and can be obtained via ELISA or a functional assay. A concentration of >19 ug/mL^{-1} suggests autoimmune PAP while <10 ug/mL^{-1} rules it out. Other biomarkers such as LDH, CEA, and KL-6 may be elevated but are not specific.

* *

Lymphoproliferative diseases are abnormal proliferations of cells by antigenic stimulation of mucosa-associated lymphoid tissue (MALT) with three entities such as follicular bronchiolitis, lymphoid interstitial pneumonia and nodular lymphoid hyperplasia; or infiltration of lung parenchyma by lymphoid cells producing primary parenchymal neoplasms such as MALT lymphomas, diffuse large B-cell lymphomas, and lymphomatoid granulomatosis.[29] The radiographic manifestations and bronchoscopic findings does not suggest that this new hypoxia is attributed to these diseases.

* *

There is no substantial evidence linking sarcoidosis with cancer yet.

Question 2: B. High-volume bronchial lavage

Whole lung lavage is indicated for immediate relief of symptoms. The procedure is performed with a double lumen endotracheal tube and rigid bronchoscopy. The patient is placed on dorsal or lateral decubitus and the lung being lavaged is placed on uppermost portion. The nonlavaged lung is ventilated. One liter of warmed saline is infused into the lung and collected by gravity after opening outflow tube. Percussion may be used to expedite drainage and up to 15 L of saline administered until fluid is less opaque. Contralateral lung can be lavaged after 24 to 48 hours. Eighty-five percent of patients show improvement with ½ requiring repeat lavages. Complications include hypoxia, convulsions, pneumothorax, pleural effusions and fever.

* *

Other treatments include GM-CSF supplementation therapy, which would take months to achieve any kind of radiographic, symptomatic and functional response. GM-CSF can be administered subcutaneously (initially 250 ug subcutaneously daily and increased to 9 ug/kg/day and after 9 months to 18 ug/kg/day) or inhaled (at 250 ug/12 h in 2 mL of saline or 125 ug inhaled twice a day for six 2-week cycles and maintenance at 125 ug once a day for an additional six 2-week cycles). Plasmapheresis

Lymphoproliferative Disorder	Definition	Radiographic Findings
Nodular lymphoid hyperplasia	Usually secondary to inflammatory conditions with median age 65 Usually asymptomatic although can present with dyspnea, cough, and pleuritic chest pain	2–3 cm solitary nodule or mass with mild focal lymphangitic extension
Follicular bronchiolitis	Benign bronchial MALT hyperplasia around bronchioles Associated with CTD, such as RA and Sjögren's syndrome, and immunodeficiencies Progressive dyspnea, cough, fever, and recurrent bronchopneumonia Treatment: steroids	Bilateral 1–3 mm centrilobular nodules, sometimes with tree in bud formation Bilateral ground glass opacities
Lymphoid interstitial pneumonia (LIP)	Interstitial polyclonal lymphocytic proliferation and follicular distribution of B cell usually associated with systemic disease such as EBV or HIV or CTD Has been suggested as an HIV defining disease particularly in children	Uniform or patchy bilateral ground glass opacities and usually associated with immunodeficiencies poorly defined centrilobular nodules usually associated with AIDS Occasional cystic lesions 1–30 mm in diameter and usually associated with Sjögren's Thickened peribronchovascular interstitium Mild interlolubar septal thickening Calcified pulmonary nodules would suggest amyloidosis
MALT lymphoma	Important differential for LIP but can be distinguished by architectural distortion, the radiographic findings, and presence of Dutcher bodies, intranuclear B-lymphocyte inclusion Good prognosis: 84–94% 5-year survival Immunohistochemistry: CD20 and CD34	Large nodules Consolidation Pleural effusions
Diffuse large B-cell lymphoma	Seen with underlying immunodeficiency Dypnea, fever, and weight loss Poor prognosis: 0–60% 5-year survival	Single or solid nodules or masses and cavitation may be present Mediastinal adenopathy
Lymphomatoid granulomatosis	EBV associated with propensity for blood vessel destruction Males 30–50 years Poor prognosis but spontaneous remission possible Lungs, CNS, kidneys Cough, dyspnea, hemoptysis	Bilateral poorly marginated nodules or mas 0.5–8 cm in diameter with basal predominance and peribronchovascular distribution Occasional cavitation Reverse halo sign Migratory nodules
Secondary pulmonary lymphoma	Mature B-cell lymphomas and identical to morphology to primary pulmonary lymphomas Hodgkin's lymphoma—parenchymal involvement usually associated with mediastinal involvement Non-Hodgkin's lymphoma isolated lung disease without mediastinal involvement	Mediastinal adneopathy Nodules <1 cm Bronchovascular thickening Cavitatin Air bronchograms Pleural effusions AIDS-related lymphoma has pleural effusions, nodules, and lymphadenopathy
Posttransplantation lymphoproliferative disorder	Associated with EBV Within 2 years of transplantation but can occur as late as 20 years which has worse prognosis Fever, lymphadenopathy, abdominal pain with diarrhea, URTI, CNS, and weight loss	Nodules 0.3–5 cm Well defined Halo sign Consolidation or ground glass Lymphadenopathy Peribronchial or subpleural distribution

might be able to remove anti–GM-CSF antibodies but results are variable. Rituximab, a monoclonal antibody against CD20 antigen of B-lymphocytes, has been shown to decrease anti–GM-CSF concentration.

CASE 7

Question 1: B. T1 helper cell response leads to production of IFN-gamma and IL-2

Granulomas are formed to contain a foreign antigen or infection from the surrounding tissue. Granuloma formation in sarcoidosis is similar to other granulomatous diseases of known cause. Inhaled antigens are phagocytosed by antigen-presenting cells such as macrophages or dendritic cells. Antigens are subsequently presented to human leukocyte antigen (HLA) Class II molecules on $CD4^+$ T cells. An intact cell-mediated immunity polarizes T lymphocytes to Th1 phenotype, followed by cellular recruitment, proliferation, and differentiation. IFN-gamma and IL-2 are excreted and augment macrophage's production of TNF-alpha and increase cellular response. A target of IFN-gamma is the STAT1 pathway. This is important in granuloma formation in sarcoidosis. Subsequently, a core of monocyte-derived epithelioid histiocytes and giant cells with scattered $CD4^+$ T lymphocytes surrounded by lymphocytes, monocytes, mast cells and fibroblasts is formed. The persistent granulomatous inflammation is in part secondary to deposition of amyloid A protein which perpetuates cytokine release via toll-like receptor 2, a dysregulation of immune response suppression, and loss of natural killer cells.

Question 2: E. All of above

The cause of sarcoidosis is unknown. Genetic basis has focused on HLA genes. HLA-DRB1*1101 and HLA-DPB1*0101 are associated with increased risk while HLA-DRB1*03 is associated with Lofgren's syndrome, which carries a good prognosis, and HLA-DQB1*0201 associated with good prognosis. Non-HLA genes associated with sarcoidosis are butyrophilin-like 2 (BTNL2) mutation, chromosomes 5p and 5q, and linkage peaks in chromosomes 12p and 9q. It has also been hypothesized that there is an infectious link with mycobacterium or propionibacterium acnes contributing to the disease. Several proteins such as mycobacterial catalase-peroxidase (mKatG) have been found in some patients with sarcoidosis. Other hypothesis suggests that deposition of serum amyloid A protein perpetuates the initial immune response through toll-like receptor 2. This

causes persistence of granulomatous inflammation. The level of serum amyloid correlates with disease activity. Another theory includes an exhausted or dysfunctional T_{reg} population.

Question 3: C. It has been implied that severity of radiographic findings has prognostic significance although interpretation has high inter-observer variability

Since the 1960s, chest radiographs have been proposed for sarcoidosis staging and prognosis. Stage 0 has no adenopathy or infiltrates, stage 1 has adenopathy with 90% resolution of radiographic findings within 2 years, stage 2 has adenopathy with infiltrates, stage 3 has infiltrates with 30% resolution of radiographic findings and stage 4 has fibrosis.[30] However, this staging has major issues with interobserver variability and no correlation with pulmonary function tests.

* *

Pulmonary function tests generally show a restrictive pattern but can have airflow obstruction secondary to endobronchial disease, stenosis, airway reactivity, or distortion from parenchymal disease. The correlation between FVC and the sensation of dyspnea is modest at best.

Question 4: A. Prednisone 40 mg PO daily for 3 months

Treatment is generally not necessary unless organ dysfunction or symptoms are present. Oral prednisone is started at 20 to 40 mg PO daily with evaluation for response after 1 to 3 months. If response is present, prednisone is tapered by 5 to 15 mg daily with additional 9 to 12 months of treatment. Since sarcoidosis is multisystemic, other immunosuppressant drugs have been used to treat these manifestations, although most of the data are anecdotal and from small studies.[30,31]

* *

Antitumor necrosis factor therapy is considered for patients with: FVC <70%, ATS dyspnea + 1 disease >2 years, significant extrapulmonary disease, lupus pernio, CNS, elevated CRP.

Question 5: E. None of the above

Generally, diagnosis of sarcoidosis is suggested by clinical features, radiographic findings, biopsy and exclusion of other causes of noncaseating granulomas via special stains and cultures for acid fast bacilli and fungus. However, there are exceptions where biopsy might not be

ORGAN INVOLVEMENT IN SARCOIDOSIS AND TREATMENT

Lungs	CXR stage 0–1 no symptoms; no systemic therapy level 1A
	CXR stage 2–4 symptomatic: prednisone 20–40 mg PO daily level 1A for 12–24 months (level 1C)
	Steroid sparing alternatives: – Methotrexate 5–15 mg once a week (level 1A) with folic acid 1 mg daily (level 1B) – Azathioprine 50–200 mg daily (level 1B) – Leflunomide 10–20 mg daily (level 1B) – Mycophenolate (level 1C)
	Refractory: Infliximab 3–5 mg kg IV and repeated 2 weeks later and then once a month level 1A
Eyes	Anterior uveitis – Topical steroid Posterior uveitis or optic neuritis – Prednisone 20–40 mg PO daily
Skin	Lupus pernio – Prednisone 20–40 mg PO daily – Hydroxycloroquine 400 mg PO daily – Methotrexate 10–15 mg/week – Thalidomide 100–150 mg daily Plaques and nodules – Prednisone 20–40 mg PO daily – Hydroxycloroquine 400 mg PO daily Erthyema nodosum – NSAID
CNS	Nerve palsies – Prednisone 20–40 mg PO daily Cerebral lesions – Prednisone 40 mg PO daily – Azathioprine 150 mg PO daily – Hydroxycloroquine 400 mg PO daily
Cardiac	Complete heart block – Pacemaker Ventricular tachycardia or fibrillation – AICD Systolic HF – AICD, prednisone 20–40 mg PO daily
Liver	Cholestatic hepatitis Prednisone 20–40 mg PO daily Ursodiol 15 mg/kg of body weight per day
Joints and Muscles	Arthralgias – NSAID Granulomatous arthritis, myositis, myopathy Prednisone 20–4 mg PO daily
Hypercalciuria and hypercalcemia	Prednisone 20–40 mg PO daily Hydroxycloroquine 400 mg PO daily

From Iannuzzi M, Rybicki BA, Teirstein AS. Sarcoidosis. *NEJM*. 2007; 357:2162.

necessary such as in Lofgren's syndrome, characterized by erythema nodosum, bilateral hilar adenopathy on chest (radiography, fever, and arthritis), Heerfordt syndrome (uveitis, parotidits, and fever) and a gallium scan with both Panda sign (parotid gland and lacrimal gland uptake) and Lambda sign (right paratracheal and bilateral hilar uptake).[31] The patient has Lofgren's syndrome.

* *

The Kveim–Siltzbach test is performed by injecting human sarcoid tissue extract intradermally, followed by the extraction of the papule that develops 4 weeks later. It is preferred in patients with primary lesions that cannot be easily biopsied and who are not on immunosuppression. Other tests such as angiotensin converting enzyme are nonspecific and are not indicated for diagnosis and determining treatment response. Although positive predictive value can reach as high as 98%, there is lack of standardization, concern for viral infections, and instability of substrate.

* *

Bronchoalveolar lavage with >15% lymphocytes and CD4:CD8 ratio of >3.5 has a specificity of 93% to 95% with a sensitivity of 53% to 59%.

CASE 8

Question 1: **A. Exaggerated immune response to a repeated exposure to an inhaled antigen involving Th1 and Th17 T cells**

The patient has chronic hypersensitivity pneumonitis based on indirect history of exposure to birds, clinical, radiologic, and physiologic findings, and BAL and surgical biopsy results. The precipitant avian antigen is related to her washing the clothes of her husband who works with birds. The pathogenesis involves an exaggerated immune response of repeated exposure to an inhaled antigen (<5 um) in predisposed patients. These patients are predisposed via genetic susceptibility through a focus within the Class II MHC genomic region and polymorphisms with HLA-DR and HLA-DQ or (PSMB8) KQ genotype – a subunit which breaks down proteins and presents to Class I MHC molecules, environmental factors such as recent respiratory viral infection, and/or abnormalities with the regulatory T cells (T_{reg}), which maintain balance between tissue damage and protection of the immune response. In subacute and chronic hypersensitivity pneumonitis, Th1 immune response is regulated under T-bet, a master regulator transcription factor. Once the antigen is presented via macrophages and dendritic cells, the CD4$^+$ T cells differentiate into subsets, such as Th1, Th2, and IL-17 which can lead to fibrosis. IL-1 and IFN-gamma directs the development of Th1 differentiation and CD34 and toll-like receptor 9 directs the granulomatous process. In acute hypersensitivity pneumonitis, immune complexes are developed.

**

The cell count of the bronchoalveolar lavage in patients with chronic hypersensitivity pneumonitis might not show the typical T-cell lymphocytes >50%. This characteristic can also be seen in smokers who develop hypersensitivity pneumonitis. Because of a higher number of CD4+ in chronic HP, it might not show a CD4$^+$/CD8$^+$ ratio <1. High numbers of mast cells can distinguish hypersensitivity pneumonitis from cryptogenic organizing pneumonia. High levels of immunoglobulin M, G, and A and immunoglobulin-free light chains are found days after antigen exposure.

**

HRCT findings in chronic HP include reticulation, ground glass changes, centrilobular nodules, interlobular septal thickening, volume loss, traction bronchiectasis, lack of lower-lobe predominance, airtrapping and honeycombing. Subacute HP predominately has ground glass opacities, nodules, and/or air trapping.

**

Diagnosis can be challenging. Circulating antibodies are markers of sensitization but not of disease. Inhalation challenges, which are not standardized, recreate the symptoms after inhalation, with a positive challenge defined as cough, fever, dyspnea, and decrease of FVC and oxygen saturation in 8 to 12 hours after exposure.

**

Acute graft versus host disease (acute GVHD) usually occurs within 100 days of allogeneic hematopoietic cell transplantation and is an exaggerated normal immune response secondary to mismatch of HLA encoded by major histocompatibility complex (MHC) and non-HLA minor histocompatibility proteins between donor T cells to genetically defined proteins on host cells. The secondary lymphoid tissues in the gastrointestinal tract are believed to be the initial site of interaction between antigen presenting cells and donor T cells.[34] Gastrointestinal damage allows upregulation of the inflammatory stimuli,

including upregulation of toll-like receptors. Donor T cells increase in response to host antigen presenting cells. These lead to increased cellular inflammation, predominantly via cytotoxic T lymphocytes and natural killer cells. There is initially skin involvement (rash), GI involvement (diarrhea), and the liver. Pulmonary involvement can be found in both acute and chronic GVHD as bronchiolitis obliterans organizing pneumonia.

**

Irritant-induced asthma (IIA) or reactive airways dysfunction syndrome is a response to multiple low-dose or single high-dose inhaled irritant without prior sensitization.[35] Reactive airways dysfunction syndrome (RADS) is considered the severe form of IIA. It consists of symptoms developing <24 hours to days after exposure and one to more high level exposures. Symptoms may persist for >3 months. Risk factors include potency of agent, level of exposure, genetics, and smoking.[35] IIA can be an occupational-related disease and cleaning solutions can trigger symptoms.

CASE 9

Question 1: A. Eosinophilic granulomatosis with polyangiitis

Eosinophilic granulomatosis with polyangiitis (EGPA) is an ANCA-associated vasculitis, although 50% of EGPA with pulmonary involvement has negative-ANCA. The American College of Rheumatology's diagnosis has a sensitivity of 85% and specificity of 99.7% if four out of the six criteria are met which include: (1) history of asthma or wheeze; (2) greater than 10% eosinophils on differential leukocyte count; (3) mononeuropathy (including multiplex) or polyneuropathy; (4) radiographically apparent migratory or transient pulmonary infiltrates; (5) paranasal sinus abnormalities; and (6) biopsy including blood vessel showing accumulation of eosinophils in extravascular space.[36-39] The Lanham criteria includes all three: asthma, peak peripheral blood eosinophilia in excess of 1,500 cells/μL, and systemic vasculitis involving two or more extrapulmonary organs.[36-39]

**

The pathogenesis is unknown although eosinophilia has a central role. Most asthmatics have mild form of eosinophilia, but eosinophilia >10% raises that question of another disease. Activated eosinophils secrete eosinophil major basic protein (MBP), eosinophil-derived neurotoxin (EDN) and peroxidase which cause tissue damage. Interleukin-3, Interleukin-5, and granulocyte-macrophage colony stimulating factor regulate the production and distribution of eosinophils. Elevated levels, whether local or systemic, can indicate a hypereosinophilic process. Other hypothesis suggested that chronic eosinophilia is secondary to prolonged survival secondary to IL-5's inhibition of eosinophilic apoptosis. CD95/CD95 Ligand system also has a role in prevention of eosinophilic apoptosis even in absence of IL-5 or IL-3. Blood eosinophilia does not correlate with tissue eosinophilia and this discrepancy has not been fully understood although genetic and local factors may be involved.

* *

There are three clinical stages: (1) asthma with eosinophilia and sinusitis; (2) tissue eosinophilia which can be presented as eosinophilic pneumonia or eosinophlic infiltration of gastrointestinal mucosa; and (3) vasculitis.

* *

Leukotriene-modifying agents (LTMA) such as zafirlukast, montelukast, panlukast, zileuton, cocaine, and omalizumab have been associated with EGPA. This is due to the unmasking of the disease as the LTMA is introduced to decrease or remove steroids. This is called forme fruste of EGPA.

* *

Given the extrapulmonary presentation, AEP and CEP are less likely the diagnosis. Loeffler's syndrome is an eosinophilic process secondary to parasitic infection. The patient's parasitic workup has been negative.

Question 2: A. Myocardial infarction

The modified Five Factor Score has been used to predict the mortality from EGPA and consists of age >65, cardiac involvement, renal insufficiency, gastrointestinal involvement, and absence of ENT involvement. A score >1 is associated with up to 45% mortality within 5 years. From the answer choices, myocardial infarction is associated with the highest mortality from this disease.

CASE 10

Question 1: C. Renal biopsy

The patient has diffuse alveolar hemorrhage as a complication of granulomatosis with polyangiitis, formerly called Wegener's granulomatosis. It is part of a group of diseases called anti-neutrophil cytoplasmic antibody

(ANCA) associated vasculitis, which includes microscopic polyangiitis, eosinophilic granulomatosis with polyangiitis formerly called Churg-Strauss syndrome, and idiopathic pauci-immune pulmonary capillaritis. ANCA promote neutrophilic migration and release of toxic metabolites in the vessel wall. The incidence is 15 to 20 cases per million per year and mortality per the European Vasculitis Study Group (EUVAS) showed 1-, 2-, and 5-year survival rates to be 88%, 85%, and 78%, respectively.[36] Poor prognostic factors include age, higher disease activity, alveolar hemorrhage, cardiac involvement, and proteinase 3 positivity.[36]

* *

GPA can affect the upper respiratory tract as otitis, sinusitis, septal perforation, mastoiditis, and saddle nose deformities; lower respiratory tract as cough, shortness of breath, chest pain, alveolar hemorrhage and radiographically present as pulmonary nodules (cavitary or noncavitary) or consolidation; and tracheobronchial disease. It can affect other organs including skin, kidneys, eyes, joints, muscles, nervous system, and heart.

* *

Prior to the development of ANCA, the American College of Rheumatology (ACR), 1990 diagnostic criteria for granulomatosis with polyangiitis could not distinguish it from microscopic polyangiitis.[36] It included nasal or oral inflammation, nodules, fixed infiltrates or parenchymal cavities on chest radiographs, abnormal urinary sediment, and granulomatosis inflammation on biopsy of an artery or perivascular area. Two or more of the criteria yielded 88% sensitivity and 92% specificity. The European Medicine Agency algorithm permitted the diagnosis of GPA in absence of biopsy if there was upper and lower airway involvement, glomerulonephritis as defined by hematuria with red cell casts or >10 dysmorphic RBCS or 2+ hematuria or 2 + proteinuria, and ANCA-positive.

* *

There are three types of pattern characterized by indirect immunofluorescence: cytoplasmic or c-ANCA, perinuclear or p-ANCA which is believed to be a technical artifact to ethanol fixation, and atypical or a-ANCA. The two target antigens are proteinase 3 (PR3) and myeloperoxidase (MPO). Immunofluorescence serves as a screening test and enzyme-linked immunosorbent assay (ELISA) is a confirmation test and can identify the target antigen

VASCULITIS AND THEIR ASSOCIATED ANCA CHARACTERISTICS

90% of patients with granulomatosis with polyangiitis	80–90% PR3-ANCA (marker of severity of disease) 10–20% MPO-ANCA 40% ANCA-negative particularly in pulmonary limited disease
70% of patients with microscopic polyangiitis	MPO-ANCA > PR3-ANCA
50% of patients with eosinophilic granulomatosis with polyangiitis	MPO-ANCA > PR3-ANCA ANCA-negative are usually with pulmonary and cardiac involvement although this is still being debated
Idiopathic pauci-immune pulmonary capillaritis	
Renal limited vasculitis	MPO-ANCA>PR3-ANCA Lysosome-associated membrane protein-2 LAMP-2 ANCA
40% of patents with anti-GBM antibody disease	MPO-ANCA > PR3-ANCA
Some have both types	
Drug-induced casculitis (Propylthiouracil, Methimazole, Carbimazole, Thiamazole, Hydralazine, Minocycline, Penicillamine, Allopurinol, Procainamide, Clozapine, Phenytoin, Rifampin, Cefotaxime, Isoniazid, Indomethacin)	MPO-ANCA Minocycline— p-ANCA against cathepsin G, elastase, and bactericidal permeability increasing protein
Rheumatologic disorders (systemic lupus erythematosus Sjögren's syndrome, rheumatoid arthritis, relapsing polychondritis, scleroderma, antiphospholipid syndrome)	p-ANCA > a-ANCA > c-ANCA
Autoimmune gastrointestinal disorders (ulcerative colitis, primary sclerosing cholangitis, Crohn's disease, autoimmune hepatitis)	p-ANCA
Cystic fibrosis	p-ANCA for bactericidal permeability increasing protein (BPI)
Levamisole contaminated cocaine	100% MPO-ANCA and 50% PR3-ANCA

(PR3 or MPO). Combination of IF and ELISA provides a sensitivity and specificity of 96% and 98.5%, respectively.

* *

Reservations for basing diagnosis and treatment response only on ANCA and their titers include: (1) no standardized value; (2) subjective interpretation of IF; and (3) no direct correlation with elevated titers and progression of disease in the absence of symptoms.

* *

Despite the availability of ANCA, it is still advised to have biopsy of organ involvement. Renal biopsy or surgical lung biopsy is preferred. The renal biopsy would show segmental crescentic necrotizing glomerulonephritis with immunoglobulin or complement deposition. It is stained with immunofluoroscent staining to exclude anti-glomerular basement membrane antibody disease which is treated with plasma exchange. Surgical lung biopsy would often show granulomas or vasculitis and exclude other diseases particularly infections. Sinus

and skin biopsy have higher rates of false-negative given the small amount of tissue.

* *

In the setting of GPA, serial ANCA may be used to determine disease activity and response to treatment.

Question 2: A. Plasmapheresis + IV cyclophosphamide + IV corticosteroids

Treatment involves two principles: the induction of remission and the maintenance of remission. The EUVAS classification of severity helps guide the appropriate medications for any ANCA-associated vasculitis and avoid unnecessary adverse effects.[36] The patient presents with a severe form of GPA with diffuse alveolar hemorrhage as suggested by the serial allioquots bronchoalveolar lavage showing progressive heme and >20% hemosiderin macrophages and renal failure. Therefore, treatment will be plasmapheresis, IV corticosteroids and IV cyclophosphamide. Plasmapheresis removes circulating factors such as ANCA, activated lymphocytes,

ANCA ASSOCIATED VASCULITIS SEVERITY AND TREATMENT

Severity	Characteristics	Medications
Limited	Isolated to upper airway disease and non-organ threatening	Topical medications, oral coritcosteroids and/or other drugs such as methotrexate, azathioprine, or mycophenolate mofetil
Early generalized	Constitutional symptoms + end-organ involvement	Cyclophosphamide or methotrexate (better tolerated, but longer to achieve remission and higher relapse rates) Alternatives: azathioprine, mycophenolate mofetil
Generalized active	Constitutional symptoms + impaired and threatened organ function	Oral cyclophosphamide + oral corticosteroids Alternative: rituximab, anti-CD20
Severe	Organ failure including severe renal impairment (Creatinine >5.7 mg/dL), alveolar hemorrhage, central nervous system involvement, cardiomyopathy, life-threatening gastrointestinal disease such as ischemia or hemorrhage	IV corticosteroids (pulse dose or 1 mg/kg/day) + IV cyclophosphamide ± plasma exchange Or IV corticosteroids (pulse dose) + rituximab ± plasma exchange
Refractory	Failure of response from a treatment	Anti-thymocyte globulin, intravenous immunoglobulin, infliximab, deoxyspergualin
Remission		Transition from oral cyclophosphamide with oral corticosteroids in 3–6 months to azathioprine, methotrexate, or mycophenolate mofetil for a duration of 18–24 months

and other inflammatory markers and is indicated to preserve renal function in rapidly progressing renal failure and diffuse alveolar hemorrhage (DAH). Rituximab may be substituted for cyclophosphamide and has been shown to be noninferior in induction of remission and superior for relapsing disease.[68]

Question 3: B. PCP prophylaxis and to eradicate *S. aureus* colonization

S. aureus nasal colonization has been associated with increased relapse in GPA.[36,40]

CASE 11

Question 1: A. Avoidance of antigen

Flock worker's lung (FWL) is an occupational-induced interstitial lung disease, primarily from Rhode Island, Massachusetts, and Ontario but case reports found in Spain and Turkey reveal that workers are exposed to inhalation of microfibers or "flock." These synthetic or natural fibers (0.2–5 mm) are cut from tow (rope of thin continuous strands) and applied to an adhesive-coated substrate. The synthetic materials include rayon, polyester, and polyolefins (polymers of propylene, ethylene, or other olefins). The method of cutting, rotational (rotary) versus gulliotine, influences the fiber size, and contribute to the disease. Rotary cut flock appears to cut fibers

faster but less precise length. IL-8 and TNF-alpha, like in other ILD, appear to be increased in this disease. Bronchoalveolar lavage can reveal eosinophilia >25%, lymphocytosis >30%, with or without neutrophilia.

* *

Patients with disease can present with pleuritic chest pain, dyspnea, and/or dry cough. Chest radiograph may be nondiagnostic and high-resolution computed tomography may reveal subtle peripheral and basal ground glass opacities, air trapping, or fibrosis with honeycombing. Pulmonary function test commonly have a restrictive deficit with reduced DLCO. Pathologically, it is characterized by lymphocytic bronchiolitis and peribronchiolitis with lymphoid hyperplasia. In most cases of FWL, it is considered NSIP but others have suggested BOOP. It is believed that FWL is not a form of hypersensitivity pneumonitis, particularly from the lack of granulomas.

* *

The natural history of the disease includes resolution, persistent restrictive deficit, persistent mixed obstructive/restrictive deficits, pulmonary fibrosis, pulmonary hypertension or death. The mixed obstructive and restrictive deficit could be attributed to the fibers inducing a concomitant occupational asthma and/or complication of smoking. The association between smoking and lung cancer in this type of ILD is still not determined. The role of steroids is also still debatable since there are cases of death in patients who have received an early course of steroids.[41-43]

CASE 12

Question 1: E. Ivermectin and abendazole

The patient has diffuse alveolar hemorrhage secondary to strongyloides hyperinfection s yndrome. Examination of the blood clot shows several filariform *Strongyloides* larvae. This is a nematode that is both infectious in humans and pets and is seen in Asia, Africa, Central and South America, Southeastern United States, and parts of Europe.[44-51] It affects between 10 and 70 million people worldwide.[44-51] There are two species: *Strongyloides stercolaris* and *strongyloides fuelleborni*. *Strongyloides* produce chronic infections, secondary to autoinfection. Because of nonspecific symptoms, *stongyloidiasis* can remain undiagnosed for many years.

* *

The life cycle consists of four larvae stages. Two stages involve newly hatched rhabditiform larvae which molt twice in the soil to evolve into filariform larvae. In this form, they can sexually reproduce rhabditiform larva or become infectious to humans. Filariform larvae penetrate the skin, pass through the lymphatics, penetrate the bloodstream, and migrate to the lungs. They pierce the alveolar membranes, ascend the tracheobronchial tree, are swallowed, and travel to the small intestine where they molt twice to become adult pathogenic females. They lay eggs which hatch rhabditiform larvae and pass out in the stool between 17 and 28 days. The larvae carry enteric bacteria and disseminate during their migration to other organs.[47] The presence of bacteria in cultures can confound the diagnosis.

* *

Strongyloides hyperinfection syndrome (SHS) involves the skin, intestines, and the lungs but can disseminate to other organs such as the brain or heart. SHS is secondary to an accelerated autoinfection. The catalyst for SHS is immunosuppression via T-cell depletion. This is due to corticosteroids, malignancy, and/or HIV. Steroids are hypothesized to increase apoptosis of TH2 cells, reduce eosinophilia, inhibit mast cell response, and increase ecdysteroid-like substances in the body. These substances act as molting signals, increasing number of infective larvae. It is unknown whether duration or dosage of corticosteroids can induce SHS. There is anecdotal evidence that cyclosporine has antihelminthic effects.[49] This is not seen with tacrolimus and mycophenolate. In transplant recipients, SHS occurs within 3 months and are due to reactivation of latent infection. It is rarely acquired from organ donors.

* *

Treatment for mild cases would be ivermectin 200 µg/kg for 2 consecutive days or 1 week apart. An alternative is abendazole 400 mg PO BID × 5 to 7 days, for severe disseminated cases.

* *

A prolonged course of ivermectin, 5 to 7 consecutive days, or ivermectin and abendazole is advised until the patient responds. Medications can be discontinued after 2 weeks of negative stool examination or negative serologies.

* *

Regarding the other answer choices, there is no indication for antifungal treatment and further immunosuppression can worsen her disease.

CASE 13

Question 1: C. Pulmonary alveolar microlithiasis

This is diffuse intra-alveolar accumulation of spherical calcium phosphate concentrations. There are less than 600 cases reported in literature, mostly in Italy, Turkey and the United States.[52-55] There is no sex predilection. It is hypothesized to be an autosomal recessive disease from a mutation of the solute carrier family 34 (sodium phosphate) member 2 gene (the SLC34A2 gene). This gene is expressed only in alveolar type II cells, which are responsible for surfactant production. Mutations lead to decreased cell uptake of phosphate, and lead to formation of microliths. Circulating levels of calcium and phosphate are usually normal. Cough and dyspnea are common symptoms.

* *

Ectopic calcium deposit occurs in two general classifications: (1) calcification in which calcium salts are deposited in tissues such as lung, kidneys, heart, and blood vessels; and (2) ossification in which bone tissue matrix occurs with or without marrow.

* *

Pulmonary calcification is further subdivided into metastatic, dystrophic, and idiopathic.[52] In metastatic pulmonary calcification, liberated $Ca_3(PO_4)_2$ and $CaCO_3$ from the bone are transported in the form of calcium hypophosphate in the blood. Calcium salts precipitate in alkaline pH and elevated calcium phosphate product >70 mg^2/dL^2 (normal 40 mg^2/dL^2). Metastatic calcification can still occur with a normal calcium phosphate product if the tissue has been primed by a calcifying factor followed by challenging agent.[52] There is a direct correlation with the calcium phosphate product and an alkaline environment in that less calcium phosphate product is required for calcification in a more alkaline environment and vice versa. Justification for an alkaline environment as a catalyst for calcification include: (1) the predominance of calcification in organs such as lung, kidneys, and stomach, that involve secretions of H+ and creating alkaline tissue; (2) upper lobes of the lung have higher V/Q ratio and pH, are predisposed to calcification compared to lower lobes with lower V/Q ratio and pH; (3) and cessation of pulmonary blood flow leads to decreased CO_2 delivery and causing tissue alkalosis.[52]

* *

In dystrophic pulmonary calcification, calcification occurs at the site of injury. Extracellular and intracellular calcium increases and activates enzymes which promote cell necrosis. Calcium binds to the free fatty acids from phospholipid degradation. The ensuing alkaline environment and involvement of collagen and calcium binding phosphoprotein osteopontin propagates the dystrophic calcification.

* *

CAUSES OF ECTOPIC CALCIFICATION

Metastatic—influenced by calcium—phosphate, alkaline phosphate, pH	Benign—ESRD, OLT, primary hyperparathyroidism, Milk Alkali syndrome, hypervitaminosis D, osteopetrosis, Paget's disease
	Malignant—parathyroid carcinoma, multiple myeloma, hematologic malignancies, squamous cell carcinoma, synovial sarcoma, breast carcinoma, choriocarcinoma
Dystrophic—influenced by injury	Granulomatous disorders, infections (viral and parasitic), amyloidosis, pulmonary vascular calcification, coal worker's pneumoconiosis, silicosis
Idiopathic	Pulmonary alveolar microlithiasis

Question 2: A. Induced sputum

Finding of microlithiasis in induced sputum is confirmation for PAM. Imaging studies are generally nonspecific for most types of pulmonary calcifications. Chest radiography is a good screening tool but unable to distinguish pulmonary calcification from infection or malignancy. With mediastinal windows on high-resolution computed tomography of the chest can help detect calcification. Typically, Hounsfield unit >100 can suggest calcification. Due to signal averaging, even Hounsfield unit <100 does not rule out calcification. Moreover, the microscopic size of the calcification may lead to a false-negative in mediastinal windows on high-resolution computed tomography. Of the imaging studies, bone scintigraphy with bone-avid radiotracer, ^{99m}Tc-MDP, can be used to confirm in equivocal cases.

* *

Unlike other forms of pulmonary calcifications, PAM has a characteristic appearance of bilateral sand-like micronodular densities that obliterate the diaphragm and mediastinal borders. However, findings of microlithiasis in induced sputum or bronchoalveolar lavage is often necessary to confirm diagnosis. Other invasive methods would include bronchoscopy with transbronchial biopsy.

Question 3: E. Lung transplantation

There is no known therapy for PAM. In severe cases, lung transplantation is the only option. There are anecdotal reports of improvement with corticosteroids, but there is no general consensus on their benefit.

CASE 14

Question 1: B. Acute hypersensitivity pneumonitis

Only 5% to 15% of individuals exposed repeatedly to an inhaled antigen, usually <5 um in diameter, develop the disease.[32] Genetics and environmental risk factors, such as concentration, duration, frequency, particle size, solubility and variability, influence the disease course. Hypersensitivity pneumonitis appears to be less prevalent in smokers, partly due to a reduced immunologic response to the antigen, but acute exacerbations in smokers generally carry a poorer prognosis.

* *

Hypersensitivity pneumonitis is not a uniform disease. It can develop different temporal patterns that do not necessarily coincide with each other.

TYPES OF HYPERSENSITIVITY PNEUMONITIS AND THEIR RADIOGRAPHIC FINDINGS

Acute hypersensitivity pneumonitis	Symptoms with 4–8 hours and resolve within 48 hours if removed from exposure.	CXR can be normal; PFT can be normal but usually shows restriction with gas transfer defect. HRCT ground glass with poorly defined nodules; recurrent episodes such as from farmer's lung can lead to obstructive disease with emphysema.
Subacute hypersensitivity pneumonitis	Symptoms can be insidious and develop within weeks to months from low-level exposure and usually the cough and dyspnea becomes persistent.	HRCT shows poorly formed nodules and ground glass opacities.
Chronic hypersensitivity pneumonitis	Symptoms can be insidious and generally do not necessary develop from acute or subacute hypersensitivity pneumonitis. Clubbing may be found and suggests poor prognosis.	HRCT shows reticular, ground glass, and centrilobular nodules associated with interlobular septal thickening, volume loss, traction bronchiectasis and honeycombing. Some, even nonsmokers, may form emphysema instead of fibrosis. Fibrotic NSIP or UIP histology shows the same prognosis as IPF. 20% of chronic HP develops pulmonary HTN.

**

Diagnostic criteria for hypersensitivity pneumonitis include (1) history of exposure to antigen as identified by history, microbiologic investigations, serum precipitins for antigen; (2) compatible (a) clinical, (b) radiographic, and (c) pulmonary function tests; (3) lymphocytosis and sometimes low CD4/CD8 ratio in the bronchoalveolar lavage; (4) positive inhalation challenge test either through (a) re-exposure to environment and (b) inhalation challenge in hospital setting; and/or (5) poorly formed non-caseating granulomas or mononuclear cell infiltrate on biopsy such as transbronchial biopsy or surgical lung biopsy in advanced cases.[32,33] Definite HP is considered if 1 to 3; 1, 2, and 4a; 1, 2a, 3, and 5; and 2, 3, and 5.[32,33] The patient has definite HP based on 1, 2, and 4a.

**

Serum precipitants are assays of IgG antibodies against antigens however it can be positive in patients exposed but do not have the disease and false-positives are high depending on the reference laboratory since they might not have all the precipitants.

**

Inhalation challenge is considered positive if there is fever, malaise, headache, crackles, neutrophilia, decreased FVC, hypoxia, and/or radiologic abnormalities within 8 to 12 hours after exposure or an initial wheeze with decreased in FEV_1 followed by fever, leukocytosis and decreased in FEV_1 and FVC 4 to 6 hours later.

**

Organic dust toxic syndrome, also called grain fever, pulmonary mycotoxicosis, and toxic alveolitis is a non-infectious febrile illness associated with chills, malaise, myalgia, dry cough, headache nausea after large dust exposure from handling grains such as corn, oats, sorghum, soybeans, or hay. It is debated whether the actual organic material or microbial contamination with resultant endotoxin actually cause the disease. It requires no prior sensitization and usually CXR and pulmonary function tests are normal. Prognosis generally is good.

**

Shrinking lungs syndrome is a rare pulmonary manifestation of SLE characterized by dyspnea, small lung volumes and elevated diaphragm.[55] Physiologic studies including maximal transdiaphragmatic pressures and electromyographic studies suggest a subclinical myositis secondary to SLE. Other hypotheses include chronic pleuritis. There has been anecdotal evidence of improvement with increasing corticosteroids or theophylline.

**

Vanishing lung syndrome is bullous paraseptal emphysematous disease usually restricted to the upper lobes, compressing the underlying lung tissue.[56] It is generally found in young, thin patients, may manifest as cough, shortness of breath and hemoptysis, and treatment is bullectomy.

CASE 15

Question 1: B. Rheumatoid arthritis

Rheumatoid factor (RF) is an immunoglobulin antibody against the Fc fragment of IG. It is present in 60% to 80% of RA but can be absent in the earliest presentation. It is also found in other connective tissue diseases, infections, autoimmune disease, and 1% to 5% of healthy persons. High levels of rheumatoid factor can be diagnostic for rheumatoid arthritis but are independent of disease progression and can remain high even in drug-induced remissions. Anticitrullinated protein antibody (ACPA or anti-CCP) appears to have equal or better sensitivity and specificity than RF with increased frequency even in the early course of the disease. It is also associated with pulmonary fibrosis and tobacco history (>25 years). It has the strongest association for development of ILD, with odds ratio of 3.8.[57]

* *

50% of patients with RA will develop pulmonary complications which can include parenchyma disease such as ILD and/or rheumatoid nodules, infectious complications, airway disease such as bronchiectasis or obliterative bronchiolitis, pleural disease (pleuritis, effusions, pneumothorax), vascular (pulmonary hypertension and alveolar hemorrphage), and diaphragm weakness or cricoarytenoid arthritis.[57,58]

* *

Patients with chronic cough or shortness of breath should obtain referral to a pulmonologist and obtain a pulmonary function test. 80% of patients will have an abnormal DLCO compared to 5% to 15% will have a restrictive defect on spirometry. Pseudo-normal pulmonary function tests can be secondary to concomitant obstructive defects. Therefore, DLCO is a more sensitive test for presence of ILD and imaging is recommended with DLCO <70% predicted.

* *

The most common histopathologic patterns in RA-ILD are UIP (56%), NSIP (33%), and organizing pneumonia (11%).[58] NSIP patterns have higher concentrations of platelet-derived growth factors AB-BB, interferon gamma, and transforming grown factor B_2 and longer duration of articular symptoms compared to UIP. Men, smokers, and a worse prognosis tend to be associated with UIP pattern. Comparing RA-ILD with UIP pattern with IPF, RA-ILD tend to have less fibroblastic foci and

increased CD4 in BAL. However, there was no significant difference in survival time between RA-ILD with UIP and IPF.[57–59]

Question 2: B. Bronchoscopy

Worsening clinical symptoms or decline in FVC 10% or DLCO 15% should warrant further investigation. Second to cardiovascular complications, infection is the second leading cause of death in RA. It is important to exclude infectious disease, particularly in patients with worsening respiratory symptoms. In RA, immunosuppression with prednisone 10 mg PO daily increases the risk for pneumonia and 15 mg PO daily increases the risk for pneumocystis pneumonia. Anti–TNF-alpha increases the risk of tuberculosis. Therefore, bronchoscopy with bronchoalveolar lavage might be employed to rule out other infectious processes. Blood cultures might not be sufficient to rule out infection, particularly with predominantly respiratory complaints.

* *

Treatment for RA-ILD, particularly for NSIP/BOOP is not standardized but a typical protocol involves glucocorticoids 0.75/mg/day prednisone during the first 4 weeks, followed by 0.5 mg/kg/day for the next 4 weeks, then 20 mg/day for 4 weeks, 10 mg/day for 6 weeks, and finally 5 mg/day for the last 6 weeks. An objective marker of response after 12 weeks is a 10% improvement in FVC or 15% in DLCO. Steroids sparing agents can also be used. Azathioprine 50 mg daily is increased to 2 to 3 mg/kg/day after thiopurine methyltransferase (TPMT) is checked to see if it is normal. If TPMT is decreased, cyclosporine at 2.5 mg/kg/day twice a day is substituted. If the PFTs are unchanged for 2 years, medical treatment is reassessed. Even in UIP, immunosuppression is attempted with the additional of N-acetylcysteine 600 mg PO TID and cyclophosphamide 2 mg/kg/day with prednisone 0.25 mg/kg/day is administered for nonresponders.

Question 3: A. Drug-induced pneumonitis

It can be difficult to determine which drug-induced pneumonitis or drug-induced interstitial lung disease (DILD) since administration of drugs overlap and sometimes there could be a delayed reaction. Methotrexate-induced lung toxicity is rare with doses 20 to 25 mg per week. Mortality is as high as 20% if it occurs within six months of administration of the drug. Preexisting pulmonary disease, DLCO <70% predicted, tobacco abuse, hypoalbumin, and previous DMARDS use are risk factors for the disease. Surgical lung biopsy would show acute and organizing diffuse alveolar damage, cellular infiltrate with or without granulomas, which differ from the normal pattern of RA-ILD NSIP and UIP picture. Leflunomide was shown to have pulmonary toxicity after receiving a loading dose of leflunomide and mortality is as high as 19%. Naproxen causes eosinophilic pneumonia. Other rheumatoid arthritis medications with pulmonary toxicity include: (1) anti–TNF-alpha (infliximab, adalimunmab, or etanercept) can cause pulmonary fibrosis; (2) gold salts which can cause ILD and diffuse alveolar hemorrhage; and (3) D-penicillamine which can cause BO, pulmonary and renal syndromes, and diffuse alveolar hemorrhage. Treatment of DILD would include cessation of the suspected drug, supportive measures, and corticosteroids. There are cases of spontaneous resolution with cessation of drug.

* *

RA-ILD exacerbation is clinical deterioration within 30 days with no radiographic abnormalities and no identifiable source (which means exclusion of infections and drugs). Diffuse alveolar damage may be observed on histologic examination. With mortality approaching 80% to 100%, pulse steroids with 1 mg/kg/day × 3 days followed by prednisolone 1 mg/kg/day is given. Cyclophosphamide (500–750 mg/m^2), cyclosporine 3 mg/kg/day, or tacrolimus 3 mg/kg/day are alternatives.

CASE 16

Question 1: A. Topoisomerase I and anti-endothelial

The patient has systemic sclerosis, or scleroderma, which is associated with endothelial dysfunction resulting in vasculopathy and fibroblast dysfunction resulting in excessive collagen production and fibrosis. Diagnosis is based on evidence of skin induration and the presence of at least one of the following: heart burn or dysphagia, hypertension or renal insufficiency, shortness of breath and/or new chest radiographic abnormalities, pulmonary hypertension, diarrhea, telangiectasis on face and hands, erectile dysfunction, and/or digital infarcts. There are three classifications of systemic sclerosis (SSc) based on skin involvement: diffuse cutaneous sclerosis, limited cutaneous sclerosis, and scleroderma sine scleroderma, which has no skin involvement. The limited cutaneous sclerosis is most closely associated with honeycombing. Pulmonary manifestations, including either interstitial lung disease and/or pulmonary hypertension, are the leading cause of the death in this disease. 90% of patients will have interstitial lung disease. Therefore screening for pulmonary disease in scleroderma is paramount. HRCT and PFT should be pursued. Normal HRCT at baseline is a good marker for development of ILD since 85% will still have normal imaging after 5 years follow-up. Serologies for systemic sclerosis include anti-topoisomerase (anti-Scl 70) and anti-endothelial cell antibodies, which target lamin, A/C, tubulin beta-chain, and vinculin.[60] These can detect which patients develop ILD. Other serologic testing such as Anticentromere and anti-RNA polymerase III are less associated with ILD. Anti-U3 ribonucleoprotein antibodies, anti-topoisomrease II alpha antibodies, and anticentromere antibodies are associated with pulmonary hypertension. These antibodies are usually mutually exclusive.

Question 2: B. Cyclophosphamide

Scleroderma Lung Study (SLS) 13 center double-blinded placebo-controlled trial showed improvement in FVC, dyspnea, and skin thickness for patients treated with 1 year of oral cyclophosphamide.[61] Another prospective trial, Fibrosis Alveolitis in Scleroderma, showed a trend toward significant improvement in FVC although no statistical differences in DLCO, HRCT, or dyspnea scores.[62] Mycophenolate mofetil can be used for maintenance. Prednisone has been shown to cause renal crisis particularly in doses greater >15 mg/day. At lower doses, it has been used in adjunct with other immunosuppressant such as cyclophosphamide. Great interest in the role of hematopoietic stem cell transplant has been generated in the recent past with studies such as the ASSIST (autologous non-myeloablative hematopoietic stem cell transplantation) showing improvement in lung function and HRCT up to 2 years after transplantation versus pulse cyclophosphamide, although in the acute setting it might not be the best option.[63]

CASE 17

Question 1: C. Idiopathic pneumonia syndrome

Hematopoietic stem cell transplantation (HSCT) is indicated for hematologic and solid malignancies as rescue therapy to restore marrow function after lethal doses of radiation and chemotherapy and to replace dysfunctional hematopoietic or lymphoreticular precursors seen in aplastic anemia, thalassemia, and immune deficiency syndromes. HSCT is subdivided by the source of the stem cells: the patient (autologous), twin (syngeneic) or nonidentical sibling, or unrelated individual (allogeneic). With allogeneic HSCT disparity between donor and recipient can precipitate graft versus host disease and host versus graft reactions; although these are also thought to improve antileukemic responses.

* *

Idiopathic pneumonia syndrome (IPS) is widespread alveolar injury with the absence of infectious, cardiac, renal, or iatrogenic etiologies occurring within the first 120 days of allogeneic HSCT.[64,65] The earliest reported median onset is at 19 days. It is seen more with allogeneic HSCT with myeloablative conditioning. Mortality rates range from 60% to 80% and >95% requiring mechanical ventilation. IPS has also been reported in autologous HSCT but responds to corticosteroids and has a better prognosis. Risk factors in allogeneic HSCT include full-intensity conditioning with total body irradiation (TBI), acute graft versus host disease (GVHD), older recipient age, and indication for HSCT include leukemia or myelodysplastic syndrome whereas risk factors for IPS in autologous HSCT include older patient age, severe oral mucositis, TBI or bischloroethylnitrosourea (BCNU)-containing conditioning regimens, radiotherapy within 14 days of HSCT, female, and diagnosis of solid tumor. The pathogenesis has been hypothesized to be secondary to the conditioning regimens, occult infections or the host flora derived LPS, and inflammatory cytokines.

* *

Three subtypes of IPS are diffuse alveolar hemorrhage (DAH), peri-engraftment respiratory distress syndrome (PERDS) which occurs within 5 days of engraftment, and delayed pulmonary toxicity syndrome (DPTS) which occurs within 45 days.

* *

Given the heterogeneous classification for IPS and the severity of symptoms, lung biopsies are not always safe to perform or helpful except to exclude infection. There are no standardized descriptions on human histopathology. In murine models, a dense mononuclear cell infiltrate around both pulmonary vessels and bronchioles with acute pneumonitis is seen. Increased levels of TNF alpha are noted in alveolar lavage.

* *

CMV pneumonitis usually results from reactivation of latent virus in seropositive recipients and in absence of CMV prophylaxis, occurs at a higher rate in allogeneic HSCT 20% to 35% compared to 1% to 6% in autologous HSCT. CMV prophylaxis decreases the incidence rate. It is rare that seronegative recipients from CMV-positive donors develop CMV pneumonitis unlike in solid organ transplant recipients. To decrease the incidence, universal prophylaxis or early treatment for subclinical viremia as detected by p65 or PCR assay has been used. Universal prophylaxis is complicated by neutropenia and has delayed incidence beyond 100 days. CMV pneumonitis is diagnosed with clinical symptoms of fever, cough, and hypoxemia, radiographic findings of consolidation, nodules, or ground glass opacities, and demonstration of viral inclusion bodies in lung tissue and/or detection of virus in alveolar lavage. Treatment is a combination of ganciclovir with CMV immunoglobulin and foscarnet with immunoglobulin for resistant cases.

* *

Pulmonary cytolytic thrombi (PCT) manifests as fever, cough, and dyspnea. HRCT shows peripheral nodules. Diagnosis is via surgical lung biopsy showing basophilic cytolytic thrombi in small to medial pulmonary vessels with monocytes. Corticosteroids have improved outcomes.

* *

Pulmonary veno-occlusive disease (PVOD) occurs after 100 days of allogeneic HSCT and manifests as dyspnea with reduced DLCO and restriction. Radiographically, it can present as nodules, ground glass opacities, septal thickening, or consolidation. CT pulmonary angiography shows no emboli and right-sided heart catheterization shows pulmonary hypertension.

Question 2: C. Solumedrol 2 mg/kg/day

There are no current standard treatments although antimicrobials, corticosteroids, and supportive measures have been used. High-dose corticosteroids (>4 mg/kg/day of methylprednisolone) have not been shown to improve mortality compared to low-dose corticosteroids (≤2 mg/kg/day) with the exception of the presence of diffuse alveolar hemorrhage (91% vs. 67%). A potential treatment is etanercept which neutralizes TNF-alpha. In conjunction with antibiotics and corticosteroids, etanercept at a dose of 0.4 mg/kg twice a week, showed decreased oxygen requirements and improved survival by day 56 of etanercept administration.

* *

Patient was not in severe respiratory distress and mechanical ventilation can be avoided. Microbiological studies show no evidence of fungal infection. There was no current role for antifungal. There is no role for diuresis in this patient.

CASE 18

Question 1: B. Asthma

Pulmonary ossification (PO) can be idiopathic or associated with another disease and is defined as bone formation with or without marrow that occurs in the interstitial and alveolar components.[66] Usually serum calcium, phosphorus, and alkaline phosphate are normal. Men >60 years of age are usually involved and the radiographic findings are lower lobe reticulonodular densities on chest radiographs or linear 1 to 4 mm calcified densities with small nodular calcifications on high-resolution computed tomography.

* *

Causes of Pulmonary Ossification

Idiopathic	
Pulmonary disorders	IPF, amyloidosis, busulfan, AIP, sarcoidosis, tuberculosis, histoplasmosis, malignancy
Cardiac disorders	Mitral stenosis, systolic heart failure, idiopathic hypertrophic subaortic stenosis
Other disorders	Hyperparathyroidism, hypervitaminosis D, pyloric stenosis

Pathogenesis is not understood. Ossification can be an end complication of a cascade of lung injury beginning with the degeneration of the arterial media, inflammation, and hyalinization of perivascular tissue. Several growth factors involved in other pulmonary diseases are involved in PO. Transforming growth factor-B, which is implicated in the pathogenesis for pulmonary fibrosis and bone morphogenic protein, which is implicated in pulmonary hypertension, are involved in PO. In addition to these factors, ionic charges, inflammation, and anoxia are involved in the transformation of fibroblasts into osteoblasts.

* *

There are two histologic types: (1) nodular, which are calcified deposits in alveolar spaces without marrow elements and are more common in preexisting cardiac conditions; and (2) dendriform, which are interstitial branching spicules of bone and marrow protruding into the alveoli.

REFERENCES

1. Travis WD, Stabel U, Hansell DM, et al. An official American thoracic society/European respiratory society statement: Update of the international multidisciplinary classification of the idiopathic interstitial pneumonias. *Am J Respir Crit Care Med.* 2013;188:733–748.

2. Souza CA, Müller NL, Flint J, et al. Idiopathic Pulmonary Fibrosis: Spectrum of High-Resolution CT Findings. *AJR Am J Roentgenol.* 2005;185:1531–1539.

3. Meyer KC, Raghu G, Baughman RP, et al. An official American Thoracic Society clinical practice guideline: The clinical utility of bronchoalveolar Lavage Cellular Analysis in Interstitial Lung Disease. *Am J Respir Crit Care Med.* 2012; 185(9):1004–1014.

4. Vij R, Strek ME. Diagnosis and treatment of connective tissue disease – associated interstitial lung disease. *Chest.* 2013;143(3):814–824.

5. Demedts M, Behr J, Buhl R, et al. High dose acetylcysteine in idiopathic pulmonary fibrosis. *N Engl J Med.* 2005;353: 2229–2242.

6. The Idiopathic Pulmonary Fibrosis Clinical Research Network. Prednisone, Azathioprine, and N-acetylcysteine for pulmonary fibrosis. *N Engl J Med.* 2012;366:1968–1977.

7. The Idiopathic Pulmonary Fibrosis Clinical Research Network. Randomized trial of Acetylcyteine in idiopathic pulmonary fibrosis. *N Engl J Med.* 2014;370:2093–2101.

8. King TE, Bradford WZ, Castro-Bernardini S, et al. A Phase 3 Trial of Pirfenidone in Patients with Idiopathic Pulmonary Fibrosis. *N Engl J Med.* 2014;370:2083–2092.

9. Richeldi L, du Bois R, Raghu G, et al. Efficacy and safety of nintedanib in idiopathic pulmonary fibrosis. *N Engl J Med.* 2014;370:2071–2082.

10. Egan JJ. Follow-up and nonpharmacological management of the idiopathic pulmonary fibrosis patient. *Eur Resp Rev.* 2011;20(120):114–117.

11. Steele M, Speer MC, Loyd JE, et al. Clinical and Pathologic Features of Familial Interstitial Pneumonia. *Am J Respir Crit Care Med.* 2005;172:1146–1152.

12. Armanios M, Chen JJ, Cogan JD, et al. Telomerase mutations in families with idiopathic pulmonary fibrosis. *N Engl J Med.* 2007;356:1317–1326.

13. Diaz de leon A, Cronkhite JT, Katzenstein AL, et al. Telomere lengths, pulmonary fibrosis, and telomerase (TERT) mutations. *PLoS One.* 2010;5(5):E10680.

14. Diaz de Leon A, Cronkhite JT, Yilmaz C, et al. Subclinical lung disease, macrocytosis, and premature graying in kindreds with telomerase (TERT) mutations. *Chest.* 2011; 140(3):753–763.

15. Hyzy R, Huang S, Myers J, et al. Acute exacerbations of idiopathic pulmonary fibrosis. *Chest.* 2007;132:1652–1658

16. Churg A, Muller N, Flint J, et al. Chronic hypersensitivity pneumonitis. *Am J Surg Pathol.* 2006;30(2):201–208.

17. Wells AU, Nicholson AG, Hansell DM, et al. Challenges in pulmonary fibrosis 4: Smoking-induced diffuse interstitial lung diseases. *Thorax.* 2007;62:904–910.

18. Ryu JH, Myers JL, Capizzi SA, et al. Desquamative interstitial pneumonia and respiratory bronchiolitis-associated interstitial lung disease. *Chest.* 2005;127:178–184.

19. Poletti V, Casoni G, Chilosi M, et al. Diffuse panbronchiolitis. *Eur Respir J.* 2006;28:862–871.

20. Davies SJ, Gosney JR, Hansell DM, et al. Diffuse idiopathic pulmonary neuroendocrine cell hyperplasia an under-recognised spectrum of disease. *Thorax.* 2007;62(3):248–252.

21. Aguayo SM, Miller YE, Waldron JA Jr, et al. Idiopathic diffuse hyperplasia of pulmonary neuroendocrine cells and airway diseases. *N Engl J Med.* 1992;327(18);1285–1288.

22. Allen J. Acute eosinophilic pneumonia. *Semin Respir Crit Care Med.* 2006;27(2):142–147.

23. Marchand E, Cordier JF. Idiopathic chronic eosinophilic pneumonia. *Orphanet J Rare Diseases.* 2006;1(11):1–4.

24. Wechsler ME. Pulmonary eosinophilic syndromes. *Immunol Allergy Clin N America.* 2007;27:477–492.

25. Bouros D, Nicholson AC, Polychronopoulos V, et al. Acute interstitial pneumonia. *Eur Respir J.* 2000;15:412–418.

26. Marchiori E, Zanetti G, Mano CM, et al. Exogenous lipoid pneumonia. clinical and radiological manifestations. *Respir Med.* 2011;105:656–666.

27. Cordier JF. Cryptogenic organizing pneumonia. *Eur Respir J.* 2006;28:422–446.

28. Borie R, Danel C, Debray MP, et al. Pulmonary alveolar proteinosis. *Eur Respir Rev.* 2011;20:98–107.

29. Hare SS, Souza CA, Bain G, et al. The radiology spectrum of pulmonary lymphoproliferative disease. *Br J Radiol.* 2012;85:848–864.

30. Iannuzzi MC, Rybicki BA, Teirstein A, et al. Sarcoidosis. *N Engl J Med.* 2007;357:2153–2165.

31. Baughman RP, Culver DA, Judson MA, et al. A concise review of pulmonary sarcoidosis. *Am J Respir Crit Care Med.* 2011;183:573–581.

32. Selman M, Pardo A, King TE Jr, et al. Hypersensitivity pneumonitis. *Am J Respir Crit Care Med.* 2012;186:314–324.

33. Bourke SJ, Dalphin JC, Boyd G, et al. Hypersensitivity pneumonitis: Current concepts. *Eur Respir J.* 2001;32:81s–92s.

34. Ferrara J, Levine JE, Reddy P, et al. Graft versus host disease. *Lancet.* 2009;373(9674):1550–1561.

35. Tarlo SM, Lemiere C. Occupational asthma. *N Engl J Med.* 2014;370:640–649.

36. Frankel SK, Schwarz MI. The pulmonary vasculitides. *Am J Respir Crit Care Med.* 2012;186(3):216–224.

37. Wechsler ME, Finn D, Gunawardena D, et al. Churg-strauss syndrome in patients receiving montelukast as treatment for asthma. *Chest.* 2000;117:708–713.

38. Hellmich B, Ehlers S, Csernok E, et al. Update on the pathogenesis of Churg-Strauss sydrome. *Clin Exp Rheumatol.* 2003;21:S69–S77.

39. Vaglio A, Buzio C, Zwerina J. Eosinophilic granulomatosis with polyangiitis(Churg-Strauss): State of the art. *Allergy.* 2013;68:261–273.

40. Stegeman CA, Tervaert JWC, DeJong PE, et al. Trimethoprim-Sulfamethoxazole for the prevention of relapses of Wegener's granulomatosis. *N Engl J Med.* 1996;335:16–20.

41. Kern DG, Kuhn C 3rd, Ely EW, et al. Flock worker's lung. *Chest.* 2000;117:251–259.

42. Atis S, Tutluoglu B, Levent E, et al. The respiratory effects of occupational polypropylene flock exposure. *Eur Respir J.* 2005;25:110–117.

43. Turcotte SE, Chee A, Walsh R, et al. Flock worker's lung disease. Natural history of cases and exposed Workers in Kingston, Ontario. *Chest.* 2013;143(6):1642–1648.

44. Williams SJ, Nunley D, Dralle W, et al. A diagnosis of pulmonary strongyloidiasis by bronchoalveolar lavage. *Chest.* 1988;94(3):643–644.

45. Siddique AA, Berk SL. Diagnosis of strongyloides stercoralis infection. *Clin Infect Dis.* 2001;33(7):1040–1047.

46. Keiser PB, Nutman TB. Strongyloides stercoralis in the immunocompromised population. *Clinical Microbiology Review.* 2004;17(1):208–217.

47. Newberry AM, Williams DN, Strauffer WM, et al. Strongyloides hyperinfection presenting as acute respiratory failure and gram negative sepsis. *Chest.* 2005;128(5):3681–3684.

48. Vadlamudi RJ, Chi DS, Krishnaswamy G, et al. Intestinal strongyloidiasis and hyperinfection syndrome. *Clin Mol Allergy.* 2006;4:1–13.

49. Patel G, Arvelakis A, Sauter BV, et al. Strongyloides hyperinfection syndrome after intestinal transplantation. *Transpl Infect Dis.* 2008;10(2):137–141.

50. Vilela EG, Clemente WG, Mira RRL, et al. Strongyloides stercoralis hyperinfection syndrome after liver transplantation: Case report and literature review. *Transpl Infect Dis.* 2009;11(2):132–136.

51. Roxby AC, Gottlieb GS, Limaye AP. Strongyloidiasis in transplant patients. *Clin Infect Dis.* 2009;49(9):1411–1423.

52. Chan ED, Morales DV, Welsh CH, et al. Calcium deposition with or without bone formation in the lung. *Am J Respir Crit Care Med.* 2002;165:1654–1669.

53. Siddiqui NA, Fuhrman CR. Best cases from the AFIP: pulmonary alveolar microlithiasis. *Radiographics.* 2011;31: 585–590.

54. Jonsson AL, Simonsen U, Hilberg O, et al. Pulmonary alveolar microlithiasis: two case reports and review of the literature. *Eur Respir Rev.* 2012;21(125):249–256.

55. Washington KJ, Moder KG, Brutinel WM. Shrinking lungs syndrome. *Mayo Clin Proc.* 2000;75(50):467–472.

56. Wang J, Liu W. Vanishing lung syndrome. *Can Respir J.* 2014;21(1):28.

57. Kim EJ, Collard HR, King TE Jr, et al. Rheumatoid arthritis-associated interstitial lung sisease. *Chest.* 2009;136: 1397–1405.

58. Lee HK, Kim DS, Yoo B, et al. Histologic pattern and clinical features of rheumatoid arthritis-associated interstitial lung diseases. *Chest.* 2005;127:2019–2027.

59. Hamblin MJ, Horton MR. Rheumatoid arthritis-associated interstital lung disease: Diagnostic dilemma. *Pulm Med.* 2011;2011:872120.

60. Solomon JJ, Olson A, Fischer A, et al. Scleroderma lung disease. *Eur Respir Rev.* 2013;22(127):6–19.

61. Tashkin DP, Elashoff R, Clements PJ, et al. Cyclophosphamide versus placebo in scleroderma lung disease. *N Engl J Med.* 2006;354:2655–2666.

62. Hoyles RK, Ellis RW, Wellsbury J, et al. A multicenter, prospective randomized double-blind, placebo-controlled trial of corticosteroids and intravenous cyclophosphamide followed by azathioprine for the treatment of pulmonary fibrosis in scleroderma. *Arthritis Rheum.* 2006;54:3962–3970.

63. Burt RK, Shah SJ, Dill K, et al. Autologous non-myeloablative haemopoietic stem cell transplantation compared with pulse cyclophosphamide once per month for systemic sclerosis (ASSIST): An open label randomized phase 2 trial. *Lancet.* 2011;378:498–506.

64. Kotloff RM, Ahya VN, Crawford SW, et al. Pulmonary complications of solid organ and hematopoietic stem cell transplantation. *Am J Respir Crit Care Med.* 2004;170: 22–48.

65. Panoskaltsis-Mortari A, Griese M, Madtes DK, et al. An official American thoracic society research statement:

Noninfectious lung injury after hematopoietic stem cell transplantation: Idiopathic pneumonia syndrome. *Am J Respir Crit Care Med.* 2011;183:1262–1279.

66. Crisosto CA, Quercia Arias O, Bustamante N, et al. Diffuse pulmonary ossification associated with idiopathic pulmonary fibrosis. *Arch Bronchopneumol* 2004;40(12):595–598.

67. Konoglou M, Zarogoulidis P, Baliaka A, et al. Lung ossification: An orphan disease. *J Thorac Dis.* 2013;5(1):101–104.

68. Stone J, Merkel PA, Spiera R, et al. Rituximab versus Cyclophosphamide for ANCA-associated vasculitis. *N Engl J Med.* 2010;363(3):221–232.

8

Cystic Lung Diseases

Daniel Greenblatt Fein MD, Stacey Verzosa MD, and Patricia Walker MD

CASE 1

A 32-year-old woman is following up with you in the clinic after presenting to the emergency department 1 week prior with a pneumothorax that was managed conservatively. On physical examination you note multiple flesh-colored papules distributed over the face, neck, and trunk. The patient notes that her mother experienced a collapsed lung on several occasions. The patient's chest computed tomography is shown below.

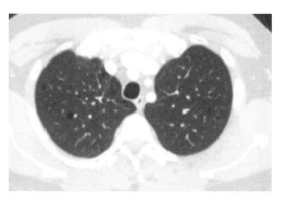

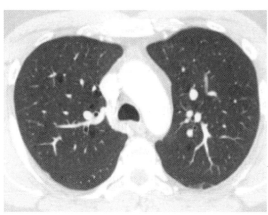

Question 1: **What is the underlying etiology of this patient's lung disease?**

A. Lymphangioleiomyomatosis

B. Birt–Hogg–Dubé syndrome

C. Smoking-related chronic obstructive pulmonary disease

D. Alpha 1 antitrypsin deficiency

E. Neurofibromatosis

Question 2: **What study can be conducted to make appropriate diagnosis?**

A. Serum alpha-1 antitrypsin level with polymerase chain reaction genotyping

B. Folliculin gene sequencing with testing for exonic deletions and amplifications

C. Reduced glucocerebrosidase activity in peripheral leukocytes

D. Whole mount platelet electron microscopy to demonstrate absent dense bodies

E. Serum anti–GM-CSF titer measurement

Question 3: **What malignancy should this patient be screened for and with what modality?**

A. Colorectal cancer with yearly colonoscopy

B. Tonsillar cancer with yearly CT scan

C. Chromophobe renal carcinoma with yearly MRI

D. Chromophobe renal carcinoma with ultrasound every 2 years

E. Multinodular goiter with ultrasound every 5 years

CASE 2

A 36-year-old woman is referred to see you in clinic after a recent admission to the hospital for spontaneous pneumothorax. She reports 3 months of exertional dyspnea and trace hemoptysis prior to the pneumothorax. Representative CT image is shown below.

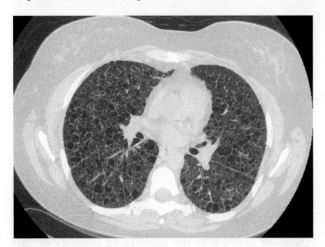

Question 1: **What test may be used to diagnose this patient?**

A. TSC1 or TSC2 mutation in nonlesional tissue
B. Vascular endothelial growth factor-D (VEGF-D) level
C. Mutation of the folliculin gene on chromosome 17p11.2
D. Germline mutation of the phosphatase and tensin homolog (PTEN) gene
E. Serum level of angiotensin converting enzyme

Question 2: **What therapy has been shown to stabilize lung function and improve quality of life in this disease?**

A. Tamoxifen
B. Estrogen containing oral contraceptive pill
C. Progesterone supplementation
D. Sirolimus
E. Smoking cessation

CASE 3

A 55-year-old woman presents to your clinic with 2 years of progressive nonproductive cough and dyspnea on exertion. Review of systems is also positive for dry eyes and mouth. Diffuse crackles are present in all lung fields. Rapid HIV testing is negative. Blood testing

is notable for positive ANA, anti-Ro and anti-La autoantibodies. CT scan of the chest is shown below.

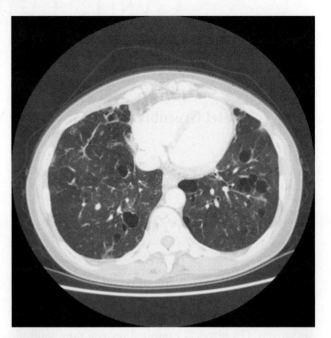

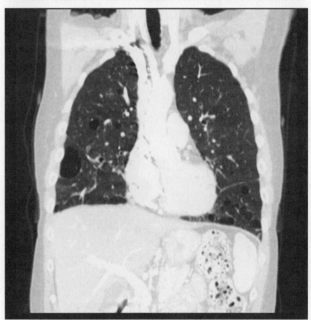

Question 1: **What is this patient's most likely pulmonary diagnosis?**

A. Pneumocystis carinii pneumonia
B. Lymphoid interstitial pneumonia
C. Hypersensitivity pneumonitis
D. Mantle cell lymphoma
E. Desquamative interstitial pneumonia

Question 2: **What further diagnostic test should this patient undergo to confirm diagnosis?**

A. Transbronchial biopsy
B. Serum protein electrophoresis
C. Open or video-assisted thorascopic biopsy
D. CD4 count
E. Low CD4 to CD8 ratio on brochoalveolar lavage

CASE 4

A 39-year-old man presents to your clinic with dyspnea on exertion, cough, and night sweats of 1-month duration. He has a history of 10 pack-years of smoking. The physical examination is unremarkable. Chest x-ray shows ill defined nodules with curvilinear reticular opacities. CT of the chest is shown below.

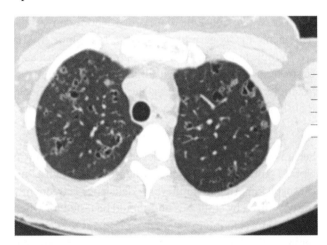

Question 1: **What is this patient's most likely diagnosis?**

A. Lymphangnioleiomyomatosis
B. Pneumocystis pneumonia
C. Langerhans cell histiocytosis
D. Cystic fibrosis
E. Multifocal low-grade adenocarcinoma

Question 2: **What would be the next appropriate diagnostic test?**

A. Bronchoscopy with bronchoalveolar lavage and staining for CD1a
B. Transbronchial lung biopsy
C. Pulmonary function testing
D. Open lung biopsy
E. Fluorodoxyglucose-PET (FDG-PET) scan

Question 3: **What intervention shows the greatest amount of evidence for clinical improvement in this patient?**

A. Smoking cessation
B. Corticosteroid administration
C. Cladribine
D. Referral for lung transplantation
E. Surgical resection

Question 4: **This condition is most commonly associated with which of the following comorbid conditions?**

A. Pleural effusion
B. Diffuse alveolar hemorrhage
C. Pulmonary arterial hypertension
D. Multiple myeloma
E. Sarcoidosis

Answers

Question 1: B. Birt–Hogg–Dubé syndrome

This patient likely has Birt–Hogg–Dubé syndrome (BHDS). BHDS is characterized by benign skin hamartomas (fibrofolliculomas), kidney neoplasms, lung pneumatocysts, and resultant spontaneous pneumothoraces.

* *

Up to 89% of patients with BHDS have lung cysts which are generally localized to the medial and lower lung zones adjacent to interlobular septa and visceral pleura.[1-3] Increased total lung cyst volume, largest cyst diameter, and largest cyst volume are all correlated with increased incidence of pneumothorax in this condition.

* *

Lung cysts seen in BHDS are generally fewer, less circular and larger than those seen in lymphangioleiomyomatosis. Lung blebs from smoking-related emphysematous lung disease are typically apical. Patients with alpha-1 antitrypsin deficiency generally present with dyspnea and often cough. Most patients with BHDS experience no symptoms from their cystic lung disease prior to pneumothorax. Lung manifestations of neurofibromatosis are very rare, and include fibrosis, upper lung bullae, or cysts. The classic skin lesions of neurofibromatosis are Café-au-lait spots and axillary freckling.

* *

Smoking is a known risk factor for the development of pneumothorax in all patients and those with BHDS should be counseled against smoking. Patients with BHDS may engage in air travel but should consult with a pulmonary physician prior to working as an airline pilot or deep sea diving.

Question 2: B. Folliculin gene sequencing with testing for exonic deletions and amplifications

Birt–Hogg–Dubé syndrome is a rare autosomal dominant genodermatosis secondary to a loss of function mutation of the folliculin (FLCN) gene. Identification of the mutation of the FLCN gene by PCR is diagnostic of BHDS. Testing should be accompanied by genetic counseling of the patient and potentially affected family members.

* *

According to the European Birt–Hogg–Dubé consortium, patients should fulfill one major and two minor criteria in order to be diagnosed with the BHDS.[2] The major criteria are at least five fibrofolliculomas or trichodiscomas or a pathogenic FLCN germline mutation. The minor criteria are multiple lung cysts without apparent cause, renal cancer or first degree relative with BHDS. The clinical manifestations of BHDS can be variable and it should be noted that skin findings are not required to make the diagnosis.

* *

Serum alpha-1 antitrypsin level is used to confirm alpha-1-antitrypsin deficiency when there is high clinical suspicion. Alpha 1-antitrypsin deficiency is frequently unrecognized by clinicians and should be tested for when emphysema is found in a patient with early onset emphysema. If the patient or family member has prominent basilar emphysema, anti-proteinase 3-positive vasculitis, history of bronchiectasis, panniculitis or unexplained liver disease alpha-1 antitrypsin should be considered.[4] The diagnosis of severe alpha-1 antitrypsin deficiency is confirmed by demonstrating serum level below 11 μmol/L in combination with a severe deficient phenotype.[4]

* *

Reduced glucocerebrosidase activity in peripheral leukocytes may be tested to confirm the diagnosis of Gaucher disease.[5-7] Gaucher disease is a lysosomal storage disease that may rarely manifest as interstitial lung disease or pulmonary hypertension.[5-7] Targeted DNA analysis may also be used to confirm this diagnosis. However failure to identify a mutation does not rule out this disorder because of genetic variability.

* *

Hermansky–Pudlak syndrome may result in pulmonary fibrosis along with oculocutaneous albinism and bleeding disorders from platelet storage deficiency.[6] Hermansky–Pudlak syndrome may be diagnosed by the demonstration of absent dense bodies on platelet whole mount electron microscopy.

* *

Pulmonary alveolar proteinosis (PAP) is a diffuse lung disease characterized by the accumulation of lipoprotein-aceous material in the alveoli.[7] Pathogenesis is believed to be related to abnormal surfactant homeostasis secondary to GM-CSF signaling. CT scan usually shows ground glass with interlobular septal thickening also known as the "crazy paving" pattern. PAP may be either congenital or acquired. In the absence of a secondary cause of PAP, an elevated serum anti–GM-CSF titer is highly sensitive and specific for the diagnosis of idiopathic PAP.

Question 3: C. Chromophobe renal carcinoma with yearly MRI

Up to 27% of patients with clinical BHDS or carriers of the Birt–Hogg–Dubé mutation may have renal tumors. The most common of these renal cancers is chromophobe renal carcinoma. Renal tumors may be multiple and bilateral. Surveillance screening is recommended for carriers of FLCN germline mutations and for at risk family members. There are no established guidelines regarding the optimum screening age, interval or modality although it has been suggested to initiate screening at age 20 with yearly MRIs to minimize cumulative radiation dosing from CT scanning.

* *

Ultrasound is too insensitive to be utilized as an effective screening modality to detect renal cancer in patients with BHDS. Colorectal cancer may occur in a subgroup of families with BHDS and periodic colonoscopy may be considered. Further research is needed before recommendations can be formally made regarding colorectal cancer screening for patients with BHDS. A range of additional benign and malignant tumors including multinodular goiter and tonsillar cancer may be associated with BHDS but surveillance for these conditions is generally not recommended.

CASE 2

Question 1: B. Vascular endothelial growth factor-D (VEGF-D) level

This patient has lymphangioleiomyomatosis (LAM). LAM is a rare pulmonary parenchymal disorder almost exclusively found in pre-menopausal woman. It is thought to be caused by abnormal smooth muscle cell proliferation leading to progressive cystic destruction of the lung with resultant airway, vascular, and lymphatic obstruction. Lymphatic obstruction may cause subsequent chylous pleural effusions. Abdominal tumors and renal angiomyolipomas also commonly are found.

* *

Characteristic CT scan findings of LAM are lung cysts which are often uniformly distributed, typically round, and have thin 1 to 2 mm smooth walls. The surrounding lung parenchyma is usually normal. These characteristics help distinguish LAM from Langerhan cell histiocytosis (LCH), a smoking-related cystic lung disease characterized by bizarre shaped and upper lung predominant cysts, and coexisting nodules.

* *

The European Respiratory Society has divided diagnostic grouping for the diagnosis of LAM into definite LAM, probable LAM and possible LAM. Definite LAM includes: (1) patients with characteristic high-resolution CT scan and a lung biopsy fitting the pathologic criteria for LAM; (2) a characteristic high-resolution CT in a patient with a chylous effusion, lymphangioleiomyoma; or (3) lymph node with LAM in a patient who has definite or probable tuberous sclerosis complex.[8] Probable LAM is characterized as a suggestive high-resolution CT scan and compatible history or CT findings or compatible CT findings with either angiomyolipoma or thoracic or abdominal chylous effusions.[8] Possible LAM includes patients with characteristic CT findings only.[8]

* *

A prospective study of 48 women with cystic lung disease found that a VEGF-D level greater than 600 pg/mL had a specificity of 97.6% for LAM and a level above 800 pg/mL was 100% specific for the diagnosis of LAM.[9] A negative VEGF-D result was not found to exclude the diagnosis of LAM.[9]

* *

LAM may be classified as either sporadic or associated with tuberous sclerosis complex (TSC).[10] TSC is an autosomal dominant disorder caused by a mutation in either the TSC1 or TSC2 gene. TSC is an inherited neurocutaneous disorder that can result in benign hamartomas of the brain, eyes, heart, lung, liver, kidney, and skin.

Because of variable disease manifestations and spontaneous mutations, the existence of tuberous sclerosis is often overlooked. In addition to a usual evaluation, a full family history as well as skin, retinal and neurologic examination should be performed in every LAM patient to evaluate for TSC.

* *

A positive test for TSC1 or TSC2 mutation from normal tissue is sufficient to make a diagnosis of tuberous sclerosis however 10% to 25% of patients with TSC have no mutation identified by conventional testing. Therefore, a normal result does not exclude the disorder. Patients should be referred to a geneticist if the diagnosis of TSC remains in question. The European Respiratory Society currently recommends against routine genetic analysis for TSC in patients with sporadic LAM.[10]

* *

A mutation of the folliculin gene (FLCN), also known as BHD, is commonly found in patients with the Birt–Hogg–Dubé syndrome.

* *

The phosphatase and tensin homolog (PTEN) gene regulates phosphatidylinositol 3-kinase-AKT and mammalian target of rapamycin (mTOR) signaling pathways. Germ line mutation of PTEN has been described in a variety of rare syndromes known as PTEN hamartoma tumor syndromes. Mutations of the PTEN gene have not been associated with the development of LAM.

* *

Sarcoidosis may be associated with lung cysts in its more advanced stages and an elevated serum angiotensin level may be found in a high proportion of patients with untreated sarcoidosis. This patient's presentation and CT findings are more characteristic of LAM. In addition, the use of serum ACE level is not thought to be a useful tool for the diagnosis of sarcoidosis due to its poor sensitivity and specificity.

Question 2: D. Sirolimus

In a randomized double blind trial of 89 patients with LAM who were given Sirolimus or placebo for 12 months, it was found that during the treatment period the patients who administered Sirolimus had improvement in FVC, FRC, serum levels of vascular endothelial growth factor D (VEGF-D), quality of life, and functional performance.[11] There was no difference between groups in 6-minute walk

or diffusing capacity. After discontinuation of sirolimus, the decline in lung function resumed in the sirolimus group and was similar to that seen in the placebo group.

* *

Although there have been case reports which describe the use of the estrogen receptor modulator Tamoxifen for the treatment of LAM, no high-quality data currently exist for the use of this therapy. For this reason, the European Respiratory Society does not recommend tamoxifen, oophorectomy, or GnRH agonists be used.[8]

* *

Estrogen containing oral contraceptive pills or hormone replacement has been associated with the progression of pulmonary LAM. For this reason, it is recommended that patients with LAM avoid estrogen containing birth control and hormone supplementation.

* *

In a report describing clinical characteristics of 243 subjects with LAM in, 55% were being actively treated with progesterone at the time of enrollment into the NHLBI national registry.[12] Despite its widespread use there are no randomized placebo-controlled trials of progesterone therapy in patients with LAM. For this reason the use of progesterone for routine use is not recommended. It is suggested that if there is a rapid decline in symptoms or lung function a trial of intramuscular progesterone may be undertaken.

* *

Cessation of smoking and avoidance of environmental tobacco smoke should be encouraged in all patients with lung disease. There has been shown to be a small increase in the risk of symptomatic disease progression in patients with LAM who smoke however unlike the cystic lung disease pulmonary Langerhans cell histiocytosis, LAM is not considered a smoking-related lung disease. Smoking cessation as monotherapy likely will not significantly alter disease progression in this patient.

CASE 3

Question 1: B. Lymphoid interstitial pneumonia

This patient likely has Sjögren's syndrome and associated lymphoid interstitial pneumonia (LIP). LIP is a rare lymphoproliferative disorder of the lungs thought due to hyperplasia of bronchiolar associated lymphoid tissue.

* *

LIP has been found to be associated with a host of auto-immune and immune deficient states including HIV.[13-15] As is the case with this patient, up to 25% of patients diagnosed with LIP are thought to have coexistant Sjögren's syndrome and 1% of patients with Sjögren's may acquire LIP during the course of their illness.[13-15] Eighty percent of patients with LIP are found to have serum dysproteinemias, the most common of which being hyper gammaglobulinemia. LIP has always been an uncommon complication of HIV infection. Its occurrence in patients with HIV has become even less frequent since the widespread implementation of HAART therapy.

* *

Typical chest x-ray findings include bilateral lower lung zone reticular or reticulonodular opacities. CT scan often shows centrilobular or subpleural nodules, ground glass opacities and interlobular septal thickening. 1 to 30 mm cysts may be seen on CT scan in up to 82% of patients with LIP. Cyst formation is thought to be due to bronchiolar compression from lymphocytic infiltrate.

* *

This patient's indolent course and negative rapid HIV testing makes Pneumocystis pneumonia less likely. Although hypersensitivity pneumonitis may be considered, a history and clinical workup suggestive of Sjögren's syndrome makes LIP more likely in this patient. Low-grade malignant lymphoma requires pathological distinction from LIP but the strong clinical picture of Sjögren's syndrome makes Mantle cell lymphoma less likely in this patient. Cysts in desquamative interstitial pneumonia (DIP) in relatively rare. Usually, the dominant CT finding in DIP is ground glass. Fibrosis and nodules are sometimes seen.

* *

The treatment of LIP is largely based on anecdotal data with the majority of reports outlining the variable response to corticosteroids, cyclophosphamide, or chlorambucil.[13-15] Suggested regimes of prednisone include 0.75 to 1.0 mg/kg/day (ideal body weight) not to exceed 100 mg/day for 8 to 12 weeks or until stabilization. The dose can slowly be tapered to 0.25 mg/kg/day for an additional 6 to 12 weeks. In patients with HIV associated disease, regression of LIP has been associated with initiation of antiretroviral therapy.

* *

Fifty to 60% of patients may show symptomatic or radiographic stabilization with regression of their disease on therapy while others advance to interstitial fibrosis despite treatment. Prognosis is poor with 33% to 50% of patients dying within 5 years of diagnosis from either progressive pulmonary fibrosis, progression to malignant lymphoma or the infectious complications of immunosuppression.

Question 2: C. Open or video-assisted thorascopic biopsy

In order to diagnose LIP, the disease needs to be distinguished from low-grade malignant lymphoproliferative diseases by the demonstration of polyclonality of B-cell infiltrates on open lung biopsy or video assisted thoracocopic biopsy. LIP is pathologically characterized by diffuse interstitial cellular infiltrates composed mostly of mature lymphocytes and plasma cells.

* *

Lymphocytic infiltration seen in LIP may be observed on transbronchial biopsy but definitive diagnosis requires surgical intervention. Although a large portion of patients with LIP have serum hypergammaglobulinemia or hypogammaglobulinemia, this finding is not sufficient to confirm diagnosis. LIP frequently coexists with Epstein Barr Virus or HIV and with the advent of highly active antiretroviral therapy the incidence of LIP is thought to have decreased. In patients with HIV there is no correlation with CD4 count and the disease is more likely to manifest when CD4 counts are within normal limits.

* *

LIP and hypersensitivity pneumonitis (extrinsic allergic alveolitis) may both show centrilobular nodules on imaging studies, however LIP tends to have a more patchy distribution. A low CD4 to CD8 ratio may be used to support the diagnosis of hypersensitivity pneumonitis but this test is generally not thought to be part of the workup for LIP.

CASE 4

Question 1: C. Langerhans cell histiocytosis

This patient likely has Pulmonary Langerhans cell histiocytosis (PLCH). PLHC is a rare disorder caused by cell proliferation and subsequent organ infiltration of the lungs, bone, pituitary gland, thyroid, liver, or lymph nodes. Pulmonary Langerhans cell histiocytosis may occur as part of a multiorgan disease or in isolation. More than 85% of cases affecting the lungs only manifest as pulmonary disease.[16,17]

* *

PLCH is frequently seen in male cigarette smokers between the ages of 30 and 50. Patients with PLCH are often asymptomatic but may present with dyspnea, cough, chest pain or constitutional symptoms such as weight loss, anorexia, fever, and night sweats. Hemoptysis is infrequent and when it does occur, coexisting bronchogenic malignancy should be investigated.

* *

Chest x-ray is frequently abnormal with early findings of micronodular or reticulonodular and interstitial infiltration mostly in the middle and upper lobes. Later in disease progression nodular lesions tend to be less frequent and cystic changes become more prominent. High-resolution CT scan generally shows nodules and bizarre shaped cysts predominately in middle and upper lobes with sparing of the costophrenic angles.

* *

Cysts are often said to have haphazard distribution in contrast to the distribution of pulmonary cysts in LAM patients who generally exhibit more uniformity. Although both men and woman may have PLCH, LAM rarely occurs in men. The surrounding lung parenchyma in patients with LAM is usually normal, whereas nodules are a common finding in PLCH. In a patient with LAM the costophrenic angles are usually not spared. This patient's indolent presentation and cystic disease on CT scan may be consistent with pneumocystis pneumonia in a patient without HIV, however he has no known risk factors for immunosuppression and CT findings of relative sparing of the costophrenic angles are more consistent with PLCH.

* *

Up to 7% of patients with cystic fibrosis may be diagnosed after age 18. Adult patients presenting with cystic fibrosis are more likely to present with gastrointestinal symptoms, diabetes and in males infertility. Chest x-ray and CT scans of patients with cystic fibrosis are more likely to exhibit signs of hyperinflation and air trapping with subsequent bronchiectasis rather than lung cysts. While low-grade adenocarcinoma can initially manifest as a complex cyst, multifocal adenocarcinoma should have more focal ground glass nodules than depicted in this case.

Question 2: **A. Bronchoscopy with bronchoalveolar lavage and staining for CD1a**

Early PLCH begins as a proliferation of Langerhans cells along the small airways. These cellular lesions expand to form nodules containing Langerhans cells, lymphocytes, macrophages, plasma cells and fibroblasts. In some cases eosinophils may be seen surrounded by a histiocytic reaction. This phenomenon has been described as an eosinophilic granuloma. The cellular lesions of PLCH may progress to form fibrotic nodules that may coalesce with other nodules to result in a distinctive honeycomb-like structure.

* *

Support for the diagnosis of PLCH in a patient with a suggestive history and CT findings includes increased numbers of Langerhans cells in bronchoalveolar-lavage fluid with CD1a staining. If greater than 5% of cells stain for CD1a in a suspected patient, then PLCH is may be confirmed.

* *

Due to the nonuniform distribution of the disease and small amount to tissue, the yield of transbronchoscopic lung biopsy ranges between 10% and 40%.[16,17] Spirometry in PLCH is often nonspecific but may show a pattern of mild obstructive or restrictive findings. Diffusing capacity may be low in 60% to 90% of patients but these findings are not specific for PLCH.[16,17]

* *

Surgical lung biopsy is considered the gold standard for diagnosis but may be deferred unless there are less than 5% of CD1a positive cells in bronchoalveolar fluid. Although elevated numbers of CD1a positive cells may be present in heavy smokers and patients with interstitial lung disease, more than 5% is thought to be specific for PLCH.

* *

Nodules in the early stages of PLCH may have abnormal uptake on FDG-PET scanning but this is nonspecific. Patients with PLCH are thought to be at higher risk for malignancy and so an FDG-PET positive lung nodule should be interpreted with caution in this patient population.

Question 3: **A. Smoking cessation**

The natural history of PLCH is variable, from progression, stabilization, or regression of their disease. Multiple case reports exist of symptom improvement and radiographic resolution following smoking cessation. Despite this literature there is no long-term data regarding progression of disease or mortality in patients with PLCH who have quit smoking.

* *

There are no well-designed clinical trials of steroids or other immune suppressive agents that control for smoking cessation to treat PLCH. Steroids may be considered after smoking cessation has failed. Further immune suppressive agents such as vinblastine, methotrexate, cyclophosphamide, etoposide, and cladribine should be reserved for patients with progressive disease that is unresponsive to smoking cessation or corticosteroids.

* *

Lung transplantation referral should be considered for patients with advanced PLCH though no clear guidelines exist for when referral should take place. Predictors of poor outcomes in patients with PLCH include older age, lower FEV1, FEV1/FVC ratio, and reduced diffusion capacity. Although often performed for early stage nonsmall cell lung cancer, surgical resection is not a treatment for LCH.

Question 4: C. Pulmonary arterial hypertension

Precapillary pulmonary hypertension is a common and severe complication of PLCH. The mechanisms are thought to include pulmonary vasculitis of arterioles and venules, vascular remodeling, and inflammation. Although no randomized data exists for the treatment of these patients, a recent retrospective study reported significant improvement in hemodynamics and a trend toward improvement in functional class among those PLCH patients treated with PAH specific therapies.[18]

* *

Although pneumothorax may occur in 15% to 25% of patients with PLCH, pleural effusion is uncommon. Hemoptysis may occur in up to 13% of patients but diffuse alveolar hemorrhage has not been reported. Hemoptysis should not be presumed to be due to PLCH until bronchogenic malignancy and aspergilloma have been excluded. A number of hematologic malignancies have been associated with PLCH including lymphoma and multiple myeloma but the frequency and association of these disorders with PLCH has not been elucidated. There is no documented association between Sarcoidosis and PLCH.

REFRENCES

1. American Thoracic Society & European Respiratory Society. American Thoracic Society/European Respiratory Society statement: standards for the diagnosis and management of individuals with alpha-1 antitrypsin deficiency. *Am J Respir Crit Care Med*. 2003;168:818–900.

2. Toro JR, Pautler SE, Stewart L, et al. Lung cysts, spontaneous pneumothorax, and genetic associations in 89 families with Birt-Hogg-Dubé syndrome. *Am J Respir Crit Care Med*. 2007;175:1044–1053.

3. Menko FH, van Steensel MAM, Giraud S, et al. Birt-Hogg-Dubé syndrome: diagnosis and management. *Lancet Oncol*. 2009;10:1199–1206.

4. Zbar B, Alvord WG, Glenn G, et al. Risk of renal and colonic neoplasms and spontaneous pneumothorax in the Birt-Hogg-Dubé syndrome. *Cancer Epidemiol Biomarkers Prev*. 2002;11:393–400.

5. Johnson SR, Cordier JF, Lazor R, et al. European Respiratory Society guidelines for the diagnosis and management of lymphangioleiomyomatosis. *Eur Respir J*. 2010;35:14–26.

6. Young LR, VanDyke R, Gulleman PM, et al. Serum vascular endothelial growth factor-D prospectively distinguishes lymphangioleiomyomatosis from other diseases. *Chest*. 2010;138:674–681.

7. Northrup H, Krueger DA. Tuberous Sclerosis Complex Diagnostic Criteria Update: Recommendations of the 2012 International Tuberous Sclerosis Complex Consensus Conference. *Pediatric Neurology*. 2013;49:243–254.

8. McCormack FX, Inoue Y, Moss J, et al. Efficacy and Safety of Sirolimus in Lymphangioleiomyomatosis. *N Engl J Med*. 2011;364:1595–1606.

9. Taylor JR, Ryu J, Colby TV, et al. Lymphangioleiomyomatosis. Clinical course in 32 patients. *N Engl J Med*. 1990;323:1254–1260.

10. Johnson SR, Whale CI, Hubbard RB, et al. Survival and disease progression in UK patients with lymphangioleiomyomatosis. *Thorax*. 2004;59:800–803.

11. Ryu JH, Moss J, Beck GJ, et al. The NHLBI Lymphangioleiomyomatosis registry: Characteristics of 230 patients at enrollment. *Am J Respir Crit Care Med*. 2006;173:105–111.

12. Strimlan CV, Roseenow EC, Weiland LH, et al. Lymphocytic interstitial pneumonitis: Review of 13 cases. *Ann Int Med*. 1978;88:616–621.

13. Swigris JJ, Berry GJ, Raffin TA, et al. Lymphoid interstitial pneumonia: a narrative review. *Chest*. 2002;122:2150–2164.

14. American Thoracic Society & European Respiratory Society. American Thoracic Society/European Respiratory Society International Multidisciplinary Consensus Classification of the Idiopathic Interstitial Pneumonias. *Am J Respir Crit Care Med*. 2002;165:277–304.

15. Shah PL, Hansell D, Lawson PR, et al. Pulmonary alveolar proteinosis: Clinical aspects and current concepts on pathogenesis. *Thorax*. 2000;55:67–77.

16. Vassallo R, Ryu JH, Colby TV, et al. Pulmonary Langerhans'-cell histiocytosis. *N Engl J Med*. 2000;342:1969–1978.

17. Vassallo R, Ryu JH, Schroeder DR, et al. Clinical outcomes of pulmonary Langerhans'cell histiocytosis in adults. *N Engl J Med*. 2002;346:484–490.

18. Le Pavec J, Lorillon G, Jaïs X, et al. Pulmonary Langerhans cell histiocytosis-associated pulmonary hypertension: clinical characteristics and impact of pulmonary arterial hypertension therapies. *Chest*. 2012;142:1150–1157.

9

Tracheal Diseases

Omar Ibrahim MD and Erik Folch MD

CASE 1

A 55-year-old man with a history of COPD and tobacco use initially presented with a productive barking cough and shortness of breath on exertion. He described a similar episode 8 months prior. While in the emergency room, he developed severe respiratory distress, an inspiratory wheeze, and stridor. During this episode, he was hemodynamically stable and his oxygen saturation remained above 95% on room air. Due to stridor and respiratory distress, he was intubated and started on positive pressure ventilation. Shortly after intubation, he was resting comfortably and able to communicate by writing. His hospital course was complicated by failed extubation on two occasions. His blood chemistry and CBC were unremarkable. He had a chest computed tomography which was shown below.

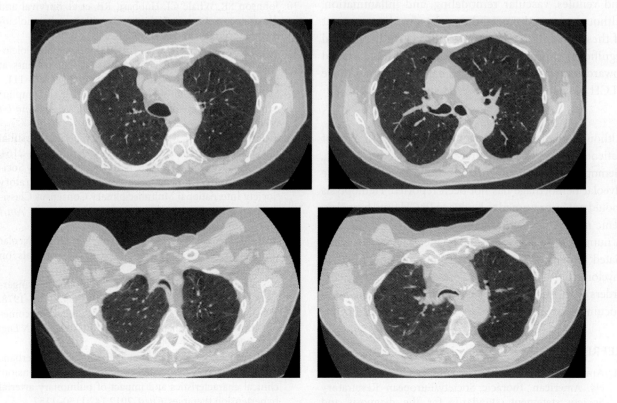

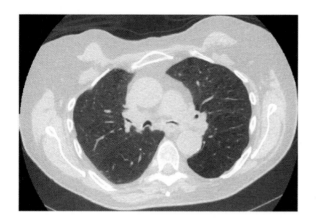

Question 1: What is the next step in management of this patient?

A. Cuff leak test
B. Extubate to CPAP
C. Tracheostomy
D. Antibiotic therapy and reassess in 3 days
E. Thoracic surgery consultation

Question 2: The GOLD standard for diagnosis of this disease is:

A. Rigid bronchoscopy
B. Flexible bronchoscopy with dynamic airway maneuvers
C. pH probe monitoring
D. Dynamic CT of the trachea
E. Spirometry

Question 3: All of the following are considered standard of care for medical management of this disease EXCEPT:

A. GERD therapy
B. Chronic antibiotics for suppressive therapy
C. Pulmonary hygiene with flutter valve
D. Mucolytic therapy
E. Pulmonary rehabilitation

Question 4: Which of the following has been associated with this disease process?

A. The atrophy of muscle and elastic tissue
B. Increased endotracheal cuff pressure associated with decreased blood flow
C. Subglottic edema associated with the endotracheal tube
D. Infiltration of cartilage with T lymphocytes and class II leukocytes antigens
E. Paradoxical movement of vocal cords

CASE 2

A 50-year-old man, nonsmoker, who was previously healthy presented with a slowly progressive onset of chest pain. He described it as midsternal pressure of moderate intensity (4/10), nonpleuritic, without radiation, and accompanied by an infrequent dry cough with minimal intermittent hemoptysis. There was no dyspnea, weight loss, or other significant respiratory disease. He had no joint pain, malaise, or fever. Upon physical examination, vital signs were normal with adequate oxygen saturation on room air. He was in no respiratory distress. Inspiratory wheezing was auscultated with right-side predominance. Wheezing was not responsive to bronchodilators and had gone unnoticed by the patient. Cardiac and abdominal examinations were normal. No digital clubbing or cyanosis was seen. Joints showed no swelling or effusions. Skin examination was normal. A bronchoscopic examination was done and shown below.

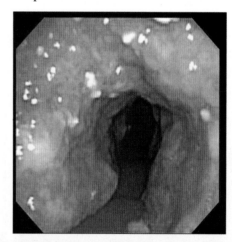

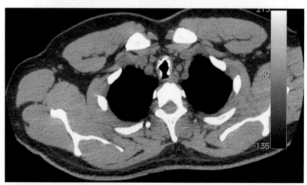

Question 1: What is the most likely diagnosis?

A. Granulomatosis with polyangiitis (formerly Wegener's granulomatosis)
B. Relapsing polychondritis
C. Amyloidosis
D. Tracheobronchomegaly
E. Tracheopathia osteochondroplastica

Question 2: The treatment of this entity includes all the following EXCEPT:

A. No treatment is needed when the patient is asymptomatic
B. Corticosteroids and immunomodulators
C. Laser therapy for hemoptysis
D. Resection for focal disease
E. Endobronchial Argon-plasma coagulation for hemoptysis

CASE 3

A 27-year-old woman presented to a new primary care physician with a 5-year history of progressive asthma. There was no history of smoking or environmental exposure to dusts, fumes, or vapors. Her physical examination was remarkable for a unilateral left wheeze that prompted referral for bronchoscopy. The results of the bronchoscopy and CT scan are seen below.

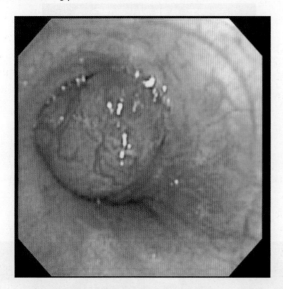

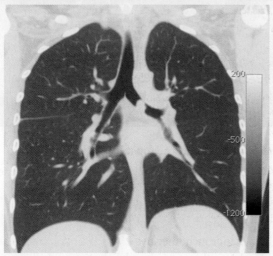

Question 1: The most common cause of a malignant tracheal tumor is:

A. Squamous-cell carcinoma
B. Adenoid-cystic carcinoma
C. Carcinoid
D. Small-cell carcinoma
E. Large-cell carcinoma

Question 2: In a young patient who has never smoked, the most likely diagnosis is:

A. Mucoepidermoid carcinoma
B. Squamous-cell carcinoma
C. Small-cell carcinoma
D. Amyloidosis
E. Lymphoma

CASE 4

A 54-year-old man with a history of smoking two packs per day for 25 years was admitted for recurrent COPD exacerbations requiring intubation and short-term tracheostomy. Six months later, the patient was admitted to the hospital with a COPD exacerbation that required intubation and failed weaning trials due to increased work of breathing. The respiratory therapist reported an absence of "cuff-leak." A flexible bronchoscopy was performed and shown below.

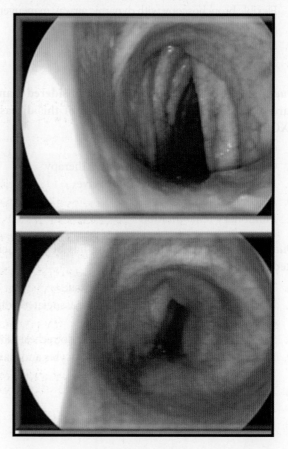

Question 1: **The most common cause of this condition is:**

A. Amyloidosis
B. Granulomatosis with polyangiitis (formerly Wegener's granulomatosis)
C. Relapsing polychondritis
D. Complication of tracheostomy
E. Secondary to untreated sarcoidosis

Question 2: **All the following apply to the treatment of this condition EXCEPT:**

A. The treatment depends on the length of involvement.
B. Some cases can be treated with endoscopic measures such as electrocautery, balloon dilation, or rigid-bronchoscopy dilation.
C. Resection with end-to-end anastomosis is possible in cases with limited involvement.
D. The use of metallic or nitinol stents is recommended to maintain airway patency.
E. Balloon dilation is very useful, but frequently short-lived.

CASE 5

A 47-year-old woman presented to her primary care physician with chronic cough and mild shortness of breath. She had a diagnosis of chronic bronchitis but had never smoked. She did not report a history of exposure to fumes, vapors, or dust. Referral to a pulmonologist for further workup yielded the following image during bronchoscopy seen below.

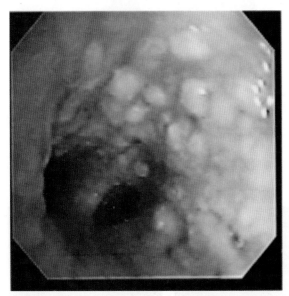

Question 1: **The most likely diagnosis is:**

A. Tracheopathia osteochondroplastica
B. Relapsing polychondritis

C. Sequelae of airway ignition
D. Airway papillomatosis
E. Amyloidosis

Question 2: **The treatment of this condition may include the following:**

A. Tracheal resection and end-to-end anastomosis
B. Endoscopic destruction of obstructing disease
C. Lung Transplantation
D. Bronchodilators and inhaled corticosteroids
E. Systemic steroids and immunomodulators

CASE 6

A 70-year-old Asian woman with a past medical history of stage IIIB squamous cell carcinoma of the lung, who had been considered to be in remission for 4 years after treatment with chemo and radiation, was referred to a pulmonologist for multiple episodes of COPD exacerbation over the previous 4 months. Each episode presented with low-grade fever, shortness of breath with a choking sensation, and a productive cough with a thick, gel-like sputum. These episodes were treated with antibiotics, oral steroids, and nebulizers. Given her recurrent symptoms and history, a CT scan of the chest was ordered and followed with a diagnostic bronchoscopy.

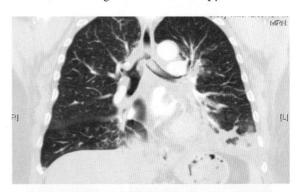

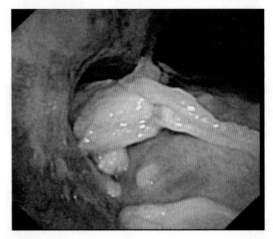

Question 1: **Based on the information provided, what is most likely to been seen upon microscopic evaluation of the obstructing lesion?**

A. Nests of tumor cells and keratin pearls
B. Filamentous organism with a weak acid-fast stain
C. Necrotizing granulomas and giant cells
D. Fibrinous exudates with septate hyphae branching at 45 degrees
E. Charcot leyden crystals

Question 2: **What is the best course of treatment for this patient?**

A. Local radiation for symptomatic control
B. Trimethoprim-sulfamethoxazole with amikacin
C. Four drug anti-tuberculosis treatment for 9-months duration
D. Voriconazole
E. Removal of the obstruction and observation

Question 3: **Which of the following causes of tracheo-bronchitis carries the greatest risk of stenosis after treatment?**

A. Aspergillus
B. Sarcoidosis
C. Amyloidosis
D. Tuberculosis
E. Inflammatory Bowel disease involving the airways

CASE 7

A 34-year-old man with a past medical history significant for 25 hospitalizations for pneumonia, upper respiratory tract infections, and bronchitis was referred for a second opinion. Each admission has significant negative impact on his quality of life, requiring him to miss multiple days at work. His last hospitalization required BIPAP, due to increased difficulty in breathing and hypoxia. He described a chronic cough, which can be productive, with thick green sputum. When these episodes occur, his primary care doctor promptly places him on antibiotics. Notably, in the intervals between infections he is relatively healthy and can perform daily activities. A chest CT and bronchoscopy findings are depicted in images below.

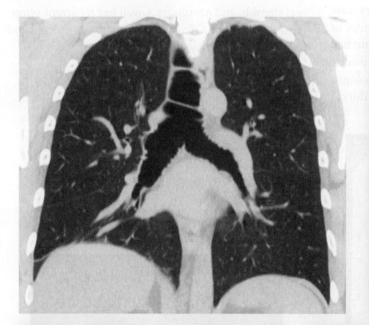

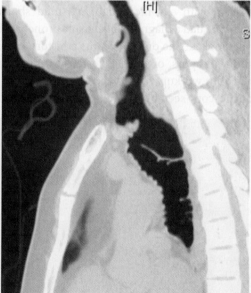

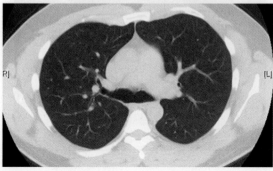

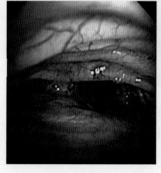

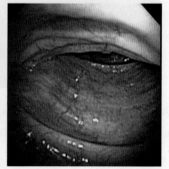

Question 1: **What is your diagnosis?**

A. Bronchiectasis
B. Trachea bronchus
C. Mounier–Kuhn syndrome
D. Williams–Campbell syndrome
E. Cystic fibrosis

Question 2: **If the above patient required an elective surgical procedure, such as a cholecystectomy, which would be the preferred approach for mechanical ventilation?**

A. Rigid bronchoscopy with jet ventilation
B. Endotracheal intubation
C. Double lumen tube
D. Laryngeal mask airway
E. Conscious sedation with airway monitoring

Question 3: **Identify from the following treatment options the one that is NOT appropriate for this disease.**

A. Tracheobronchoplasty
B. Pulmonary hygiene with flutter valve
C. Lung transplantation
D. Mucolytic therapy
E. Pulmonary rehabilitation

CASE 8

A 77-year-old man with a history of COPD presented to the emergency department with respiratory distress and oxygen saturation of 82% on a nonrebreather mask. After nebulizers, intravenous steroids, and a trial of BIPAP his respiratory status worsened and mechanical ventilation was started. Shortly after a first year resident performed the intubation, under the supervision of a qualified physician, the ventilator began to alarm with decreased tidal volumes. The patient developed worsening respiratory distress and significant subcutaneous emphysema. Urgent radiologic images were shown below.

Question 1: **What is the cause and site of this injury?**

A. Rupture of emphysema bullae in the upper lobes
B. Rupture of emphysema bullae secondary to increased PEEP
C. Mechanical ventilation and auto-PEEP
D. Traumatic injury at the lateral aspect of the trachea
E. Traumatic injury at the posterior membrane of the trachea

Question 2: **A right-sided chest tube is placed, what is the next urgent step in management?**

A. Call thoracic surgery for emergent consultation
B. Prophylactic left chest tube placement
C. Advance endotracheal tube 3 cm.
D. Bronchoscopy-guided repositioning of the ETT
E. Emergency tracheostomy

Question 3: **Which of the following is NOT an indication for acute surgical management?**

A. Bilateral pneumothorax
B. Failure of supportive care
C. Esophageal involvement
D. Injury at level of the carina
E. Mediastinitis

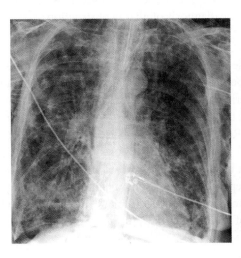
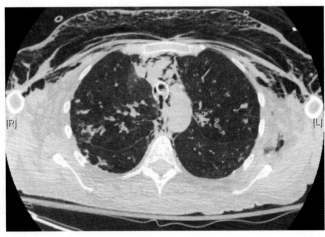

Answers

CASE 1

Question 1: B. Extubate to CPAP

This case is a classic description of a patient presenting with exacerbation of tracheobronchomalacia (TBM). TBM is often seen in patients with COPD caused by concomitant smoking history, but unlike COPD, it is episodic and its exacerbations may be self-limited with use of nonpharmacological therapy. Tracheobronchomalacia is a disease caused by malacia or "softening" of the cartilage that supports the trachea and helps maintain its natural horseshoe shape.[1-6] The causes of this disease process can be divided into congenital or acquired. The acquired TBM is more common in adults, and may be related to chronic inflammation of the airway, COPD and other airway diseases.

**

The morphology of the trachea can be described as saber-sheath trachea, crescent shape, or circumferential. The prevalence in patients with chronic bronchitis has ranged from 12.7% to as much as 44% in some reports.[1] The symptoms of TBM are a consequence of the lack of tracheal wall integrity and wall collapse. This leads to an inability to take deep breaths during episodes of shortness of breath, thus leading to an increased respiratory rate and worsening the cycle of a hyperdynamic airway collapse. Consequently, the inability to clear secretions, due to the malacia, results in increasing rates of infection. A new inflammatory cascade perpetuates the cycle.

**

The patient presents with inspiratory wheeze. Symptoms are resolved with positive pressure ventilation, thus making COPD exacerbation less likely. Positive pressure ventilation allows for airway stabilization of the dynamic airway and opens up the trachea during the entire respiratory cycle.[2] A cuff leak test prior to extubation, while useful in patients with upper airway edema, would be less useful in our patient due to limited intubation time and thus unlikely to be the cause of extubation failure and presenting symptoms. Tracheostomy may ease the

need for mechanical ventilation at a later date and may even mechanically tent the airways open; however, less aggressive measures should be attempted first. While antibiotic therapy may be needed in some exacerbations of TBM, it would have little impact on the patient's current condition. A trial of extubation to CPAP would provide positive pressure and alleviate the paradoxical airway movement; therefore, B is the correct answer.

CAUSES OF TRACHEOBRONCHOMALACIA

Primary (congenital)	Secondary (acquired)
Genetic	Emphysema/COPD
Idiopathic	Chronic infection/bronchitis
Giant trachea or Mounier–Kuhn syndrome	Chronic inflammation
	Extrinsic compression of the trachea
	Relapsing polychondritis
	Malignancy
	Post-intubation
	Post-tracheotomy

Question 2: B. Flexible bronchoscopy with dynamic airway maneuvers

In the patient's current condition (acute illness), a definitive diagnosis of TBM would not be possible. Once he has been extubated and stabilized, a more definite diagnosis can be made. A pH probe monitor is useful in TBM as GERD is a frequent comorbidity. However, it has no role in the diagnosis of airway obstruction.

**

The use of dynamic CT scan of the trachea has been described to establish the diagnosis of TBM. In a small case series, it was shown to make the correct diagnosis in 97% of the cases. However, no standardization currently exists. Rigid bronchoscopy causes a mechanical opening of the airway, and while it is used in placing a Y-silicone stent, it has no role in diagnosis.[3] Furthermore, the need for deep sedation or general anesthesia during rigid bronchoscopy, it is likely to mask the excessive collapsibility of the malacic airways.

**

Flexible bronchoscopy with local anesthetic (lidocaine) and mild sedation will allow the patient to have spontaneous respiration and cooperate with instructions, thus eliciting dynamic collapse of airways in excess of 50% of lumen. Some studies have shown an overlap of asymptomatic patients with 50% of dynamic airway collapse, with symptomatic patients that have similar airway collapse. However, some experts use a threshold of 75% or even 90% of airway collapse to confirm the diagnosis of TBM and to recommend treatment. The patient's symptoms, findings on CT scan and bronchoscopic appearance are all taken into consideration to estimate the probability of the presence of TBM. However, it is also the therapeutic response to the airway stent that confirm if these nonspecific symptoms resolve or significantly improve whenever patency of the airway is achieved.

Question 3: B. Chronic antibiotics for suppressive therapy

Medical management of this disease has been supported by all but chronic antibiotic therapy. Mucolytic and flutter valves provide increased clearance of secretions and likely result in a decreased rate of infections. Pulmonary rehabilitation can aid in the overall improvement of the pulmonary status and function. As previously described, reflux therapy can decrease the severity of the disease, although the benefits of all these therapies are anecdotal and limited to case series.

**

Those patients with confirmed TBM may follow one of the following three scenarios: First, some patients continue their current conservative management and are likely to have episodic exacerbations. Secondly, some patients receive noninvasive mechanical ventilation at home in the form of CPAP. Thirdly, some patients receive a Y-stent trial and if they show improvement, they may be considered for surgical tracheoplasty.[4,5]

Question 4: A. The atrophy of muscle and elastic tissue

While the exact pathophysiology is not entirely understood, studies have shown that in congenital as well as acquired TBM, elastic integrity of the cartilage is compromised, whether from an autoimmune infiltrative process or lack of development in the normal cartilage matrix. One of the most common forms of acquired TBM is seen in post intubation caused by microvascular ischemia from endotracheal tube cuff pressure.

CASE 2

Question 1: E. Tracheopathia osteochondroplastica

The bronchoscopic image of tracheopathia osteochondroplastica (TOC) consists of normal mucosa with a "rock garden and cobble stone appearance."[7,8] Histologically, bronchial cartilage with areas of mineralization is displayed under H & E stain. The CT scan demonstrates tracheal cartilage with irregular nodules studding the trachea involving the lateral and anterior walls but always sparing the posterior membrane.

**

This benign, rare disease affects the trachea and major bronchi. The presence of multiple submucosal cartilaginous nodules is projected into the airway lumen, while sparing the posterior wall are pathognomonic. There is a male to female predilection. However, given the rarity of this condition it is yet unclear.

**

The etiology of this condition is poorly understood. The possibility of congenital origin has been disputed by a case report where a patient developed the disease in an interval of 15 years between two bronchoscopies.

Question 2: B. Corticosteroids and immunomodulators

Treatment of symptomatic patients with TOC can be challenging. The most urgent need for treatment is hemoptysis and airway obstruction. Hemoptysis can be managed by endoscopic techniques such as laser therapy or argon plasma coagulation. Hemoptysis usually presents due to calcified nodules rubbing together and causing erosion of the normal surrounding mucosa. Whenever significant hemoptysis occurs, it is usually the result of erosion into larger vessels. These focal complications may require surgical intervention. The role of antibiotics is limited but may be necessary if a secondary infection is noted due to disruption of the mucosa. There is presently no role for corticosteroids (systemic) or immunomodulators. At this time, it is still unclear what the pathophysiology of this disease entails. Immune-suppressive therapy may lead to a predisposition to infection in an already compromised airway.

CASE 3

Question 1: A. Squamous cell carcinoma

Wheeze is a very common pulmonary symptom with a broad differential diagnosis. In the patient above, we have a 27-year-old with a new diagnosis of asthma 5 years prior without a clear environmental exposure history and with a focal wheeze. Asthma is a diffuse process and thus a focal wheeze is a red flag requiring further evaluation. The bronchoscopic image demonstrates a nearly complete obstruction of the left main stem bronchus with an endobronchial mass. The corresponding CT image demonstrates the mass in the left main stem, but there is clearly no collapse and thus it is providing some ventilation to the left lung.

* *

According to the Surveillance, Epidemiology, and End Results (SEER) program of the National Cancer Institute (NCI) database, the most common type of tracheal tumor by far is a squamous cell carcinoma.[9] In the data collected from 1973 to 2004, squamous cell carcinoma is accounted for approximately 44% of all tracheal tumors, followed by adenoid cystic at 16%.[9] Tracheal tumors favored men over women by 55.7% and 44.3%, respectively.[9]

Question 2: A. Mucoepidermoid carcinoma

The images are not characteristic of any particular type of cancer but given the history of the patient, the most likely answer is mucoepidermoid carcinoma. In the absence of any other symptoms and without significant lymphadenopathy, lymphoma is very unlikely to present, especially as a focal tracheal tumor. Without a significant smoking history and given her young age, carcinoma such as small cell and squamous cell are not likely. While mucoepidermoid carcinoma is rare and only accounts for less than 2% of all tracheal tumors,[10,11] this is the correct answer. It is common in younger patients without a significant smoking history and given the likelihood that her "wheeze" was caused by this, it is a fairly slow growing tumor and could have been present for 5 years.

CASE 4

Question 1: D. Complication of tracheostomy

Tracheal stenosis is an uncommon but potentially life-threatening complication of many diseases. It can be insidious in its presentation, as symptoms will only present once a minimum of 50% to 75% obstruction has been reached. Clinical symptoms can range from asymptomatic to respiratory failure, but a physical examination is usually consistent with central wheeze and/or stridor. Tracheal stenosis can be defined as simple versus complex stenosis. Simple tracheal stenosis has favorable outcomes due to being focal in nature, usually limited to one tracheal ring, and not associated with any malacia or chondritis. Complex tracheal stenosis is associated with longer length, surrounding damage to cartilage, and may have a significant dynamic component.

* *

The images show what is classically known as an "A"-shaped deformity. This is seen in post-tracheostomy patients and thought to be secondary to fracture of the tracheal ring. The other diseases have been known to cause tracheal stenosis but are usually associated with diffuse disease and more concentric stenosis.

Question 2: D. The use of metallic or nitinol stents is recommended to maintain airway patency.

In general, the use of metallic or nitinol stents should be avoided in the treatment of benign tracheal stenosis. The other treatment options are appropriate in this case.

* *

Treatment for post tracheostomy stenosis is driven by the length of airway involvement. Simple limited stenosis can usually be treated with endoscopic techniques which produce good outcomes and have sustained benefits. Surgery is the definitive treatment for those who are good surgical candidates with few to no comorbidities. Balloon dilation alone has a very limited role in treatment of "A"-shaped tracheal stenosis. The dilation will usually push the lateral walls back, usually due to the flexible nature of the walls. Silicone stents have been used for tracheal stenosis with good results; however, metallic stents or nitinol stents have been shown to have complication rates of up to 48%.[12-14] Metallic and nitinol stents can cause a significant amount of reactive granulation in tissue, leading to worsening of stenosis. The complication rate is so high and significant that the Food and Drug Administration (FDA) has issued a warning for metallic and nitinol stents in benign airway disease.[12-14] The warning states that they should only be used when all other options have been exhausted and in the hands of experienced bronchoscopists able to treat the complications that may occur. For this reason, the use of metallic or nitinol stents in benign disease is considered a last resort.

CASE 5

Question 1: D. Airway papillomatosis

The image is most consistent with airway papillomatosis. This can be seen with wart-like projections into the airway. More commonly seen in the upper respiratory tract, it can be seen in the trachea as well. It is considered as a benign disease because less than 1% will convert to malignant disease.[15] It has been associated with the human papilloma virus and has over a 100 serotypes but types 6 and 11 are the most common. There are many classification systems but the Derkay classification system is the most widely accepted because it accounts for clinical symptoms and grades the lesion by location and involvement (from none to bulky).[15,16]

Question 2: B. Endoscopic destruction of obstructing disease

Treatment of airway papillomatosis can be challenging due to the recurrent nature of the disease. Given their viral etiology (HPV), the role of definitive surgical management is limited. Resection of involved areas has conflicting results and has mostly been abandoned.[15-17] Even with the apparent removal of all clinically evident papilloma, latent virus remains in adjacent tissue. The mortality rate associated with airway papillomatosis is low. However, the associated suffering and need for recurrent medical care lead initiatives for better understanding of this disease. The routine use of immunosuppressive therapy such as steroids and immunomodulators is not recommended for treatment of recurrent respiratory papillomatosis. While treatment with antiviral agents and vaccination attempts has shown promising results in the cervical and anogenital tract, they have not shown significant benefit in the respiratory tract.[18] At the present time, the mainstay of treatment is endobronchial management for obstructing disease. This can be done with thermal therapy (i.e., Laser) and endoscopic microdebrider. Lasers such as CO_2, KTP, and Nd-YAG have replaced most surgical procedures as they provide precision vaporization of papilloma lesions in the airways. The major drawbacks include: (1) the risk of airway fire in the presence of high concentrations of oxygen, which can be mitigated by using FiO_2 lower than 40%; and (2) the concerns over laser smoke or "plume" that can contain active viral DNA and extend infection locally or transmit to the medical provider. Some experts have turned to the microdebrider or "shaver" in order to minimize these risks. The microdebrider is used through a rigid bronchoscope or suspension laryngoscopy. It has three components: disposable blade, handpiece, and a console. The rotating blade is coupled with a suction catheter that allows tissue to be drawn into the blade aperture with simultaneous suctioning of the removed tissue and blood. This technique was compared against CO_2 laser for removal of vocal cord papillomas. The postoperative results were better for the microdebrider group, achieving superior postoperative voice outcomes.

CASE 6

Question 1: D. Fibrinous exudates with septate hyphae branching at 45 degrees

The patient presents with recurrent respiratory tract infection symptoms, but of particular note is her productive cough of gelatinous material. The CT scan shows an obstructing mass-like lesion, with a bronchoscopic examination demonstrating a thick exudative material, which appears to be nonadherent to the walls of the airway. These findings would be most consistent with Aspergillus tracheobronchitis. Aspergillus is classically described as septate hyphae branching at 45 degrees. While Aspergillus has been described in a variety of diseases, ranging from allergic bronchopulmonary aspergillosis to invasive aspergillosis, there are three airway presentations: Obstructive aspergillus tracheobronchitis, pseudomembranous aspergillus tracheobronchitis, and ulcerative aspergillus tracheobronchitis (see table below).[19-22] Answer A would be associated with a recurrence of the squamous cell carcinoma, and a CT image could be considered if the bronchoscopic images did not show a mass. Answer B refers to infection with Nocardia that typically presents with a parenchymal pulmonary process, not airway involvement. Tuberculosis tracheobronchitis would give nectrotizing granulomas as described in C, but without a history of night sweats, weight loss, or recent exposure, TB would be less likely in this.

TYPES OF *ASPERGILLUS* TRACHEOBRONCHITIS

Obstructive aspergillus tracheobronchitis	Thick mucous plug with extensive *Aspergillus spp.* without macroscopic evidence of bronchial inflammation
Pseudomembranous aspergillus tracheobronchitis	Extensive inflammation of the tracheobronchial tree with a membrane overlying the mucous containing Aspergillus, seen in neutropenic patients
Ulcerative aspergillus tracheobronchitis	Limited involvement of tracheobronchial tree and typically seen in suture line of lung transplant patients

Question 2: D. Voriconazole

Voriconazole is the mainstay of treatment for aspergillus infections, but for severe disease amphotericin can also be used. While debulking the fibrinous exudative material may be necessary for relieving the central airway obstruction, without antifungal therapy recurrence is likely. The course of treatment can be altered by performing an endobronchial biopsy to monitor if invasion of the bronchial wall can be seen.

Question 3: D. Tuberculosis

While tracheal or bronchial stenosis can arise from any degree of inflammation, it has been reported that up to 90% of patients with tracheobronchial tuberculosis develop stenosis, despite appropriate and timely antituberculosis therapy. This is thought to be secondary to the stages that tuberculosis, from endobronchial infiltration, infection, ulceration, and eventually granulation tissue formation. Sarcodiosis tends to cause stenosis secondary to extrinsic compression from hilar or mediastinal lymph nodes. Inflammatory bowel disease tracheobronchitis is extremely rare, and will present with diffuse sclerosing.

CASE 7

Question 1: C. Mounier–Kuhn syndrome

Mounier–Kuhn syndrome (MKS, or tracheobronchomegaly) is defined as a marked enlargement of the central airways (trachea and main bronchi), with recurrent respiratory infections, dyspnea, and occasionally hemoptysis. By definition, MKS must meet a tracheal diameter of 21 mm in coronal dimension and 23 mm in sagittal dimension in females, and 25 mm in coronal dimension and 27 mm in sagittal dimension in males. It is almost eight times more common in males than females, and often presents in the third decade of life.[23,25] It is thought to be congenital in nature, with the histological features being thinning of the muscular mucosa, and atrophy of muscle and elastic fibers in the main airways. The prevalence of the disease has been reported to be between 0.4% and 1.6% of patients with pulmonary disease.[23,25]

* *

Bronchiectasis is acquired as well as congenital, but classically involves the distal airways.

* *

A tracheal bronchus refers to an additional bronchus originating from the trachea, which is usually 2 cm above the main carina.

* *

Cystic fibrosis involves a defect in the CF transmembrane conductance regulator (CFTR which regulates sodium-chloride transport across the epithelium, it does cause bronchiectasis later in life but the central airways size is unchanged).

* *

Williams-Campbell syndrome is a congenital disorder which causes bronchial dilation, but only presents at the minimum of the fourth order division of the bronchi; while often confused with the Mounier–Kuhn syndrome, this patient has tracheal and main bronchial dilatation.

Question 2: C. Laryngeal mask airway

Recent studies have shown that the use of the Laryngeal mask airway can be effective in managing a patient with Mounier–Kuhn syndrome (tracheobronchomegaly).[26,27] Once seated correctly in the hypopharynx, it can provide a proper seal and avoid some potentially catastrophic consequences. While endotracheal intubation is not contraindicated, the following complications can be seen: it is very common to see out-pouching of the airway and diverticula in patients with Mounier–Kuhn syndrome. If the distal end of an endotracheal tube is placed in one of these blind pouches, ventilator complications can easily occur. The diameter of the airway is markedly enlarged, thus improper sealing and air leaks may be seen, or increased cuff pressures can lead to possible stenosis. Conscious sedation for any procedure in patients with MKS should proceed with extreme caution as these patients have dynamic airways, secondary to malacia, which can cause respiratory distress.[26,27] Double lumen intubation and jet ventilation do not serve any role in routine ventilator support in these patients.

Question 3: C. Lung transplantation

Lung transplantation is not indicated in the management of Mounier–Kuhn syndrome.

* *

The mainstay of treatment for Mounier–Kuhn syndrome is supportive care. While no randomized trials have been done, due to the low prevalence of the disease, the standard care consists of mucolytic therapy, pulmonary hygiene, including flutter valve and postural chest physical therapy. While only limited cases of tracheobronchoplasty have been reported, the outcomes are promising. According to recent publications, only two cases of lung transplantation have been documented in patients with Mounier–Kuhn syndrome, and both died shortly after transplantation.

CASE 8

Question 1: E. Traumatic injury at the posterior membrane of the trachea

Tracheal laceration is seen in this patient: after intubation he developed subcutaneous emphysema, decreased tidal volume, and worsening respiratory distress. The CT scan shows injury to the posterior membrane of the trachea. This is the most common site of injury for tracheal laceration. Our patient also experienced the most common cause of injury, iatrogenic injury from intubation. Incidence of injury increases with emergency intubation and decreased level of experience in intubation.[28–30]

Question 2: D. Bronchoscopy-guided repositioning of the ETT

The endotracheal tube will need to be advanced in order to bypass the area of the injury.

* *

While bypassing the level of injury is the most important initial step in managing a tracheal laceration, it is important to use direct visualization, via the bronchoscope. Blind advancement of the endotracheal tube can cause worsening of the tear, as well as the possibility of advancing the tube into the mediastinum. Chest tube placement is only needed if the patient develops a pneumothorax, if the patient was for some reason not intubated, a pneumothorax of less than 2 cm could be observed, but under mechanical ventilation a chest tube is required.

Question 3: A. Bilateral pneumothorax

Bilateral pneumothorax in itself is not sufficient reason to proceed to surgical repair. A classification system created by Cardillo and colleagues best describes the injury (see chart below).[28] The two approaches to management are conservative management and surgical management. It is reasonable to treat all injuries other than level IIIb injuries conservatively. Injury of the esophagus increases the risk of mediastinitis and fistula formation, and thus surgery is recommended in patients who can tolerate the procedure.

* *

Conservative management consists of:

- Bronchoscopy
- Cuff of ET tube below laceration
- Drainage of pneumothorax (if present)
- Prophylactic antibiotics
- Rule out esophageal involvement
- Daily bronchoscopy and limited blind suction via ET tube

* *

Surgical management should be undertaken when:

- Injury occurs in OR setting
- Laceration is more than 2 cm, or distal 3rd of trachea involving the carina
- Esophageal involvement
- Patient fails to respond to conservative management

GRADE AND TYPE OF TRACHEAL INJURY

Grade	Type of Injury
Level I	Injury to the mucosal or submucosal tracheal with no mediastinal emphysema and no esophageal injury
Level II	Injury to the tracheal as deep as the muscular wall with subcutaneous or mediastinal emphysema and no injury to the esophageal or signs of mediastinitis
Level IIIa	Laceration to the tracheal wall causing esophageal or mediastinal soft-tissue to herniate into airway but without esophageal injury or mediastinitis
Level IIIb	Laceration of the tracheal wall with esophageal injury or mediastinitis

REFERENCES

1. Ernst A, Odell D, Michaud G, et al. Central airway stabilization for tracheobronchomalacia improves quality of life in patients with COPD. *Chest.* 2011;140(5):1162–1168.
2. Ferguson GT, Benoist J. Nasal continuous positive airway pressure in the treatment of tracheobronchomalacia. *Am Rev Respir Dis.* 1993;147(2):457–461.
3. Ernst A, Majid A, Feller-Kopman D, et al. Airway stabilization with silicone stents for treating adult tracheobronchomalacia: a prospective observational study. *Chest.* 2007; 132(2):609–616.
4. Wright CD, Grillo HC, Hammoud ZT, et al. Tracheoplasty for expiratory collapse of central airways. *Ann Thorac Surg.* 2005;80(1):259–266.
5. Majid A, Guerrero J, Gangadharan S, et al. Tracheobronchoplasty of severe tracheobronchomalacia: a prospective outcome analysis. *Chest.* 2008;134(4):801–807.
6. Majid A, Sosa AF, Ernst A, et al. Pulmonary function and flow-volume loop patterns in patients with severe tracheobronchomalacia. *Respir Care.* 2013;58(9):1521–1526.
7. Barros-Casas D, Fernandez-Bussy S, Folch E, et al. Nonmalignant central airway obstruction. *Arch Bronconeumol.* 2014; 50(8):345–354.

8. Leske V, Lazor R, Coetmeur D, et al; Groupe d'Etudes et de Recherche sur les Maladies "Orphelines" Pulmonaires (GERM"O"P). Trachopathia osteochondroplastica: a study of 41 patients. *Medicine (Baltimore)*. 2001;80:378–390.

9. Urdaneta AI, Yu JB, Wilson LD. Population based cancer registry analysis of primary tracheal carcinoma. *Am J Clin Oncol*. 2011;34(1):32–37.

10. Heitmiller RF, Mathisen DJ, Ferry JA, et al. Mucoepidermoid lung tumors. *Ann Thorac Surg*. 1989;47(3):394–399.

11. Zhu F, Liu Z, Hou Y, et al. Primary salivary gland-type lung cancer: clinicopathological analysis of 88 cases from China. *J Thorac Oncol*. 2013;8(12):1578–1584.

12. Plojoux J, Laroumagne S, Vandemoortele T, et al. Management of benign dynamic "A-shaped" tracheal stenosis: a retrospective study of 60 patients. *Ann Thorac Surg*. 2015; 99(2):447–453.

13. Dutau H. Airway stenting for benign tracheal stenosis: what is really behind the choice of the stent? *Eur J Cardiothorac Surg*. 2011;40:924–925.

14. FDA Public Health Notification: Complications from Metallic Tracheal Stents in Patients with Benign Airway Disorders http://www.fda.gov/MedicalDevices/Safety/AlertsandNotices/PublicHealthNotifications/ucm062115.htm

15. Derkay CS, Wiatrak B. Respiratory papillomatosis. *Laryngoscope*. 2008;118:1236–1247.

16. Derkay CS. Task force on recurrent respiratory papillomatosis. A preliminary report. *ArchOtolarngol Head Neck Surg*. 1995;121:1386–1391.

17. Holler T, Allergro J, Chadha NK, et al. Voice outcomes following repeated surgical resection of larngeal papillomata in children. *Otolaryngol Head Neck Surg*. 2009;141(4): 522–564.

18. Vandepapeliere P, Barrasso R, Meijer CJ, et al. Randomized controlled trial of an adjuvanted human papillomavirus (HPV) Type 6L2E7 vaccine. *Infection of external anogenital warts with multiple HPV types and failure of therapeutic vaccination*. 2005;192:2099–2107.

19. Kradin RL, Mark EJ. The pathology of pulmonary disorders due to Aspergillus spp. *Arch Pathol Lab Med*. 2008;132: 606–614.

20. Denning, DW. Commentary: unusual manifestations of aspergillosis. *Thorax*. 1995;50(7):812–813.

21. Tasci S, Glasmacher A, Lentini S, et al. Pseudomembranous and obstructive Aspergillus tracheobronchitis: optimal diagnostic strategy and outcome. *Mycoses*. 2006;49:37–42.

22. Fernández-Ruiz M, Silva JT, San-Juan R, et al. Aspergillus tracheobronchitis: report of 8 cases and review of the literature. *Medicine*. 2012;91(5):261–273.

23. Kang EY. Large airway disease. *J Thorac Imaging*. 2011;26 (4):249–262.

24. Collins J, Stern EJ. *Chest Radiology*. Lippincott Williams & Wilkins; 2007.

25. Krustins E, Kravale Z, Buls A. Mounier-Kuhn syndrome or congenital tracheobronchomegaly: a literature review. *Respir Med*. 2013;107(12):1822–1828.

26. Min JJ, Lee JM, Kim JH, et al. Anesthetic management of a patient with Mounier-Kuhn syndrome undergoing off-pump coronary artery bypass graft surgery -a case report. *Korean J Anesthesiol*. 2011;61(1):83–87.

27. Imashuku Y, Kitagawa H, Fukushima Y, et al. Anesthesia with the proSeal laryngeal mask airway for a patient with Mounier-Kuhn syndrome. *J Clin Anesth*. 2010;22:154.

28. Cardillo G, Carbone L. Tracheal lacerations after endotracheal intubation: a proposed morphological classification to guide non-surgical treatment. *Eur J Cardiothorac Surg*. 2010;37:581–587.

29. Borasio P, Ardissone F. Post-intubation tracheal rupture. A report on ten cases. *Eur J Cardiothorac Surg*. 1997;12:98–100.

30. Gabor S, Renner H. Indications for surgery in tracheobronchial ruptures. *Eur J Cardiothorac Surg*. 2001;20:399–404.

10

Mediastinal Diseases

George Cheng MD and Colleen Keyes MD

CASE 1

A 25-year-old woman with a history of polycystic ovary syndrome on oral contraceptive pills presented with two-and-half weeks of sudden onset, pleuritic left chest pain associated with dry cough and progressive dyspnea on exertion. She denied any associated fever, chills, night sweats, weight loss or hemoptysis. She was a lifelong nonsmoker. Her vital signs were within normal limits. Examination showed diminished breath sounds on the left hemithorax. Chest radiograph revealed a large left-sided pleural effusion with corresponding mediastinal shift (Figure A). Follow up computed tomography (CT) of the chest showed a large anterior mediastinal mass, left pleural nodules, and an enlarged internal mammary node measuring 1.8 cm (Figure B). The thyroid was normal on scan.

Question 1: What is the most likely diagnosis for this patient?

A. Thymic cyst
B. Lymphoma
C. Metastatic ovarian cancer
D. Primary adenocarcinoma of the lung
E. Tuberculosis

Question 2: What is the most likely diagnosis if the mass is located in the posterior mediastinal compartment?

A. Aortic aneurysm
B. Metastatic ovarian cancer
C. Neurogenic tumor
D. Esophageal cancer
E. Lymphoma

Question 3: The patient was given the appropriate workup and diagnosis. As she was about to begin her treatment, she asked, "What are the considerations if I were to require intubation in the future?"

A. Given the anterior mediastinal mass, she is considered high risk for intubation.
B. Given the large pleural effusion, she is considered a high risk for intubation.
C. Given her young age, she is at a less risk of intubation.
D. She is at normal risk with intubation.
E. It depends on her response to her treatment.

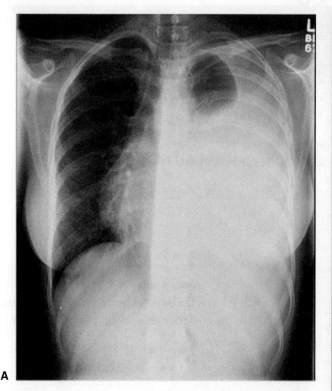

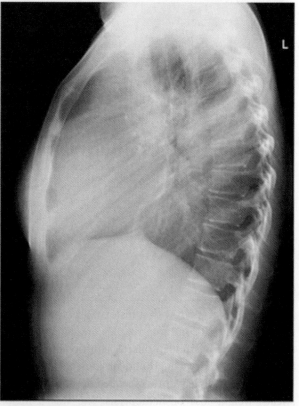

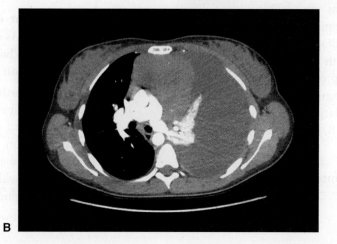

CASE 2

A 41-year-old woman arrives for a 1-month post-partum visit. She reports a dry cough that was present around the time of conception, but since delivery it has continued to worsen. Review of systems is otherwise negative. Vital signs are within normal limits, and physical examination is unremarkable. Basic laboratory tests during pregnancy are normal, including HIV testing. A chest x-ray is performed (see top of page 181).

Question 1: **Which of the following is NOT true?**

A. A cervical mediastinoscopy reaches fewer lymph node stations when compared to endobronchial ultrasound guidance (EBUS).

B. The lack of symptoms in this patient makes a diagnosis of Castleman's disease unlikely.

C. Breastfeeding should be stopped while a woman is being treated for tuberculous lymphadenitis, to avoid drug toxicity to the newborn.

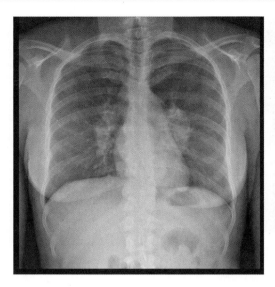
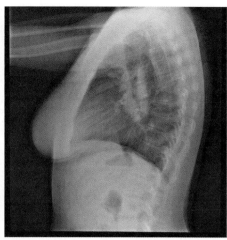

D. Central America is endemic for Histoplasmata capsulatum infection.

E. None of the above.

Question 2: What is true about sarcoidosis?

A. African Americans show an increased incidence compared to the general population.

B. The natural course of disease confined to the mediastinum is progressive and debilitating.

C. The disease has been associated with occupational farming.

D. The presence of hypercalcemia makes tissue diagnosis unnecessary.

E. None of the above.

Question 3: What is NOT true regarding lymphomas?

A. Diffuse B-cell lymphoma shows a bimodal distribution of age at presentation.

B. NK/T-cell lymphoma does not commonly involve the lung.

C. Direct vascular invasion is responsible for non-Hodgkin lymphoma-associated superior vena cava syndrome.

D. Prior history of mononucleosis increases the risk for developing Hodgkin lymphoma.

E. Lymph node involvement on both sides of the diaphragm increases the stage per the Ann Arbor classification system.

CASE 3

A 72-year-old woman with hypertension and 70 pack-years smoking history underwent recent resection and BCG/IFN treatment for recurrent high grade T1 bladder cancer. During her workup, CT torsal demonstrated a thoracic mass note addition of: (see next page). She denied hemoptysis, fever, chills, weight loss, diplopia, or muscle weakness. Her home medications include atenolol, lisinopril, nifedipine ER, aspirin, pravastatin, omeprazole, and oxybutynin ER.

**

Physical examination revealed stable vital signs, elderly female in no acute respiratory distress. Lung evaluation was unremarkable; trachea was midline, no adenopathy. Laboratory study was notable for hemoglobin of 10.6 g/dL, normal MCV, white count, and platelets.

Question 1: What is the most likely diagnosis?

A. Metastatic bladder cancer

B. Lipoma

C. Thymoma

D. Bronchogenic cyst

E. Lymphoma

Question 2: What other syndromes are associated with this mass?

A. Addison's syndrome

B. Red cell aplasia

C. Myasthenia gravis

D. Hypogammaglobulinemia

E. All of the above

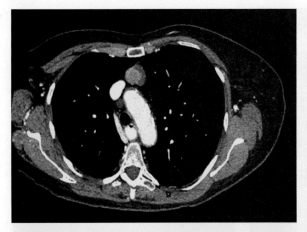

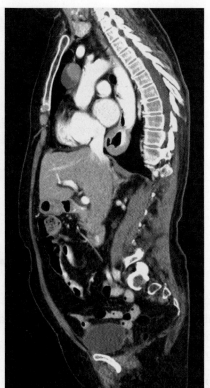

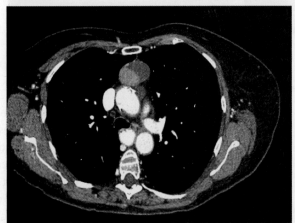

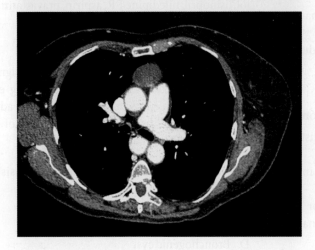

Question 3: **What is the next step in management?**

A. Surgical resection

B. Bronchoscopic needle aspiration

C. Chemotherapy

D. Radiation therapy

E. Palliative care

CASE 4

A 53-year-old man with history of atrial fibrillation on coumadin recently underwent chest MRA in preparation for pulmonary vein ablation. He was a lifelong non-smoker. There was an incidental finding shown on the imaging. He has been asymptomatic, denied any dyspnea, cough, chest pain.

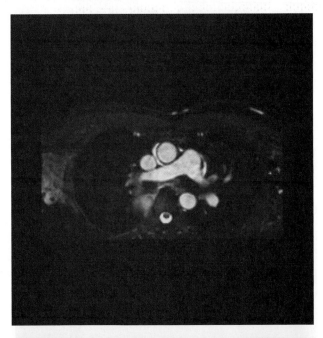

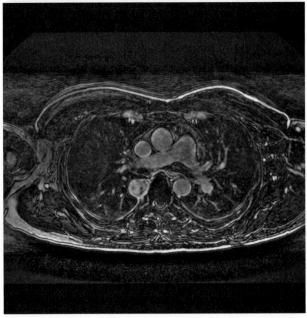

Question 1: **What is the most likely etiology of the lesion?**

A. Schwannoma
B. Lymphoma
C. Bronchogenic carcinoma
D. Thymoma
E. Germ cell tumor

Question 2: **What is the next step of his management?**

A. MRI of the involved spine region
B. Chemotherapy
C. CT-guided biopsy
D. Surgical resection
E. Radiation therapy

CASE 5

A 61-year-old woman with history of Crohn's disease, OSA, and hypertension presented with acute onset of chest pain and shortness of breath to the emergency room. She reported sudden onset, severe substernal chest pain, radiating to the back, which was accompanied by shortness of breath. At the time, she was walking around at a technology sales show. She never had symptoms like this before. She was not dizzy or lightheaded. She denied fever, chills or cough. After arrival to the ED, her chest pain resolved after 15 minutes, although the shortness of breath persisted. ECG showed nonspecific ST changes, cardiac enzymes were negative. She underwent CTA of chest to r/o aortic dissection and PE. CT of chest showed anterior mediastinal mass shown in figures on the next page.

Question 1: **What is the next step in management?**

A. Refer to PCP for outpatient management
B. Repeat CT chest in 12 months
C. PET-CT as soon as possible
D. CT-guided biopsy as soon as possible
E. Comparing to a prior CT scan

Question 2: **What is the most likely diagnosis?**

A. Teratoma
B. Bochdaleck hernia
C. Lymphoma
D. Thymoma
E. Morgagni hernia

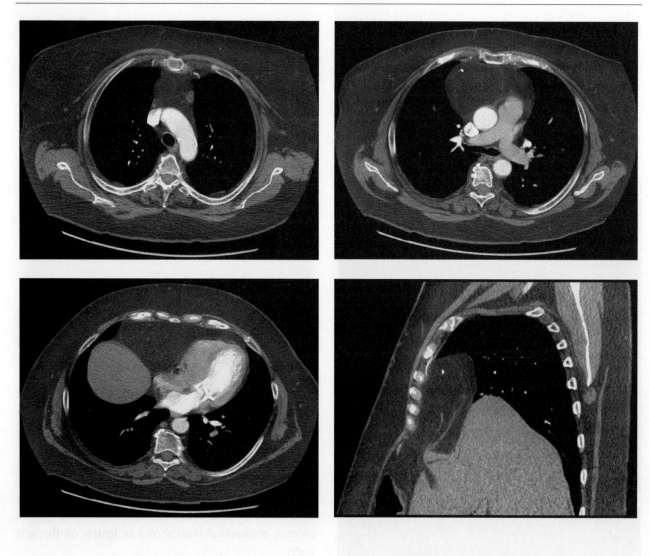

CASE 6

A 26-year-old man of South-East Indian descent (born in the United States) with no past medical history presented with cough and hemoptysis for 1-week duration. He was in his usual state of health until a week ago when he returned from a camping trip to Acadia national park. He reported fatigue, weakness, and had a cough productive of yellow sputum. Approximately 4 days into his course, he developed chest pain with cough, which he described as splinting. Fever, chills, night sweats, loss of appetite and hemoptysis shortly followed. He reported bright red blood streaks with his sputum. He worked as a computer programmer for a local pharmaceutical company. He denied any recent sick contact, smoking history, drug abuse, or prior TB exposure. He had not been sexually active in the past 3 years. He had dog at home but no other pets.

On physical examination, he had stable vitals. Slight sinus tenderness, posterior pharynx had slight erythema and but no exudate. Enlarged inguinal lymph nodes were appreciated. Pulmonary examination was benign. Rest of the examination was unremarkable. Laboratory findings were significant for lactate dehydrogenase (LDH) level of 1850 u/L; otherwise, normal CBC and chemistries. Results of a urinalysis were normal. CT scan (see following page) showed multiple bilateral nodules of variable sizes with the largest measuring up to 2 cm.

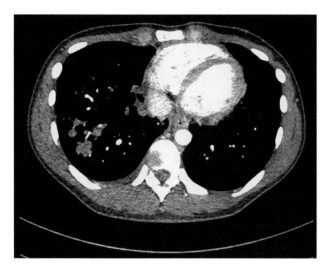 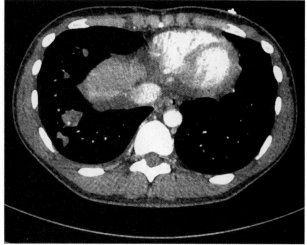

Question 1: **What is the best next step in management of this patient?**

A. Bronchoalveolar lavage with biopsy
B. Transthoracic needle aspiration
C. Focused testicular examination and ultrasound
D. Blood cultures and initiate broad-spectrum antibiotics
E. MRI of the chest

Question 2: **What is the blood test that is useful for diagnosis?**

A. D-dimer
B. AFB
C. Beta-hCG
D. IgE
E. ANCA

Question 1: **What is the most likely diagnosis?**

A. Pulmonary vein stenosis due to prior PVI
B. Pulmonary vein stenosis due to fibrosis mediastinitis
C. Pulmonary vein stenosis due to cancer compression
D. Pulmonary vein stenosis due to foreign body aspiration
E. Pulmonary vein stenosis due to cancer

Question 2: **What is the best next step in management of this patient?**

A. Get more history to see if there is bat-cave exploration
B. Send for anti–GM-CSF antibody
C. Perform flexible bronchoscopy with stent insertion
D. Start antifungal medications
E. Send for IR for pulmonary vein stenting

CASE 7

A 66-year-old man with a history of refractory atrial fibrillation status post-radiofrequency ablation 5 years prior (left upper, middle and right upper PVI), presented with hemoptysis. He has worked for an engineering company, lived and moved mostly in the mid-west states. He has a 30 pack-years smoking history, quit 18 years ago. Initial studies were notable for negative urine histoplasma antigen, serum galactomannan, 1,3 beta-glucan, blastomyces antibody, hepatitis panel, and HIV serology. He underwent CT scan of chest and ventilation perfusion for the hemoptysis which is shown on the following page.

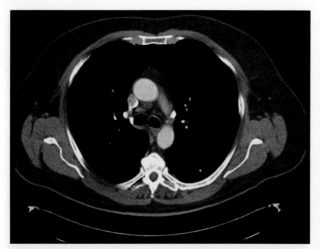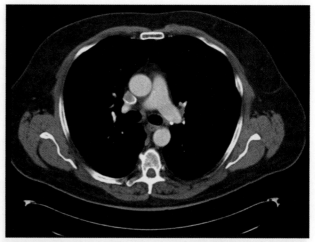

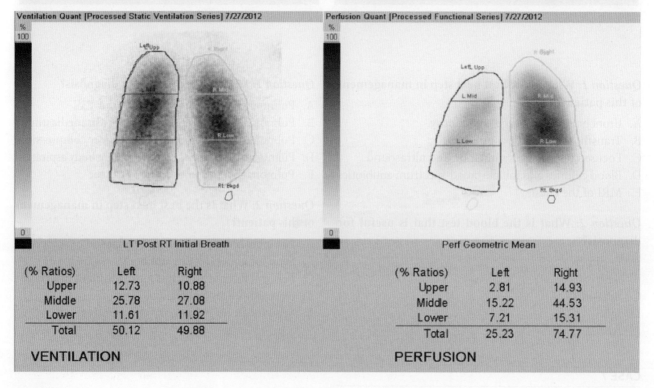

(% Ratios)	Left	Right
Upper	12.73	10.88
Middle	25.78	27.08
Lower	11.61	11.92
Total	50.12	49.88

VENTILATION

(% Ratios)	Left	Right
Upper	2.81	14.93
Middle	15.22	44.53
Lower	7.21	15.31
Total	25.23	74.77

PERFUSION

Answers

CASE 1

Question 1: B. Lymphoma

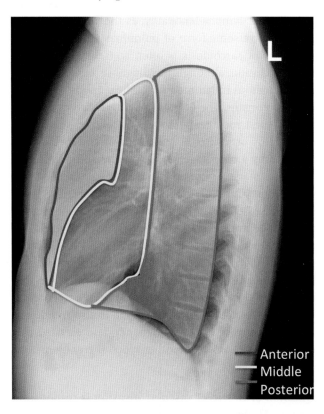

Mediastinal borders are defined by thoracic inlet superiorly, the diaphragm inferiorly, the sternum anteriorly, and the spine posteriorly, with pleural spaces laterally.[1-3] Three major anatomical compartments are anterior (sternum to great vessel and anterior pericardium), middle (anterior pericardium to thoracic spine) and posterior (spine to costovertebral sulci). Lesions that occur in the anterior compartment are often referred to as the "terrible T's": Thymoma, Teratoma, "Terrible" lymphoma, and Thyroid tissue. The most common lesion in the middle compartment is lymphadenopathy due to lymphoma, sarcoid, or metastatic lung cancer. Neurogenic tumors are the most common causes of lesions in the posterior compartment.[1]

DIFFERENTIAL FOR MEDIASTINAL MASSES

Anterior	Middle	Posterior
Goiter	Lymphoma	Neurogenic tumor *50%*
Ascending aortic aneurysm	Lymph node hyperplasia	Aortic aneurysm
Parathyroid tumor	Bronchogenic tumor	Enteric cyst
Esophageal tumor	Bronchogenic cyst	Hiatal hernia
Angiomatous tumor		Esophageal tumor
Teratoma		Bronchogenic tumor
Thymic neoplasm *Most Common**		Paraspinal abscess
Pericardial cyst *LOS.*		Extramedullary hematopoiesis
Lymphoma		
Morgagni hernia *— Congenital ® sm Ant*		
Lipoma		

(handwritten annotations: foot @ Bdachek; Histal hernia)

* *

In adults, the most common lesion in the anterior compartment is thymoma then lymphoma and germ cell tumors (teratoma). While thymoma is common, thymic cysts, congenital or acquired, are rare. Thymic cysts appear as a simple homogenous cyst on CT chest which is not seen in this patient. A history of PCOS does carry an increased risk of developing endometrial cancer; the risk of developing ovarian cancer is not well defined. Adenocarcinoma of the lung with an anterior mediastinal mass in a young nonsmoker is an unlikely diagnosis. While tuberculosis can present as an anterior mass, the lack of systemic symptoms and risk factors for exposure argues against this choice. Given our patient's young age, lymphoma and germ cell tumors, usually presenting between the second and fourth decade of life, are the most likely diagnosis for the anterior mediastinal mass.

Question 2: C. Neurogenic tumor

Neurogenic tumors account for over 50% of posterior mediastinum masses. These lesions are classified based upon their neural cell of origin. In adults, 90% of the neurogenic tumors arise from the intercostals nerve sheath and are benign schwannomas or neurofibromas.[1-4]

romas, which occur more commonly in young are benign lesions that arise from the sympathetic glia; whereas, neuroblastomas and ganglioneuroblastomas are malignant tumors that occur most commonly in children. Lesions that arise from paraganglionic cells include pheochromocytomas and paragangliomas. Some neurogenic tumors involve posterior mediastinal and intraspinal compartments; thus, resection usually requires a combined approach with neurosurgery and thoracic surgery.

Question 3: A. Given the anterior mediastinal mass, she is considered high risk for intubation.

When managing a patient with a large anterior mediastinal mass complicated by a large pleural effusion, one must evaluate the extent of airway obstruction and pericardial involvement. At induction, patient may experience airway obstruction due to anterior compression of the airway by the mass effect. Thus, it is important to evaluate for tracheobronchial compression that can occur distal to the end of the ETT.[5] Patients who are at high risk should be considered for local or regional anesthesia to undergo diagnostic and therapeutic procedures. Awake intubation of the trachea before induction can be done in adults, especially if there is a specific area of compression that can be bypassed by the endotracheal tube.

CASE 2

Question 1: C. Breastfeeding should be stopped while a woman is being treated for tuberculous lymphadenitis, to avoid drug toxicity to the newborn.

The four drugs commonly used to treat tuberculosis in the antimycobacterial era—rifampin, isoniazid, pyrazinamide, and ethambutol—are all safe to use in breastfeeding women, as the dose in breast milk is just a small fraction of the normal dose used to treat infants with disease.[6] Breastfeeding infants should receive pyridoxine supplementation, though, and breastfeeding would be contraindicated in the need for treatment with rifabutin or a fluoroquinolone.[6] Interestingly, in the United States, pyrazinamide is not used as a first-line agent in pregnant women due to unclear effects on the fetus.[7]

Question 2: A. African Americans show an increased incidence compared to the general population.

Sarcoidosis is a granulomatous disease of still unknown etiology, however a genetic linkage has long been suggested. Cluster analyses among African Americans have

been estimated to exhibit a three- to fourfold increased incidence of sarcoid, with an increased familial relative risk compared to Caucasian Americans.[7-10] An environmental link has also been postulated, however, an occupational link to farming has not been found. A similar disease presentation is with chronic beryllium exposure, which would include work that commonly involves the development of nuclear weapons and military aircraft, or the manufacturing or recycling of electronic or computer components.

**

The disease is commonly suspected when a chest x-ray reveals hilar lymphadenopathy, as the vast majority of patients have some form of pulmonary involvement. A diagnosis of sarcoidosis is often considered a diagnosis of exclusion, although the diagnosis can be made if granulomatous inflammation can be demonstrated in at least two organs. The original staging, based on evaluation of chest roentgenograms, is as follows: stage 0: no adenopathy or infiltrates; stage 1: hilar and mediastinal adenopathy alone; stage 2: adenopathy and pulmonary infiltrates; stage 3: pulmonary infiltrates alone; and stage 4: pulmonary fibrosis. About 90% of those diagnosed with stage 1 disease will show spontaneous resolution; stage 3 patients are much less likely to show such at 2 years. The activated macrophages present in sarcoid granulomas produce calcitriol independent of the normal renal feedback mechanisms, and parathyroid hormone-related peptide production has also been suspected to contribute to hypercalcemia. This hormone is also implicated in the hypercalcemia of malignancy, and elevated calcium levels can be seen in other types of granulomatous diseases.

Question 3: C. Direct vascular invasion is responsible for non-Hodgkin lymphoma-associated superior vena cava syndrome.

Superior vena cava (SVC) syndrome is a condition that is most commonly associated with malignant invasion or external compression, and can often present with cough and dyspnea, along with facial or arm swelling. Our patient did not suffer from this problem, but it is important to understand its presentation and management. Over 90% of cases are caused by lung cancers, with just a minority caused by Non-Hodgkin lymphoma (NHL), despite NHL's frequent association with mediastinal, and head and neck lymphadenopathy. When SVC syndrome is associated with NHL, it occurs from external compression, not vascular invasion.[1]

Table 10–1   MASAOKA STAGING SYSTEM FOR BOTH THYMOMAS AND THYMIC CARCINOMAS[1,11]

Stage	Histological/Anatomical Findings	Treatment	5-yr Survival
I	Macroscopically and microscopically completely encapsulated	Surgery	94–100%
II	A: Microscopic transcapsular invasion B: Macroscopic invasion into surrounding fatty tissue or grossly adherent to but not through the mediastinal pleura or pericardium	Surgery and adjuvant RT	86–95%
III	A: Macroscopic invasion into pericardium or lung without great vessel invasion B: Macroscopic invasion into pericardium or lung with great vessel invasion	Neoadjuvant chemotherapy, surgery, adjuvant RT	56–69%
IV	A: Pleural or pericardial dissemination B: Lymphogenous or hematogenous metastases	Chemotherapy	11–50%

CASE 3

Question 1: C. Thymoma

Computed tomography (CT) scan reveals an anterior mediastinum mass of mixed solid and cystic components. There is no mediastinal, hilar, or axillary lymph node enlargement. Heart, pericardium, and great vessels are within normal limits. Comprising approximately 20% of mediastinal neoplasms, thymomas are the most common anterior mediastinal masses. Therefore, they are the most likely diagnosis of an anterior mediastinal mass in adults. Thymomas are well-defined tumors with smooth margins located adjacent to the great vessels. Typically they present as incidental findings on thoracic imaging studies in an asymptomatic patient (50–60%). Localized symptoms are due to compression of the adjacent structures, or due to paraneoplastic syndrome evaluation.

* *

Metastatic bladder cancer is not likely as patient did not have invasive disease (T1). Lipoma and bronchogenic cysts are usually uniform density on CT scan of fat and fluid respectively. This is not the case for our patient. Other common causes of anterior mediastinal masses include lymphomas and germ cell tumor/teratoma. Lymphomas are more common in younger patients and often present with airway obstruction and associated systemic symptoms.

Question 2: E. All of the above

Thymomas, typically present in 40 to 60 age group with a slight male predominance, are strongly associated with paraneoplastic findings in up to 60% of patients, including myasthenia gravis in 30% to 40% of cases.[11]

Myasthenia gravis arises from the presences of autoantibodies to acetylcholine receptors leading to symptoms such as weakness, easy fatigability, diplopia, ptosis, and dysphagia. Thymic production of autoantibodies also can lead to hypogammaglobulinemia, Addison syndrome, and pure red cell aplasia. Not mentioned in the answer choices is thymoma-associated multiorgan autoimmunity (TAMA), which mimics graft-verse-host disease and can present with symptoms such as skin rash, diarrhea, and elevated liver enzymes.

Question 3: A. Surgical resection

Given our patient's localized disease, she will benefit from surgical resection. Thymomas can be benign or malignant. The Masaoka staging system uses anatomical involvement and histological invasiveness (See Table 10-1). About 60% of thymomas are benign and contained within a capsule and without any spread. These are treated with surgery and have an excellent prognosis. In contrast, malignant thymomas are invasive and are treated with surgery and radiation. These carry a poor prognosis. Overall, prognosis correlates with level of invasiveness, histology, and staging.

CASE 4

Question 1: A. Schwannoma

Posterior mediastinum contains thoracic descending aorta, esophagus, thoracic duct, proximal intercostals neurovascular bundles, the spinal ganglia, the sympathetic chain, lymphatic and connective tissue. It is defined as the anatomical space bounded anteriorly by the posterior pericardium, posteriorly by the vertebral bodies, laterally

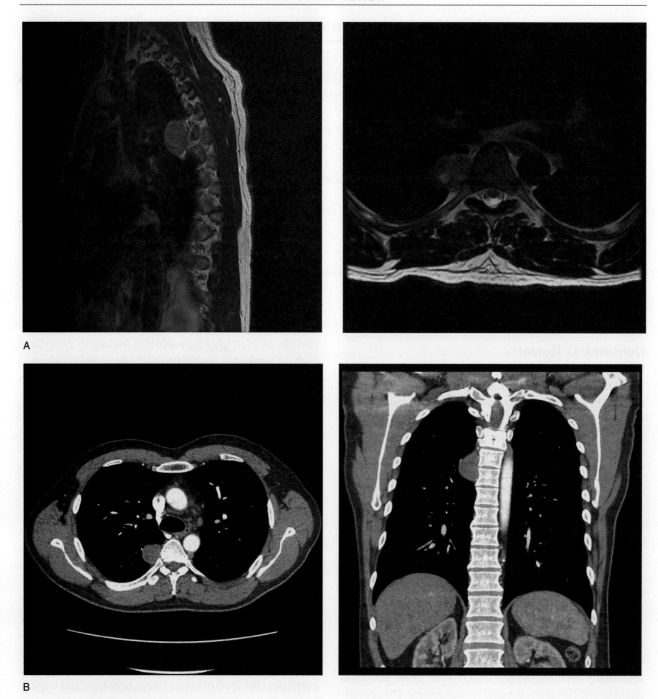

Figure: A Cardiac MRI representative slices. B. CT scan.

by the mediastinal pleura. The large posterior mediastinum mass most likely is schwannoma. Neurogenic tumors make up approximately 60% of posterior mediastinal masses. Peripheral nerves give rise to schwannomas, neurofibromas, and malignant tumors of the nerve. Sympathetic ganglia give rise to ganglioneuromas, ganglioneuroblastomas, and neuroblastomas. Schwannomas and neurofibromas affect male and female equally, with peak incidence usually in the 30 to 40 years of age.

Thymomas are located in the anterior mediastinum. Germ cell tumor usually affects the anterior mediastinum and is present in an earlier age group with male predominance. Lymphoma can affect all three compartments; however, it mostly affects the middle compartment. Bronchogenic carcinoma in a life-long nonsmoking male is highly unlikely.

Question 2: **A. MRI of the involved spine region**

About 90% of neurogenic tumors in adults occur in the posterior mediastinum. Majority of the tumors are slow growing and amenable to surgical intervention. Often, the tumors are found incidentally as patients are mostly asymptomatic. Schwannomas usually arise as single benign lesions in the costovertebral sulcus, but multiple lesions have been described. In approximately 10% of schwannomas, the tumor may extend to the spinal canal (dumbbell tumors). T1-weighted MRI is helpful in evaluation of vertebral column and spinal cord involvement by the tumor. Dumbbell tumors will require combined resection approach with neurosurgery and thoracic surgery.

CASE 5

Question 1: **E. Comparing to a prior CT scan**

The mass-abnormality with questionable calcification located in the anterior compartment is concerning for a teratoma. However, given the history of sudden onset of patient's chest pain, comparison to a prior film if available would provide valuable information. As shown below, the mass was not present 3 months prior on a CT abdomen and pelvis. This makes teratoma a highly unlikely possibility. Referral to PCP and repeat CT scan of chest are not great options given patient's symptoms and the large abnormality. PET-CT and CT-guided biopsy would not lead to a diagnosis, are costly, and expose the patient to the risk of either radiation or complications of an invasive procedure.

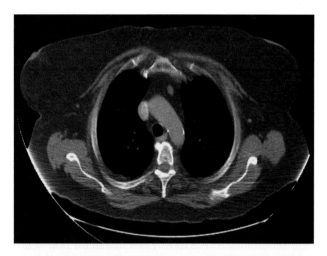

Question 2: **E. Morgagni hernia**

The mass-like abnormality with questionable calcification seen in the standard CT scan is a Morgagni hernia. Having the coronal and sagittal reconstruction will help to trace the origin of the hernia. Comparing with the prior CT scan will likely give an appreciation of recent development of the hernia. Morgagni hernia usually occurs anteriorly on the right with loops of bowel herniating through the foramen of Morgagni. In adults, these hernias develop as a result of trauma or persisting congenital abnormality.[12,13] Bochdaleck hernia occurs posteriorly on the left with loops of bowel herniating through the foramen of Bochdaleck. Given their respective locations, stomach, ileum, colon, and spleen most commonly are associated with herniating through Bochdaleck hernia. With Morgagni hernia, the liver or right kidney may herniate in addition to the bowel. Symptomatic hernias in adults are usually surgically corrected.

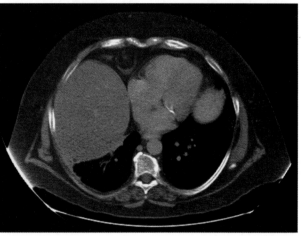

CASE 6

Question 1: **C. Focused testicular examination**

Testicular cancer should be considered in a young male who presents inguinal lymphadenopathy, hemoptysis, and radiographic findings of multiple nodules of varying size and shape. History is not suggestive of infection (born in the United States, no TB exposure, no recent sick contact), no risk factors for HIV infection or IV drug use, no fever or white count, and normal vital signs. Thus, blood culture and broad-spectrum antibiotics are not the best next step. Given the concern of testicular cancer, a focused thorough testicular examination and ultrasound should be performed.

* *

MRI of the chest, TTNA, BAL, and biopsy will put the patient through unnecessary costly procedures without achieving any definitive diagnosis.

Question 2: **C. Beta-hCG**

According to NCI, in 2014, there are more than 8,800 new cases of testicular cancer diagnosed in the United States, comprising of 0.5% of all new cancer cases, with a 5-year survival rate of 95%.[14,15] Germ cell tumors are the most common solid tumors in men between the ages of 15 and 34 years of age.[14,15] Germ cell tumors include seminoma and nonseminoma. Nonseminomatous tumors include embryonal cell carcinoma, choriocarcinoma, yolk sac tumor, and teratoma. Nonseminoma has a more aggressive behavior. There are several tumor markers for germ cell tumor. Beta-hCG, AFP, and LDH are often elevated. Beta-hCG is elevated in both seminoma and non-seminoma. AFP is mostly elevated in the non-seminoma subtype. Thus, an elevated beta-hCG in this patient will support the diagnosis of metastatic germ cell tumor.

CASE 7

Question 1: **B. Pulmonary vein stenosis due to fibrosis mediastinitis**

The CT images are consistent with fibrosing mediastinitis resulting from excessive fibrotic reaction in the mediastinum resulting in airway and vascular compromise and associated symptoms related to the location and extent of fibrosis. Fibrosing mediastinitis is associated with histoplasmosis infection. *Histoplasma capsulatum*, a dimorphic fungus, is endemic in the central, southeastern, and the mid-Atlantic United States.[16] Infection with *H. capsulatum* ranges from asymptomatic to fibrosing mediastinitis. *H. capsulatum* inoculates via the lung, then disseminates to the mediastinal lymph nodes and other reticuloendothelial organs where cell-mediated immunity contains the fungus. The involved mediastinal lymph nodes can form a mediastinal granuloma or can lead to a sclerosing process called fibrosing mediastinitis.

Question 2: **E. Send for IR for pulmonary vein stenting**

Patient hemoptysis is likely the effect of fibrosing mediastinitis. Pulmonary vein stenting will help reduce pulmonary pressure and reduce hemoptysis. History of bat cave exploration only supports the diagnosis but does not address hemoptysis.[17] Anti–GM-CSF antibody is associated with pulmonary alveolar proteinosis; it is not associated with DAH or hemoptysis.[17] Antifungal medications have not been shown to be effective in treating fibrosing mediastinitis. Patient did not have airway compression but rather vascular compression. Thus, bronchoscopy with stent will not change the course for the patient.

REFERENCES

1. Duwe BV, Sterman DH. Msani AI Tumors of the mediastinum. *Chest.* 2005;128(4):2893–2909.
2. Kim JY, Hofstetter WL. Tumors of the mediastinum and chest wall. *Surg Clin North Am.* 2010;90(5):1019–1040.
3. Strollo DC, Rosado-de-Christenson ML, Jett JR. Primary mediastinal tumors: Part 2. Tumors of the middle and posterior mediastinum. *Chest.* 1997;112:1344–1357.
4. Marchevsky AM. Mediastinal tumors of peripheral nervous system origin. *Semin Diagn Pathol.* 1999;16:65–78.
5. Gothard JW. Anesthetic considerations for patients with anterior mediastinal masses. *Anesthesiol Clin.* 2008;26(2): 305–314.
6. Loto OM, Awowole I. Tuberculosis in pregnancy: A review. *J Pregnancy.* 2012;2012:379271.
7. Baughman RP, Culver DA, Judson MA. A concise review of pulmonary sarcoidosis. *Am J Respir Crit Care Med.* 2011;183(5):573–581.
8. Rybicki BA, Major M, Popovich J Jr, et al. Racial differences in sarcoidosis incidence: A 5-year study in a health maintenance organization. *Am J Epidemiol.* 1997;145(3):234–241.
9. Iannuzzi MC, Rybicki BA, Teirstein AS. Sarcoidosis. *N Engl J Med.* 2007;357(21):2153–2165.
10. Statement on sarcoidosis. Joint Statement of the American Thoracic Society (ATS), the European Respiratory Society (ERS) and the World Association of Sarcoidosis and Other Granulomatous Disorders (WASOG) adopted by the ATS Board of Directors and by the ERS Executive Committee, February 1999. *Am J Respir Crit Care Med.* 1999;160(2): 736–755.
11. Falkson CB, Bezjak A, Darling G, et al. The management of thymoma: A systematic review and practice guideline. *Thorac Oncol.* 2009;4(7):911–919.
12. Schumacher L, Gilbert S. Congenital diaphragmatic hernia in the adult. *Thorac Surg Clin.* 2009;19(4):469–472.
13. Nasr A, Fecteau A. Foramen of Morgagni hernia: Presentation and treatment. *Thorac Surg Clin.* 2009;19(4): 463–468.
14. Bokemeyer C, Nichols CR, Droz JP, et al. Extragonadal germ cell tumors of the mediastinum and retroperitoneum: Results from an international analysis. *J Clin Oncol.* 2002;20(7):1864–1873.
15. Albany C, Einhorn LH. Extragonadal germ cell tumors: Clinical presentation and management. *Curr Opin Oncol.* 2013;25(3):261–265.
16. Peikert T, Colby TV, Midthun DE, et al. Fibrosing mediastinitis: Clinical presentation, therapeutic outcomes, and adaptive immune response. *Medicine (Baltimore).* 2011;90(6):412–423.
17. Thiessen R, Matzinger F, Seely J, et al. Fibrosing mediastinitis: Successful stenting of the pulmonary artery. *Can Respir J.* 2008;15(1):41–44.

11

Pleural Diseases

Oleg Epelbaum MD and Irene Galperin MD

CASE 1

A 56-year-old man presents to the emergency department with progressively worsening dyspnea on exertion since his discharge 2 weeks earlier after thymectomy for thymic carcinoma, which included freeing the left subclavian artery of adherent tumor. His postoperative course is complicated by pulmonary embolism, and the patient is discharged on low–molecular-weight heparin. There has been no fever, cough, or interval trauma. He is afebrile with normal vital signs. Physical examination is notable for decreased breath sounds and dullness to percussion in the lower left chest. Laboratory evaluation reveals a peripheral leukocyte count of 16,000/μL and a platelet count of 600,000/μL. The serum lactate dehydrogenase (LDH) level is 217 U/L (normal range 90–225 U/L), the serum total protein (TP) level is 6.1 g/dL (normal range 6.5–8.5 g/dL), and the serum glucose level is 102 g/dL (normal range 74–110 g/dL). His chest radiograph is shown right. Diagnostic and therapeutic thoracentesis is performed and yields pleural fluid with the following characteristics:

Parameter	Result
Appearance	Milky/bloody
pH	7.50
Leukocyte count	3,000/μL (47% lymphocytes)
Red blood cell (RBC) count	125,000/μL
LDH	257 U/L
TP	3.6 g/dL
Glucose	107 mg/dL
Triglycerides (TG)	504 g/dL
Cholesterol	59 mg/dL
Gram stain	Negative

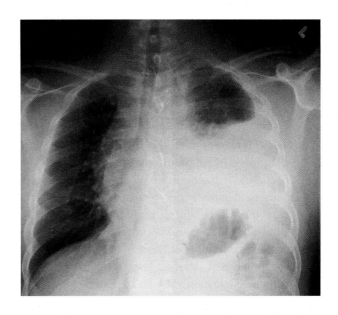

* *

Bacterial culture and cytology ultimately return negative. Serum total cholesterol is 133 mg/dL, and the serum TG level is 256 mg/dL.

Question 1: **Which of the following laboratory findings in this patient favors the diagnosis of chylothorax over a chyliform effusion (pseudochylothorax)?**

A. Pleural fluid triglyceride level >110 mg/dL and pleural fluid cholesterol < serum cholesterol
B. Pleural fluid triglyceride level >110 mg/dL and pleural fluid glucose > serum glucose
C. Pleural fluid triglyceride level >110 mg/dL and pleural fluid TP < serum TP
D. Pleural fluid cholesterol level >40 mg/dL but < serum cholesterol

E. Pleural fluid cholesterol level >40 mg/dL and pleural fluid glucose > serum glucose

Question 2: Which of the following etiologies has NOT been associated with chylothorax?

A. Kaposi's sarcoma
B. Trauma
C. Idiopathic pulmonary fibrosis (IPF)
D. Lymphangioleiomyomatosis (LAM)
E. Lymphoma

Question 3: Which of the following choices correctly pairs a specific treatment option for chylothorax with its main disadvantage?

	Treatment	Disadvantage
A.	Pleuroperitoneal shunt	General anesthesia
B.	Thoracic duct ligation	Invasiveness
C.	Medium-chain TG diet	Hypoglycemia
D.	Intravenous hyperalimentation	Thrombosis
E.	Somatostatin (Octreotide)	Nephrotoxicity

Question 4: Which of the following laboratory scenarios is diagnostic of a hemothorax?

A. Pleural fluid hematocrit >10% of serum hematocrit
B. Pleural fluid hematocrit >50% of serum hematocrit
C. Pleural fluid LDH >5x serum LDH
D. Pleural fluid RBC count >1 million with a drop in serum hematocrit of >10% in 24 hours
E. Pleural fluid RBC count >1 million with a drop in serum hematocrit of >50% in 24 hours

Question 5: Which of the following is the most common cause of hemothorax?

A. Iatrogenic
B. Anticoagulation
C. Thrombocytopenia
D. Trauma
E. Endometriosis

CASE 2

A 68-year-old man is referred to the pulmonary clinic for a pleural effusion discovered on abdominal imaging 1 week ago. His past medical history is significant for stage IIB adenocarcinoma of the pancreas and he is status post distal pancreatectomy and splenectomy 6 months earlier. He has completed adjuvant chemotherapy and radiation. He also has a history of hypertension, diabetes mellitus, and chronic kidney disease (CKD) stage 5 with a baseline serum creatinine level of approximately 3.5 mg/dL and an estimated glomerular filtration rate (EGFR) of 15 mL/min/1.73 m^2. He requires hemodialysis transiently in the postoperative period and is now receiving furosemide. Upon evaluation in the clinic, he is hypertensive but saturating 98% on room air and is breathing comfortably. He is emaciated with no jugular venous distention. Cardiac examination is unremarkable. He has decreased breath sounds at the left base with dullness to percussion and reduced fremitus. The abdominal surgical scar is healing well. There is no edema. Laboratory evaluation is significant for a serum creatinine level of 4.1 mg/dL, glucose 225 mg/dL (normal range 74–110 mg/dL), albumin 2.5 g/dL (normal range 3.5–5.0 g/dL), lactate dehydrogenase (LDH) 166 U/L (normal range 90–225 U/L), and total protein (TP) 7.3 g/dL (normal range 6.5–8.5 mg/dL). The chest radiograph (CXR) obtained during the current visit is shown in Figure 11–1. His preoperative CXR is normal. No other postoperative chest imaging is available. Results of recent echocardiography are reviewed and are notable for left ventricular hypertrophy with impaired relaxation. The patient is scheduled for a routine ultrasound-guided left thoracentesis, which yields the following values:

Parameter	Result
Appearance	Clear yellow
pH	7.42
Leukocyte count	600/μL (65% neutrophils)
Glucose	203 mg/dL
LDH	220 U/L
TP	3.1 mg/dL
Cholesterol	41 mg/dL
Amylase	16 U/L
Cytology	Negative

Question 1: Which of the following is most accurate about the nature of this patient's pleural effusion?
A. It is classified as a transudate by Light's criteria.
B. It is a discordant exudate by Light's criteria.
C. It is the result of esophageal rupture.
D. It is the result of pancreatic inflammation.
E. Repeat pleural cytology is likely to be positive.

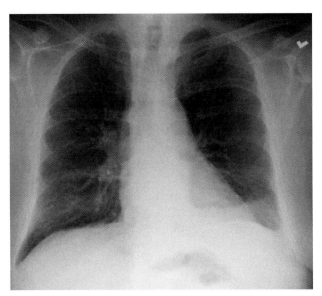 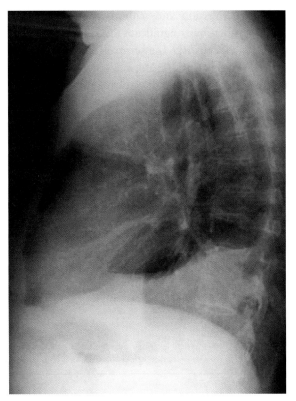

Figure 11–1 Posterior-anterior view and lateral view of chest radiograph for patient in Case 2.

Question 2: **Which of the following additional tests on this patient's pleural fluid would be most helpful in confirming the etiology of his effusion?**
A. Albumin level
B. Triglyceride level
C. Adenosine deaminase level
D. Flow cytometry
E. Fungal cultures

Question 3: **Which of the following is the most accurate description of the <u>principal</u> mechanism of the accumulation of pleural fluid in this patient?**
A. Decreased fluid drainage due to obstruction of pleural lymphatics
B. Increased pleural capillary permeability
C. Reduced pleural capillary oncotic pressure
D. Reduced central venous pressure
E. Increased pulmonary capillary hydrostatic pressure

Question 4: **Which of the following is true about N-terminal pro-brain natriuretic peptide (NT-proBNP) measurements in the evaluation of pleural effusions in the setting of heart failure?**
A. NT-proBNP is cleared by the liver and thus its levels need to be interpreted with caution in advanced hepatic disease.

B. Pleural and serum NT-proBNP levels are elevated only in congestive heart failure with reduced ejection fraction.
C. Serum NT-proBNP levels are highly correlated with those of pleural fluid in a given patient.
D. Pleural NT-proBNP is inferior to the serum-pleural protein gradient in correctly classifying discordant exudates identified by Light's criteria.
E. The high negative predictive value of clinical signs of heart failure obviates the need for NT-proBNP measurement in their absence when evaluating pleural effusions.

CASE 3

A 69-year-old man without significant past medical history presents with 5 days of cough productive of yellow sputum with occasional blood streaking. He describes associated fevers and chills. He is a light smoker and works as a limousine driver. His vital signs are notable for a pulse of 104 beats/min, a respiratory rate of 22 breaths/min, and an oxygen saturation of 95% on 2 L/min of oxygen via nasal cannula. The patient appears dyspneic and diaphoretic. Lung examination reveals diminished breath sounds in the left lower chest with dullness to percussion and without egophony. Initial laboratory evaluation is significant for a blood leukocyte count of 26,000 cells/μL. The serum lactate dehydrogenase (LDH) level is 139 U/L (normal range 90–225 U/L), serum total protein is 6.6 g/dL (normal range 6.5–8.5 g/dL), and serum glucose is 81 g/dL (normal range 74–110 g/dL). The patient's chest radiograph (CXR) and a representative chest computed tomography (CT) image are shown in Figure 11–2A and B. The following results are obtained upon thoracentesis:

Parameter	Result
Appearance	Clear yellow
Cell count	660 cells/μL with 88% neutrophils
pH	7.08
LDH	1,249 U/L
Total protein	4.6 g/dL
Glucose	25 g/dL
Gram stain	Gram+ cocci in pairs and chains

Question 1: Which of the following options correctly pairs the most appropriate terminology to describe this patient's pleural effusion with an appropriate single management strategy?

	Terminology	Management
A	Simple parapneumonic effusion	Thoracotomy
B	Simple parapneumonic effusion	Video-assisted thoracoscopic surgery (VATS)
C	Complicated parapneumonic effusion	Antibiotics
D	Complicated parapneumonic effusion	VATS
E	Empyema	Thoracotomy

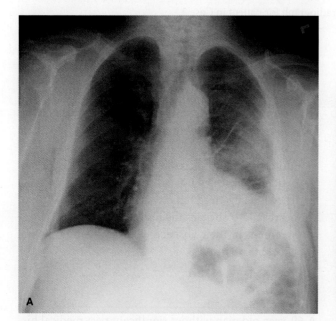

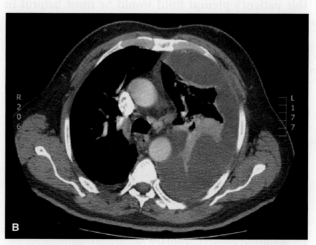

Figure 11–2   **A.** Posterior-anterior view of chest radiograph for patient in Case 3. **B.** Computed tomography of the chest for patient in Case 3.

Question 2: **Which of the following procedural factors is most likely to reduce the risk of iatrogenic pneumothorax during the performance of this patient's initial thoracentesis?**

A. Diagnostic versus therapeutic procedure
B. Greater operator experience
C. The use of real-time ultrasound guidance
D. Lower number of needle passes
E. Initial versus repeat procedure

Question 3: **Which of the following advantages can be expected from the insertion of a small-bore (i.e., 14Fr) chest tube rather than a large-bore (i.e., 32Fr) chest tube for the drainage of the infected pleural space?**

A. Reduced hospital stay
B. Reduced pain upon insertion
C. Reduced mortality at 1 year
D. Reduced need for surgery at 1 year
E. Reduced radiographic abnormality at 3 months

Question 4: **Which of the following options contains valid conclusions from <u>both</u> the MIST1 and MIST2 trials of intrapleural thrombolytic therapy for pleural space infection?**

	MIST 1	MIST 2
A	Streptokinase does not reduce mortality or the need for surgery.	Combination of tissue plasminogen activator (tPA) and DNase does not facilitate radiographic resolution.
B	Streptokinase reduces mortality and the need for surgery.	Combination of tPA and DNase facilitates radiographic resolution.
C	Streptokinase does not reduce mortality or the need for surgery.	tPA alone facilitates radiographic resolution.
D	Streptokinase reduces mortality and the need for surgery.	DNase alone facilitates radiographic resolution.
E	Streptokinase does not reduce mortality or the need for surgery.	tPA alone does not facilitate radiographic resolution.

Question 5: **Which of the following is true of pleural fluid analysis in pleural space infection?**

A. Inoculation of blood culture media has not been shown to increase microbiologic yield.
B. Pleural fluid pH can be falsely reduced by delays in processing.

C. Pleural fluid pH may vary in multi-loculated parapneumonic effusions depending on the loculation being sampled.
D. Empyema is not associated with an elevated pleural adenosine deaminase (ADA) level.
E. Empyema fluid remains uniformly opaque after centrifugation.

CASE 4

A 56-year-old woman presents to the emergency department with left-sided chest pain beginning 1 week prior. The pain is described as severe, constant, and associated with dyspnea. She denies fevers, night sweats, and weight loss. She has been a smoker since the age of 18. There is no history of tuberculosis. Since immigrating to the United States from Trinidad and Tobago 10 years earlier, she has not traveled to any foreign country and has done clerical work. She has been a teacher in her home country. She is afebrile with a blood pressure of 167/100 mm Hg, heart rate 96 beats/min, respiratory rate 22 breaths/min, and an oxygen saturation of 96% on room air. Physical examination reveals a well-nourished female in no acute distress with diminished breath sounds over the left chest with dullness to percussion and reduced tactile fremitus. Her chest radiograph shows near-total opacification of the left hemithorax with slight contralateral displacement of the mediastinum. Bedside pleural ultrasonography confirms the presence of an effusion. Results of the subsequent thoracentesis are summarized below:

Parameter	Result
pH	7.43
Lactate dehydrogenase (LDH)	1,068 U/L
Total protein	4.7 g/dL
Differential cell count	46% lymphocytes, 20% mesothelial cells

* *

Pleural fluid cytology is positive for malignant cells, favoring adenocarcinoma pending immunohistochemical stains.

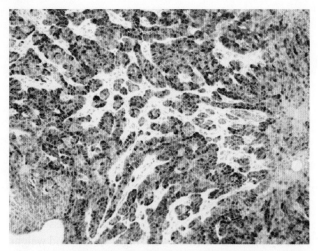

Figure 11–3 Immunohistochemical staining result for calretinin of this patient's pleural fluid cell block (original magnification × 100).

Question 1: Which one of the following clinical features of this case is most supportive of the diagnosis of malignant pleural mesothelioma (MPM) over lung adenocarcinoma?

A. Pleural fluid LDH >1,000 U/L
B. Lack of asbestos exposure history
C. History of smoking
D. Severe constant chest pain
E. Duration of symptoms

Question 2: The result of this patient's immunohistochemical stain of the pleural fluid cell block for calretinin is shown in Figure 11–3. Positivity for which of the following additional immunohistochemical markers would favor the diagnosis of MPM over lung adenocarcinoma?

A. WT-1
B. Thyroid transcription factor 1 (TTF-1)
C. Napsin A
D. Carcinoembryonic antigen (CEA)
E. P63

Question 3: Which of the following is true about the diagnosis of MPM?

A. Surgical pleural biopsy does not increase diagnostic yield over guided cutting needle biopsy.
B. The serum biomarkers megakaryocyte potentiation factor (MPF) and osteopontin exhibit sensitivities of <50% for MPM.
C. Finding sarcomatoid histology in a patient with MPM is a favorable prognostic indicator.
D. The TNM staging system cannot be applied to the prognostication of MPM.
E. Male gender portends a favorable prognosis in MPM.

Question 4: Which of the following is true about treatment options in MPM?

A. Extrapleural pneumonectomy (EPP) has been shown to significantly improve survival compared to pleurectomy/decortication (P/D).
B. Adjuvant radiation therapy has been shown to improve survival following EPP.
C. Patients with the sarcomatoid subtype of MPM appear to derive greater benefit from surgery.
D. Platinum-based combination chemotherapy is the standard of care in both definitive and neoadjuvant settings.
E. MPM commonly exhibits activating mutations of the epidermal growth factor receptor (EGFR).

CASE 5

A 62-year-old man presents to a pulmonary clinic with dyspnea on exertion. He reports increasing difficulty performing activities of daily living due to shortness of breath since returning home from the hospital 2 weeks earlier. He denies fevers, chills, cough, or sputum production. He reports no associated palpitations or chest discomfort. He has a history of diabetes mellitus, atrial fibrillation, and hypertension. His medications include metformin, amiodarone, metoprolol, and warfarin. Approximately 3 weeks ago, he underwent uncomplicated coronary artery bypass surgery (CABG) with both internal mammary artery (IMA) and saphenous vein grafting (SVG) after cardiac catheterization revealed 3-vessel coronary artery disease. The patient has immigrated to the United States from Mexico and works in construction. He is a lifelong smoker. On examination, he appears comfortable at rest with a temperature of 97.2°F, blood pressure 138/70 mm Hg, pulse 74 beats/min, respiratory rate 16 breaths/min, and oxygen saturation 95% on room air. His neck is supple and without JVD or palpable lymphadenopathy. The midline post-sternotomy scar exhibits granulation without evidence of infection, inflammation, or dehiscence. The heart rate and rhythm are irregular without murmurs or rubs. Lung examination reveals diminished breath sounds over the lower left chest with associated dullness to percussion and decreased tactile fremitus. There is no egophony or pleural rub. There is no hepatojugular reflux, and the extremities are warm and nonedematous. Routine laboratory evaluation reveals the following values:

Parameter	Result	Normal Range
Leukocyte (WBC) count	9,600/μL (normal differential)	4,500–11,000/μL
Hemoglobin	11.3 g/dL	12–16 g/dL
Platelet count	420,000/μL	130,000–400,000/μL
Serum glucose	156 mg/dL	74–110 mg/dL
Serum lactate dehydrogenase (LDH)	290 U/L	90–225 U/L
Serum total protein (TP)	7.2 g/dL	6.5–8.5 g/dL
International normalized ratio (INR)	1.8	N/A
B-type natriuretic peptide (BNP)	85 pg/mL	N/A

WBCs (50% neutrophils, 10% lymphocytes, 10% monocytes, 30% eosinophils), pH 7.52, glucose level 80 mg/dL, LDH 720 U/L, and TP 3.7 mg/dL. The post-thoracentesis CXR is shown below.

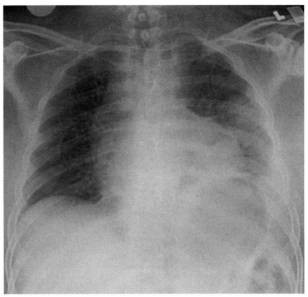

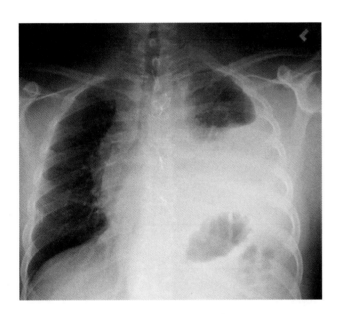

Question 1: **Which of the following is the <u>most appropriate</u> next step in the management of this patient?**

A. Thoracentesis

B. Computed tomography angiography (CTA) of the chest

C. Aggressive diuresis with furosemide

D. Broad spectrum respiratory antibiotics

E. Nonsteroidal anti-inflammatory drugs (NSAIDs)

* *

The patient undergoes thoracentesis, and 650 mL of hemorrhagic fluid is drained without complications. The patient experiences significant symptomatic relief. Pleural fluid analysis reveals 800,000 red blood cells, 9,000

Question 2: **Which of the following is true about this type of effusion?**

A. It is associated with antimyocardial antibodies.

B. Incidence is increased with an IMA graft versus an SVG.

C. It will resolve spontaneously with discontinuation of the culprit medication.

D. Pleural fluid adenosine deaminase level should be obtained to exclude tuberculous pleuritis.

E. Prophylactic post-CABG colchicine can reduce the likelihood of developing such an effusion.

* *

The patient is discharged home and is subsequently lost to follow-up. He returns to the clinic 2 years later seeking to re-establish care. He is active and able to walk on a treadmill for 20 minutes at home. He does not experience chest pain. On examination, his vital signs are normal with an oxygen saturation of 96% on room air at rest. Diminished breath sounds are again noted over the left lung base with associated dullness to percussion and decreased tactile fremitus. There is no egophony or rub. The remainder of the physical examination is unremarkable. Serum LDH, TP, and glucose are within the normal range. CXR is obtained and shows a moderate left pleural effusion. After drainage of 350 mL of serosanguinous fluid by thoracentesis, the procedure is aborted due to the patient's complaint of significant chest discomfort, which resolves upon termination of the procedure. His vital signs and saturation are unchanged compared to initial triage. Pleural fluid analysis reveals 315 WBCs (12% neutrophils, 53% lymphocytes, 35% monocytes), pH 7.34, TP 2.8 mg/dL, LDH 99 U/L, and glucose 74 mg/dL. Shortly after the post-thoracentesis CXR is performed, there is a phone call from the radiology reading room reporting a left hydropneumothorax without mediastinal shift.

Question 3: **Which of the following choices correctly pairs the best explanation for this patient's post-thoracentesis CXR abnormality with the associated pleural elastance curve (A, B, or C in Fig. 11–4)?**

	Explanation for CXR Abnormality	Pleural Elastance Curve
A	Hydropneumothorax	Curve A
B	Hydropneumothorax	Curve B
C	Hydropneumothorax	Curve C
D	Trapped lung	Curve A
E	Trapped lung	Curve C

Question 4: **Which of the following is the <u>most appropriate</u> next step in management of this patient?**
A. Tube thoracostomy followed by talc pleurodesis
B. Indwelling pleural catheter (IPC) insertion
C. Medical pleuroscopy with pleural biopsy
D. Surgical decortication
E. Observation

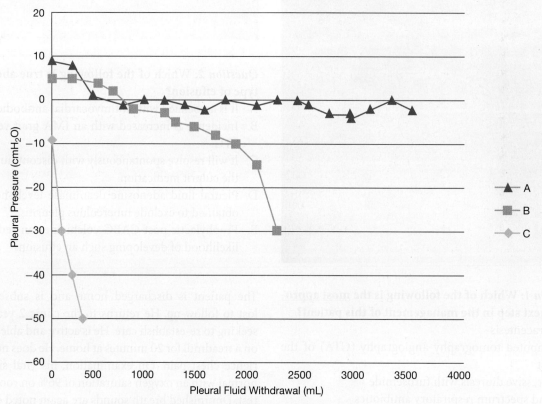

Figure 11–4 Pleural pressure (cmH₂O) over pleural volume (ml) graph.
Modified with permission from Huggins JT, Sahn SA, Heidecker J, et al. Characteristics of trapped lung: pleural fluid analysis, manometry, and air-contrast chest CT. *Chest.* 2007;131(1):206–213.

CASE 6

A 59-year-old man presents to the emergency department (ED) with sudden onset of dyspnea and sharp right-sided chest pain while driving. His past medical history is significant for interstitial lung disease of undetermined etiology about which no further information is available. He has a history of smoking but had quit about 20 years prior. He is not taking any medications. In the ED, he has a blood pressure of 160/87 mm Hg, pulse 116 beats/min, respiratory rate 26 breaths/min, and oxygen saturation 82% while breathing room air, improving to 95% on supplemental oxygen at 4 L/min via nasal cannula. The patient's breathing is labored with use of accessory muscles noted. Breath sounds are decreased over the right chest. The trachea is palpated in the midline. The remainder of the physical examination is normal as is a complete blood count and basic metabolic panel. Arterial blood gas analysis with the patient breathing supplemental oxygen reveals a pH of 7.28, pCO_2 of 55 mm Hg, and a PaO_2 of 70 mm Hg. Electrocardiogram shows sinus tachycardia. The patient's chest radiograph (CXR) appears below.

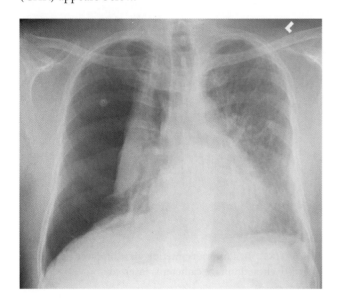

Question 1: **Which of the following is the most appropriate next step in the management of this patient?**
A. Immediate video-assisted thoracoscopic surgery (VATS)
B. Needle aspiration
C. Large-bore (i.e., 32Fr) surgical tube thoracostomy
D. Medical thoracoscopy
E. Small-bore (i.e., 14Fr) tube thoracostomy

Question 2: **Which of the following is true about the initial radiologic evaluation of pneumothorax?**
A. Pleural ultrasonography is less sensitive than chest radiography in the detection of occult pneumothorax in trauma patients.
B. Expiratory chest radiography should be routinely obtained as part of the evaluation of spontaneous pneumothorax.
C. Chest radiography is more accurate than chest computed tomography in the calculation of pneumothorax size.
D. The presence of the "sliding lung" sign on pleural ultrasonography excludes the presence of pneumothorax at the location of the probe with a negative predictive value of >90%.
E. Intrinsic lung pathology has not been associated with false negativity of the "sliding lung" sign on pleural ultrasonography.

* *

The patient undergoes successful bedside tube thoracostomy. Subsequent computed tomography of the chest reveals full re-expansion of the right lung and fibrocystic changes in the upper lobes bilaterally. By hospital day 3, an air leak is no longer appreciated. You decide that the patient had a secondary spontaneous pneumothorax (SSP) and thus warrants an intervention to minimize the likelihood of ipsilateral recurrence.

Question 3: **Which of the following choices correctly pairs the most effective intervention for SSP recurrence prevention with the closest estimate of the likelihood of post-procedure recurrence?**

A	Pleurodesis via VATS	5%
B	Pleurodesis via tube thoracostomy	5%
C	Pleurodesis via VATS	15%
D	Pleurodesis via tube thoracostomy	15%
E	Pleurodesis via VATS	50%

Question 4: **In which of the following options are both of the listed characteristics known predisposing factors for *primary* spontaneous pneumothorax?**
A. Presence of subpleural blebs and increased pleural porosity
B. Presence of subpleural blebs and decreased pleural porosity

C. Subclinical interstitial lung disease and increased pleural porosity

D. Subclinical interstitial lung disease and decreased pleural porosity

E. Female gender and increased pleural porosity

CASE 7

A 37-year-old woman presents to the emergency department with worsening dyspnea for approximately 1 week. She is diagnosed with receptor-negative breast adenocarcinoma 6 months prior and is status post right mastectomy followed by adjuvant chemotherapy and radiation. She is born and raised in the Northeastern United States and has not traveled abroad. On presentation, she is afebrile with a blood pressure of 119/70 mm Hg, pulse 113 beats/minute, respiratory rate 20 breaths/minute, and oxygen saturation of 97% on room air. Her physical examination reveals decreased breath sounds over the right chest with dullness to percussion and reduced tactile fremitus. Initial laboratory evaluation is remarkable only for a microcytic anemia. Her admission chest radiograph (CXR) is shown in Figure 11–5A. Diagnostic and therapeutic thoracentesis is performed without manometry, after which the patient experiences symptomatic relief, and her CXR markedly improves. The pleural fluid characteristics are consistent with a lymphocyte-predominant exudate with a pH of 7.33. A 60-mL sample of pleural fluid sent for cytology ultimately returns negative.

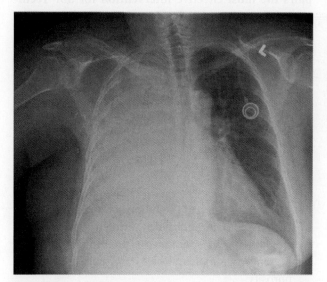

Figure 11–5 **A.** Posterior-anterior view of chest radiograph for patient on admission.

Question 1: **Which of the following is the most appropriate next __diagnostic__ maneuver?**

A. Blind closed needle biopsy of the pleura

B. Thoracoscopy

C. Whole-body positron emission tomography (PET)

D. Repeat thoracentesis for additional cytology

E. Measurement of pleural fluid adenosine deaminase (ADA) level

* *

Four days after her initial thoracentesis, she complains of worsened dyspnea. Repeat CXR is identical to the admission film shown in Figure 11–5A. An ultrasound-guided 14Fr chest drainage catheter is inserted percutaneously at the bedside. The postinsertion CXR and CT images are shown in Figures 11–5B and C.

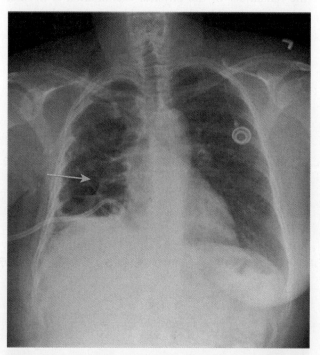

Figure 11–5 **B.** Posterior-anterior view of chest radiograph after 14F chest drainage catheter is inserted.

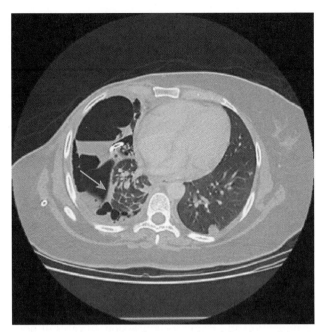

Figure 11–5   **C.** Computed tomography of the chest after 14F chest drainage catheter inserted.

Question 2: Which of the following is the best explanation for the CT findings?

A. Hemothorax
B. Iatrogenic pneumothorax
C. Spontaneous pneumothorax
D. Entrapped lung
E. Re-expansion pulmonary edema

Question 3: Assuming the etiology of the patient's pleural effusion is eventually confirmed to be her breast adenocarcinoma for which only outpatient salvage chemotherapy is being offered, which of the following is the most appropriate next intervention?

A. Pleurodesis via the chest tube
B. Medical thoracoscopy with pleurodesis
C. VATS with pleurodesis
D. Serial thoracentesis
E. Indwelling pleural catheter (IPC)

Question 4: Which of the following is true regarding talc pleurodesis in malignant pleural effusions?

A. Talc poudrage may be more effective than slurry in cases of lung and breast malignancy.
B. Doxycycline is more effective than talc as a pleurodesis agent.
C. Graded large-particle talc is associated with a higher incidence of ARDS than is nongraded talc.
D. Talc pleurodesis becomes more cost-effective than IPC insertion as the patient's life expectancy decreases.
E. The success rate of talc pleurodesis is under 50%.

Question 5: Which of the following is true about vascular endothelial growth factor (VEGF) in the context of pleural effusions?

A. VEGF is found at high levels in malignant pleural effusions but not in empyemas.
B. VEGF antagonism in the laboratory inhibits formation of malignant effusions in animal models.
C. The ability of VEGF to induce vascular permeability is weaker than that of histamine.
D. VEGF is believed to promote the formation of malignant effusions by interfering with pleural lymphatic drainage.
E. Hypoxia and transforming growth factor beta (TGF-β) inhibit VEGF production.

Answers

CASE 1

Question 1: A. Pleural fluid triglyceride level >110 mg/dL and pleural fluid cholesterol <serum cholesterol

A chylothorax results from the accumulation of chylomicron-rich lymphatic fluid in the pleural space caused by the interruption or blockage of the thoracic duct.[1] The principal component of these chylomicrons is triglycerides. A milky pleural effusion that remains opaque following centrifugation is suspicious for a chylothorax, a diagnosis which is supported by a fluid triglyceride concentration of >110 mg/dL.[2] Further distinction needs to be made between chylothorax and pseudochylothorax (or chyliform effusion). The latter occurs when a long-standing pleural effusion associated with chronic changes to the pleural lining acquires a high cholesterol concentration by mechanisms that are not completely understood.[3] To exclude this entity, the diagnostic criteria for chylothorax also require a pleural fluid to serum cholesterol ratio of <1. This ratio is reversed in pseudochylothorax. If any doubt about the diagnosis of chylothorax persists, the fluid can be analyzed for the presence of chylomicrons, which are not found in pseudochylothorax.[1]

Question 2: C. Idiopathic pulmonary fibrosis (IPF)

Most cases of chylothorax are caused by traumatic or iatrogenic damage to the thoracic duct or by malignant obstruction to the flow of chyle, primarily by lymphoma. Pulmonary lymphangioleiomyomatosis (LAM) is a cystic lung disease that occurs exclusively in females and is associated with chylothorax. Pathologic proliferation of immature smooth muscle in this condition can cause lymphatic obstruction in the chest as well as abnormal tone of the thoracic duct's smooth muscle layer.[4] Kaposi's sarcoma is a known, albeit rare, cause of chylothorax in the immunocompromised host.[1] Idiopathic pulmonary fibrosis (IPF) has not been associated with chylothorax.

Question 3:

B	Thoracic duct ligation	Invasiveness

Following thoracentesis or tube thoracostomy for the immediate relief of symptoms associated with chylothorax, various methods of resolving the chyle leak ought to be considered. Prolonged external drainage of chylothorax is inadvisable due to the resultant potential for malnutrition and immunosuppression. In cases of non-traumatic chylothorax, addressing the predisposing condition is recommended if possible. Specific therapeutic approaches progress from the least to the most invasive. Medium chain triglycerides (MCTs) offer the theoretical advantage of being directly absorbed from the intestine into the bloodstream without passing through lymphatics. However, the efficacy of restricting lipid intake to MCTs is controversial while poor gastrointestinal tolerance and palatability rather than hypoglycemia are the main drawbacks.[1] Complete cessation of oral nutrition in favor of total parenteral nutrition effectively reduces chyle flow, but intravenous hyperalimentation predisposes to bloodstream infections (not to thrombosis).[5] The use of somatostatin and its analogues such as octreotide is based on its ability to reduce the flow of chyle by several hypothetical mechanisms.[6] Evidence for its efficacy is thus far sparse, and so this therapy remains largely unproven. Gastrointestinal disturbances rather than nephrotoxicity are the main side effects. Both pleuroperitoneal shunting and thoracic duct ligation are effective ways of abrogating chyle entry into the pleural space.[5] The advantage of the former is that it can be placed under local anesthesia and subsequently removed. Thoracic duct ligation is definitive therapy but, unlike pleuroperitoneal shunting, requires general anesthesia whether performed via thoracoscopy or thoracotomy.[1]

Question 4: B. Pleural fluid hematocrit >50% of serum hematocrit

In addition to peritoneal fluid (hepatic hydrothorax), urine (urinothorax), and chyle (chylothorax), another bodily fluid capable of entering the pleural space is blood. A significant collection of blood in the pleural space is called a hemothorax, which is defined by a pleural fluid hematocrit >50% of serum hematocrit. In the absence of a hematocrit measurement, dividing the pleural fluid red blood cell count by 100,000 can be used to estimate its hematocrit.[1] Parameters listed in the other choices are not part of the laboratory definition of hemothorax.

Question 5: D. Trauma

Trauma is the most common etiology of hemothorax, which can also occur spontaneously in association with thrombocytopenia and anticoagulation.[1] Hemothorax is also a known complication of vascular and pleural procedures. The rare entity called catamenial hemothorax occurs in the presence of endometrial implants on the pleural surface usually as part of pelvico-abdominal endometriosis.[7] A more common manifestation of the so-called "thoracic endometriosis syndrome" is catamenial pneumothorax, which should be considered in the evaluation of recurrent pneumothorax in females of reproductive age. The typical pathologic finding in these patients is endometrial pleural implants in conjunction with diaphragmatic defects.[7] Treatment is usually with surgical pleurodesis with or without diaphragmatic repair and with or without adjunctive hormonal therapy.

CASE 2

Question 1: B. It is a discordant exudate by Light's criteria

This patient presents a common clinical dilemma. There are factors in this case that promote the formation of a transudative pleural effusion, such as advanced CKD, diastolic heart failure, and hypoalbuminemia. On the other hand, the effusion is not bilateral and there is worrisome history of pancreatic malignancy. The best characterization of the biochemistry of this effusion is that it is a discordant exudate according to Light's criteria, meaning that it fulfills exudative criteria by LDH (>0.6 × serum LDH, fluid LDH >2/3 the upper limit of normal for serum LDH) but not by protein (<0.5 × serum protein).[1] This is an expected consequence of Light's criteria having been designed to have great sensitivity for exudates (97%) at the expense of misclassifying 15% to 25% of actual transudates as exudates.[8] When this is the case, the patient usually meets exudative criteria by only one parameter and marginally so while receiving diuretic therapy. Both esophageal rupture (Boerhaave's

syndrome) and pancreatitis are associated with elevated pleural fluid amylase levels and the former with a very low pH. Malignant effusions are expected to be lymphocyte-predominant and fully exudative.

Question 2: A. Albumin level

When faced with the discordant exudate by Light's criteria in a patient clinically suspected of having a transudate, the most immediate option available to the physician is the calculation of the serum-pleural protein gradient. A value >3.1 g/dL has been shown to correctly reclassify a substantial percentage (62%) of such effusions as transudates.[9] The additional measurement of pleural fluid albumin allows the calculation of an analogous albumin gradient wherein a value of >1.2 g/dL has superior performance characteristics, correctly reclassifying >80%.[10] In a very recent systematic review, the lowest negative likelihood ratio for the exclusion of an exudate belonged to a pleural cholesterol level <55 mg/dL.[11] This patient's protein gradient and pleural cholesterol level both favor a transudative process. The other options listed would not refine the classification of this effusion.

Question 3: E. Increased pulmonary capillary hydrostatic pressure

The major culprit in the pathophysiology of this patient's effusion is his diastolic heart failure with additional contributions from low oncotic pressure and hypervolemia due to renal insufficiency. The current hypothesis regarding pleural fluid accumulation in left ventricular dysfunction implicates elevated pulmonary capillary hydrostatic pressure, which leads to migration of fluid into the lung interstitium and then across the visceral pleura into the pleural space. Pleural capillaries, even if their oncotic pressure is reduced by concomitant hypoalbuminemia, are now thought to add relatively little fluid to the pleural space in this scenario. Increased central venous pressure may compound the problem by providing an unfavorable pressure gradient for the emptying of lymphatics. Increased pleural capillary permeability underlies fluid formation in exudative phenomena such as infection and inflammation while pleural lymphatic obstruction is caused by malignant implants.

Question 4: C. Serum NT-proBNP levels are highly correlated with those of pleural fluid in a given patient

Brain natriuretic peptides comprise a family of neurohormones released by cardiac myocytes in response to increased ventricular filling pressures as may be seen in the setting of systolic or diastolic left ventricular dysfunction. NT-proBNP and its cleavage product, BNP, are both renally cleared, which can affect their utility in advanced kidney disease.[12] The accuracy of pleural fluid NT-proBNP in discriminating between effusions caused by heart failure and those that are not exceeding 90% and is superior to that of BNP.[13] Although measurement of these peptides in pleural fluid is not widely available, studies have demonstrated such an excellent correlation between pleural and serum levels that serum testing can be substituted without sacrificing performance characteristics.[14] Additionally, pleural fluid NT-proBNP is similar to the albumin gradient and superior to the protein gradient in the ability to correctly identify cardiac effusions misclassified as exudates by Light's criteria.[14] The physical examination in heart failure is not sufficiently sensitive to obviate biochemical testing in cases of suspected cardiac effusion, though normal cardiac size on the chest x-ray is inconsistent with that diagnosis.[1]

CASE 3

Question 1:

| D | Complicated parapneumonic effusion | VATS |

Pleural involvement related to pneumonia is a prevalent phenomenon that runs the gamut from sterile, free-flowing fluid generated by increased pleural capillary permeability (simple parapneumonic effusion) to actual extension of the infection into the pleural space with possible fluid loculation (complicated parapneumonic effusion) to frank pleural pus (empyema). Simple parapneumonic effusions, once sampled, do not require drainage as they are expected to resolve uneventfully with appropriate antibiotic therapy alone. Complicated parapneumonic effusions (CPE) are tantamount to a closed-space infection and thus mandate drainage in addition to antibiotics (see Table 11-1). This patient's effusion is classified as a CPE based on the pH, LDH, and positive Gram stain. The ACCP guidelines also consider fluid loculation as a criterion for labeling a parapneumonic effusion as complicated.[15] In current practice, both image-guided tube thoracostomy as well as VATS are viewed as appropriate initial drainage options for CPE; approaches vary according to specific patient and institutional factors. Empyemas require immediate evacuation, which will usually be accomplished via VATS, but a trial of chest tube drainage can be attempted, especially in poor operative candidates.

Question 2: C. The use of real-time ultrasound guidance

The use of portable pleural ultrasonography for the guidance of thoracentesis has been shown to reduce serious procedural complications, of which pneumothorax is the most common (~6%). A 2010 meta-analysis revealed that, of the factors listed, only real-time sonographic guidance is unequivocally associated with a reduced risk of iatrogenic pneumothorax.[18] A very recent systematic review casts some doubt on that assertion but is likely inapplicable to cases of loculated pleural fluid as in this patient.[11]

Question 3: B. Reduced pain upon insertion

Although Poiseuille's law and experimental results suggest that large-bore chest tubes ought to be superior to small-bore ones for the drainage of viscous pleural infection, clinical evidence indicates otherwise.[19] Rahman et al. reviewed available chest tube pain score data from the MIST1 trial and found that larger drains were associated with higher pain scores.[20] Furthermore, the use of larger drains did not lead to improvement in hospital stay, mortality, the need for surgical intervention, or radiographic appearance.

Table 11–1 TYPES OF PARAPNEUMONIC EFFUSIONS WITH THEIR FLUID CHARACTERISTICS

Parameter	Simple	Complicated	Empyema
Appearance	Clear	Clear or cloudy	Pus
pH	>7.20	<7.20	Not required
LDH	<1,000 U/L	>1,000 U/L	Not required
Glucose	>40 mg/dL	<40 mg/dL	Not required
Microbiology	Negative	+/–Gram stain/culture	+/–Gram stain/culture
Management	Antibiotics	Antibiotics + drainage	Antibiotics + drainage

Modified from the work of Davies et al.[16] and Heffner et al.[17]

Question 4:

E	Streptokinase does not reduce mortality or the need for surgery	tPA alone does not facilitate radiographic resolution

The MIST1 (2005) and MIST2 (2011) trials are both randomized, controlled studies from the United Kingdom have greatly influenced clinical practice with regard to thrombolytic therapy in pleural infection. MIST1 randomized 454 patients to receive either streptokinase or placebo via chest tube for 3 days.[21] The primary end-point was a composite one of death or the need for surgical drainage at 3 months, and there was no difference between the two groups in that regard or with respect to any of the secondary end-points. MIST2 investigators compared the combination of tissue plasminogen activator (tPA) and DNase (a mucolytic) to double-placebo and to each agent alone administered for 3 days via chest tube for pleural infection.[22] The primary end-point was radiographic reduction in pleural opacity; secondary end-points included surgery and length of hospitalization. Intrapleural tPA and DNase in combination—but not individually—led to greater radiographic improvement and reduced the need for surgery and the length of stay. No significant difference in adverse events was observed in either trial.

Question 5: **C. Pleural fluid pH may vary in multi-loculated parapneumonic effusions depending on the loculation being sampled**

An important consideration in the management of multi-loculated pleural infections is that the fluid pH, a very important parameter for decision-making, can vary among different pleural locules to a clinically significant extent.[23] In addition, it has been shown that delays in pleural pH processing, which must be done by a blood gas analyzer, can lead to falsely elevated values as can residual air in the heparinized syringe and an admixture of lidocaine.[24] Of note, pleural fluid glucose was not influenced by these factors in the same study. The yield of standard bacterial pleural cultures, which is typically quite low (<40%), can be increased by about 20% with the additional inoculation of aerobic and anaerobic blood culture bottles.[25] Empyemas are associated with some of the highest reported levels of pleural fluid ADA.[26] Besides empyema, the differential diagnosis of milky pleural fluid includes chylothorax, pseudochylothorax, and rheumatoid pleurisy, which can be cholesterol-rich. The suspended cellular debris that makes empyema fluid turbid precipitates out upon centrifugation, leaving a clear supernatant. The other milky effusions remain opaque after centrifugation.[1]

CASE 4

Question 1: **D. Severe constant chest pain**
Malignant pleural mesothelioma (MPM) is an uncommon primary malignancy of the pleural lining that is intimately associated with asbestos exposure, which may have occurred in the distant past or unbeknownst to the patient. Unlike lung adenocarcinoma, MPM does not have an established causal relationship with cigarette smoking. MPM patients tend to become symptomatic insidiously and it is therefore typical for them to present after months of symptoms; this patient's presentation after one week of symptoms would be more consistent with a rapidly accumulating pleural effusion from adenocarcinoma. The chest pain that occurs with MPM classically becomes very severe and, unlike the pleuritic chest pain from metastatic pleural malignancy, is often described as constant. In both malignancies, the pleural fluid is a lymphocyte-predominant exudate capable of exhibiting LDH levels of >1,000 U/L.

Question 2: **A. WT-1**
The diagnosis of MPM is hindered by the difficult distinction between malignant and reactive mesothelial cells on cytology and by the tendency of MPM to mimic a variety of other neoplasms on biopsy. A hematoxylin & eosin (H&E)-stained tissue sample from this patient's pleura is shown in Figure 11–6. One can appreciate the nonspecific histology of MPM. Therefore, immunohistochemical staining is an integral part of issuing a definitive diagnosis of this malignancy. Because of the potential for great morphologic similarity, one of the most important distinctions to make is that between MPM and lung adenocarcinoma. Calretinin and WT-1 are very useful markers in this setting because they are very specific for MPM and are not expressed in lung adenocarcinoma.[27] TTF-1, Napsin A, and CEA, on the other hand, are specific adenocarcinoma markers. P63 is specific for squamous cell carcinoma, which can also create diagnostic confusion with MPM.

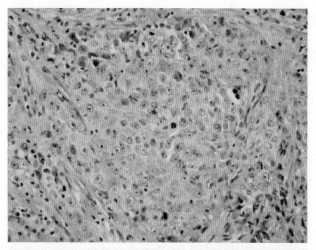

Figure 11–6 Pleural biopsy from this patient showing an invasive neoplasm with non-specific morphology ultimately diagnosed as epithelioid MPM (H&E, original magnification × 400).

Question 3: B. The serum biomarkers megakaryocyte potentiation factor (MPF) and osteopontin exhibit sensitivities of <50% for MPM

For reasons outlined earlier, the yield of pleural fluid cytology and even guided needle biopsy of the pleura in MPM is far inferior to that of surgical pleural biopsy. Pleural biopsy via video-assisted thoracoscopic surgery (VATS) is the optimal diagnostic modality for MPM and also allows for easier histologic subtyping into the epithelioid, sarcomatoid, and mixed variants, which has prognostic and treatment implications. The TNM staging system as well as a number of scoring systems can all be used to prognosticate MPM patients. When the latter are applied, sarcomatoid histology invariably emerges as an unfavorable prognostic indicator. In the independently validated MPM scoring system derived by the European Organization for Research and Treatment of Cancer, male gender is associated with worse outcome.[28] Efforts are ongoing to develop useful serum biomarkers that would inform diagnosis, prognosis, and treatment selection. Among three emerging biomarkers, namely MPF, osteopontin, and soluble mesothelin-related peptide (SMRP), only SMRP exhibited a sensitivity of >50% (73%) for MPM in a comparison study.[29]

Question 4: D. Platinum-based combination chemotherapy is the standard of care in both definitive and neoadjuvant settings

The approach to the treatment of MPM is usually based on multi-modality therapy. Extrapleural pneumonectomy (EPP) is a highly morbid operation performed by a select group of experienced centers in an attempt to cure MPM. Its combination with induction platinum-based chemotherapy with or without radiotherapy has yielded median survival in the range of 18 to 20 months in contemporary series.[30] Platinum-based combination regimens are the accepted standard in both neoadjuvant and definitive chemotherapeutic applications. The role of adjuvant radiotherapy following EPP is improvement of local control—overall survival is unaffected.[28] Recent data indicate that P/D, a more conservative surgical intervention for MPM, produces similar outcomes to EPP with a lower rate of operative complications.[31] Nonepithelioid histology has been consistently associated with inferior surgical outcomes, so much so that surgery is virtually never offered to patients with the sarcomatoid subtype. Unlike lung adenocarcinoma, MPM rarely exhibits activating EGFR mutations, rendering tyrosine kinase inhibitors erlotinib, and gefitinib ineffective in this disease.[28]

CASE 5

Question 1: A. Thoracentesis

Well over half of patients undergoing CABG will develop a pleural effusion at some point in their postoperative course.[32] The majority of post-CABG effusions are small, left-sided, and asymptomatic. The relatively uncommon large, symptomatic post-CABG effusion warrants a diagnostic and therapeutic thoracentesis in order to characterize the fluid, exclude other competing diagnoses—such as heart failure, chylothorax, and infection—and provide symptom relief.[33] Most post-CABG effusions will not recur following one or a short series of thoracenteses, so the initial therapeutic tap may be the only required intervention. Because the clinical and radiographic picture in this case is not suggestive of heart failure, empiric administration of furosemide would not be appropriate. Nor is there sufficient evidence for pleural infection to justify empiric antibiotic therapy prior to fluid sampling. The differential diagnosis in this patient does include pulmonary embolus (PE) for which CTA would be the study of choice, but pleural effusions associated with PE—though mostly left-sided—are usually small in size. It would be best to first sample and drain the pleural effusion. CTA is considered if dyspnea persisted. NSAIDs may have a role in hastening the resolution of certain post-CABG effusions but would not be the appropriate initial step prior to a diagnostic evaluation.

Table 11–2 THE MOST COMMON KNOWN ETIOLOGIC CATEGORIES OF EOSINOPHILIC (≥10%) PLEURAL EFFUSIONS WITH NOTABLE EXAMPLES OF EACH[38]

Etiology	Example
Malignancy	Lung carcinoma
Infection	Parapneumonic, parasitic
Post-CABG	Early hemorrhagic
Drug-induced	Nitrofurantoin
Hemo/pneumothorax	Trauma, procedures
Occupational	Benign asbestos pleural effusion (BAPE)

Question 2: B. Incidence is increased with an IMA graft versus an SVG

Pleural effusions directly related to CABG can be separated into those occurring early (<30 days postoperatively) and late (>30 days postoperatively); this somewhat arbitrary division facilitates their characterization.[32] The early post-CABG effusion (seen in this case) is classically a hemorrhagic exudate with eosinophils as the predominant cell type—presumably the result of blood in the pleural space (Table 11–2 lists the most common etiologies of pleural eosinophilia).[34] A number of investigators have found an association between IMA grafting and the incidence of such effusions, giving rise to the hypothesis that they result from pleural injury during the harvesting process.[35] The typical patient presents with dyspnea in the absence of inflammatory signs or leukocytosis. In the vast majority of cases, this type of effusion resolves following one or more therapeutic taps.[36] Despite a lack of evidence to support this practice, NSAIDs are often given in an attempt to accelerate resolution.

* *

The late post-CABG effusions come in two distinct but likely related flavors. The first is part of the so-called post-cardiac injury syndrome (PCIS), also known as Dressler's syndrome. This is believed to be an immune-mediated process associated with the presence of antimyocardial antibodies and triggered by violation of the pericardium.[32] The affected patient presents with dyspnea and chest pain in the setting of fever, pleuropericarditis, and parenchymal lung infiltrates. The pleural fluid in such cases is frequently hemorrhagic with neutrophils predominating in the early stages with subsequent conversion to lymphocytes. Clinical experience indicates that this syndrome responds well to anti-inflammatory therapy whether steroidal or nonsteroidal. A recent study has shown that a prophylactic course of colchicine in the early postoperative period can significantly reduce the incidence of this complication (number needed to treat = 10).[37]

* *

The other late post-CABG effusion directly attributable to the surgery is a lymphocyte-predominant nonhemorrhagic exudate in a patient presenting with bland dyspnea. Some experts consider this to be a less inflammatory and thus less symptomatic version of PCIS.[32] The differential diagnosis includes tuberculous pleuritis, as it does in the case of PCIS, so measurement of pleural fluid ADA has clinical utility when confronted with these effusions. Drug-induced pleural effusion should also be considered in the appropriate clinical setting (e.g., dantrolene, ergot alkaloids, dasatinib, valproic acid, clozapine) but is not applicable in this patient's case.[1] Table 11–3 summarizes the features of the three types of post-CABG effusions discussed above.

Question 3:

E	Trapped lung	Curve C

Trapped lung is a form of unexpandable lung wherein aberrant healing of the visceral pleura following an insult results in the development of a fibrous pleural peel that prevents expansion of the subjacent lung.[39] This

Table 11–3 COMPARISON OF THE THREE MAJOR CLASSES OF POST-CABG EFFUSIONS

Type	Timing	Clinical	Appearance	Cell type	Autoantibody	Treatment
Early	<30 days	Dyspnea	Hemorrhagic	Eosinophil	None	Tap +/− NSAIDs
PCIS	>30 days	Fever, chest pain	Hemorrhagic	Neutrophil lymphocyte	Antimyocardial	NSAIDs +/− steroids
Late	>30 days	Dyspnea	Clear	Lymphocyte	None	Conservative +/− tap/steroids

occurs as a delayed complication of pleural inflammation, and post-CABG effusions are likely the commonest cause of trapped lung.[1] While a history of remote pleural disease can suggest this diagnosis, in practice trapped lung is usually first suspected after one or more characteristic features is noted during the initial thoracentesis for a persistent unilateral pleural effusion. The failure of the underlying lung to re-expand as pleural fluid is withdrawn leads to a precipitous drop in intrapleural pressure, effectively creating a vacuum inside the pleural space. Radiographically, this vacuum has the appearance of a pneumothorax (or hydropneumothorax) and can cause diagnostic confusion even though the pathophysiology of pneumothorax and trapped lung is entirely different: only in the former and not in the latter is there is air in the pleural space. Sometimes, the term "pneumothorax-ex-vacuo" is applied to the radiographic appearance of trapped lung, which is a reminder of both the similarities and the differences between these two conditions. The rapid fall in intrapleural pressure associated with trapped lung results in extreme patient discomfort after the removal of a relatively small volume of fluid, leading to the premature termination of the procedure. If pleural manometry is performed, trapped lung is characterized by an initially negative intrapleural pressure that falls further with each aliquot of drained fluid (Fig. 11–4, curve C), indicating a pleural elastance (Δpressure/Δvolume) much higher than that of fully expandable lung (curve A) and lung entrapment (curve B).[40] The pleural fluid classically associated with trapped lung is a paucicellular transudate, having been essentially "sucked out" of the pleural capillaries to fill the resultant pleural vacuum. In lung entrapment, on the other hand, there is active pleural inflammation, so the accompanying pleural fluid is exudative.

Question 4: E. Observation

The symptomatology, if any, of a patient with trapped lung is primarily a function of the resultant restrictive lung physiology. The pleural fluid component can, however, cause discomfort in its own right, which is the only scenario in which it needs to be addressed. Asymptomatic patients such as the one in this case do not require any intervention for trapped lung. The definitive solution for this condition is operative decortication, which usually requires thoracotomy and can be performed at any point in the disease course. The alternative for poor surgical candidates who have symptoms attributable to the pleural effusion caused by trapped lung is IPC placement since pleurodesis will be ineffective when pleural apposition cannot be achieved.

CASE 6

Question 1: E. Small-bore (i.e., 14Fr) tube thoracostomy

Although Poiseuille's law states that flow through a tube increases exponentially with increasing diameter, there are compelling data to support the notion that clinical outcomes are no different with large-bore versus small-bore chest drains in pleural infection and malignancy with the added advantage of greater patient comfort with smaller catheters.[41,42] Similar evidence exists for SSP, and so the British Thoracic Society guidelines published in 2010 recommend the use of small-bore chest tubes in the management of this condition.[20,43] Needle aspiration is less likely to be a durable solution in SSP compared to primary spontaneous pneumothorax (PSP) and is thus not the initial procedure of choice in most cases. It does have a role in the emergency decompression of an unstable tension SSP, and can also be attempted in the stable patient in whom avoidance of tube thoracostomy is of high priority. Video-assisted thoracoscopic surgery (VATS) is the most effective means of recurrence prevention but is not a practical initial treatment option. Medical thoracoscopy does not yet have an established role in pleural disease therapeutics.

Question 2: D. The presence of the "sliding lung" sign on pleural ultrasonography excludes the presence of pneumothorax at the location of the probe with a negative predictive value of >90%

Pleural ultrasonography is a widely available tool for the evaluation of suspected pneumothorax at the bedside.[44] The presence of sonographic "lung sliding" at a given intercostal space has a very high negative predictive value (>90%) for the exclusion of pneumothorax at that location and may reach 100% if comet-tail artifacts are also observed.[45] The sensitivity of ultrasound for the diagnosis of pneumothorax is approximately 90%, a value far superior to that of chest radiography.[46] False negativity of the "sliding lung" sign can be encountered in the presence of lung pathology, including pneumonia, massive atelectasis, and ARDS.[47] Ultrasound is also more sensitive than chest radiography for the detection of occult pneumothorax in emergency room trauma patients (92% vs. 52%).[48] Chest computed tomography remains the gold standard for both the diagnosis of pneumothorax and the calculation of its size. Expiratory chest radiographs are not routinely recommended in the evaluation of pneumothorax.[43]

Question 3:

A.	Pleurodesis via VATS	5%

Without intervention, recurrence rates of SSP approach 50%, and these episodes are not well-tolerated by patients with underlying chronic lung disease.[49] Recurrence prevention is paramount in this condition. The most effective option is surgical pleurodesis—nowadays done mostly via VATS—with stapling or ligation of any visible bullae. This can reduce the risk of recurrence to 5% or less.[1] Those unfit for surgery can undergo chemical pleurodesis via tube thoracostomy, which has been shown to reduce the rate of recurrence to as low as 15%, a number still significantly inferior to operative intervention.[1] Nonsurgical candidates with persistent air leaks and failure of full lung re-expansion can be managed with Heimlich valves, though the use of endobronchial valves and sealants such as fibrin glue is being increasingly reported.

Question 4: A. Presence of subpleural blebs and increased pleural porosity

Male gender, tall stature with low body-mass index, and smoking are among the traditionally identified predisposing factors for PSP. The advent of high-resolution chest CT has enabled the identification of subpleural bullae and blebs, so-called "emphysema-like" changes (ELC), in about 80% of PSP cases in what would have previously been labeled as normal lungs.[50] No similar association with subclinical interstitial lung disease has been reported. When the pleural spaces of PSP patients were studied using fluorescein-enhanced autofluorescence thoracoscopy, leaks of inhaled fluorescein into the pleural space were detected, suggesting increased pleural porosity.[51] This phenomenon was not observed in control subjects. Of note, these leak sites were noted to be distinct from areas of identifiable ELC, which could mean that air escape in PSP is a more complex phenomenon than simple rupture of a bleb or bulla. One of the hypotheses to explain the increased pleural porosity in PSP implicates the disruption of normal mesothelial cells and their replacement by a less air-tight fibroelastic layer.[51]

CASE 7

Question 1: B. Thoracoscopy

In this case scenario, all evidence points to malignancy as the etiology of this patient's undiagnosed lymphocytic exudate. After the initial pleural fluid cytology returns negative, the next best diagnostic intervention would be thoracoscopic biopsy, whether performed surgically or medically depending on local expertise. The expected yield of either approach in malignant pleural disease exceeds 90%.[52] One of the advantages of thoracoscopy is the ability to perform both a biopsy and, if malignancy is obvious, a therapeutic intervention such as pleurodesis, indwelling pleural catheter (IPC) insertion, and lysis of adhesions.[53] While the yield of blind-needle biopsy of the pleura in malignancy is approximately 50%, making it an inferior option, ultrasound- or CT-guided needle biopsy of the pleura can achieve a yield comparable to that of thoracoscopy in experienced centers.[54] In a recent large series examining pleural effusions, pleural fluid cytology was diagnostic in <60% of malignant cases including those with serial aspirations.[55] PET scans, while potentially relevant as a guidance modality for needle biopsies of the pleura, suffer from false positivity in pleural malignancy and, of course, do not produce a laboratory diagnosis.[56] The highest pleural fluid ADA levels among lymphocytic exudates are seen in tuberculous effusions; levels >70 U/L in a lymphocyte-predominant exudate are practically diagnostic of pleural tuberculosis.[57] Levels <40 U/L can be used to exclude pleural tuberculosis in low-prevalence settings. Because that diagnosis is not a serious consideration in the present case, an ADA measurement would not be informative.

Question 2: D. Entrapped lung

The post-thoracostomy CXR shows volume loss in the right hemithorax despite adequate pleural fluid drainage and suggests the presence of a pneumothorax. The corresponding CT reveals what has been referred to as a "pneumothorax-ex-vacuo," that is, an apparent pneumothorax which in reality is actually a vacuum resulting from the failure of the lung to fully re-expand despite drainage of the ipsilateral pleural effusion. The CT also demonstrates thickening of the visceral pleura, which is responsible for the unexpandable lung in this patient (the CT did not reveal endobronchial obstruction). The underlying lung is likely entrapped by active pleural malignancy in this patient. Pleural manometry can aid in the differentiation of lung entrapment, which is caused by an active pleural process, from trapped lung, which occurs if pleural inflammation persists and then heals in the form of a visceral pleural rind.[58,59] Effusions associated with trapped lung, as opposed to the current case, are transudative.

Question 3: **E. Indwelling pleural catheter (IPC)**

In light of this patient's limited chemotherapeutic options and the relief provided by thoracentesis, interventional management of her malignant pleural effusion (MPE) would be appropriate at this point.[60] Because of her unexpandable lung, pleurodesis by whatever route would not be expected to succeed due to the inability of the visceral and parietal pleural surfaces to oppose. Serial thoracentesis can be an option for selected patients with very limited life expectancy in a hospice setting but is impractical for those expected to receive further treatment and remain at home. Symptomatic MPEs complicated by unexpandable lung are best palliated with an IPC as its success is not predicated on pleural apposition. In MPEs with full lung expansion, the choice between pleurodesis and IPC remains a patient-driven one. Available evidence indicates that IPCs reduce the length of stay and the need for repeat pleural procedures compared to pleurodesis with no difference in symptom improvement.[61] The main drawbacks of IPCs are the need for patient involvement and catheter-related complications, including infection, occlusion, and tract metastases. In the majority of cases, these can be addressed with minimal additional invasiveness, and the incidence of each of these complications is <10%.[62] Of note, spontaneous pleurodesis after several weeks to months of IPC drainage is an increasingly recognized phenomenon with reported rates of approximately 50%, allowing for the eventual removal of the IPC in those cases.[61]

Question 4: **A. Talc poudrage may be more effective than slurry in cases of lung and breast malignancy**

Talc is widely accepted as the most effective pleurodesis agent currently in clinical use, superior to alternatives such as doxycycline and bleomycin. Its success rate can be conservatively estimated as at least 70%.[63] Concern persists over reports of ARDS connected to the instillation of talc into the pleural space, though very few such cases have been reported with the use of graded large-particle talc routinely employed outside the United States. The theory is that there is less systemic absorption of the larger talc particles.[1] As a result, the use of ungraded talc is not recommended. A seminal study by Dressler et al. compared thoracoscopic talc insufflation (poudrage) to talc slurry via chest tube and found no overall difference in efficacy.[64] However, subgroup analysis revealed greater success of poudrage in cases of breast and lung malignancy. Cost-effectiveness analyses comparing talc pleurodesis to IPC placement have concluded that the former

is the more expensive of the two options in patients with a short life expectancy (e.g., <14 weeks).[65]

Question 5: **B. VEGF antagonism in the laboratory inhibits formation of malignant effusions in animal models**

Both MPEs and empyemas are characterized by markedly elevated levels of pleural fluid VEGF, a much more potent mediator of vascular permeability than is histamine.[66] VEGF is thought to be elaborated by malignant cells in the pleural space and contribute to pleural fluid accumulation by increasing pleural capillary permeability. Hypoxia and TGF-β are the strongest known inducers of VEGF release.[67] A number of animal models employing various methods of VEGF antagonism have demonstrated inhibition of malignant pleural and ascitic fluid formation.[67] Human data in support of the efficacy of VEGF inhibition as a treatment approach for MPEs are currently lacking.

REFERENCES

1. Light RW. *Pleural Diseases.* 5th ed. Philadelphia, PA: Lippincott Williams & Wilkins; 2007:306–339.
2. McGrath EE, Blades Z, Anderson PB. Chylothorax: aetiology, diagnosis and therapeutic options. *Respir Med.* 2010; 104(1):1–8.
3. Huggins JT. Chylothorax and cholesterol pleural effusion. *Semin Respir Crit Care Med.* 2010;31(6):743–750.
4. Almoosa KF, McCormack FX, Sahn SA. Pleural disease in Lymphangioleiomyomatosis. *Clin Chest Med.* 2006;27:355–368.
5. Maldonado F, Cartin-Ceba R, Hawkins FJ, et al. Medical and surgical management of chylothorax and associated outcomes. *Am J Med Sci.* 2010;339(4):314–318.
6. Kalomenides I. Octreotide and chylothorax. *Curr Opin Pulm Med.* 2006;12(4):264–267.
7. Visouli AN, Zarogoulidis K, Kougioumtzi I, et al. Catamenial pneumothorax. *J Thorac Dis.* 2014;6(S4):S448–S460.
8. Romero-Candeira S, Hernandez L, Romero-Brufao S, et al. Is it meaningful to use biochemical parameters to discriminate between transudative and exudative pleural effusions? *Chest.* 2002;122:1524–1529.
9. Porcel JM. Identifying transudates misclassified by Light's criteria. *Curr Opin Pulm Med.* 2013;19:362–367.
10. Bielsa S, Porcel JM, Castellote J, et al. Solving the Light's criteria misclassification rate of cardiac and hepatic transudates. *Respirology.* 2012;17:721–726.
11. Wilcox ME, Chong CAKY, Stanbrook MB, et al. Does this patient have an exudative pleural effusion? *JAMA.* 2014;311:2422–2431.
12. Porcel JM, Martinez-Alonso M, Cao G, et al. Biomarkers of heart failure in pleural fluid. *Chest* 2009;136:671–677.
13. Kolditz M, Halank M, Schiemanck S, et al. High diagnostic accuracy of NT-proBNP for cardiac origin of pleural effusions. *Eur Respir J.* 2006;28:144–150.

14. Porcel JM. Pleural effusions from congestive heart failure. *Semin Respir Crit Care Med.* 2010;31:689–697.

15. Colice GL, Curtis A, Deslauriers J, et al. Medical and surgical treatment of parapneumonic effusions: an evidence-based guideline. *Chest.* 2000;118:1158–1171.

16. Davies CWH, Gleeson FV, Davies RJO, et al. BTS guidelines for the management of pleural infection. *Thorax.* 2003;58(Suppl II):ii18–28.

17. Heffner JE, Klein JS, Hampson C. Interventional management of pleural infections. *Chest.* 2009;136:1148–1159.

18. Gordon CE, Feller-Kopman D, Balk EM, et al. Pneumothorax following thoracentesis. *Arch Intern Med.* 2010; 170:332–339.

19. Park JK, Kraus FC, Haaga JR. Fluid flow during percutaneous drainage procedures. *AJR Am J Roentgenol.* 1993;160: 165–169.

20. Rahman NM, Maskell NA, Davies CWH, et al. The relationship between chest tube size and clinical outcome in pleural infection. *Chest.* 2010;137:536–543.

21. Maskell NA, Davies CWH, Nunn AJ, et al. U.K. controlled trial of intrapleural streptokinase for pleural infection. *N Engl J Med.* 2005;352:865–874.

22. Rahman NM, Maskell NA, West A, et al. Intrapleural use of tissue plasminogen activator and DNase in pleural infection. *N Engl J Med.* 2011;365:518–526.

23. Maskell NA, Gleeson FV, Darby M, et al. Diagnostically significant variations in pleural fluid pH in loculated parapneumonic effusions. *Chest.* 2004;126:2022–2024.

24. Rahman NM, Mishra EK, Davies HE, et al. Clinically important factors influencing the diagnostic measurement of pleural fluid pH and glucose. *Am J Respir Crit Care Med.* 2008;178:483–490.

25. Menzies SM, Rahman NM, Wrightson JM, et al. Blood culture bottle culture of pleural fluid in pleural infection. *Thorax.* 2011;66:658–662.

26. Porcel JM, Esquerda A, Bielsa S. Diagnostic performance of adenosine deaminase activity in pleural fluid: a single-center experience with over 2100 consecutive patients. *Eur J Intern Med.* 2010;21:419–423.

27. Husain AN, Colby T, Ordonez N, et al. Guidelines for pathologic diagnosis of malignant mesothelioma: 2012 update of the consensus statement from the international mesothelioma interest group. *Arch Pathol Lab Med.* 2013;137:647–667.

28. Ray M, Kindler HL. Malignant pleural mesothelioma: an update on biomarkers and treatment. *Chest.* 2009;136:888–896.

29. Creaney J, Yeoman D, Demelker Y, et al. Comparison of osteopontin, megakaryocyte potentiating factor, and mesothelin proteins as markers in the serum of patients with malignant mesothelioma. *J Thorac Oncol.* 2008;3:851–7.

30. Bovolato P, Casadio C, Bille A, et al. Does surgery improve survival of patients with malignant pleural mesothelioma?: a multicenter retrospective analysis of 1365 consecutive patients. *J Thorac Oncol.* 2014;9(3):390–396.

31. Flores RM, Pass HI, Seshan VE, et al. Extrapleural pneumonectomy versus pleurectomy/decortication in the surgical management of malignant pleural mesothelioma: results in 663 patients. *J Thorac Cardiovasc Surg.* 2008;135 (3):620–626.

32. Heidecker J, Sahn SA. The spectrum of pleural effusions after coronary artery bypass grafting surgery. *Clin Chest Med.* 2006;27:267–283.

33. Light RW, Rogers JT, Cheng D, et al. Large pleural effusions occurring after coronary artery bypass grafting. *Ann Intern Med.* 1999;130:891–896.

34. Sadikot RT, Rogers JT, Cheng D, et al. Pleural fluid characteristics of patients with symptomatic pleural effusions after coronary artery bypass graft surgery. *Arch Intern Med.* 2000;160:2665–2668.

35. Labidi M, Baillot R, Dionne B, et al. Pleural effusions following cardiac surgery. *Chest.* 2009;136:1604–1611.

36. Light RW, Rogers JT, Moyers JP, et al. Prevalence and clinical course of pleural effusions at 30 days after coronary artery and cardiac surgery. *Am J Respir Crit Care Med.* 2002;166:1567–1571.

37. Imazio M, Brucato A, Rovere ME, et al. Colchicine prevents early postoperative pericardial and pleural effusions. *Am Heart J.* 2011;162:527–532.

38. Krenke R, Nasilowski J, Korczynski P, et al. Incidence and aetiology of eosinophilic pleural effusion. *Eur Respir J.* 2009;34:1111–1117.

39. Pereyra MF, Ferreiro L, Valdes L. Unexpandable lung. *Arch Bronconeumol.* 2013;49:63–69.

40. Huggins JT, Sahn SA, Heidecker J, et al. Characteristics of trapped lung. *Chest.* 2007;131:206–213.

41. Tattersall DJ, Traill ZC, Gleeson FV. Chest drains: does size matter? *Clin Radiol.* 2000;55(6):415–421.

42. Tsai WK, Chen W, Lee JC, et al. Pigtail catheters vs large-bore chest tubes for management of secondary spontaneous pneumothoraces in adults. *Am J Emerg Med.* 2006; 24(7):795–800.

43. MacDuff A, Arnold A, Harvey J, et al. Management of spontaneous pneumothorax: British Thoracic Society Pleural Disease Guideline 2010. *Thorax.* 2010;65(Suppl 2): ii18–31.

44. Yarmus L, Feller-Kopman D. Pneumothorax in the critically ill patient. *Chest.* 2012;141(4):1098–1105.

45. Ding W, Shen Y, Yang J, et al. Diagnosis of pneumothorax by radiography and ultrasonography. *Chest.* 2011;140 (4):859–866.

46. Alrajhi K, Woo MY, Vaillancourt C. Test characteristics of ultrasonography for the detection of pneumothorax: a systematic review and meta-analysis. *Chest.* 2012;141(3):703–708.

47. Soldati G, Testa A, Sher S, et al. Occult traumatic pneumothorax: diagnostic accuracy of lung ultrasonography in the emergency department. *Chest.* 2008;133(1):204–211.

48. De Luca C, Valentino M, Rimondi MR, et al. Use of chest sonography in acute-care radiology. *J Ultrasound.* 2008; 11(4):125–134.

49. Light RW, O'Hara VS, Moritz TE, et al. Intrapleural tetracycline for the prevention of recurrent spontaneous pneumothorax. Results of a Department of Veterans Affairs cooperative study. *JAMA.* 1990;264:2224–2230.

50. Grundy S, Bentley A, Tschopp JM. Primary spontaneous pneumothorax: a diffuse disease of the pleura. *Respiration.* 2012;83:185–189.

51. Noppen M, Dekeukeleire T, Hanon S, et al. Fluorescein-enhanced autofluorescence thoracoscopy in patients with primary spontaneous pneumothorax and normal subjects. *Am J Respir Crit Care Med.* 2006;174(1):26–30.

52. Azzopardi M, Porcel JM, Koegelenberg CFN, et al. Current Controversies in the management of malignant pleural effusions. *Semin Respir Crit Care Med.* 2014;35:723–731.

53. Reddy C, Ernst A, Lamb C, et al. Rapid pleurodesis for malignant pleural effusion. *Chest.* 2011;139(6):1419–1423.

54. Koegelenberg CFN, Diacon AH. Pleural controversy: closed needle pleural biopsy or thoracoscopy—which first? *Respirology.* 2011;16:738–746.

55. Porcel JM, Esquerda A, Vives M, et al. Etiology of pleural effusions: analysis of more than 3,000 consecutive thoracenteses. *Arch Bronconeumol.* 2014;50:161–165.

56. Porcel JM, Hernandez P, Martinez-Alonso M, et al. Accuracy of fluorodeoxyglucose-PET imaging for differentiating benign from malignant pleural effusions. *Chest.* 2015; 147:502–512.

57. Ferreiro L, San Jose E, Valdes L. Tuberculous pleural effusion. *Arch Bronconeumol.* 2014;50:435–453.

58. Huggins JT, Doelken P, Sahn SA. The unexpandable lung. *F1000 Med Rep.* 2010;2:77 doi:10.3410/M2-77.

59. Feller-Kopman D, Parker MJ, Schwartzstein RM. Assessment of pleural pressure in the evaluation of pleural effusions. *Chest.* 2009;135:201–209.

60. Thomas R, Francis R, Davies HE, et al. Interventional therapies for malignant pleural effusions: the present and the future. *Respirology.* 2014;19:809–822.

61. Davies HE, Mishra EK, Kahan BC, et al. Effect of an indwelling pleural catheter vs chest tube and talc pleurodesis for relieving dyspnea in patients with malignant pleural effusion: the TIME2 randomized controlled trial. *JAMA* 2012;307:2383–2389.

62. Ost DE, Jimenez CA, Lei X, et al. Quality-adjusted survival following treatment of malignant pleural effusions with indwelling pleural catheters. *Chest.* 2014;145:1347–1356.

63. Tan C, Sedrakyan A, Browne J, et al. The evidence on the effectiveness of management for malignant pleural effusion: a systematic review. *Eur J Cardiothorac Surg.* 2006;29: 829–838.

64. Dresler CM, Olak J, Herndon JE, et al. Phase III intergroup study of talc poudrage vs talc slurry sclerosis for malignant pleural effusion. *Chest.* 2005;127:909–915.

65. Penz ED, Mishra EK, Davies HE, et al. Comparing the cost of indwelling pleural catheter vs talc pleurodesis for malignant pleural effusion. *Chest.* 2014;146:991–1000.

66. Thickett DR, Armstrong L, Millar AB. Vascular endothelial growth factor (VEGF) in inflammatory and malignant pleural effusions. *Thorax.* 1999;54:707–710.

67. Grove CS, Lee YCG. Vascular endothelial growth factor: the key mediator in pleural effusion formation. *Curr Opin Pulm Med.* 2002;8:294–301.

12

Pulmonary Vascular Diseases

Luis D. Quintero, DO and Roxana Sulica, MD

CASE 1

A 43-year-old woman with no past medical history is seen in an urgent care setting for a 2-week history of leg swelling. She states her left leg is swollen and she notices edema around her calf. She has seen her primary care physician 1 week ago and he prescribed Bactrim. She has no travel history and she is a teacher. She is gravid 2 para 2 abortus 0. Vital signs are stable and the patient breaths 100% on ambient air. Her left leg has 2/4 edema compared to her right leg with some mild erythema. Dorsalis pedis and posterior tibialis are felt on her left leg and there is no tenderness to her left calf when squeezed. An ultrasound of her left leg shows a thrombus in her deep vein.

Question 1: What would be the most appropriate initial treatment?

A. Coumadin
B. Enoxaparin
C. Dabigatran
D. Heparin
E. Argatroban

Question 2: Given the patient's medical history, what is the minimum amount of time the patient should be anticoagulated?

A. 6 weeks
B. 12 weeks
C. 6 months
D. 12 months
E. Indefinite

Question 3: Which of the following has the correct drug with its mechanism of action?

A. Coumadin—Binds to antithrombin III
B. Enoxaparin—Inhibit vitamin K-dependent coagulation factor synthesis
C. Argatroban—Reversibly interact with platelet ADP receptor
D. Apixaban—Selectively blocks factor Xa
E. Dabigatran—Directly reversibly inhibits factor VII

CASE 2

A 95-year-old woman with history of CAD, chronic renal insufficiency, and hypertension is seen complaining of hemoptysis. Her vital signs are significant for a heart rate of 120, blood pressure of 100/60, respiratory rate of 24, and oxygen saturation of 90% on room air. A CT scan with IV contrast did show the following:

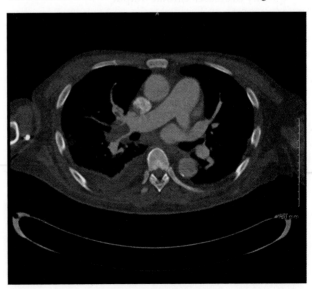

215

* *

Transthoracic echocardiogram is done which shows right ventricular strain. She is transferred to the ICU for further management.

Question 1: Based on the patients' history and examination, this patient would be classified into what prognostic category?

A. Low-risk pulmonary embolism
B. Medium to high risk pulmonary embolism
C. High-risk pulmonary embolism
D. Massive pulmonary embolism
E. Submassive pulmonary embolism

Question 2: Which of the following treatment plan is appropriate if the patient's blood pressure no longer responds to fluid bolus?

A. Milrinone
B. Norepinephrine
C. Furosemide
D. Thrombolytics
E. Antibiotics

Question 3: Which of the following is the correct pathophysiology that describes hypotension in pulmonary embolism?

A. Persistent hypoxia that results in systemic vasoconstriction followed by vasodilation
B. Inhibits forward flow at the level of the pulmonary artery
C. Inhibits forward flow by decreasing left ventricular size and thus cardiac output
D. Acute hypoxia that results in arrhythmia and subsequently decreases cardiac output
E. None of the above

CASE 3

A 65-year-old man with a past medical history significant for pancreatic cancer status post Whipple procedure comes to the emergency room for a sudden onset of pain in his left lower extremity. The pain began 6 hours prior to his ED visit and since that time his left leg has swollen and turned a deep purple. His pain is 10/10. His vital signs are 180/97, pulse 122, oxygen saturation 100% on ambient air. Physical examination reveals a large swollen

left leg with 4/4 pitting edema and a bullae noted on the anterior thigh. The leg has a purple discoloration with left toe nails blue. No dorsalis pedis or posterior tibialis is felt. There is also decreased sensation on his right foot all the way up to his thigh. Tactile pain is also out of proportion when light touch is done on the left leg.

* *

Ultrasound of the left lower extremity indicates a thrombus in the deep and superficial venous system with Doppler indicating a low-flow state in the left leg.

Question 1: Which of the following is the best diagnosis to fit the patient's condition?

A. Pyoderma gangrenosum
B. Acute arterial embolism
C. Phlegmasia alba dolens
D. Phlegmasia cerulean dolens
E. Venous gangrene

Question 2: Which of the following is the most appropriate initial treatment?

A. Fasciotomy
B. Thrombectomy
C. Catheter-directed thrombolysis
D. Amputation
E. Coumadin

Question 3: Which of the following describes the pathophysiology of this condition?

A. Acute arterial emboli lodged in the arterial system
B. Infection causing large volume exudates causing increased pressure in extremity
C. Mass compressing the proximal venous system causing increased hydrostatic pressure in extremity
D. Extensive thrombus formation in venous system causing increased hydrostatic pressure
E. None of the above

CASE 4

A 69-year-old man with a past medical history of hypertension presented to the emergency room for dyspnea. He was given a diagnosis of pulmonary arterial hypertension 3 months ago and was started on bosentan 2 weeks ago. CXR showed the following:

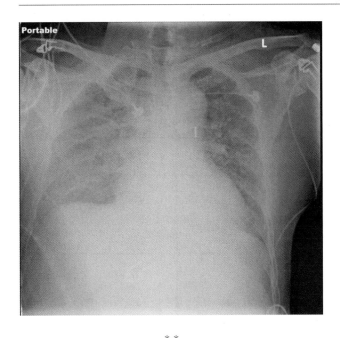

* *

While in the hospital, the patient underwent VQ scan which showed large perfusion/ventilation defects at left lower lobe anterior basal segment and at left apex with several other medium size perfusion/ventilation mismatched defects at the right lung. A right heart catheterization was done with measurement of three different pulmonary wedge pressures at three different locations.

Right Heart Catheterization

PCW	Mean	10	Mean	13	Mean	18
PA	Systolic	70	Diastolic	30	Mean	44
RV	Systolic	74	Diastolic	8	End-diastolic	10
RA	a-wave	15	v-wave	13	Mean	11

All values in mm Hg.

Pulmonary angiogram showed no evidence of chronic thromboembolic disease. Bosentan was discontinued and a combination of diuresis and thoracentesis improved the patient's dyspnea. Concerned for a rapidly progressing pulmonary artery pressures and failed bosentan treatment, the patient was referred to a transplant center.

Question 1: **What is the most likely diagnosis?**

A. Idiopathic pulmonary arterial hypertension
B. Chronic thromboembolic pulmonary hypertension
C. Systemic sclerosis-induced pulmonary hypertension
D. Pulmonary venous hypertension due to left heart disease
E. Pulmonary veno-occlusive disease

Question 2: **Which of the following methods would lead to accurate diagnosis of this disease?**

A. Pro-BNP
B. Bronchoscopy
C. Right heart catheterization
D. Lung biopsy
E. CT scan with IV contrast

Question 3: **The pathophysiology of this disease differs from all others in its class by affecting which portion of the cardiopulmonary system?**

A. Pulmonary arterial branches
B. Pulmonary capillary beds
C. Pulmonary venous branches
D. Right ventricular musculature
E. Left ventricular musculature

CASE 5

A 65-year-old woman with no significant past medical history come the office for evaluation of dyspnea on excursion. She was in her usual state of health until 9 months ago when her exercise tolerance had decreased. She was an avid marathon runner but now she cannot finish more than half a mile without having shortness of breath. Initial evaluation showed a loud P2 and her transthoracic echocardiogram showed an estimated pulmonary arterial systolic pressure of 70 mm Hg. Workup for pulmonary hypertension revealed a normal chest radiograph, pulmonary function test with mildly decreased DLco, and radioisotope ventilation/perfusion scan showed the following:

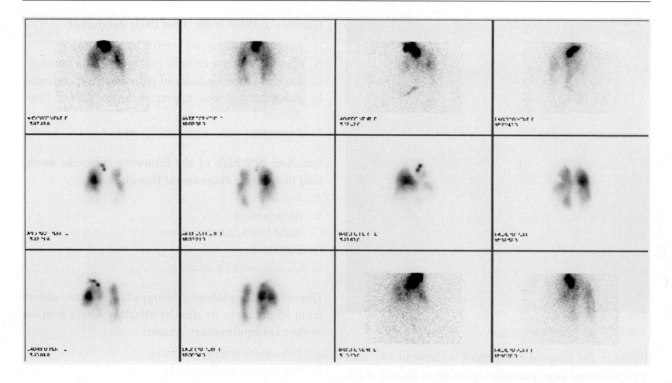

Question 1: **Which of the following is the most sensitive test to help screen for this particular type of pulmonary hypertension?**

A. CT pulmonary angiography
B. MR of the pulmonary vessels
C. Transthoracic echocardiogram
D. Lung ventilation–perfusion scan
E. D-dimer

Question 2: **Which of the following is the best therapeutic option for this patient?**

A. Riociguat
B. Pulmonary thromboendarterectomy
C. Coumadin
D. Percutaneous pulmonary angioplasty
E. Enoxaparin

Question 3: **Which of the following treatment modality has shown promise to reduce the occurrence of this disease?**

A. Altaplase
B. Pulmonary wedge resection
C. Azithromycin
D. Apixaban
E. All of the above

CASE 6

A 45-year-old woman presents to clinic for evaluation of chronic dyspnea. She states her dyspnea occurs after a few minutes of exercise and her tolerance has decreased over the last 6 months. She is able to walk four flights of stairs without stopping and walks at brisk pace in the park on inclines for at least 5 minutes before becoming short of breath. She has no significant past medical history. She is not sure of her family history but knows her mother passed away in her 50s from a heart problem. Initial examination reveals the following:

**

Vital Signs: 112/70, pulse 80, respiratory rate 16, 96% O$_2$ on ambient air. She is well appearing, under no acute distress. On physical examination she has a loud P2 and RV heave and a systolic murmur at the left lower sternal level.

**

During a 6-minute walk test she is able to walk 420 m without desaturation. She has had a right heart catheterization which showed the following:

Right Heart Catheterization					
PCW	Mean	12			
PA	Systolic	65	Diastolic	40	Mean	50
RV	Systolic	62	Diastolic	10	End-diastolic	8
RA	a-wave	15	v-wave	13	Mean	16

Mean PAP Pre-Nitric Oxide	Mean PAP Post-Nitric Oxide
50	35

All values in mm Hg.

* *

Cardiac output and systolic blood pressure did not change with the inhalation of 40 ppm of nitric oxide during right heart catheterization. A VQ scan done shortly after RHC was not significant.

Question 1: **Based on the patient's clinical symptoms and new diagnosis of pulmonary hypertension, what World Health Organization function class would the patient be identified as?**

A. WHO Function Class I
B. WHO Function Class II
C. WHO Function Class III
D. WHO Function Class IV
E. WHO Function Class V

Question 2: **Based on the patient's clinical symptoms and right heart catheterization, what would be the best medication to begin in order to optimize the patient's functional status?**

A. Sildenafil
B. Nifedepine
C. Epoprostenol
D. Digoxin
E. Pulmonary thromboendarterectomy

Question 3: **According to the REVEAL registry, which of the following risk factors has a greater impact on the prognostic factor for a newly diagnosed patient with pulmonary hypertension?**

A. WHO Class I
B. Pericardial effusion on echocardiogram
C. Pulmonary function test which shows percent predicted DLco >80
D. Baseline heart rate greater than 92 bpm
E. Hereditary pulmonary arterial hypertension

CASE 7

This is a 50-year-old man with past medical history of alcoholism and cirrhosis of the liver, with a Child-Pugh class B and MELD score of 20, who is evaluated for persistent shortness of breath.

* *

He is able to walk five blocks without any chest pain or shortness of breath 6 months ago but now he cannot walk more than one block. His initial examination demonstrates oxygen saturation of 94% in ambient air. Physical examination reveals sclera icterus, jugular venous distension, loud P2 noticed in right sternal boarder, crackles at the lung bases bilaterally, abdominal distention, and ¾ pitting edema in lower extremities. Chest radiograph illustrates clear lungs with distended pulmonary artery.

* *

As part of the initial workup an ABG shows mild hypoxemia, pulmonary function testing has found a restrictive pattern with a percent predicted DLco of 55%, and echocardiogram demonstrates distended right ventricle.

Question 1: **Which of the following transthoracic echocardiogram criteria should be used when screening this patient for pulmonary hypertension?**

A. Using a right ventricular systolic measure of greater than 50 mm Hg
B. Right ventricular end diastolic diameter greater than 3.3 cm
C. Unremarkable left ventricular function
D. Contrast TTE that is negative intracardiac shunts
E. All of the above

Question 2: **Which of the following should be used in the treatment of this patient?**

A. Nifedipine
B. Enoxaparin
C. Sildenafil
D. Iloprost
E. Nadolol

Question 3: **Which of the following is indicative of a diagnosis of hepatopulmonary syndrome?**

A. Normal to mild hypoxemia on ABG
B. Pulmonary vascular resistance greater than 240 dyn s/cm^5
C. Loud P2 on cardiac examination
D. Transthoracic Echocardiogram which demonstrates intrapulmonary shunting (in 3–6 cardiac cycles.)
E. Cyanosis

CASE 8

A 51-year-old woman is admitted to the hospital for worsening dyspnea and chest pain. She has a history of pulmonary hypertension and has failed multiple treatments. She was placed on continuous intravenous epoprostenol 6 months ago with good response. She is in her usual state of health until 2 days ago when she experiences increased dyspnea with exertion and finally dyspnea at rest.

**

Vital signs are the following: 100/65, pulse 110, respiration 20/min, and 89% on 4L nasal cannula. Her physical examination demonstrates stone facies, sclerodactyly with pitting finger nails, telangiectasia, 2/4 pitting edema in lower extremity, loud P2 with systolic murmur at left second intercostal area, and a fine crackles in lower lungs bilaterally.

**

Chest radiograph shows alveolar filing and increased interstitial marking with a prominent aortic knob. The patient is started on broad spectrum antibiotics, while her steroids and diuresis were increased.

Question 1: **Which of the following profile predisposes this patient to pulmonary hypertension?**

A. Anti-topoisomerase antibodies
B. Anti–U3-RNP
C. Anti-Ro and anti-La
D. Scl-70
E. Anti-double stranded-DNA

Question 2: **Which of the following treatment has been shown to be effective in the treatment of connective tissue disease–associated pulmonary hypertension?**

A. Sildenafil
B. Bosentan
C. Epoprostenol
D. Treprostinil
E. All of the above

Question 3: **Which treatment has recent studies demonstrated to have improvement in patients with pulmonary hypertension and systemic scleroderma?**

A. Nifedepine
B. Imatinib
C. Dexamethasone
D. Torsemide
E. Cyclosporine

CASE 9

A 67-year-old African-American man presented for evaluation of dyspnea. He had a past medical history of "eye problems" which had gotten worse recently, in addition to a family history of "lung problems" for which his father passed away when he was 55-year-old. The patient stated he has noticed decrease exercise tolerance for the last year. Previous cardiac workup had been negative. His physical examination was significant for fine bibasilar crackles. Pulmonary function testing showed restrictive physiology and a decrease in diffusion capacity. Echocardiogram and right heart catheterization showed moderate pulmonary hypertension with right heart dysfunction. He was started with bosentan with modest improvement. The patient had the following CT scan demonstrating hilar adenopathy and interstitial fibrotic changes most pronounced in the upper lobes.

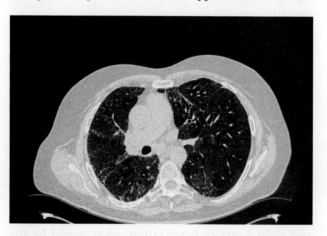

**

He subsequently had bronchoscopy with EBUS. His medical treatment for dyspnea was changed once his lung biopsies returned and demonstrated marked improvement.

Question 1: **Which of the following findings warrant screening for pulmonary hypertension?**

A. Bibasilar crackles bilaterally
B. Restrictive lung pattern on PFTs
C. CT scan results
D. Low diffusion capacity on PFTs
E. Family history of lung problems

Question 2: **Based on the patient's primary diagnosis, what would be first choice of treatment?**

A. Bosentan
B. Prednisone
C. Epoprostenol
D. Infliximab
E. Treprostinil

Question 3: **A patient, like the one in this case, presents to the emergency room with similar complaints. The diagnosis of this patient is the same as the one in the case study except for the following right heart catheterization:**

Right Heart Catheterization

PCW	Mean	30				
PA	Systolic	60	Diastolic	40	Mean	42
RV	Systolic	60	Diastolic	10	End-diastolic	8
RA	a-wave	15	v-wave	13	Mean	11

All values in mm Hg.

Which of the following pathologies explain the patient's symptoms and catheterization?

A. Idiopathic pulmonary hypertension
B. Pulmonary fibrosis
C. Cardiomyopathy
D. Tricuspid stenosis
E. Ventricular septal defect

CASE 10

A 72-year-old woman with past medical history of hypertension was admitted to the hospital for hemoptysis. The patient admits she has a history of hemoptysis for several years but recently has been coughing up a cup of blood a day for the last week. Her sister has similar complaints of bleeding but from the rectum. CT scan with IV contrast shows a single feeding artery and draining vein in the right lower lobe. Bronchoscopy did not demonstrate active bleeding but several areas of clots.

Question 1: **Which of the following diseases is associated with the patient's symptoms?**

A. Hereditary hemorrhagic telangiectasia
B. Hepatopulmonary syndrome
C. Bidirectional cavopulmonary shunt
D. Pulmonary malignancy
E. Pulmonary tuberculosis

Question 2: **Which of the following test could have been done in order to screen for intrapulmonary shunting?**

A. Chest x-ray
B. Bleeding scan
C. Transthoracic contrast echocardiography
D. Blood gas before and after exertion
E. All of the above

CASE 11

An 18-year-old man is for chronic cough. He has tried several OTC and prescription remedies with minimal improvement. His past medical history is unremarkable except for several hospitalizations for pneumonia when he was a child. His medical records indicate a negative sweat chloride test, and treatment for pseudomonal pneumonia 1 year ago. Previous CT scans do not suggest bronchiectasis or dextrocardia. An ultrasound of his lung reveals an echodense homogeneous mass and Dopplers demonstrate blood flow from lung mass to aorta. An MRA is ordered which confirm the ultrasound/Doppler results.

Question 1: **In which part of the lung is this pathology generally found?**

A. Medial basal segment of right lung
B. Posterior basal segment of left lung
C. Apical segment of right lung
D. Anterior segment of left lung
E. Bilateral lower lobes

Question 2: **Which of the following is the most appropriate treatment assuming the mass is intrapulmonary?**

A. No intervention needed
B. Chronic antibiotic use
C. Investigational bronchoscopy
D. Bronchodilators
E. Lobectomy

Question 3: **Which of the following is the pathophysiology for the creation of this mass?**

A. Accessory lung bud that develops from the ventral aspect of the primitive foregut
B. Proliferation of bronchial cells
C. Proliferation of pleural cells
D. Accessory esophagus bud that develops from the ventral aspect of the primitive foregut
E. Displacement and proliferation of cardiac cells

Answers

CASE 1

Question 1: B. Enoxaparin

Enoxaparin is the best option for a healthy patient with new onset DVT. Meta-analysis and Cochrane reviews suggest low molecular weight heparin (LMWH), such as enoxaparin, is superior in a patient with good renal function and no contraindication to heparin.[1]

* *

These studies explain that LMWH molecules are more stable and their pharmacokinetics are more predictable when compared to unfractionated heparin. These studies suggest lower mortality, fewer recurrent thromboembolic events, and a decrease incidence of major bleeding. However, LMWH is less desirable in patients who are obese (greater than 165 kg), have low body weight (less than 45 kg in women and less than 57 kg in men), and have renal insufficiency (creatinine clearance less than 30 mL/min).[1,2] These make anti-Xa levels unpredictable and testing for anti-Xa is not readily available.

* *

Advantages to the use of intravenous unfractionated heparin (IVUFH) include: (1) no reservations regarding its use in renal failure and obese patients; (2) easily monitored with partial prothrombin time every 6 hours; and (3) short half-life so can be easily.[1,2]

* *

The use of heparin can be given in patients with upper extremity DVTs (UEDVT). These types of DVTs have a greater risk of thoracic outlet obstruction and limb ischemia. Therefore the recommendation for heparin is used only in patients in whom UEDVT is chronic (<2 weeks) and not causing ischemia.[1,2] If the UEDVT is less than 2 weeks or causing ischemia, it is recommended that the patient undergoes thrombolysis or surgical decompression.[1,2]

* *

Regardless of which type of heparin patients are exposed to, there is always the possibility of heparin induced thrombocytopenia (HIT). Heparin-induced thrombocytopenia type I demonstrates a transient decrease of platelets roughly 2 days after exposure to heparin, which is relieved shortly after discontinuation of heparin.[3] This decrease appears to be due to platelet aggregation. Heparin induced thrombocytopenia type II is a more aggressive phenomenon that results in antibodies to platelet factor IV.[3] This heparin-antibody complex can cause acute drop (50%) of platelets if they had prior exposure to heparin in the last 30 days or at least 5th day of initiation of heparin. This may cause thrombosis and limb ischemia.[3] A high clinical suspicion is needed because a prompt discontinuation of heparin may save a limb and decrease morbidity.

* *

If HIT is suspected or confirmed, the type of anticoagulation should be changed to a nonheparin option. Argatroban is a competitive direct thrombin inhibitor that reversibly binds to thrombin active site.[3,4] It is difficult to initiate and maintain and not generally part of everyday practice, therefore, argatroban is reserved to those who have HIT or cannot tolerate heparin for any other reason.

* *

Coumadin is drug that works on inhibiting vitamin K and thus inhibiting all coagulation factors that are associated with vitamin K. This would be appropriate treatment for long-term anticoagulation but inappropriate for a new onset DVT. Low molecular weight heparin or IVUFH is generally used first as a bridge to Coumadin because it takes approximately 5 days in order to obtain a therapeutic INR. Since LMWH and IVUFH are fast acting agents, they are used prior to initiation of Coumadin in order to prevent cutaneous necrosis. Once the INR is at a therapeutic range, heparin is discontinued in favor of monotherapy with Coumadin.

**

Dabigatran has been approved for the prophylaxis and treatment of DVT and PE treatment. The FDA recently considered Dabigatran to have a favorable benefit to risk profile compared to Coumadin, but is still not recommended as the first line treatment.

Question 2: B. 12 weeks

The decision on how long to treat a DVT or subsequent pulmonary embolus is a decision that is multifactorial. In 2012 the American College of Chest Physicians released their recommendations on how long a patient should be treated with anticoagulation for DVT/PE.[1] The recommendation comes from analysis of several studies performed throughout the years.

**

The ACCP divides patients into several categories: surgical patients, provoked patients, and unprovoked (idiopathic) patients. There is also a section regarding anticoagulation and cancer. The following is a chart that illustrates those recommendations:[1]

Recommendations for the Duration of Anticoagulation Therapy for DVT	
Risk factor for DVT/PE	Duration of treatment
Transient risk factor	3 months—Minimum treatment
Unprovoked	Indefinitely—Maximum treatment
• Minimal treatment: Isolated distal DVT, or first proximal DVT/PE and a high/moderate risk of bleeding, or a patient's wish to stop	3 months—Minimum treatment
Active malignancy	Indefinitely—Maximum treatment
• Minimal treatment: Very high risk of bleeding, isolated distal DVT, or an additional major transient risk factor for PE/DVT	Consider stopping therapy at 3 months or when the cancer becomes inactive

All patients with DVT/PE should be anticoagulated for at least 3 months. Since she had an unprovoked episode of DVT, her risk for developing a PE/DVT after completing treatment with anticoagulation is 10% and 30% within 5 years, it is recommended to be treated indefinitely.

Question 3: D. Apixaban—Selectively blocks factor Xa

Drug	Mechanism of Action
Coumadin	Inhibits vitamin K–dependent coagulation factor synthesis (II, VII, XI, X, protein C and S)
Enoxaparin	Binds to antithrombin III and accelerates activity, inhibiting thrombin and factor Xa
Argatroban	Competitive direct thrombin inhibitor that reversibly binds to thrombin active site
Apixaban	Selectively blocks active site of factor Xa (factor Xa inhibitor)
Dabigatran	Directly, reversibly inhibits thrombin

CASE 2

Question 1: E. Submassive pulmonary embolism

The European Society of Cardiology and American Heart Association have classified pulmonary embolism into three different categories depending on their vital signs, echocardiogram findings and prognosis.[5,6] The three categories are divided into high-risk (massive) PE, intermediate risk (submassive) PE, and low risk (nonmassive PE). According to the International Cooperative Pulmonary Embolism Registry (ICOPER), the 90-day mortality for massive PE was 52% compared to 15% in the submassive category.[5,6] The following describes how to categorize PEs.

Classification of PE into Prognostic Categories by the European Society of Cardiology and American Heart Association

Category	Definition
High-risk (Massive) pulmonary embolus	1. Arterial hypotension (systolic BP <90 mm Hg or a decrease of >40 mm Hg) for more than 15 minutes or requiring inotropic support, which is not caused by a new onset arrhythmia 2. Cardiogenic shock (oliguria, lactic acidosis, cool extremities, or altered level of consciousness) 3. Circulatory collapse, in patients with syncope or undergoing cardiopulmonary resuscitation
Intermediate-risk (submassive) pulmonary embolus	1. Systolic blood pressure greater than 90 mm Hg 2. Echocardiograph evidence of RV dysfunction or pulmonary hypertension 3. Presence of increased markers of MI
Low-risk (nonmassive) pulmonary embolus	1. Systolic blood pressure greater than 90 mm Hg 2. No evidence of RV dysfunction or hypertension 3. No evidence of MI

Question 2: B. Norepinephrine

Since the patient is classified as having a submassive pulmonary embolism, treatment of the patient is geared toward hemodynamic stability without overloading the right ventricle and causing right ventricular failure. As with any hemodynamically unstable patient, fluid bolus or challenge should be attempted. However, patients with submassive PEs have right heart dysfunction due to pulmonary artery resistance caused by the embolus. Continuous fluid administration in a patient that does not respond should alert the physician that right heart overload is occurring and the patient should be switched to another medical therapy. Though decreasing fluid overload on the right heart with furosemide may be an option for patients with chronic pulmonary hypertension and elevated RV preload, the patient in this case study has acute RV dysfunction with likely normal preload and is not hemodynamically stable and thus diuresis is not an option.

* *

An appropriate next option would be positive RV inotropic support with a medication like dobutamine; however, milrinone has a significant systemic hypotensive effect and may worsen her hemodynamic instability. Thrombolysis is not routinely indicated in submassive pulmonary embolism. Though antibiotics would be given in any patient with hypotension of unknown cause (e.g., sepsis) the patient in this question has a reason to be hypotensive thus antibiotics would not be given.

* *

Since her blood pressure is not responding to fluid bolus a vasopressor, such as norepinephrine or dopamine, is the best option to maintain perfusion.

Question 3: C. Inhibits forward flow by decreasing left ventricular size and thus cardiac output

The pathophysiology of massive and submassive pulmonary embolus is complex and multifactorial. The embolus causes a mechanical obstruction which inhibits blood flow from the pulmonary artery to the left ventricle. This ultimately increases right ventricular strain which can lead to RV overload. When the right ventricle expands, it displaces the interventricular septum toward left heart. This decreases the left ventricular volume capacity. This can cause a decrease in cardiac output and cardiogenic shock.

* *

In addition to mechanical obstruction, persistent resistance in the right ventricle and pulmonary artery causes a release of vasoactive substances such as thromboxane A2 and serotonin which causes vasoconstriction in the pulmonary arteries, increase in pulmonary resistance, and increase in VQ mismatch.

* *

Persistent hypoxia has shown to cause vasoconstriction, which is the reason why patients with pulmonary hypertension are given oxygen if their oxygen saturation is less than 90% in ambient air. Acute persistent hypoxia can cause arrhythmia due to ultimate myocardial infarction, but this is toward the end of the disease process and not the central aspect of this disease progression.

CASE 3

Question 1: D. Phlegmasia cerulean dolens

The patient is experiencing complications of a venous thrombus formation called phlegmasia cerulean dolens

(PCD). The milder form is called phlegmasia alba dolens (PAD) and this condition is observed when a patient develops thrombosis in the major deep venous system of an extremity. Patients with PAD present with edema of the affected extremity, pain, and blanching of the skin without signs of cyanosis.

* *

Phlegmasia cerulean dolens is a severe condition with complete obstructive of venous outflow from thrombosis in the major deep venous system and the collateral veins.[7-9] This causes massive venous congestion and fluid sequestration which can cause compromise of oxygen to the affected limb. The large volume fluid sequestration can also cause circulatory collapse and shock. PCD present with a classic triad of edema, pain out of proportion to physical examination, and cyanosis. Large venous congestion can cause blebs or bullae formation.

* *

The most severe complication of venous thrombosis is venous gangrene. The clinical presentation is like PCD with arterial compromise to the affected limb. This is caused by an increase in pressure from the venous congestion which leads to compartment syndrome followed by ischemia. Phlegmasia cerulean dolens and venous gangrene continue to have a large morbidity and mortality rates regardless of medical and surgical advances. Amputation rates are seen in 12% to 50% are seen is those who survive the condition.[9]

* *

Arterial embolism can cause edema, pain, and cyanosis in those limbs affected. However, arterial emboli usually affect only one portion of the limb or digits on the limb and not the whole limb. The classic case is a patient with endocarditis with dry gangrene to the first digit on the lower extremity.

* *

Pyoderma gangrenosum is a disorder associated with other systemic diseases (e.g., inflammatory bowel disease and leukemia) that presents as a large ulcerative lesion that generally begins as small red papule or pustule. The progression of the disease varies but physical examination demonstrates normal peripheral pulses and a large ulceration in the affected area.

* *

Several risk factors have been associated with the development of thrombus formation, but not all of these risk factors apply to patients who develop PCD. Below is a list of risk factors with the greatest increase on the top to the lowest risk at the bottom.

Risk Factors for Phlegmasia Cerulean Dolens
Malignancy
Hypercoagulable state
Venous stasis
Contraceptive agents
IVC filter
May–Thurner syndrome
Aneurysm
Previous DVT
Trauma

Question 2: C. Catheter-directed thrombolysis

Treatment of PCD and venous gangrene has mixed results over the years. Unfortunately it still maintains a high morbidity and mortality rate. Vascular surgeons used to perform manual thrombectomy to the proximal veins and some of the distal veins as well. This treatment has not been successful due to the fact that smaller thrombi would be left in distal and collateral veins and therefore would not fix the entire problem.

* *

Fasciotomy was used in the past with dismal results. Undergoing only fasciotomy did not address the underlying problem of massive thrombus formation and increased fluid sequestration. The fasciotomy itself had a high rate of infection and poor healing prognosis. Today, fasciotomy is only used if compartment syndrome is suspected as this will buy time before additional interventions are done. Finally, amputation is a last resort if the patient develops venous gangrene.

* *

Recently, there have been two treatments that have been used to help with PCD. The first is using anticoagulation, such as heparin, in order to prevent clot formation.[8,10] This method has been used in conjunction of limb elevation and fluid resuscitation. The treatment is indicated for PAD and PCD and has success in those patients with PCD who are not yet in danger of venous gangrene. The idea behind the treatment is to use heparin to prevent any additional clot formation thus preventing the progression from PCD to venous gangrene. Limb elevation is used to help decrease edema and thus decrease the compartment pressure. Fluid resuscitation is used in case the sequestration of fluid in the limb is large enough to cause circulatory collapse. It should be noted that if the patient does not improve over 8 hours or shows progression of disease then a surgical option is mandated.

**

Currently, catheter-directed thrombolysis is thought to be the best surgical option for those patients suffering from PCD.[8,9,10] The idea is to direct thrombolytic therapy to the affected limb and not only manage the proximal thrombus but also the more distal thrombi that cannot be manually removed. This method also has been shown to preserve the patency of venous collateral circulation. Catheter-directed thrombolysis has been attempted from the venous circulation and from the arterial circulation. Both methods have been successful with the arterial side being slightly better. The major complication of thrombolysis is the dislodging of a thrombus and causing a pulmonary embolus. Currently, it is recommended that any patient who undergoes catheter-directed thrombolysis have an IVC filter inserted prior to the procedure.

**

Coumadin is the treatment of choice to help clear the overall clot burden after catheter-directed thrombolysis is done. Coumadin works by inhibiting vitamin K and thus inhibiting all coagulation factors that are associated with vitamin K. Achieving a therapeutic INR allows the body to break down chronic clots in the affected limb thus decreasing the overall clot burden overtime. Depending if this is the first or second episode of PCD will dictate how long that patient will need to be on Coumadin.

Question 3: D. Extensive thrombus formation in venous system causing increased hydrostatic pressure

Since the patient in the case has phlegmasia cerulean dolens, the thrombus formation is located in the major deep veins in addition to collateral and small veins. This thrombus formation can involve the capillaries which ultimately lead to venous gangrene. The thrombus in the capillaries increases the hydrostatic pressure beyond the oncotic pressure causing fluid sequestration in the interstitium. In the lower extremities, the legs can hold up to 10 liters of fluid which can cause circulatory collapse and shock. Simple thrombectomy of the proximal veins is not sufficient in patients with severe PCD because the pressure from the collateral veins and capillaries cannot be removed.

**

Acute arterial emboli lodged in the arterial system are seen in endocarditis. Infection causing large volume exudates causing increased pressure in extremity is seen in sepsis and at time DIC. Mass compressing the proximal venous system causing increased hydrostatic pressure in extremity can cause marked edema and even lymphedema but the condition itself only manifests the proximal veins and lymphatics, leaving the capillaries and collateral veins intact.

CASE 4

Question 1: E. Pulmonary veno-occlusive disease

The case illustrated is of a patient with pulmonary veno-occlusive disease (PVOD). PVOD is thought to represent approximately 5% to 10% of all cases diagnosed with idiopathic pulmonary arterial hypertension (IPAH).[11-13] A rare disease with a poor prognosis and limited treatment plan, PVOD is definitively diagnosed with a biopsy of the pulmonary vasculature. Unlike IPAH, PVOD affects the pulmonary venous system and causes fibrous intimal proliferation that mostly involves the pulmonary venules and small veins. Although controversial, the presence of segmental mismatched perfusion defects with normal pulmonary angiogram has been described in PVOD.[11-13]

**

One of the characteristics of PVOD is the inability to use IPAH treatment due to the risk of abrupt and potentially life-threatening deterioration. Most patients develop pulmonary edema when started on IPAH specific therapy such as bosentan, sildenafil, or even epoprostenol. Because of the lack of appropriate medical treatment available, few patients survive longer than 2 years. The only curative measure known is lung transplantation, but finding an appropriate surgical candidate is difficult and thus studies have recently been geared toward early identification of PVOD.

**

Identifying risk factors for PVOD has been challenging given the small number of patients confirmed with the disease post-mortem. PVOD is seen in several different diseases that affects IPAH such as connective tissue diseases, sarcoidosis, pulmonary Langerhans cell histiocytosis, and HIV infection.

＊ ＊

There are isolated case reports of PVOD who have been exposed to chemotherapy agents such as bleomycin, bis-chloronitrosourea, and mitomycin after bone marrow transplantation. The only known risk factor that has been identified is tobacco exposure. This is of interest because tobacco exposure is not a known risk factor for the development of IPAH and is a risk factor for PVOD.

Question 2: D. Lung biopsy

PVOD is a rare disease that is difficult to diagnose because only surgical biopsy of the pulmonary vascular system can accurately diagnose the disease. Since lung transplant is the only curative measure, it is important to distinguish the disease from IPAH as these patients should be referred to a transplant center as soon as possible. This would increase the chances that a patient would be a good candidate for transplantation. The following table describes differences between IPAH and PVOD:

Selected Characteristics of Idiopathic Pulmonary Arterial Hypertension and Pulmonary Veno-Occlusive Disease		
Testing	**IPAH**	**PVOD**
Pulmonary function tests	Normal (possible restrictive pattern)	Normal (possible mild restrictive pattern)
Diffuse capacity (DLco/VA)	Often reduced	Lower than IPAH
PaO$_2$ at rest	Often reduced	Lower than IPAH
High-resolution CT scan	Lungs normal, enlarged pulmonary artery	Centrilobular ground-glass opacities, septal lines and lymph node enlarged, pleural disease
Bronchoalveolar lavage	Normal	Possible occult alveolar hemorrhage

＊ ＊

Bronchoalveolar lavage has recently been studied since occult pulmonary hemorrhage regularly occurs in PVOD rather than IPAH.[13] The Golde score, which has been used in leukemia patients suffering from pulmonary hemorrhage, is being studied as a way to quantify hemorrhage in PVOD. The Golde score takes BAL samples and looks at the number of intra-alveolar

siderin-laden macrophages. They are given a coefficient of 1 to 4 based on the staining intensities. This allows for a qualitative assessment in cell count. Patients with PVOD generally have a Golde score greater than 100. Golde score suggests pulmonary hemorrhage but is not specific to one particular disease.

＊ ＊

Pro-BNP is nonspecific to both diseases and right heart catheterization is the gold standard to diagnose pulmonary hypertension but cannot distinguish the different types of pulmonary hypertensions. Although controversial, the presence of segmental mismatched perfusion defects with a CT scan or V/Q scan with normal pulmonary angiogram has been described in PVOD. However, the gold standard for the diagnoses of PVOD continues to be a lung biopsy.

Question 3: C. Pulmonary venous branches

Pulmonary veno-occlusive disease is different from other forms of pulmonary hypertension because it affects the post-capillary and venous branches in the pulmonary vascular system. This is unlike IPAH, which affects the pre-capillary and pulmonary arterial system. Histologic examination reveals post-capillary lesions in septal veins and preseptal venules consisting of loose, fibrous remodeling of the intima.

＊ ＊

Decompensation in patients with PVOD using IPAH medical therapy is thought to be related to the vasodilation of the pre-capillary resistance vessels greater than the pulmonary capillaries and veins. This increases blood flow and increases hydrostatic pressure that leads to increase transudate and thus pulmonary edema. Surgical biopsies also demonstrate that PVOD involves the lymphatic system thus making resolution of pulmonary edema less likely. Case reports suggest that medications, such as epoprostenol, can be used cautiously in patients who are awaiting transplant. Patients started on these types of medications should be given low doses and increased in small increments in order to prevent rapidly accumulating pulmonary edema.

CASE 5

Question 1: D. Lung ventilation–perfusion scan

According to the American College of Chest Physicians, as part of the workup for pulmonary hypertension, patients should undergo a lung ventilation–perfusion (V/Q) scan in order to detect segmental or larger unmatched perfusion defects, which is the screening test for CTEPH.[14] Compared with CTPA, V/Q scan has a higher sensitivity (97.4%) in detecting CTEPH.[14,15]

* *

CT pulmonary angiography (CTPA) is routinely used in order to help diagnose acute pulmonary emboli, but this method should not be used in order to detect CTEPH. Since the pathogenesis of CTEPH is from chronic and unresolving clots, CTPA has a difficulty differentiating chronic thrombus with thickened vascular wall, erratic filling defects, sudden vessel narrowing, and intraluminal webs. Because of this, the sensitivity is variable depending on who reads the CTPA. Current studies have the sensitivity between 51% and 94% for detecting CTEPH.[14,15]

* *

MRI of the pulmonary vessels (MRPV) is a rapidly growing method to help diagnose CTEPH. The usefulness of MRPV comes from the ability identifying chronic clots at the segmental level but and also assesses right ventricular anatomy and function. MRPV has the added benefit of no radiation or iodine contrast. Though MRPV is relatively new, a recent study has the sensitivity of MRPV at 97% if done correctly.[15]

* *

Transthoracic echocardiogram (TTE) does not play a role in the diagnosis of CTEPH and can only identify those individuals who have elevated pulmonary pressures. It is recommended that patients who have an acute pulmonary embolus undergo a TTE 6 to 12 weeks after the initial TTE in order to determine if the mean pulmonary pressures remain elevated even in the setting of anticoagulation.

* *

Though D-dimer test is used to rule out DVT, it has little value to determine thrombus formation in the pulmonary vasculature. Therefore D-dimer test has little value as a screening tool for determining CTEPH.

Question 2: B. Pulmonary thromboendarterectomy

The patient in this scenario has chronic thromboembolic pulmonary hypertension (CTEPH), as suggested by VQ scan. A formal pulmonary angiogram is required for diagnostic confirmation. The disease is characterized by organized, nonacute thrombus in the pulmonary vascular bed causing a mean pulmonary arterial pressure greater than 25 mm Hg. Initially, CTEPH was thought that in order to have the disease, the patient needed to have a symptomatic pulmonary embolism. It is now known that approximately 60% to 75% of patients with CTEPH have a documented PE with the rest having silent thrombus formation in the pulmonary vasculature.[14-16] This chronic unresolving clot formation leads to pathological changes in the large vessels and distal small vessel arteries causing increasing pulmonary pressure.

* *

The diagnosis of CTEPH is critical in a patient with pulmonary hypertension because the optimal treatment is surgical rather than medical therapy. Once CTEPH is diagnosed, surgical candidates should be identified rapidly in order to halt the progression of the disease. The ideal surgical candidate is one who has proximal organized thrombi or isolated segmental disease with distal obstruction. In addition, patients who achieve the greatest benefit from this surgical procedure have preoperative pulmonary vascular resistance less than 1,000 dyn/s/cm[5].[15,16] Severe lung disease is contraindicated to surgery because of the potential reperfusion damage and worsening hypoxemia. Currently, pulmonary thromboendarterectomy (PTE) is the best therapy for those who are surgical candidates.[33]

* *

Medical therapy used on other pulmonary hypertension diseases is left only to those who are not considered surgical candidates or who have undergone surgery but continue to have elevated pulmonary pressures. Most patients who undergo medical therapy share the same benefits as seen in those with idiopathic pulmonary hypertension (improvement in 6-minute walk and improved pulmonary hemodynamics). Bosentan was used in the BENEFIT (Bosentan Effects in Inoperable Forms of chronic Thromboembolic pulmonary hypertension) trial and was found to improve pulmonary hemodynamics but not overall exercise capacity.[17] Sildenafil has also seen mixed results in patients with inoperable CTEPH but in one major open label trial, patients treated with sildenafil experienced improved symptoms and better 6-minute walk. The newer agent riociguat is the only medication specifically approved for CTEPH, but only in inoperable cases or residual pulmonary hypertension after PTE. In a double-blind placebo-controlled multicenter trial riociguat has improved exercise capacity and hemodynamics in patients with inoperable or residual CTEPN.[18] It should, however, not be administered instead of preoperative evaluation and PTE.

* *

Percutaneous pulmonary angioplasty has a history of mixed results. Studies done in the late 1990s and early 2000s demonstrated no improvement in cardiac index or hemodynamics and actually developed significantly more reperfusion lung injury when compared to PTE. Recently, pulmonary angioplasty has gained interest due to success in decreasing pulmonary arterial pressure without the increase in adverse events. This is partially due to modified procedure of the angioplasty, the use of smaller catheters, and the use of ultrasound guided placement of catheters. Currently this method is being studied on patients who are inoperable, the preliminary studies are promising, but it is restricted to a few centers of expertise.

* *

Enoxaparin is a low molecular weight heparin that should be used in order to help treat acute DVT/PE or chronic anticoagulate to prevent reoccurring PEs. Though most patients with CTEPH have an increased clot burden, enoxaparin is used only to help prevent additional perfusion mismatch and prevent worsening pulmonary arterial pressure.

* *

Coumadin (warfarin) interferes with synthesis of vitamin K–dependent clotting factors as well as protein C and protein S. It is generally used in conjunction with enoxaparin or heparin during initiation of Coumadin. This long-term anticoagulation helps decrease the overall clot burden which may help decrease overall pulmonary artery pressure. The use of Coumadin also helps prevent any additional clot burden, which would increase pulmonary artery pressure in the future. However, the use of Coumadin is limited to the prevention of additional thrombus formation in an already overburdened pulmonary vasculature.

Question 3: A. Altaplase
Two recent studies suggest that patients who present with an initial right ventricular systolic pressure of greater than 60 mm Hg at the time a massive pulmonary embolism occurs have a significantly higher probability of developing CTEPH 6 to 9 months after the initial echocardiogram. However, a retrospective study done by Thomas and Limbrey in 2012 suggested those patients with increased pulmonary pressures during PE and received thrombolytics had a significantly lesser chance of developing CTEPH versus those who did not receive lytics.[19] This same concept was discovered in 2009 by Kline et al. who enrolled 200 patients who were identified as having acute PE and increased pulmonary pressures.[20] All patients in the study received heparin for treatment, but those patients that received altaplase had a significantly lower pulmonary pressure 6 months after their acute PEs compared to those who did not receive alteplase.

* *

These two studies suggest two things. First, if the PE is removed quickly, there is less chance for sustained pulmonary pressures and thus would decrease the chance for CTEPH to develop. Second, the use of thrombolytics during an acute PE would not only help remove the massive clot, but would also remove distal clots as well thus decreasing the overall perfusion mismatch and remodeling of the pulmonary arterial system. Though the evidence is scarce, there may be a future role in using thrombolytics in those patients with increased pulmonary pressures in the setting of an acute PE.

CASE 6

Question 1: B. WHO Function Class II
Patients with pulmonary hypertension are grouped into a functional class defined by the WHO.[14] This functional class is important because it can help guide clinicians to appropriate treatment options.

WHO Functional Classification	Description
WHO Function Class I	No resulting limitation of physical activity
WHO Function Class II	Comfortable at rest and ordinary physical activity results in fatigue or dyspnea, chest pain, or heart syncope
WHO Function Class III	Comfortable at rest but can only undergo less than average physical activity due to fatigue, dyspnea, chest pain, or heart syncope
WHO Function Class IV	Inability to carry on any physical activity without symptoms; signs and symptoms of right heart failure or fatigue at rest

Based on the patient's new onset exercise tolerance and new diagnosis of pulmonary hypertension, the patient would be WHO Function Class II.

Question 2: **B. Nifedipine**

Pulmonary hypertension should be approached in a stepwise fashion in order to determine the etiology of the disease and treatment. If clinical suspicion is high for pulmonary hypertension, a noninvasive test, such as echocardiogram, should be performed. If the echocardiogram shows elevated right ventricular pressure then other noninvasive testing, such as VQ scan, overnight oximetry, blood testing for HIV/ANA/liver function tests, and pulmonary function testing should be done first. These tests attempt to identify the cause of elevated pulmonary pressure. If an underlying disease is identified as the cause of elevated pulmonary arterial pressure then treatment is geared toward addressing that particular disease process rather than solely focusing on decreasing the elevated pulmonary arterial pressures.

* *

Right heart catheterization, with pulmonary arterial pressure ≥25 mm Hg and a normal pulmonary capillary wedge pressure ≤15 mm Hg, is the gold standard for the diagnosis of pulmonary hypertension.[14] This method helps determine a more accurate pulmonary artery pressure since an echocardiogram can under or overestimate the actual pressure. If the pulmonary capillary wedge pressure is elevated, this indicates that the increased pressure is due to left heart dysfunction and not from the pulmonary artery itself. As in the patient's case, her PCWP is normal while her mean pulmonary artery pressure is 50 mm Hg, thus suggesting pulmonary hypertension.

* *

According to the 2014 pulmonary hypertension guidelines from the American College of Chest Physicians, patients who have newly diagnosed pulmonary hypertension and are symptomatic should undergo a right heart catheterization with acute vasoreactivity testing using a short-acting agent.[21] Patients are given epoprostenol, adenosine, or nitric oxide. Responders are defined as patients who experience a decrease in mean pulmonary arterial pressure (mPAP) of at least 10 mm Hg to an absolute mPAP <40 mm Hg without a decrease in cardiac output. This vasoreactivity testing is chosen because those patients that respond are considered candidates for calcium channel blocker therapy. This recommendation comes from two large prospective uncontrolled studies which showed that approximately 10% of patients with pulmonary hypertension, who responded

to vasoreactivity testing, have significant reduction in pulmonary arterial pressure and pulmonary ventricular pressure when high-dose calcium channel blockers were used. Of the calcium channel blockers studied amlodipine, nifedipine, and diltiazem have been used with good response.

* *

Sildenafil is a phosphodiesterase inhibitor which enhances the effects of nitric oxide. This in turn increases cGMP and decreases pulmonary arterial pressures. The 2014 guidelines state that sildenafil 20 mg three times a day should be attempted for patients with WHO Functional Class II who are nonvasoreactive.[21]

* *

Epoprostenol is a continuous infusion drug that vasodilates the pulmonary artery. It has been studied in patients with WHO Functional Classes III and IV. A landmark-controlled trial in IPAH patients has shown survival benefit and an increase in exercise capacity in patients with IPAH.[22] Given the fact that she is in WHO Functional Class II, IV epoprostenol would not be the first choice.

* *

Pulmonary thromboendarterectomy is the treatment of choice with those individuals diagnosed with chronic thromboembolic pulmonary hypertension. Since this patient has a normal VQ scan, which is the screening test for CTEPH, the use of pulmonary thromboendarterectomy is not appropriate for this patient.

Question 3: **E. Hereditary pulmonary arterial hypertension**

The Registry to Evaluate Early and Long-Term Pulmonary Arterial Hypertension Disease Management (REVEAL) registry is the largest registry of patients with pulmonary hypertension to date with 3,515 patients.[23,24] The data from the participants were used to create an algorithm-predicted survival with Kaplan–Meier estimates for five riskiest groups.

* *

The REVEAL risk calculator used nine risk indicators in order to help determine prognosis.[23,24] Each risk indicator is subdivided based on category and each category is assigned an equivalent point based on the risk. A version of the risk score calculator is viewed below.

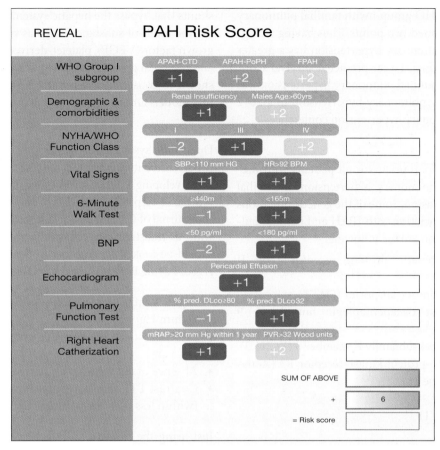

Reproduced with permission from Benza RL, Gomberg-Maitland M, Miller DP, et al: The REVEAL Registry risk score calculator in patients newly diagnosed with pulmonary arterial hypertension. *Chest.* 2012;141(2):354–362.

FPAH– Familial pulmonary arterial hypertension
PoPH—Portopulmonary hypertension
APAH-CTD—Associated pulmonary arterial hypertension due to connective tissue disease

* *

The score is between 1 and 22. Points were assigned based on risk and their related increase in morbidity and mortality. Inversely, a negative score was given for those categories that increased the likelihood for survival. The risk calculator divides patients to low-risk groups, average-risk groups, moderately high-risk group, and high-risk group based on their score. Below is a table that illustrates points, risks, and predicted 1-year survival.

Risk Group	Score	Percent Survival (%)
Low	1–7	95–100
Average	7–8.5	90–95
Moderate–high	8.5–9.5	85–90
High	9.5–11	70–85
Very high	>11	<70

* *

Of the choices given above, WHO Function Class I subtracts two points from the total score, pulmonary function test with a percent predicted DLco >80 subtracts one point from the total score, pericardial effusion adds one point, and a WHO group I with familial pulmonary hypertension is allotted two points. Thus having a diagnosis of familial pulmonary hypertension has a greater impact on the REVEAL 1-year predicted survival score. Recently, the term familial pulmonary hypertension was renamed hereditary pulmonary hypertension in a 2012 international pulmonary hypertension conference.

* *

Genetic testing is appropriate for all patients with presumed idiopathic pulmonary hypertension or familial pulmonary hypertension. Some of the genetic mutations that have some association with IPAH and familial pulmonary hypertension are the following:

- Bone Morphogenetic protein receptor type II (BMPR2)
- 5-hydroxytryptaimin transporter (5HTT)
- Mothers against decapentaplegic homologue 9 (SMAD9)
- Potassium channel subfamily K member 3 (KCNK3)
- Serine/threonine-protein kinase receptor R3 (Activin-like kinase type 1)
- Endoglin (ENG)
- Caveolin 1 (CAV1)

CASE 7

Question 1: E. All of the above
The patient in this scenario raises concern for portopulmonary hypertension (PoPH). PoPH is defined as a patient with portal hypertension due to liver disease, which causes pulmonary arteriopathy. It is thought that PoPH has a prevalence of 2% among patients with liver disease and can be as high as 6% in those being evaluated for liver transplant.[25-27] It is important to identify these patients because morbidity and mortality is high compared to those with other hepatic pulmonary syndromes.

* *

The definitive diagnosis of PoPH is a right heart catheterization (RHC) with increased mean pulmonary arterial pressures (mPAP), normal pulmonary capillary wedge pressure (PCWP), variable cardiac output (CO), and increased pulmonary vascular resistance (PVR). It is difficult to identify patients with PoPH because these patients have portal hypertension which increases the amount of vasoactive chemicals in the blood leading to a decrease in systemic resistance and increase in cardiac output. The increase in portal hypertension creates

shunts that bypass the hepatic system. There are increasing the levels of substances such as vascular endothelial grown factor (VEGF), platelet-derived growth hormone, and placental growth factor. These substances have been shown to cause pulmonary arterial remodeling in animal models and in some case reports.

* *

Due to the systemic changes associated with pulmonary hypertension it is difficult identifying those patients at risk for developing PoPH. Current guidelines released by the Journal of Hepatology, Annals of Hepatology, and American Journal of Cardiology suggest screening these patients with a transthoracic echocardiogram. Several factors should be looked for in order to determine the patient's risk of having PoPH. These risk factors are the following:

- Right ventricular systolic pressure greater than 50 mm Hg
- Presence of RV dilation (RV end diastolic diameter >3.3 cm)
- Absence of left ventricular disorder
- Contrast TTE that is negative for intracardiac shunts (within less than three cardiac cycles)

Just using the first two risk factors has a sensitivity of 100% and a specificity of 93%.[25-27] It is recommended that those patients who fit the first two risk factors be evaluated with an RHC.

Question 2: C. Sildenafil
The 2014 American College of Chest Physicians guideline regarding the treatment of those with pulmonary hypertension, states that the first line therapy should be a calcium channel blocker in those individuals who respond to the acute vasoreactive testing.[21] With individuals who have PoPH, the use of calcium channel blockers is contraindicated. This is because this calcium channel blockers promote mesenteric vasodilation which increases hepatic venous pressure and thus increasing portal hypertension.

* *

Identification of PoPH is critical in the treatment modality of this patient. A ventilation-perfusion scan should be done in order to evaluate for chronic thromboembolic disease in this patient because given his liver cirrhosis he is *hypercoagulable*. This increases his chances of having pulmonary hypertension due to chronic thromboembolic disease rather than having PoPH. This is critical because the use of anticoagulation, such as enoxaparin, is contraindicated in PoPH due to the increased risk of hemorrhagic complications from the liver cirrhosis.

* *

The use of beta blocker on patients with PoPH is being debated. In PoPH, beta blockers should not be used if varices have a low likelihood to rupture. The use of a beta blocker, like propranolol, causes chronotropic suppression and can overload the right ventricle in individuals with an already dysfunctional right ventricle.

* *

The use of other pulmonary hypertension medications, such as phosphodiesterase-5 inhibitors and endothelin receptor antagonist, can be used in patients with PoPH. The use of endothelin receptor antagonist such as bosentan and ambrisentan have been studied and well tolerated in this population of patients.[51–54] Savale et al. demonstrated significant hemodynamic response with bosentan in patients with PoPH and Child-Pugh class A.[52] This hemodynamic response was increased in patients with Child-Pugh class B.[52] It is thought that those patients with worse hepatic function had a higher level of bosentan in the blood, thus increasing the clinical benefit from the same dose of drug. Because of this, hepatic function is mandated monthly in bosentan. The use of sildenafil has been studied with good response and low side effect profile with patients with PoPH.[55] It is currently the only phosphodiesterase-5 inhibitor that has been studied in PoPH. Neither bosentan nor sildenafil has been shown to be superior and thus no recommendation is given on which drug should be started first.

* *

The use of prostacyclin analogs such as epoprostenol and iloprost are currently the only class of drugs that have been shown to have sustained improvement in symptoms and New York Heart Association function class.[21] Iloprost is a newer prostacyclin analog, that unlike its predecessor epoprostenol is an inhaled drug that has a couple of open-label studies that have increased patient's 6-minute walk test in addition to improve their symptoms.[28,29] There is a concern that patients with PoPH already have elevated levels of endogenous prostacyclin. Adding medications like epoprostenol and iloprost can cause an overdose state. For this reason, other treatment modalities should be attempted first before prostacyclin analogs are used.

* *

The identification of liver transplant patients is imperative as this has been shown to improve some patients with PoPH. Initial liver transplantation had a mortality rate of 65% to 100% within the first 2 weeks after transplant.[25–27] With the advancement of surgical management and pulmonary hypertension treatment there have been patients who survived the transplant and have halted the progression of pulmonary arteriopathy. Though most of these patients required PH medical management post-transplantation, their quality of life improves by eliminating the complications of liver disease and stabilizing pulmonary pressures. Nevertheless, there are some patients which liver transplant exacerbates their pulmonary hypertension.

* *

Early identification of patients with PoPH has led to the possibility of better transplant candidates. In the United States, the Organ Procurement and Transplantation Network policy states that candidates should have the following criteria in order to be eligible:

- 10% mortality equivalent increase in 3 months
- Pulmonary artery pressure below 35 mm Hg
- Pulmonary vascular resistance less than 400 dyn s/cm^5 (<5 wood units)

It should be noted that this criteria is MELD independent and as long as the patient has all three criteria, any patient is eligible for transplant.

Question 3: A. Normal to mild hypoxemia on ABG

When evaluating a patient with liver dysfunction and pulmonary hypertension it is important to know the difference between PoPH and hepatopulmonary syndrome (HPS) because HPS is three times more common and the prognosis is better than that of PoPH. Hepatopulmonary syndrome is defined a patient who has the following problems: liver disease, impaired oxygenation, and intrapulmonary vascular abnormalities. Patients generally present with liver dysfunction, hypoxemia, orthodeoxia, and platypnea. Currently there are no effective medical therapies for patients with HPS but liver transplantation is generally curative with resolution of pulmonary symptoms within 6 months.

* *

Below is a table that illustrates the fundamental difference between PoPH and HPS.

A Comparison of PoPH and HPS

	PoPH	HPS
Symptoms	Dyspnea Chest pain Syncope	Dyspnea Platypnea
Signs	Loud P2 RV Heave Lower extremity edema	Cyanosis
Arterial blood gas	Normal to mild hypoxemia	Moderate to severe hypoxemia A-a gradient >20
Contrast TTE	Negative or + intracardiac shunt (positive within <3 cardiac cycles)	Positive for intrapulmonary shunting (3–6 cardiac cycles)
Hemodynamics	PVR>240 dyn s/cm^5 (>3 woods units)	Normal or low PVR
Role of LT	Consider in selected patients if mPAP <35 mm Hg	Indicated exception points granted if room air Pao$_2$ <60 mm Hg

TTE, transthoracic echocardiogram; PVR, pulmonary vascular resistance; Pao$_2$, partial pressure of oxygen in arterial blood; LT, liver transplant.

CASE 8

Question 1: B. Anti–U3-RNP

Connective tissue diseases (CTD) are known to cause systemic disease and some have a higher prevalence of pulmonary hypertension than others. Epidemiologic studies suggest that there are certain CTDs that have a higher incidence and prevalence and thus a worse morbidity and mortality.[30] Some of the CTDs that are known to have an association with PHT are shown below. They have been matched with their associated autoantibodies.

Autoimmune Disorder	Autoantibody
Systemic lupus erythematosus	Anti-double stranded-DNA
Mixed connective tissue disease	Anti–U1-RNP
Scleroderma	Anti-topoisomerase (Scl-70) Anti–U3-RNP
Sjögren's syndrome	Anti-Ro/SSA and anti-La/SSB

Those individuals who only had anti-double stranded DNA, anti-Ro/SSA, and anti-La/SSB had a low probability of developing pulmonary hypertension. Those patients with lupus or Sjögren's syndrome who ended up developing PH secondary to pulmonary damage rather than arteriopathy had better outcomes when their underlying disease were treated.

* *

Recent retrospective studies have identified that having the anti–U3-RNP (fibrillarin) antibody or the anti-centromere antibodies has a higher risk to develop PH. In contrary, having the anti-topoisomerase antibody tends to be protective in developing PH, but does increase the risk of having interstitial lung disease. Other autoantibodies associated with systemic sclerosis and PHT include angiotensin-II type I receptor antibodies and endothelin-1 receptor type A antibodies.

Question 2: E. All of the above

The patient in question has a CTD-associated pulmonary hypertension that has not responded to initial treatment. Those patients who have a diagnosis of CTD and PH should have a trial of either an endothelin receptor antagonists (ERA) or phosphodiesterase type 5 inhibitors (PDE-5). This recommendation comes from studies that were done on patients with idiopathic PH. The Bosentan Randomized Trial of Endothelin Antagonist Therapy Trial (BREATHE) showed that patients with CTD-PH showed some improvement with therapy after 12 weeks.[31] The same was seen in the ambrisentan in pulmonary arterial hypertension randomized, double-blinded, placebo-controlled, multicenter, efficacy study (ARIES).[32] Those patients with CTD-associated PH had some effect with ambrisentan compared to those with idiopathic PH.

* *

Sildenafil is the phosphodiesterase type 5 inhibitor that has been studied the most. Like the BREATHE and ARIES trials, data on the efficacy is compared to those with idiopathic PH. Though the data is few, initial results range from slight improvement of symptoms to no change in symptoms. Though additional studies are needed to see if PDE-5 inhibitors have no benefit, their low cost and easy to administer properties make them a tempting option as a first line therapy.

* *

Main therapy for autoimmune disorders and CTD continues to be immunosuppression with steroids or other immunomodulating drugs like methotrexate. However, those patients with systemic sclerosis, scleroderma, or anti–U3-RNP and anti-centromere have a low probability of responding to immunosuppression in regard to their pulmonary hypertension. Small case studies have shown success of aggressive immunosuppression in patients with SLE and MCTD with favorable results.[30,34] These case studies used high-dose steroids or cyclophosphamide and had some success in halting the progression of PH with improvement of their symptoms.[30,34]

* *

The only class of medication that has been consistently proven to improve symptomatology and hemodynamics are the prostacyclin agonist such as epoprostenol and treprostinil. Epoprostenol is used only when all other options have been exhausted due to the complexity of the medication regimen and the continuous intravenous infusion that is required. In addition, most patients with CTD have deformed hands, which make handling the IV pump difficult to maneuver. Treprostinil is a newer prostacyclin analog that vasodilates both pulmonary and systemic arterial vascular beds while also inhibiting platelet aggregation. Its advantage has been the use of several administration methods (pill, oral inhalation, and injectable). Though more studies are needed to confirm the efficacy of treprostinil, the initial results are promising.

* *

Therefore patients with CTD-associated PAH should continue to abide by the same step wise fashion of treatment as idiopathic pulmonary hypertension with the addition of immunomodulators.

Question 3: B. Imatinib

With the advancements in medicine and the creation of genetically altered immunomodulators, antifibrotic therapies have been of interest in the field of CTD-PH. Studies on CTD suggest that TGF-B plays a role in developing fibrosis and the current thought is that if one can control this signal, then perhaps the advancement of CTD and thus PH would be altered. Imatinib is a tyrosine kinase inhibitor that down-regulates c-Abl protein and thus should decrease TGF-B signaling pathway. In a study done by Gorden et al., patients with systemic sclerosis who used imatinib in an open label trial had improvements

in skin scores and some improvement in PFTs.[35] It is unclear if further studies are to be done, given the results of the IMPRES study, where imatinib was associated with increased incidence of intracerebral bleeds.[35]

* *

Most patients with scleroderma-associated PAH are nonvasoreactive and calcium channel blockers (CCBs) are contraindicated. However, CCBs are used for other symptoms such as Raynaud phenomenon, it is not recommended for the treatment of most patients with CTD-PH.

* *

Torsemide is a loop diuretic that is commonly used with patients who have PH. Torsemide helps reduce the right ventricular strain by decreasing preload. Though torsemide or other loop diuretics do not alter the progression of the disease, it does decrease symptoms of dyspnea and right heart dysfunction.

* *

As stated in a previous question, steroid, like dexamethasone, has not been shown to alter the progression of pulmonary arteriopathy and thus should not be used as part of the pulmonary hypertension treatment regimen.

* *

Cyclosporine is an immune modulator drug that suppresses cellular and humoral immunity. It is used for the aggressive forms of systemic sclerosis or those that have failed conventional treatment. Though cyclosporine can be used to slow the progression of the disease, studies are inconclusive on whether cyclosporine can alter the progression of pulmonary arteriopathy.

CASE 9

Question 1: D. Low diffusion capacity on PFTs

Sarcoidosis-associated pulmonary hypertension (SAPH) has recently been recognized as having a large impact in morbidity and mortality.[36–40] Though the mechanism for this development is not clear, it is thought to be composed of two different pathophysiologic mechanisms. First, sarcoidosis causes pulmonary parenchymal destruction and thus causes hypoxia. This hypoxia causes vasoconstriction which can increase pulmonary pressures. The second mechanism involves compression of central hilar and mediastinal vessels due to enlarged lymph nodes or enlarged pulmonary vessels. This compression causes pulmonary resistance which causes pulmonary hypertension over time.

* *

Several studies have looked at patients with sarcoidosis who develop SAPH and those that do not. The idea is to create a screening tool that will help identify patients at risk for SAPH and begin treatment sooner.[36-40] Though there is no consensus, there are expert opinion recommendations on who should get screened for SAPH. The following is a list of items that help identify those who are at risk to develop SAPH:

- Radiographic scadding stage III and IV disease
- Decrease FVC or total lung capacity
- Arterial oxygen desaturation during ambulation
- Disproportionate decrease in diffusion capacity
- Those with dyspnea despite immune modulation therapy

Of the list above, the patient has disproportionate decrease in diffusion capacity and this risk factor alone would qualify him to undergo an echocardiogram.

Question 2: B. Prednisone

Patients with pulmonary sarcoidosis generally do not need treatment because the majority of granulomatous disease regresses before major damage is done to the lungs. However, for those patients which damage is noticed and progressing, it is appropriate to start a dose of corticosteroids in order to halt the progression of the disease. Initial treatment with prednisone 20 to 40 mg daily for 3 months is used in order to determine if steroids will affect the disease process. If the pulmonary sarcoidosis responds to steroids, a minimum of 12 months of steroids are used in order to slow the progression.

* *

According to the recommendations set by American College of Chest Physicians in 2014, Bosentan is an appropriate medication for patients who have WHO class III pulmonary hypertension symptoms.[21] Bosentan has been shown to decrease hospitalizations related to pulmonary hypertension and also improve overall cardiopulmonary hemodynamics. The drug works by binding to endothelin receptors thus blocking *vasoconstrictive* effects of endothelin-1. This helps reduce pulmonary vascular resistance. Since this patient suffers from pulmonary hypertension secondary to sarcoidosis, it is appropriate to treat the underlying disease before starting the patient on pulmonary hypertension specific treatments.

* *

Epoprostenol is a medication that directly dilates peripheral vessels and inhibits platelet aggregation. It has been studied extensively with patients with poorly controlled and end stage pulmonary hypertension. The 2014 American College of Chest Physician recommendations state that epoprostenol should be considered for patients with WHO Function Class III who have progression of the disease or markers of poor prognosis despite the treatment with one or two class agents.[21] Epoprostenol is also recommended for WHO Function Class IV. As noted before, the patient does meet WHO Function Classes III or IV and thus this would not be an appropriate treatment at this time.

* *

Treprostinil is a newer prostacyclin analog that vasodilates both pulmonary and systemic arterial vascular beds while also inhibiting platelet aggregation. Its advantage has been the use of several administration methods (pills, oral inhalation, and injectable). Like epoprostenol, it should be used in patients with at least a WHO Function Class III. Given the available studies, treprostinil seems promising as a treatment option that can be tried before committing someone to epoprostenol.

* *

Medications that block the effect of TNF-a have been shown to be beneficial in treating sarcoidosis. It is thought that TNF-a accelerates the inflammatory process and helps maintenance of the granuloma. Drugs such as infliximab, adalimumab, etanercept, and golimumab have all shown some success, but most of the studies have been with infliximab.[41] In a double-blinded trial done at the University of Cincinnati, evaluation at 24 and 52 weeks into treatment, low-dose infliximab showed an increase in predicted forced vital capacity compared to baseline.[42] Though anti-TNF a shows promise to halt the progression of sarcoidosis, this option is left after the patient has exhausted steroid use and other immune modulating agents such as methotrexate, azathioprine, and leflunomide.

Question 3: C. Cardiomyopathy

Given the patient's clinical symptoms and biopsy this patient most likely suffers from sarcoidosis. Sarcoidosis has several manifestations and depending on the severity. SAPH and cardiac sarcoidosis (CS) can have similar symptoms and can be difficult to distinguish. Cardiac sarcoidosis involves infiltration of the myocardium that has a predilection for the basal ventricular septum and left ventricular free wall.[43] Symptoms of concern with CS include atrioventricular block, severe ventricular arrhythmia, and sudden death due to asystolic arrest. In addition to electrical disturbance, CS can also cause dilated cardiomyopathy which can cause left heart dysfunction. Cardiac sarcoidosis–induced dilated cardiomyopathy acts similar to congestive heart failure and symptoms are identical (e.g., dyspnea, exercise intolerance, edema, JVD).

* *

Echocardiogram or right heart catheterization is able to distinguish CS from SAPH. In the right heart catheterization given, the patient has a pulmonary capillary wedge pressure (PCWP) of 30 mm Hg. This measurement is an indirect measurement of left ventricular end diastolic pressure (LVEDP). As such, an elevated LVEDP is associated with left ventricular failure (i.e., congestive heart failure). Since the circulatory system is a closed circuit, elevated LVEDP would result in an elevated PCWP, pulmonary arterial pressure, right ventricular pressure, and right atrial pressure. The option of ventricular septal defect would not cause an increase in PCWP because the high pressure in the left ventricle would cause fluid to shift to the right ventricle causing an increase in right ventricular and right atrial pressure but preserving PCWP.

* *

Treatment of CS is similar to the treatment of SAPH with the prevention of fatal arrhythmias. Patients with a high probability of arrhythmias (e.g., previous episode of ventricular tachycardia, heart block) benefit from antiarrhythmic medications, pacemaker, or implantable defibrillator. Aggressive diuresis is helpful for symptomatic relieve in patients with dilated cardiomyopathy. Early identification of patients with CS is crucial because early immunotherapy can help alter the progression of CS and decrease morbidity and mortality.

CASE 10

Question 1: **A. Hereditary hemorrhagic telangiectasia**
The patient in this question has pulmonary arteriovenous malformation (PAVM), which occurs between 2 and 3 per 100,000 patients.[44-47] PAVMs cause a shunt that connects the pulmonary artery to the pulmonary vein, bypassing the pulmonary capillaries. Normal pulmonary shunting occurs between the bronchial artery and veins and generally is less than 5%. Patients with PAVM can have up to 20% shunting at rest and up to 90% shunting during exercise. In addition to dyspnea and cyanosis, patients present with occasional hemoptysis and have a higher rate of CVA and brain abscesses.[47] Classic clinical symptoms include orthodeoxia, platypnea, clubbing, and occasional bruits in the pulmonary artery. Normally PAVMs occur in the lower lung fields and have a nodular imaging on CT scan and chest radiograph. The gold standard to detect PAVM is pulmonary angiography, but this is rarely used today. CT scans with IV contrast or MRA are acceptable measures to view PVMs.

* *

Eighty to ninety-five percent of PAVM patients have hereditary hemorrhagic telangiectasia (HHT), which is a heterogeneous disease with penetrance roughly 97% by the age of 45 years.[44-46] Genetic studies are not yet conclusive but the disease appears to be multifactorial and with different severity among family members. In order to diagnose HHT there must be at least three of the following symptoms:

1. Spontaneous and reoccurring epistaxis
2. Multiple sites with telangiectases
3. Visceral telangiectases lesions
4. Family history of a first degree relative with HHT

Hepatopulmonary syndrome can also present with vascular abnormalities such as PAVM. In order to diagnose hepatopulmonary syndrome the patient needs to have portal hypertension independent of cirrhosis, hypoxemia, and intrapulmonary vascular dilation. The patient in this question does not have a history suggestive of cirrhosis or pulmonary hypertension and therefore does not have hepatopulmonary syndrome.

* *

Bidirectional cavopulmonary shunt is a surgical procedure that is used in order to treat complex cyanotic heart disease. In order to correct the cyanosis, anastomoses are created between the vena cava and pulmonary arteries. This surgical procedure is known to cause PAVM several years later. This is corrected by ensuring hepatic blood flow to both lungs equally. The patient in this question does not have a history of cyanotic heart disease and thus has not undergone bidirectional cavopulmonary shunt.

* *

Neither pulmonary malignancy nor pulmonary tuberculosis has been shown to cause creation of AVMs.

* *

Complications include CVA, cerebral abscess and migraines, decreased exercise tolerance, and pulmonary hemorrhage. The gold standard treatment is percutaneous transcatheter embolization (PTE) is the gold standard. Candidates for PTE have PAVM with a feeding artery of >3 mm in diameter. Other options to treat PAVMs include the use of steel or platinum coils or surgical resection.

Question 2: C. Transthoracic contrast echocardiography

Identifying a PAVM is a tedious process and the clinician should have a high suspicion before testing occurs. Initial testing that would raise suspicion for PAVM would be desaturation at rest and with exertion and focal and round opacity on imaging studies. In order to screen for an intrapulmonary shunt a transthoracic contrast echocardiogram can be performed. The transthoracic contrast echocardiogram, also known as a bubble study, uses agitated saline and monitors the bubbles on echocardiogram. If bubbles originally seen in the right heart are seen in the left heart after four cardiac cycles, there is 100% sensitivity and 91% specificity that an intrapulmonary shunt is present. This is because bubbles injected into the right heart are normally removed by the pulmonary capillaries and the presence of the bubbles on the left side indicates a shunt that bypasses those pulmonary capillaries.

* *

A bleeding scan does not indicate whether a PAVM is present but would light up if a PAVM is actively bleeding. Therefore, this test is not recommended for the identification of a PAVM.

CASE 11

Question 1: B. Posterior basal segment of left lung

The patient in the vignette has pulmonary sequestration. This is a congenital condition that is composed of nonfunctioning tissue that does not communicate with the tracheobronchial tree and has a systemic blood supply. In the United States, it affects 6% of all congenital pulmonary malformations.[48–51] There are two types of pulmonary sequestration based on its location. The first is extrapulmonary sequestration which is completely encased in its own pleural sac but can be located anywhere above or below the diaphragm. It is generally found in the left side of the body with the majority of its placement in the costophrenic sulcus on the left. It may also be found in the mediastinum, pericardium, or in the

abdomen. Extrapulmonary sequestration is generally found incidentally on an examination of the GI tract as some patients may present with more GI symptoms than pulmonary symptoms. Removal of the sequestration is generally uneventful.

* *

The patient in this vignette has intrapulmonary sequestration which is composed of nonfunctioning primitive tissue that does not communicate with the tracheobronchial tree and has anomalous systemic blood supply. Intrapulmonary sequestration should be suspected in a child or adolescent who has a consolidation on chest radiograph after treatment of pneumonia. Though there is no gold standard in the diagnosis of pulmonary sequestration, the use of Doppler and ultrasounds is a good noninvasive method to identify an echogenic mass within the lung with a blood supply independent of the surrounding parenchyma. A CT or MRA is done to attempt and identify the sequestration borders and also the overall arterial and venous system.

* *

The majority of patients with intrapulmonary sequestration are located in the posterior basal segment of the left lung but they can also be found anywhere in the lower lobes of either lung. They are seldom found bilaterally.

Question 2: E. Lobectomy

Intrapulmonary sequestration can have different presentations based on its location, size, and whether it has a communication with other bronchi or lung parenchyma. The majority of patients present with a chronic cough and depending on how big the sequestration is, it can cause atelectasis in the adjacent lung parenchyma. If the sequestration has communication with the bronchi, infection is possible and may be difficult to treat. For these reasons, treatment to remove the intrapulmonary sequestration is suggested by most pulmonologist and CT surgeons.

* *

The standard of practice currently is surgical removal of the intrapulmonary sequestration before it becomes chronically infected or large enough to cause respiratory compromise.[48–51] Lobectomy in childhood or young adolescence has been described as having low surgical complications and low morbidity/mortality. If an intrapulmonary sequestration is removed that is chronically infected or causing atelectasis of adjacent parenchyma, a larger lobectomy is needed and there is an associated increase risk of hemorrhage from arteriovenous anastomosis.

* *

Investigational bronchoscopy does not play a role in the management of intrapulmonary sequestration unless a foreign object is suspected to be lodged in the area. Interventional bronchoscopy with balloon occlusion or embolization can be used in order to eliminate shunting toward the sequestration and this would immediately help hemodynamics in addition to decrease surgical complications once a lobectomy occurs. Though this is not routine some surgeons are opting for patients to undergo this procedure. Prolong antibiotics does not play a role in the treatment of intrapulmonary sequestration but may be used in order to clear reoccurring infection of the area.

Question 3: A. Accessory lung bud that develops from the ventral aspect of the primitive foregut

The development of the pulmonary sequestration is thought to be part of a malfunction in the migration of primitive structures in the evolution of the lung. It is thought that accessory lung bud develops from the ventral aspect of the primitive foregut and migrates in a caudal direction receiving its blood supply from the aorta. Intrapulmonary sequestration occurs in the visceral pleura of the lung and thus shares the parietal pleura with the normal lung parenchyma. Extrapulmonary sequestration migrates outside of the visceral pleura and is encased in its own pleural sac. It is associated with GI abnormalities and can communicate with the structures such the diaphragm, esophagus and intestines. The blood supply is not necessarily from the aorta but does arise from the systemic arteries and veins.

REFERENCES

1. Al-Naamani N, Roberts KE. Portopulmonary hypertension. *Clin Chest Med.* 2013;34:719–737.
2. Badesch DB, Champion HC, Sanchez MA, et al. Diagnosis and assessment of pulmonary arterial hypertension. *Am Coll Cardiol.* 2009;54(1 Suppl):S55–S66.
3. Badesch DB, Raskob GE, Elliott CG, et al. Pulmonary arterial hypertension: baseline characteristics from the REVEAL Registry. *Chest.* 2010;137(2):376–387.
4. Baughman RP, Lower EE, Drent M. Inhibitors of tumor necrosis factor (TNF) in sarcoidosis: who, what, and how to use them. *Sarcoidosis Vasc Diffuse Lung Dis.* 2008;25(2):76–89.
5. Becattini C, Agnelli G, Schenone A, et al. Aspirin for preventing the recurrence of venous thromboembolism. *N Engl J Med.* 2012;366(21):1959–1967.
6. Benza RL, Gomberg-Maitland M, Miller DP, et al. The REVEAL registry risk score calculator in patients newly diagnosed with pulmonary arterial hypertension. *Chest.* 2012;141(2):354–362.
7. Bird RL, Hamilton G. Treatment options for phlegmasia cerulea dolens. *J Vasc Surg.* 1995;21(6):998–999.
8. Bourbonnais JM, Samavati L. Clinical predictors of pulmonary hypertension in sarcoidosis. *Eur Respir J.* 2008;32:296–302.
9. Brighton TA, Eikelboom JW, Mann K. Low-dose aspirin for preventing recurrent venous thromboembolism. *N Engl J Med.* 2012;367(21):1979–1987.
10. Cartin-Ceba R, Swanson KL, Krowka MJ. Pulmonary arteriovenous malformation. *Chest.* 2013;144(3):1033–1044
11. Chapelon-Abric C. Cardiac sarcoidosis. *Curr Opin Pulm Med.* 2013;19:493–502.
12. Chinsakchai K, Duis KT, Moll FL, de Borst GJ. Trends in management of phlegmasia cerulea dolens. *Vasc Endovascular Surg.* 2011;45(I) 5–14.
13. Corbett HJ, Humphrey GM. Pulmonary sequestration. *Paediatr Respir Rev.* 2004;5(1):59–68.
14. Cordova FC, D'Alonzo G. Sarcoidosis-associated pulmonary hypertension. *Curr Opin Pulm Med.* 2013;19:531–537.
15. Cottin V, Plauchu H, Bayle JY, et al. Pulmonary arteriovenous malformations in patients with hereditary hemorrhagic telangiectasia. *Am J Respir Crit Care Med.* 2004;169(9):994–1000.
16. Darren BT, Ornelas J, Chung L, et al. Pharmacologic therapy for pulmonary arterial hypertension in adults: CHEST guidelines and expert panel report. *Chest.* 2014;146(2):449–475.
17. Diaz-Guzman E, Farver C, Parambil J, et al. Pulmonary hypertension caused by sarcoidosis. *Clin Chest Med.* 2008;29:549–563.
18. Forfia PR, Trow TK. Diagnosis of pulmonary arterial hypertension. *Clin Chest Med.* 2013;34:665–681.
19. Galie N, Olschewski H, Oudiz RJ, et al. Ambrisentan for the treatment of pulmonary arterial hypertension: results of the ambrisentnan in pulmonary arterial hypertension, randomized, double-blind, placebo-controlled, multicenter, efficacy (ARIES) study 1 and 2. *Circulation.* 2008;117:3010–3019.
20. Gezer S, Tastepe I, Sirmali M, et al. Pulmonary sequestration: a single-institutional series composed of 27 cases. *J Thorac Cardiovasc Surg.* 2007;133(4):955–959.
21. Goldberg A. Pulmonary arterial hypertension in connective tissue disease. *Cardiology in Review.* 2010;18(2):85–88.
22. Gordon J, Mersten J, Spiera RF, et al. Imatinib mesylate (Geevec) in the treatment of systemic sclerosis: interim results of a phase IIa, one year, open label clinical trial. Poster and Lecture presented at: ACR Scientific Meeting; October 18, 2009; Philadelphia, PA. Abstract 606.
23. Guyatt GH, Akl EA, Crowther M, et al. American College of Chest Physicians Antithrombotic Therapy and Prevention of Thrombosis Panel. *Executive Summary: Antithrombotic Therapy and Prevention of Thrombosis.* 9th ed. American College of Chest Physicians Evidence-Based Clinical Practice Guidelines. *Chest.* 2012;141(2 suppl):7S–47S.

24. Handa T, Nagai S, Ueda S, et al. Significance of plasma NT-proBNP levels as a biomarker in the assessment of cardiac involvement and pulmonary hypertension in patients with sarcoidosis. *Sarcoidosis Vasc Diffuse Lung Dis.* 2010; 27:27–35.

25. Hostettler KE, Studler U, Tamm M, et al. Long-term treatment with infliximab in patients with sarcoidosis. *Respiration.* 2012;83(3):218–224.

26. Huertas A, Girerd B, Dorfmuller P, O'Callaghan D, et al. Pulmonary veno-occlusive disease: advances in clinical management and treatment. *Expert Rev Resp Med.* 2011; 5(2):217–231.

27. Jaff MR, McMurtry MS, Archer SL, et al. Management of massive and submassive pulmonary embolism, iliofemoral deep vein thrombosis, and chronic thromboembolic pulmonary hypertension: a scientific statement from the American Heart Association. *Circulation.* 2011;123(16):1789–1793.

28. Jais X, D'Armini A, Jansa P, et al. Bosentan for treatment of inoperable chronic thromboembolic pulmonary hypertension: BENEFIT (Bosentan effects in iNopErable Forms of chronic Thromboembolic pulmonary hypertension), a randomized, placebo-controlled trial. *J Am Coll Cardiol.* 2008;52:2127–2136.

29. Kline J, Steuerwald M, Marchick M, et al. Prospective evaluation of right ventricular function and functional status 6 months after acute submassive pulmonary embolism: frequency of persistent or subsequent elevation in estimated pulmonary arterial pressure. *Chest.* 2009;136(5):1202–1210.

30. Laberge JM, Bratu I, Flageole H. The management of asymptomatic congenital lung malformations. *Paediatr Respir Rev.* 2004;5(Suppl A):S305–S312.

31. Lee GM, Arepally GM. Diagnosis and management of heparin-induced thrombocytopenia. *Hematol Oncol Clin North Am.* 2013;27:541–563.

32. Krowka MJ, Swanson KL, Frantz RP, et al. Portopulmonary hypertension: results from a 10-year screening algorithm. *Hepatology.* 2006;44(6):1502–1510.

33. Madani MM, Auger WR, Pretorius V, et al. Pulmonary endarterectomy: recent changes in a single institution's experience of more than 2,700 patient. *Ann Thorac Surg.* 2012;94:97–103.

34. Mahomed A, Williams D. Phlegmasia caerulea dolens and venous gangrene. *Br J Surg.* 1996;83(8):1160–1161.

35. Marshall PS, Kerr KM, Auger WR. Chronic thromboembolic pulmonary hypertension. *Clin Chest Med.* 2013;34: 779–797.

36. McDonald J, Bayrak-Toydemir P, Pyeritz RE. Hereditary hemorrhagic telangiectasia: an overview of diagnosis, management, and pathogenesis. *Genet Med.* 2011;13(7): 607–616.

37. McGoon M, Gutterman D, Steen V, et al. Screening, early detection, and diagnosis of pulmonary arterial hypertension: ACCP evidence-based clinical practice guidelines. *Chest.* 2004;126(Suppl 1):14S–34S.

38. Montani D, Achouh L, Dorfmuller P, et al. Pulmonary veno-occlusive disease: clinical, functional, radiologic, and hemodynamic characteristics and outcomes of 24 cases confirmed by histology. *Medicine (Baltimore).* 2008;87(4): 220–233.

39. Moorjani N, Price S. Massive pulmonary embolism. *Cardiol Clin.* 2013;31 503–518.

40. Morris TA. New synthetic antithrombotic agents for venous thromboembolism: Pentasaccharides, direct thrombin inhibitors, direct Xa inhibitors. *Clin Chest Med.* 2010;31(4):707–718.

41. Pendleton RC, Rodgers GM, Hull RD. Established venous thromboembolism therapies: heparin, low molecular weight heparins, and vitamin K antagonist, with a discussion of heparin-induced thrombocytopenia. *Clin Chest Med.* 2010;31(4):695–705.

42. Porres-Aguilar M, Zuckerman MJ, Figueroa-Casas JB, et al. Portopulmonary hypertension: state of the art. *Ann Hepatol.* 2008;7(4):321–330.

43. Rabiller A, Jais X, Hamid A, Resten A. Occult alveolar haemorrhage in pulmonary veno-occlusive disease. *Eur Resp J.* 2006;27(1):108–113.

44. Rapti A, Kouranos V, Gialafos E, et al. Elevated pulmonary arterial systolic pressure in patients with sarcoidosis: prevalence and risk factors. *Lung.* 2013;191:61–67.

45. Rubin LJ, Badesch DB, Barst RJ, et al. Bosentan therapy for pulmonary arterial hypertension. *N Engl J Med.* 2002;346: 896–903.

46. Sanchez O, Sitbon O, Jais X, et al. Immunosuppressive therapy in connective tissue diseases-associated pulmonary arterial hypertension. *Chest.* 2006;130:182–189.

47. Sellers MB, Newby LK. Atrial fibrillation anticoagulation fall risk and outcomes in elderly patients. *Am Heart J.* 2011;161(2):241–246.

48. Sersar Sameh I, El Diasty M, Ibrahim Hammad R, et al. Lower lobe segments and pulmonary sequestrations. *J Thorac Cardiovasc Surg.* 2004;127(3):898–899.

49. Shovlin CL, Jackson JE, Bamford KB, et al. Primary determinants of ischemic stroke/brain abscess risks are independent of severity of pulmonary arteriovenous malformation in hereditary haemorrhagic telangiectasia. *Thorax.* 2008;63(3):259–266.

50. Simonneu G, Robbins IM, Beghetti M, et al. Updated clinical classification of pulmonary hypertension. *J Am Coll Cardiol.* 2009;54(Suppl. 1):S43–S54.

51. Steen V, Medsger TA Jr. Predictors of isolated pulmonary hypertension in patients with systemic sclerosis and limited cutaneous involvement. *Arthritis Rheum.* 2003;48: 516–522.

52. Thomas D, Limbrey R. P145 Thrombolysis of acute PE patients reduces development of subsequent CTEPH. *Thorax.* 2012;67:A125.

53. Torbicki A, Perrier A, Konstantinides S, et al; ESC Committee for Practice Guidelines (CPG). Guidelines on the diagnosis and management of acute pulmonary embolism: the Task Force for the Diagnosis and Management of Acute Pulmonary Embolism of the European Society of Cardiology (ESC). *Eur Heart J.* 2008;29(18) 2276–2283.

54. Wells PS, Owen C, Doucette S, et al. Does This Patient Have Deep Vein Thrombosis? *JAMA.* 2006;295(2):199–207.

55. Woodhead F, Wells AU, Desai SR. Pulmonary complications of connective tissue diseases. *Clin chest med.* 2008;8: 149–164.

13

Lung Cancer

Ronaldo Collo Go MD

CASE 1

A 60-year-old woman with 30 pack-year history and COPD complains of weakness, particularly in the legs and more pronounced when climbing up the stairs or rising from a seated position. She also complains of a dry throat and noticed that her symptoms were worse after a recent bout of pneumonia (for which she was treated with levaquin). Physical examination is unremarkable.

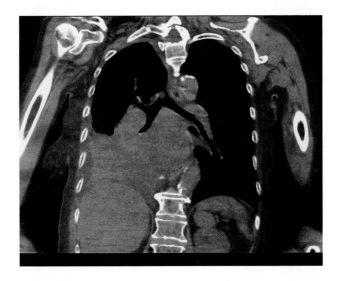

Sodium	145 mmol/L
Potassium	4.8 mmol/L
Chloride	105 mmol/L
CO_2	27 mmol/L
Urea nitrogen	10 mg/dL
Creatinine	0.58 mg/dL
Glucose	123 mg/dL
Anion gap	13 mmol/L
Magnesium	1.4 mg/dL
Calcium	9.5 mg/dL
WBC count	10.5 k/uL
Hemoglobin	11.0 g/dL
Hematocrit	33.5%
Platelet count	156 k/uL
RBC	3.99 M/uL
MCV	83.8 fL
MCH	27.5 pg
MCHC	32.9 g/dL
RDW	14.4%
MPV	11.6 fL
Troponin I	<0.012 ng/mL
	<0.012 ng/mL
Creatine kinase	111 U/L
B-type natriuretic peptide	9.1 pg/mL Cortisol level

* *

Chest radiograph is obtained which prompts the chest computed tomography seen on the previous page. It shows right lower lobe consolidation with pleural effusion and a 2.5-cm subcarinal lymph node.

* *

Endobronchial biopsy of the lesion at the distal portion of the bronchus intermedius shows small size, scant cytoplasm, >11 mitoses/2 mm², large zone necrosis CD56 +

Synaptophysin positive
TTF-1 positive
Cytokeratin AE 1/3 negative
Cytokeratin 8/18 negative
EBUS-FNA Level 7:
TTF-1 positive
Chromogranin-A positive
Synaptophysin positive
CD56 positive
CK7 positive
CK20 negative

Further radiographic imaging does not show any additional lesions.

Question 1: **Which of the following helps with the diagnosis of her weakness?**

A. Anti-VGCC
B. Anti-AchR
C. Perivascular or interfascicular muscle fiber inflammation with perifascicular atrophy
D. Secretion of adrenocorticotrophic hormone
E. Secretion of parathyroid hormone-related protein

Question 2: **What is your diagnosis?**

A. Small cell lung carcinoma
B. Atypical neuroendocrine carcinoma
C. Typical neuroendocrine carcinoma
D. Adenocarcinoma
E. Squamous cell carcinoma

Question 3: **What stage is your patient?**

A. Limited stage
B. Extensive stage
C. T3N0M0
D. T4N0M0
E. T2N1M1a

Question 4: **What is your treatment?**

A. Surgical resection with adjunct cisplatin and etoposide for four cycles
B. Carboplatin with irinotecan for four cycles with prophylactic cranial irradiation
C. Cisplatin and etoposide for four cycles with consolidative thoracic radiotherapy and prophylactic cranial irradiation
D. Surgical resection with doxorubicin, cyclophosphamide, and etoposide for six cycles
E. Topotecan

CASE 2

A 50-year-old woman with a smoking history of 1 PPD × 15 years (and stopped 2 years ago) was diagnosed with abdominal liposarcoma 2 years ago. She had resection with chemotherapy and radiation therapy. During serveillance computed tomography, 2-cm pulmonary nodule is noted.

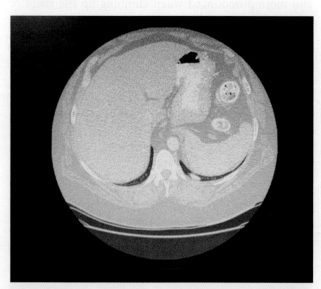

Question 1: **The patient has been reluctant for an aggressive management. What is the next best step?**

A. Repeat CT scan after 6 weeks
B. PET
C. CT-guided transthoracic needle biopsy (TTNB)
D. Endobronchial ultrasound (EBUS)
E. Wedge resection

CASE 3

A 55-year-old man with diabetes and hypertension is seen for a routine physical examination. He currently has no complaints. He lives with his wife, works in an office and has smoked 1 pack per day for 20 years. He has a family history of lung cancer in both of his parents.

Question 1: **What would be the next best step?**

A. Low-dose computed tomography of his chest for lung cancer screening
B. Sputum cytology
C. Smoking cessation
D. Lung cancer chemoprevention
E. Chest radiograph

* *

He has continued to smoke. Two years later, he complains of submassive hemoptysis. Chest computed tomography is below:

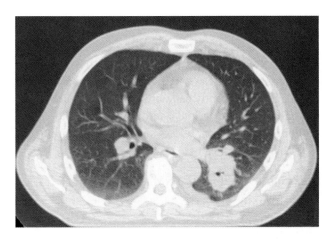

He subsequently has a bronchoscopy with transbronchial biopsy. Pathology shows keratin pearls with intracellular bridges. Immunohistochemistry shows:

    AE-1/AE-3 +
    P63 +
    CK5/6 +
    CK7 +
    TTF-1 –
    Napsin-A –
    CK20 –

Question 2: **What is your diagnosis?**

A. Atypical carcinoid
B. Small cell lung carcinoma
C. Adenocarcinoma
D. Squamous cell carcinoma
E. Gastric cancer

Question 3: **For central airway malignancies, what is the initial transformation that leads to invasive carcinomas?**

A. Hyperplasia
B. Metaplasia
C. Mild dysplasia
D. Moderate dysplasia
E. Severe dysplasia

Question 4: **With the data that is available at this point, what would be an indication for white light bronchoscopy and autofluorescence bronchoscopy for this patient?**

A. For evaluation of sputum atypia
B. Predetermine surgical margins
C. Serial evaluation for CIS
D. For evaluation of curative therapy
E. For endobronchial therapy

CASE 4

A 40-year-old woman, nonsmoker, has a pre-employment physical examination. She has no complaints but is noted to have a wheeze on physical examination which prompts a chest radiograph. A subsequent computed tomography with IV contrast shows a well-circumscribed 2.5-cm nodule in the right upper lobe. She subsequently has a bronchoscopy and transbronchial biopsy which indicated cells in nesting pattern with a prominent vascular stroma. The cells had a moderate amount of eosinophilic cytoplasm and granular nuclear chromatin with no necrosis or mitosis seen.

* *

Immunohistochemistry reveals:

    TTF +
    Chromogranin +
    CD56 +
    Synaptophysin +
    Estrogen +

Question 1: **What is your diagnosis?**

A. Large cell carcinoma
B. Breast cancer
C. Typical carcinoid
D. Aypical carcinoid
E. Mucoepidermoid carcinoma

Question 2: What is the next step?

A. Wedge resection
B. Somatostatin receptor scintigraphy
C. CT/PET
D. Neoadjuvant chemotherapy
E. Neoadjuvant radiotherapy

Question 3: Further radiographic investigation does not show additional lesions. What TNM stage is this patient?

A. T1aN0M0
B. T1bN0M0
C. T2aN0M0
D. T2bN0M0
E. T1aN1M0

CASE 5

A 65-year-old woman, nonsmoker, recently treated for pneumonia now complains of progressive shortness of breath on exertion. She denies any fevers and is not noted to be hypoxic on room air. The computed tomography of the chest shows collapse of the entire left lung. Hilar adenopathy appears to be present but margins are hard to discern. There appears to be invasion of the trachea and great vessels. She subsequently has a bronchoscopy that reveals an endobronchial lesion <2 cm from the carina. The endobronchial biopsy and EBUS of 10 L FNA shows: TTF-1+, CK7+, and CK20−.

Question 1: What is the TNM stage?

A. Stage IIA
B. Stage IIB
C. Stage IIIA
D. Stage IIIB
E. Stage IV

Question 2: What is the suggested treatment?

A. Radiotherapy
B. Concurrent chemoradiotherapy
C. Sequential chemoradiotherapy
D. Surgical resection with complete lymphadenectomy
E. Doublet chemotherapy

Question 3: Before the initiation of the treatment, the patient returns complaining of worsening shortness of breath. Laboratory results show INR 2, LDH 300, and platelets 80. CTA is negative. Echocardiogram shows severe pulmonary hypertension. She subsequently expires. Autopsy shows tumor cells with intimal hyperplasia of the pulmonary arteries and arterioles. What is the diagnosis?

A. Pulmonary embolism
B. Pulmonary tumor thrombotic microangiopathy
C. Chronic pulmonary embolism
D. Pulmonary hypertension
E. Metastatic adenocarcinoma

CASE 6

A 50-year-old man with no history of smoking is noted to have multiple pulmonary nodules <5 mm on CT scan.

Question 1: What is the next best step?

A. Surgical resection
B. No surveillance CT scan
C. Surveillance CT scan in 3 months
D. Surveillance CT scan in 2 years
E. Surveillance CT scan in 1 year

CASE 7

A 60-year-old African-American man with 30 pack-year history is noted to have RUL atelectasis and 5-cm RUL mass. He subsequently has a bronchoscopy which shows an endobronchial lesion 4 cm away from the carina. Endobronchial biopsy shows squamous cell carcinoma. CT/PET and CT head are negative.

Question 1: What is the TNM stage?

A. T1bN0M0
B. T2aN0M0
C. T2bN0M0
D. T3aN0M0
E. T3bN0M0

Question 2: What is the optimum treatment?

A. Concurrent chemoradiotherapy
B. Radiology
C. Radiotherapy
D. Surgical resection followed by adjunct chemotherapy
E. Surgery

Question 3: The preoperative pulmonary evaluation indicates PPO FEV_1 >60% predicted and DLco <50% predicted. What is the next step?

A. Stair-climbing test
B. CPET
C. Patient can go for surgery

D. Treatment is surgery but the patient is not a candidate for surgery
E. Treatment is not surgery

CASE 8

A 50-year-old Japanese woman who is a nonsmoker, complains of weight loss and cough. Her past medical history includes atrial fibrillation, hypertension, and hypertension. She is on aspirin 81 mg daily, amiodarone 400 mg daily that has been started 1 month ago, and metoprolol 25 mg twice a day. She has a chest radiograph with subsequent computed tomography showing a left apical spiculated mass 3 cm × 2 cm, 1.5 cm 4R, and 1 cm right lower lobe nodule.

Question 1: **With the assumption that all CT findings are related to the same malignancy, what is the TNM stage?**

A. T3N2M1a
B. T2aN3M1b
C. T2bN3M1a
D. T1aN3M1b
E. T1bN3M1a

Question 2: **Patient has EBUS-guided FNA of 4R and transbronchial biopsy of left apical mass. Pathology shows glandular differentiation with tubules and immunostaining TTF1+, CK7+, CK20−, EGFR+, KRAS−. CT head is negative and performance status is excellent. CT/PET shows elevated SUV in the left apical mass, 4R, and RLL nodule. What is the first line of treatment?**

A. Crizotinib
B. Concurrent platinum-based chemotherapy with radiation therapy
C. Erlotinib
D. Carboplatin with paclitaxel with bevacizumab
E. Carboplatin with gemcitabine

Question 3: **What would the maintenance treatment be?**

A. Pemetrexed
B. Continuation maintenance with platinum-based chemotherapy
C. Erlotinib
D. Carboplatin with paclitaxel
E. No maintenance treatment

Question 4: **A week after chemotherapy, she complains of shortness of breath. She is noted to have oxygen saturation of 86% on room air, afebrile, and chest radiograph shows bilateral infiltrates. WBC 10, BNP 100, and arterial blood gas shows PO₂ 60 on 100% nonrebreather. She gets intubated. Bronchoscopy is done and there is no evidence of hemorrhage. The cell count from bronchial alveolar lavage shows neutrophilia. She is started on empirical antibiotics and cultures are negative. All home medications are discontinued and corticosteroids are started. Clinical and radiographic improvements follow. What is the mechanism of action of her disease?**

A. Reactive oxygen species
B. Decreased metabolism of neuropeptides
C. Increased phospholiposis
D. Unknown
E. Cardiogenic

CASE 9

A 77-year-old man is noted to have a persistent peripheral 4-cm ground-glass opacity and shortness of breath.

Question 1: **The patient has a CT-guided biopsy which shows neoplastic lesions along alveolar structures with no stromal, vascular, or pleural invasion. What is your diagnosis?**

A. Bronchioloalveolar carcinoma (BAC)
B. Adenocarcinoma in situ (AIS)
C. Minimally invasive adenocarcinoma in situ (MIA)
D. Lepidic predominant invasive adenocarcinoma, nonmucinous (LPA)
E. Invasive mucinous adenocarcinoma

Question 2: **Patient is referred for preoperative surgical evaluation. What would be included in your pre-evaluation assessment?**

A. Cardiac risk assessment and pulmonary function test
B. Pulmonary function test
C. CPET
D. Low-risk assessment
E. Patient is not a candidate for surgery because of his age

Question 3: **What is the correct association?**

A. EGFR = erlotinib, gefitinib
B. KRAS = EGFR
C. EML4-ALK = crizotinib, afatinib
D. HER2 = afatinib
E. BRAF = HER2

CASE 10

A 65-year-old man, current smoker, complains of sub-massive hemoptysis. He has a chest radiograph and chest computed tomography which show 5-cm right upper-lobe peripheral mass with invasion of the chest wall and left hilar adenopathy. He has a transbronchial biopsy which shows keratin pearls, intracellular bridges, and elements of cartilage. Immunostains show TTF-1+, CK7+, CK20−, P63+, and CK5/6+.

Question 1: **What is your diagnosis?**

A. Sarcomatoid carcinoma
B. Mucoepidermoid carcinoma
C. Large cell lung carcinoma
D. Adenosquamous carcinoma
E. Squamous cell carcinoma

Question 2: **What is the stage?**

A. Stage IIA
B. Stage IIB
C. Stage IIIA
D. Stage IIIB
E. Stage V

CASE 11

A 68-year-old woman with history of breast cancer complains of cough and fever. She has a chest radiograph which shows a peripheral 2-cm well-circumscribed nodule. She is a former smoker and has a strong family history of colorectal adenocarcinoma. She previously had surveillance computed tomography, colonoscopy, and mammograms 2 years ago which were negative.

Question 1: **For cancer of unknown primary (CUP), immunohistochemistry is key in identifying the malignancy. Which is *NOT* the correct association?**

A. GCDFP-15—Breast cancer
B. Napsin A—Lung adenocarcinoma
C. CDX2—Gastric cancer
D. TTF-1—Thyroid cancer
E. CD20—Melanoma

Question 2: **For which of the following malignancies is pulmonary metastasectomy less indicated?**

A. Soft tissue sarcoma
B. Breast cancer
C. Colorectal carcinoma
D. Renal carcinoma
E. Melanoma

Question 3: **Which of the following presentations of NSCLC have benefited from surgical resection?**

A. Multiple ground-glass opacities
B. Lung mass with solitary brainstem lesion
C. Apical lung mass infiltrating the subclavian vessels
D. Lung nodule in the left lower lobe with lung nodule in right lower lobe in a patient with good lung reserve
E. All of the above

CASE 12

A 50-year-old woman with Stage IIA lung adenocarcinoma has a surgical resection, R0, with curative intent.

Question 1: **What surveillance would you recommend?**

A. CT at 3 months
B. CT at 6 months
C. Biomarkers
D. Bronchoscopy at 6 weeks
E. Bronchoscopy at 1 month

CASE 13

A 70-year-old man is noted to have a 2.5-cm nodule. The biopsy is positive for lung adenocarcinoma. He has a wedge resection and stereotactic body radiation therapy (SBRT) because margins were inadequate.

Question 1: **Which is NOT true of radiation induced lung injury?**

A. Straight-line effect on radiograph is typically seen in conformal radiation therapy, stereotactic body radiation therapy, and gamma knife therapy.
B. Symptoms may precede radiographic evidence of radiation-induced lung injury.
C. Symptomatic improvement plateau at 18 months
D. Risk factor includes 20 Gy.
E. Corticosteroids are a treatment.

Answers

CASE 1

Question 1: A. Anti-VGCC

Paraneoplastic syndromes may indirectly suggest the presence of malignancy and are listed below[1]:

SIADH: Small cell lung cancer (SCLC)	Production of antidiuretic hormone and atrial natriuretic peptide
Hypercalcemia: Squamous cell carcinoma	Production of parathyroid hormone-related protein (PTHrP)
Cushing syndrome: SCLC and carcinoids	Production of corticotropin releasing factor
Limbic encephalitis: SCLC, thymoma, teratoma, lymphoma	Anti-Hu, anti-Ma2, anti-CRMP5, anti-amphiphysin
Paraneoplastic cerebellar degeneration: SCLC, lymphoma, breast cancer	Anti-Yo, anti-Hu, anti-CRMP5, anti-Ma, anti-Tr, anti-Ri, anti-VGCC, anti-MGluR1
Lambert-Eaton: SCLC	Anti-VGCC (presynaptic)
Myasthenia gravis: thymoma	Anti-AchR (postsynaptic) MuSK protein
Autonomic neuropathy: SCLC, thymoma	Anti-Hu, anti-CRMP5, anti-nAchR, anti-amphiphysin
Subacute sensory neuropathy: SCLC, sarcomas, lymphomas, breast	Anti-Hu, anti-CRMP5, anti-amphiphysin
Dermatomyositis: ovarian, breast, lung, lymphoma	Mixed B- and T-cell perivascular migration and perifascicular fiber atrophy
Hypertrophic osteoarthropathy: lung cancer	Vascular endothelial growth factor, platelet-derived growth factor and prostaglandin E2 causing periostosis and subperiosteal new bone formation

* *

The patient appears to have Lambert-Eaton syndrome (LES), with onconeural antibodies to voltage gated calcium channel type P/Q, targeting the presynaptic junction. Clinical manifestations consist of (1) proximal extremity weakness, greatest in the lower extremities, that might worsen with temperature or exercise; (2) ptosis or diplopia less pronounced than in myasthenia gravis; and (3) autonomic dysfunction such as dry mouth and eyes, urinary retention, constipation, and postural hypotension. Respiratory failure is possible but rare. Reflexes are usually absent but can be provoked by contracting the muscle for at least 10 seconds prior to reflex test. There is a paradoxical eyelid elevation after persistent upward gaze. Symptoms may be exacerbated by certain medications including aminoglycosides, fluoroquinolones, erythromycin, quinine, quinidine, procainamide, and beta-adrenergic blocking agents. Diagnosis is identification of onconeural antibodies; although they are neither sensitive nor specific. On EMG, the baseline compound muscle action potential (CMAP) is reduced but high-frequency stimulation shows a marked increase in CMAP amplitude. This is defined as postactivation facilitation. An increase of CMAP amplitude >100% after this high-frequency or postexercise stimulation suggests presynaptic junction disorder. Treatment consists of replenishing acetylcholine (guanidine, 3,4-diaminopyridine, and pyridostigmine) and to reduce the antibodies via immunosuppression (IVIG, azathioprine, prednisone, or plasma exchange).

* *

Myasthenia gravis (MG) has onconeural antibodies against acetylcholine receptors that target the postsynaptic junction. Clinical manifestations consist of (1) ptosis and diplopia; (2) generalized fatigue that is worse with activity and improves with rest; (3) paralysis of respiratory muscles; and (4) dysarthria and dysphagia. Diagnosis includes identification of onconeural antibodies in the serum, decremental response to repetitive peripheral nerve stimulation, ice test which consists of applying ice to muscles with improvement of strength; and edrophonium test which consists of improvement of ocular weakness after application of edrophonium chloride or neostigmine. Treatment consists of thymectomy, pyridostigmine, prednisone, azathioprine, cyclosporine, tacrolimug, rituximab, cyclophosphamide, plasma exchange, or IVIG. AchR-Ab negative MuSK-Ab positive MG generally have an oculobulbar form, no thymic pathology, and are less responsive to acetylcholinesterase inhibitors. Anti-striated muscle antibodies might suggest the presence of thymoma.

* *

Dermatomyositis (DM) is an inflammatory myopathy with proximal muscle weakness and dermatologic manifestations (gottron's papules, heliotrope eruption, facial erythema, photodistributed poikiloderma, periungual abnormalities, and calcinosis cutis), interstitial lung disease, esophageal muscle weakness, and myocarditis. It can be part of antisynthetase syndrome, which includes interstitial lung disease, inflammatory myopathy, and polyarthritis, and can have positive antibodies to aminoacyl-transfer ribonucleic acid (tRNA) synthetase enzymes. Diagnosis includes: (1) elevated muscle enzymes such as CK, LD, aldolase, AST, and ALT; and (2) autoantibodies such as TRNA synthetases antibodies (anti–Jo-1), SRP antibodies, Mi-2 antibodies, anti–MDA-5, anti-p155/140, and anti-MJ. Muscle pathology would consist of perifascicular atrophy and fibrosis, perimysial CD4+ inflammatory infiltrate, and no invasion of nonnecrotic fibers. Treatment is with immunosuppression with corticosteroids or steroid sparing agents.

* *

Hypercalcemia in squamous cell carcinoma is secondary to secretion of parathyroid hormone-like protein. Clinical manifestations include neurologic (altered mental status, anxiety, depression, cognitive abnormalities, and coma), cardiovascular (short QT interval); gastrointestinal (constipation, anorexia, and nausea), muscle weakness, and renal (nephrogenic diabetes insipidus, nephrolithiasis, renal tubular acidosis, and renal failure). After hypercalcemia is confirmed with the calcium level corrected for albumin, other labs are ordered which include parathyroid hormone, PTH-related protein, 25-hyroxyvitamin D (25[OH]D) which is elevated from vitamin D intoxication, and 1,25-dihydroxyvitamin D, which is elevated by increased intake, extra-renal production such as granulomatous disease and lymphoma, or increased renal production. Aggressive treatment is usually reserved when the serum calcium is >14. Treatment includes saline hydration, calcitonin which reduces calcium by increasing renal excretion and decreasing bone resorption, and bisphosphonates, which inhibit calcium release from bones by interfering with osteoclast function.

* *

Syndrome of inappropriate antidiuretic hormone (SIADH) is typically caused from tumor cell production of antidiuretic hormone with atrial natriuretic peptide and causes euvolemic hyponatremia. Clinical manifestations include weakness, headaches, memory difficulties, seizures, and coma. Diagnosis involves determination of euvolemia with normal vital signs, blood urea, uric acid, urea nitrogen, urinary sodium >40 mmol/L and urine osmolality >100 mOsm/kg of water. Treatment involves fluid restriction, administration of hypertonic fluids, demeclocycline, or conivaptan.

* *

Hypertrophic osteoarthropathy is not only associated with lung cancer, particularly adenocarcinoma, but also can be seen in pulmonary fibrosis, inflammatory bowel disease, Graves' disease, and endocarditis. It is secondary to proliferation of vascular endothelial growth factor, platelet-derived growth factor, and prostaglandin E2. It is defined by new bone formation along the shaft of long bones and phalanges.

Question 2: A. Small cell lung carcinoma
Signs, symptoms, and radiographic findings are nonspecific for a particular type of malignancy. Often histologic characteristics with immunohistochemistry are necessary to diagnose the type of cancer.

Question 3: A. Limited stage
Evaluation for metastatic disease takes precedence in a patient with newly diagnosed cancer. CBC, renal and liver studies, LDH, and imaging studies are routinely ordered (Grade 1B).[2] In SCLC, 15% to 30% have bone marrow metastases; patients with cytopenia should be evaluated with a bone-marrow biopsy. Brain metastases should be evaluated with an MRI, which can detect 10% to 15% of metastatic disease in asymptomatic patients.

* *

The Veterans Administration Lung Study Group (VALSG) has previously classified the clinical staging of small cell lung carcinoma into limited (LS) and extensive (ES).[2] LS was determined as a region that can be irradiated with a single port. LS is confined to

Type of Cancer	Histopathology	Immunohistochemistry
Small cell carcinoma	Small size, scant cytoplasm, ≥11 mitoses/2 mm², large zone necrosis	AE1/AE3. Chromogranin, CD56, synaptophysin, 80–100% proliferation by Ki-67 staining 70–80% have + TTF-1
Typical neuroendocrine carcinoma	≥0.5 cm with organizing nest pattern with prominent vascular stroma, <2 mitoses/2 mm², lack of necrosis	Chromogranin, CD56, synaptophysin, ≤5% proliferation by Ki-67 staining
Atypical neuroendocrine carcinoma	≥0.5 cm with organizing nest pattern with prominent vascular stroma, 2–10 mitoses/2 mm², OR punctate necrosis	Chromogranin, CD56, synaptophysin, 5–20% proliferation by Ki-67 staining
Large cell carcinoma	Organizing nest pattern, ≥11 mitoses/2 mm², large zone necrosis, large cell size, low nuclear cytoplasmic ratio, fine chromatin, and multiple nuclei	Chromogranin, CD56, synaptophysin, 50–100% proliferation by Ki-67 staining 41–75% have + TTF-1
Squamous cell carcinoma	Keratin pearls and intracellular bridges	P63, cytokeratin 5/6, CK7+, CK20–
Lung adenocarcinoma	Heterogeneous	TTF-1, mucin, napsin-A, surf-A, surf-B
Adenosquamous cell carcinoma	>10% adenocarcinoma features + >10% squamous cell features	
Mucoepidermoid carcinoma	Mucous secreting, squamous, and intermediate cell types	
Lymphoma	Reed steinberg cells	CLA, CD45, CD20, CD3, CD138, CD30
Colorectal carcinoma		CK7, CK20, CDX2
Prostate carcinoma		PSA
Breast carcinoma		Mammaglobin, ER, CA125, CK7
Pancreatic carcinoma		CA125, Mesothelin, CK7, CDX2, CK20
Gastric carcinoma		
Melanoma	Atypical melanocytes	S100, melan-A, HMB45
Sarcoma		Vimentin, actin, desmin, S100, c-kit
Mesothelioma		EMA, WT1, calretinin, mesothelin-1, cytokeratin 5–6, HBME-1

a hemithorax including primary and regional lymph nodes with no extrathoracic metastases except for ipsilateral supraclavicular lymph node. ES includes malignant pleural and pericardial effusions, contralateral lymph node involvement, and hematogenous metastases. This staging has been modified by the International Association for the Study of Lung Cancer (IASLC) where LS is expanded to include contralateral mediastinal and supraclavicular lymph node and ipsilateral pleural effusions (Grade 1B).[2] However, most have used a hybrid of the classifications by considering contralateral mediastinal adenopathy and ipsilateral supraclavicular LN in LS since they can be included in radiotherapy port.

* *

Despite retrospective studies supporting TNM staging in SCLC, it has less prognostic significance compared to NSCLC. However, it is advocated for patients that might benefit from surgical resection (up to T2N0). LS is equivalent to T any, N any, M0 (except T3–T4) and ES is T any, N any, M1a/b or T3–T4 (Grade 1B).[2]

PRIMARY TUMOR (T)

TX means that tumor cannot be assessed or presence of malignant cells but no visualized via bronchoscopy or radiographic imaging.

T0 no evidence of tumor
Tis carcinoma in situ

TNM STAGING AND 5 YEAR PROGNOSIS

	Primary Tumor (T)	Regional LN (N)	Distant Met (M)	5-Year Survival for NSCLC (%)
Stage 0	Tis	N0	M0	
Stage IA	T1a	N0	M0	60–80
	T1b	N0	M0	
Stage IB	T2a	N0	M0	60–80
Stage IIA	T2b	N0	M0	60–80
	T1a	N1	M0	N1 = 25–50
	T1b	N1	M0	
	T2a	N1	M0	
Stage IIB	T2b	N0	M0	25–50
	T3	N1	M0	
Stage IIIA	T1a	N2	M0	N0–N1 = 25–40
	T1b	N2	M0	N2 = 10–30
	T2a	N2	M0	
	T2b	N2	M0	
	T3	N1	M0	
	T3	N2	M0	
	T4	N0	M0	
	T4	N1	M0	
Stage IIIB	T1a	N3	M0	<5
	T1b	N3	M0	
	T2a	N3	M0	
	T2b	N3	M0	
	T3	N3	M0	
	T4	N2	M0	
	T4	N3	M0	
Stage V	Any T	Any N	M1a	<5
	Any T	Any N	M1b	

T1 ≤3 cm, surrounded by lung or visceral pleural without bronchoscopic evidence more proximal than lobar bronchus

T1a ≥2 cm
T1b >2–3 cm

* *

T2 >3–7 cm or with any of the following: involves main bronchus, ≥2 cm distal to the carina; visceral pleural (PL1 or PL2); atelectasis or obstructive pneumonitis extending to hilar region but not entire lung

T2a >3–5 cm
T2b >5–7 cm

* *

T3 >7 cm or any of the following: parietal pleural invasion (PL3), chest wall (including superior sulcus tumors), diaphragm, phrenic nerve, mediastinal pleura, parietal pericardium, or <2 cm distal to carina without involvement of the carina, atelectasis, or obstructive pneumonitis involving entire lung or separate nodules in same lobe.

* *

T4 any size and invasion of mediastinum, heart, great vessels, trachea, recurrent laryngeal nerve, esophagus, vertebral body, carina, separate nodules(s) in different ipsilateral lobe.

REGIONAL LYMPH NODES (N)

Nx Regional LN cannot be assessed

N0 No regional LN metastases

N1 Ipsilateral peribronchial and/or hilar LN and intra-pulmonary nodes

N2 ipsilateral mediastinal and/or subcarinal LN

N3 contralateral mediastinal, hilar, ipsilateral or scalene LN or supraclavicular LN

DISTANT METASTASIS (M)

M0 no metastasis

M1 distant metastasis

M1a separate nodules in contralateral lobe, pleural nodules, malignant pleural, or pericardial effusion

M1b extrathoracic metastasis

Question 4: C. Cisplatin and etoposide for four cycles with consolidative thoracic radiotherapy and prophylactic cranial irradiation

Staging will guide treatment. Surgical resection with curative intent, particularly for clinical stage I, is preferred over nonsurgical treatment (Grade 2C) with adjuvant chemotherapy (Grade 1C).[2] The value of surgical resection in SCLC has been investigated in analysis on two large population databases and found that patients with T1/T2 who have had surgical resection had better survival for both localized and regional diseases. Using the TNM staging, this patient does not meet these criteria.

* *

The platinum-based chemotherapy for either limited stage or extensive stage is four to six cycles of either cisplatin or carboplatin plus either etoposide or irinotecan (Grade 1A).[2] The choice of which chemotherapy to use may differ in terms of refractory/resistant and relapsed/sensitive SCLC, which is defined as progression or recurrence within 3 months of treatment and recurrence >3 months after initiation of treatment respectively (Grade 1B).[2] Hematologic abnormalities are greater with the combination therapy. Patients with relapse >6 months from completion of initial chemotherapy can be treated with initial regimen.

* *

There is limited data on patients greater >70 years of age and chemotherapy despite 43% of patients with SCLC >70 years of age because of poor enrollment in trials. With current data available, it has been suggested that patients >70 years of age with good performance status (ECOG 0–2) can be treated with platinum-based chemotherapy plus TRT for limited stage disease (Grade 2B) and carboplatin-based chemotherapy for extensive stage disease

(Grade 2A).[2] If performance status is poor secondary to SCLC, chemotherapy is still advocated (Grade 2C).[2]

* *

There are three types of radiation therapy in SCLC, TRT, prophylactic cranial irradiation (PCI), and palliative RT. Cumulative data has suggested that the concurrent TRT with chemotherapy has improved survival (Grade 1A).[2] Complications include esophagitis, and occurrence is higher with BID TRT. TRT may also benefit patients with extensive disease but have complete remission outside of the chest (Grade 2C).[2] PCI is beneficial since the blood brain barrier prevents chemotherapy from reaching the CNS. Brain metastases is common in SCLC therefore PCI is recommended for limited and extensive disease (Grade 1B).[2] Leukoencephalopathy is a complication of PCI and more common if PCI is administered concurrently with chemotherapy and at large doses. Other complications include headache, nausea, and vomiting. Recommended dose of PCI is 25 Gy in 10 fractions.

CASE 2

Question 1: C. CT-guided transthoracic needle biopsy (TTNB)

Radiographic evaluation of a pulmonary nodule includes size, number, and degree of opacification. A nodule is defined as ≤3 cm, and has no associated atelectasis, hilar adenopathy, or pleural effusion. >3 cm are called masses and are presumed to be malignant unless proven otherwise. Subcentimeter nodule, ≤8 mm, are further distinguished because they are usually benign, difficult to characterize radiographically, and difficult to approach without a surgical biopsy. Diffuse nodules are defined as >10 nodules. With multiple nodules, suspicion for malignancy is focused on the nodule with increasing size.

* *

Benign characteristics includes diffuse, central, laminated, and popcorn calcifications. Intranodular fat density and popcorn calcification is specific for hamartoma. Malignant characteristics include spiculated margins, vascular convergence, dilated bronchus leading to nodule, air bronchiolograms, and thick and irregular cavitation. Evaluation of most types of pulmonary nodules usually requires comparison with prior films (Grade 1C).

* *

Subcentimeter nodules (≤8 mm) are further characterized as solid, part solid, or pure ground glass. From the baseline low-dose CT screening of US Trials, <1% of solid nodules <5 mm are malignant and 2.3% to 6% of solid nodules 6 to 9 mm are malignant. According to the current ACCP guidelines for subcentimeter solid nodules with no risk factors for lung cancer, CT chest surveillance is dictated below.[3]

≤8-mm solid nodule without lung cancer risk	≤8-mm solid nodule with lung cancer risk
≤4-mm follow-up optional	≤4 mm 12 month; if stable no add. Follow-up
4–6 mm 12 months; if stable no follow-up	4–6 mm 6–12 months; if stable at 18–24 months
6–8 mm 6–12 months; if stable follow-up at 18–24 months	6–8 mm 3–6 months; if stable then at 9–12 months and then 24 months

* *

Subsolid nodules, those with varying degrees of attenuation resulting in ground glass with or without solid components, appear to be more concerning for malignancy than solid nodules. ≤10 mm ground-glass nodules could represent atypical adenomatous hyperplasia (AAH), or adenocarcinoma in situ (AIS). AIS and invasive adenocarcinoma are more prevalent if with >50% solid components. Growth or development of solid component warrants further investigation and/or resection. Functional studies via PET are not advocated for solid components ≤8 mm. Solid components >1.5 mm warrant further investigation with PET, nonsurgical biopsy, or resection. CT surveillance is described in the table ACCP Guidelines on Pulmonary Nodules Surveillance[3].

ACCP GUIDELINES ON PULMONARY NODULES SURVEILLANCE

Pure Ground-Glass Nodule	Part Solid Nodule
≤5 mm—No further evaluation >5 mm—CT in 3 months and then annual surveillance for >3 years	≤8 mm—CT surveillance at 3, 12, and 24 months followed by annual CT for 1–3 years >8 mm—CT at 3 months followed by PET, nonsurgical biopsy, or resection if persistent

* *

For solid indeterminate >8 mm nodules, the next step is assessment for surgical risk. If it is high, surveillance or nonsurgical biopsy is advised. If the surgical risk is low, assessment of malignant probability is based on a validated model is such as the one used by Mayo Clinic. It identifies clinical independent predictors of malignancy for nodules 4 to 30 mm. These include: older age (OR 1.04 per year), current or past smoking history (OR 2.2), extrathoracic cancer >5 years before nodule detection (OR 3.8), nodule diameter OR 1.14 per millimeter), spiculation (OR 2.8), and upper-lobe location (OR 2.2).

$$\text{Probability of malignancy} = e^x /(1 + e^x)$$
$$X = -6.8272 + (0.0391 \times \text{age}) + (0.7917 \times \text{smoke})$$
$$+ (1.3388 \times \text{cancer}) + (0.1274 \times \text{diameter})$$
$$+ (1.0407 \times \text{spiculation}) + (0.7838 \times \text{location})$$

These clinical factors are combined with FDG-PET, surgical biopsy, and CT scan surveillance to assess the probably of risk, which is seen in the table below, Probability of Malignancy.

	Probability of Malignancy		
Assessment Criteria	**Low (<5%)**	**Intermediate (5–65%)**	**High (>65%)**
Clinical factors alone (determined by clinical judgment and/or use of validated model)[a]	Young, less smoking, no prior cancer, smaller nodule size, regular margins, and/or non–upper-lobe location	Mixture of low and high probability features	Older, heavy smoking, prior cancer, larger size, irregular/spiculated margins, and/or upper-lobe location
FDG-PET scan results	Low–moderate clinical probability and low FDG-PET activity	Weak or moderate FDG-PET scan activity	Intensely hypermetabolic nodule
Nonsurgical biopsy results (bronchoscopy or TTNA)	Specific benign diagnosis	Nondiagnostic	Suspicious for malignancy
CT scan surveillance	Resolution or near-complete resolution, progressive or persistent decrease in size,[b] or no growth over ≥2 years (solid nodule) or ≥3–5 years (subsolid nodule)	NA	Clear evidence of growth

Reproduced with permission from Tomblyn M, Chiller T, Einsele H, et al: Guidelines for preventing infectious complications among hematopoietic cell transplantation recipients: a global perspective. *Biol Blood Marrow Transplant.* 2009;15(10):1143–1238.

**

Because the typical doubling time of solid nodules is within 400 days, it is recommended that solid indeterminate nodules >8 mm have surveillance noncontrast low-dose chest computed tomography at 3 to 6 months, 9 to 12 months, and 18 to 24 months if the clinical probability is low. This surveillance computed tomography is also recommended if the functional imaging is negative, the needle biopsy is nondiagnostic with a nonhypermetabolic lesion via PET, and/or the patient prefers nonaggressive approach (Grade 2C).[3] If there is improvement with the size or resolution, it should still follow the full 2 years. A solid indeterminate nodule that shows stability for at least 2 years requires no further evaluation (Grade 2C).[3]

**

Functional imaging such as dynamic contrast-enhanced CT, dynamic MRI, or PET with fluorodeoxyglucose, is advocated for solid indeterminate nodule >8 to 30 mm with a low to moderate pretest probability or when clinical pretest probability and CT scan results are discordant (Grade 2C).[3] Dual-time FDG-PET has a pooled sensitivity of 85% add (95% CI 82% to 89%) and specificity 77% (95% CI 72–81%). False negatives are seen in lepidic growth adenocarcinomas, mucinous adenocarcinomas, and carcinoid tumors. False positives are from infections or other inflammatory disorders. FDG uptakes inversely correlated with survival. Characterization via functional imaging for a solid indeterminate nodule with high pretest probability of malignancy is not necessary (Grade 2C).[3]

**

Nonsurgical lung biopsy via CT-guided transthoracic needle biopsy (TTNB) is correct for this patient. Nonsurgical lung biopsy such as TTNB, endobronchial ultrasound (EBUS), bronchoscopy with transbronchial biopsy with fluoroscopy, electromagnetic navigation bronchoscopy (ENB), and virtual bronchoscopy navigation (VBN) is recommended for >8 mm solid indeterminate nodules if the clinical probability of malignancy is low to moderate, discordance between clinical probability and imaging tests, benign etiology is suspected, or patient desires proof of malignancy (Grade 2C).[3] Given the peripheral location of the lesion and the patient's desire for the least invasive approach, CT-guided TTNB is preferred. For TTNB, sensitivity for diagnosis is >90% but only 70% to 82% if lesions ≤15 mm.

If the patient is aggressive with her pursuit of a diagnosis, and given the patient's high clinical probability of malignancy, wedge resection via thoracoscopy is recommended (Grade 1C).[3]

CASE 3

Question 1: C. Smoking cessation

The modifiable risk factor for lung cancer is smoking, with a 10-fold increased risk of cancer compared to never smokers (<100 cigarettes in a lifetime). After 10 years of smoking cessation, the risk decreases up to 50%. However, former smokers will still carry a risk compared to nonsmokers.

**

The high incidence of death related to lung cancer is in part secondary to the advanced stage of the disease at the time of initial presentation. Lung cancer screening is difficult due to heterogeneous nature of lung cancer and the complications from screening. Serial chest radiographs (Grade 1A) and sputum cytology (Grade 2B) are not advocated as screening tools by the recent ACCP guidelines.[4] The National Lung Cancer Screening Trial (NLST) advocates annual screening with low-dose CT over chest radiograph in patients aged 55 to 74 years for smokers or former smokers with at least 30 pack-year who continue to smoke or have quit within the past 15 years (Grade 2B).[4,5] The patient does not meet these criteria. The basis of this recommendation is secondary to a 20% reduction in mortality in patients screened with LDCT compared to CXR (RR 0.80; 95% CI 0.73–0.93; $P = 0.04$).[5]

**

Concerns for screening via LDCT include the high incidence of nonmalignant abnormalities. There was a higher rate of death or complication due to the investigation of these benign lesions. Another concern is the amount of radiation. However, according to the NLST, the risk of radiation induced cancer is one death in 2,500 screened patients.[5] Chemoprevention with B carotene, Vitamin E, retinoids, N-acetylcysteine, isotretinoin, aspirin, selenium, prostacyclin analogs, cyclooxygenase-2 inhibitors, anethole dithiolethione, inhaled steroids, pioglitazone, tea extract, or metformin are not recommended.[6]

Question 2: **D. Squamous cell carcinoma**
Squamous cell carcinoma is the second most common type of lung carcinoma. It is believed to arise from molecular airway epithelium alterations.

Question 3: **A. Hyperplasia**
Bronchial Intraepithelial Neoplasia (BIN) is a central airway carcinomas that arises from a stepwise fashion from normal epithelium to dysplastic tissue. An example of this type of neoplasm is squamous cell carcinoma. The transformation to preinvasive lesions begins with hyperplasia, metaplasia, mild dysplasia which has mild atypia limited to lower 1/3 of the epithelium, moderate dysplasia, which has atypia limited to two-thirds of the epithelium, and severe dysplasia which shows high degree of cellular atypia and some cell maturation. Carcinoma in situ (CIS) shows marked cytologic abnormalities but does not infiltrate the basement membrane unlike invasive squamous cell carcinoma.

Question 4: **B. Predetermine surgical margins**
White light bronchoscopy (WLB) with autofluorescence bronchoscopy (AFB) as an adjunct has been shown to have increased sensitivity (43–100%) but decreased specificity (4–94%)compared to WLB, sensitivity 0% to 85% and specificity 36% to 94% respectively, in identifying precursors to BIN.[7] The rationale behind AFB is that dysplasia, carcinoma in situ, and invasive carcinoma have different fluorescence patterns (weaker green and red fluorescence via 380–440 nm) than normal tissues.

* *

Other methods to evaluate airway mucosa are narrow band imaging (NBI) and optical coherence tomography. In terms of lung cancer extension, NBI and AFB show higher sensitivity and specificity than WLB alone.

* *

According to the ACCP guidelines 2013,[7] indications for the use of WLB and AFB include:

(1). Evaluation for endobronchial lesions in patients with severe dysplasia or CIS in sputum cytology but no localizing chest imaging (Grade 2C)

(2). Follow-up WLB for patients with known severe dysplasia or CIS in central airways on biopsy (Grade 2C)

(3). Delineation of tumor margins and assessment of synchronous lesions (Grade 2C)

(4). Curative endobronchial therapy to treat CIS or early central lung cancer (Grade 2C)

CASE 4

Question 1: **C. Typical carcinoid**
Typical carcinoid is a low-grade neuroendocrine (NE) tumor, and represents 1% to 2% of all invasive lung cancers.[8,9] Neuroendocrine pulmonary malignancies represent 20% to 25% of all pulmonary malignancies. These tumors arise from the kulchitzky cells or enterochromaffin cells present in the bronchial mucosa and are from the foregut. Two-thirds of these tumors have neuron-like properties and are able to secrete and decarboxylate amine precursors. There are several types of NE tumors with the well differentiated cancers which usually have better prognosis and can be treated with surgery whereas the poorly differentiated cancers have worse prognosis and the main treatment is chemotherapy.

* *

There is no age or sex predilection although compared to the poorly differentiated NE tumors, carcinoids tend to occur in young nonsmokers. There are other lesions such as tumorlets which are similar to typical carcinoid except ≤0.5 cm and surrounded by fibrotic parenchyma and diffuse idiopathic pulmonary neuroendocrine cell hyperplasia (DIPNECH) which are proliferation of single or multiple neuroendocrine bodies. DIPNECH is thought to be a precursor to both typical and atypical carcinoid. Patients with multiple endocrine neoplasia type I (MEN I) have high incidence of these tumors.

* *

Clinical manifestations depend on the location. Central lesions can manifest with chest pain, cough, and dyspnea whereas peripheral lesions can be clinically silent.

* *

Often the diagnosis is dependent on pathology and immunohistochemistry. Carcinoids can have a positive estrogen immunostaining.

Question 2: **B. Somatostatin receptor scintigraphy**
Eighty percent of typical carcinoids have positive somatostatin receptors and somatostatin receptor scintigraphy (SRS) may be used to evaluate for extrapulmonary metastases. However, less than 5% of carcinoids have extrapulmonary metastases and SRS is nonspecific, being positive in granulomatous diseases, other tumors, and autoimmune diseases. Due to this, some would forego SRS and proceed to resection. Unlike other types of carcinoid, the risk of carcinoid syndrome is lower

in bronchial carcinoid. Carcinoid syndrome and crisis occur secondary to the release of serotonin and other amines and lead acute symptoms such as flushing, diarrhea, hypertension or hypotension, tachycardia, and bronchospasm and chronic complications such as valvular heart disease and retroperitoneal fibrosis. Because of the low probability of occurrence in bronchial NE, prophylactic administration of octreotide prior to resection is generally not recommended. Positron emission tomography has low sensitivity in detecting metastatic disease for carcinoids, as well as adenocarcinoma is situ and mucinous adenocarcinoma due to low FD uptake. There is currently no role for neoadjuvant chemotherapy or radiotherapy in typical carcinoids.

Question 3: B. T1bN0M0

Refer to the TNM table in Case 1 *Question 3* for explanation of staging.

CASE 5

Question 1: C. Stage IIIA

Refer to the TNM stable in Case 1 *Question 3* for explanation of staging.

Question 2: B. Concurrent chemoradiotherapy

As per ACCP guidelines, Stage III NSCLC treatment is dependent on the discernibility of the N2 lymph nodes, weight loss, and performance status.[10] There are three subclasses: (1) Infiltrative Stage III disease where lymph nodes are bulky and cannot be distinguished; (2) N2 disease determined preoperatively through radiographic evaluation such as CT/PET; and (3) N2 disease identified perioperatively.

* *

For infiltrative Stage III disease, platinum-based chemotherapy concurrently with radiotherapy at 60 to 70 Gy has been shown to improve tumor rate and prolong survival compared to radiotherapy alone (Grade 1A).[10] Despite this, the rate of systemic metastases is high. However, induction and consolidation chemotherapy (Grade 1C) and prophylactic cranial irradiation (Grade 2C) are currently not recommended.[10]

* *

The current ACCP guidelines also emphasize that chemoradiotherapy should be avoided and palliative radiotherapy should be treatment of choice if the patient is symptomatic with performance status 3–4, comor-

bidities, or disease is too extensive (Grade 1C). Platinum-based doublet chemotherapy is suggested if performance status is 0—1 (Grade 2C).[10]

* *

For N2 disease that is identified preoperatively, chemoradiotherapy or induction therapy followed by surgery is recommended (Grade 1A).[10] For N2 disease which is identified via frozen section perioperatively or after pathology, systemic mediastinal lymph node sampling or complete mediastinal lymph node dissection (Grade 1B) or complete lung resection and mediastinal lymphadenectomy is recommended (Grade 2C).[10]

Question 3: B. Pulmonary tumor thrombotic micro-angiopathy

The patient has pulmonary tumor thrombotic microangiopathy (PTTM) which is an embolic disease with pulmonary arteries or arterioles proliferation. It is associated with adenocarcinomas and pulmonary hypertension.[11,12] Clinically, signs and symptoms are nonspecific with cough and dyspnea. Computed tomography is nonspecific. Diagnosis is often confirmed postmortem with fibrocellular intimal hyperplasia of pulmonary arteries and clumps of tumor cells on histopathology. Suggested treatment is chemotherapy.

CASE 6

Question 1: B. No surveillance CT scan

In patients with multiple pulmonary nodules, each nodule should be assessed individually. However, in patients with pure ground glass <5 mm nodules, surveillance computed tomography is not indicated.

CASE 7

Question 1: B. T2aN0M0

Refer to the TNM table found in Case 1 *Question 3* for further discussion on staging.

Question 2: C. Surgical resection followed by adjunct chemotherapy

According to the 2013 ACCP guidelines, surgical resection is recommended Stage I and II NSCLC (Grade 1B) via a board certified thoracic surgeon, whose practice consists of >75% thoracic procedures with >4 anatomic surgical resections per month (Grade 1B) with systemic mediastinal lymph node sampling or dissection at the time of resection (Grade 1B).[13] Pulmonary resection through minimally invasive approach such as video-assisted thoracic surgery is preferred for Stage I NSCLC (Grade 2C).[13] If the patient is a candidate for complete resection, sleeve or bronchoplastic resection is preferred over pneumonectomy (Grade 2C) although lobectomy is preferred over sublobar resection (Grade 1B).[13] Sublobar resection is preferred if (1) increased risk of perioperative mortality or comorbidities or (2) clinical stage I with predominantly ground-glass opacities (GGO) ≤2 cm (Grade 2C). Wedge resection with stereotactic body radiation therapy (SBRT) is preferred over no therapy for clinical Stage I NSCLC over no therapy (Grade 2C).[13]

* *

No adjuvant chemotherapy is necessary for Stage I NSCLC. Completely resected Stage IIA, B(N1) with good performance status, postoperative platinum-based chemotherapy is recommended (Grade 1A).[13]

* *

The benefit from surgery is also dependent on the degree of resection. Complete resection implies negative microscopic margins and systemic LN dissection with no extracapsular nodal extension and most distant LN disease and is designated as R0. Microscopic evidence if malignancy is designated R1. Macroscopic evidence of malignancy is designated R2. After surgery, chemotherapy is not recommended for completely resected NSCLC Stage IA or IB but is recommended for Stage IIA, B(N1). Postoperative radiation therapy is recommended if resection is R1 (Grade 2C).[13]

Question 3: A. Stair-climbing test
For patients being evaluated for lung resection, if either a PPO FEV_1 or PPO DLco are <60% predicted but both are >30% predicted, stair-climbing test or shuttle-walk test (SWT) is recommended (Grade 1C).[18] If SWT <25 shuttles (<400 m), <22 m with symptom-limited stair-climbing test (Grade 1C), PPO FEV_1 <30% or PPO DLco <30% predicted (Grade 1B) a formal CPET is recommended. If the VO_2 max <10 mL/kg/min or <35% predicted, minimally invasive surgery, sublobar resection or nonoperative treatment is advised (Grade 1C).[18]

CASE 8

Question 1: E. T1bN3M1a
Patient has Stage IV disease. Refer to the TNM table found in Case 1 *Question 3* for further discussion on staging.

Question 2: C. Erlotinib
Patients with known EGFR mutations are recommended to have tyrosine kinase inhibitors (TKI) such as erlotinib or gefitinib as first-line treatment in NSCLC Stage IV (Grade 1A).[14] Somatic mutations in EGFR render the cancer cell highly sensitive to TKIs. These mutations are more prevalent in East Asians, adenocarcinoma, and nonsmokers. Four randomized control studies, including IPASS, WJTOG, North-East Japan Study Group 002 trial, and the OPTIMAL study, compared doublet platinum-based chemotherapy over TKI, gefitinib or erlotinib (in OPTIMAL study) and show improved progression free survival (9–14 months) but didn't show improved overall survival. Authors of the latest ACCP guidelines hypothesize that this could be in part secondary to the introduction of TKIs after platinum-based doublet chemotherapy in some of the study patients. Rash and diarrhea were common complications in TKIs.

* *

Platinum-based doublet chemotherapy, such as carboplatin with gemcitabine is advised for patients who are EGFR—and good performance status (Grade 1A).

* *

Studies such as ECOG 4599 have shown that Bevacizumab, an anti-vascular endothelial growth factor (VEGF), improve progression free survival, overall survival, and response rates in combination with platinum-based doublet chemotherapy as first line for NSCLC lung cancer (Grade 1A) with the following prerequisites: nonsquamous cell histology, no brain metastases, and no hemoptysis because of the high risk of bleeding. Patients with brain metastases that were treated at least 3 months ago via radiation therapy, radiosurgery such as gamma knife, linear particle accelerator, or neurosurgery, can receive bevacizumab (Grade 2B). Recommendation cannot be made on patients on full anticoagulation and poor performance status.

* *

Despite 30% of NSCLC having brain metastases, prophylactic cranial irradiation has not been beneficial.

* *

Crizotinib is the TKI for EML4-ALK. Anaplastic lymphoma kinase fusion oncogene is associated with never or light smokers (<10 pack-year), young age, and adenocarcinoma with signet ring or acinar histology. It is mutually exclusive from EGFR or KRAS. These TKI have not shown improvement in overall survival but have been shown to prolong progression free survival, improved response rate, and quality of life in treatment naive patients assigned to chemotherapy with crizotinib. Another EML4-ALK TKI is ceritinib and used if disease progressed on crizotinib.

Question 3: C. Erlotinib

Maintenance therapy is implemented on patients who have had a stable or improved response after 4 to 6 cycles of platinum-based chemotherapy with a goal to improve PFS or OS. There are two approaches to maintenance therapy: (1) continuation in which the nonplatinum-based chemotherapy is continued until toxicity or disease progression; or (2) switch in which a third agent is added. As per ACCP guidelines, maintenance therapy for nonsquamous histology is with pemetrexed. It is the only agent shown to improve OS, even if the first-line chemotherapy is doublet platinum-based with pemetrexed (Grade 2B).[14] Toxicities from platinum-based chemotherapy are predominantly hematologic. However, studies on maintenance EGFR TKI therapy such as SATURN and C-TONG have suggested the use of TKI as maintenance therapy with erlotinib showing improved PFS and OS (Grade 2B).[14]

Question 4: D. Unknown

Patient most likely has erlotinib-induced pneumonitis as suggested by the normal BNP, echocardiogram, and neutrophilia from the bronchioalveolar lavage. Although it has been postulated that it can be secondary to decreased type II pneumocytes response to injury, its true mechanism is unknown. The other answer choices suggest other DILD. Reactive oxygen species could be related to bleomycin and oxygen administration, decreased metabolism of neuropeptides causing cough is secondary to ACEI, and increased phospholiposis is secondary to amiodarone. Treatment usually is drug withdrawal and corticosteroids although spontaneous resolution has been known to occur. In certain instances such as amiodarone, decreasing the dose and addition of corticosteroids can improve symptoms.

* *

Drug-induced lung diseases (DILD) is a diagnosis of exclusion. Over 380 drugs have been associated with a pulmonary complication. Risk factors include age (childhood and elderly >70 years of age), female sex, dose (particularly in amiodarone 400 mg for at least 2 months, bleomycin >450–500 total units, hydralazine >400 mg/dL, aspirin <35 mg/dL causes respiratory alkalosis and >45 mg/dL causes noncardiogenic pulmonary edema and metabolic acidosis, and BCNU at >1,500 mg/m^2), oxygen therapy such as in bleomycin if fraction of inspired oxygen >0.25 or in mitomycin C if fraction of inspired oxygen >0.5, drug

interaction, radiation therapy, and underlying disease.[15,16] Pulmonary manifestations of this disease include: (1) parenchymal disease such as pulmonary edema, interstitial lung diseases, alveolar hemorrhage, and pulmonary nodules; (2) pleural diseases; (3) airway disease from cough to reactive airway diseases; (4) pulmonary vascular diseases; (5) mediastinal diseases such as mediastinal adenopathy to lymphoproliferative diseases; and (6) neuromuscular dysfunction.

* *

Mechanisms include: (1) disruption of antioxidant/oxidant balance particularly with reactive oxygen

DRUG ASSOCIATED LUNG DISEASES AND THEIR ETIOLOGIES

Pulmonary Disease	Etiologies
Interstitial lung diseases	Rituximab, everolimus, temsirolimus, erlotinib, gefitinib, etanercept, infliximab, adalimub, methotrexate, amiodarone, amphoterin B, nitrofurantoin, sulfasalazine, paclitaxel, gold, interferon alfa, interferon beta, sirolimus
Noncardiogenic pulmonary edema	Heroin, cocaine, methotrexate, hctz, cyclophosphamides, terbutaline, albuterol, ritodrine
Pulmonary hypertension	Amphetamines, fenfluramine, beta-blockers, mitomycin C
Diffuse alveolar hemorrhage	Penicillamine, amiodarone, cocaine, hydralazine, mitomycin, nitrofurantoin, abciximab, methotrexate, carbamazepine, rituximab
Bronchospasm	Calcium channel blockers, beta-blockers, amphoterin B, amiodarone, ACEI, dipyridamole, nitrofurantoin, penicillamine, pentamidine, aspirin, cetuximab, panitumumab, trastuzumab
Asthma	Aspirin, NSAID
Drug induced lupus	Hydralazine, isoniazid, penicillamine, procainamide, quinidine
Mediastinal adenopathy	Phenytoin, bleomycin, carbamazepine
Mediastinal lipomatosis	Corticosteroids
Pleural disease	Methotrexate, nitrofurantoin, amiodarone, procarbazine, carmustine, cyclophosphamide, phenytoin, hydralazine, procainamide, mitomycin C
Thromboembolic disease	Bevacizumab

species; (2) disruption of pulmonary vasculature from increased permeability with increased hydrostatic pressure, impaired homeostasis, and direct occlusion of the vasculature; (3) accumulation of phospholipids in the lysosomes such as in amiodarone; (4) immune mediated lung toxicity; and (5) central nervous system depression.

CASE 9

Question 1: **D. Lepidic predominant invasive adenocarcinoma, nonmucinous (LPA)**

According to ACCP guidelines, the term bronchioloalveolar carcinoma (BAC) is no longer used since it encompasses a heterogeneous group of tumors and cannot distinguish those with good from poor prognosis.[17] In general, mucinous adenocarcinomas have worse prognosis and are associated with KRAS mutation unlike nonmucinous adenocarcinomas.[17]

* *

There are two preinvasive lesions: atypical adenomatous hyperplasia (AAH) and adenocarcinoma in situ (AIS). Their squamous cell counterparts would be squamous dysplasia and squamous cell carcinoma in situ, respectively. AAH is a ≤0.5 cm proliferation of clara cells and/or type II pneumocytes lining alveolar walls and the cells are separated by gaps. Radiographically they appear as ground glass. AIS is ≤3 cm of neoplastic cells along alveolar structures (lepidic growth) lacking stromal, vascular, or pleural invasion. It is mostly nonmucinous and there is an absence of papillary or micropapillary patterns and intraalveolar cells.

* *

Minimally invasive adenocarcinoma (MIA) is mostly nonmucinous, ≤3 cm with lepidic pattern, ≤5 mm invasion but no invasion of lymphatics, blood vessels or pleural, and no necrosis. With complete resection, there is 100% disease-specific survival.[17]

* *

There is insufficient data to support 100% disease-specific survival for lesions >3 cm, therefore they are termed lepidic predominant adenocarcinoma (LPA).[17] LPA should also be termed if there is invasion of the lymphatics, blood vessels, or pleura and/or contains necrosis.

* *

Invasive adenocarcinoma subtypes include acinar, papillary, micropapillary or myofibroblastic stroma, and solid. Acinar consists of glands surrounded by tumor cells. Papillary consists of glandular growth along fibrovascular cores. Micropapillary implies tumor cells growing in papillary tufts. Micropapillary growth carries a poor prognosis. Solid pattern shows tumor cells forming sheets. Nonmucinous usually appears as ground glass, CK7+, CK20−, TTF+, and EGFR+.

* *

Invasive mucinous adenocarcinoma has columnar and/or goblet cells with abundant intracytoplasmic mucin that may follow lepidic, acinar, papillary, micropapillary, and solid patterns. They are usually >3 cm, multiple nodules with military spread to adjacent areas; therefore tend to be more diffuse. Mixed mucinous and nonmucinous adenocarcinoma is possible, if there is at least 10% of each component. Radiographically, they appear as consolidation with air bronchograms. For phenotypes, they are CK7+, CK20+, TTF−, and KRAS+.

* *

Variants of adenocarcinoma include: (1) colloid adenocarcinoma with mucin within airspaces, well-differentiated glandular epithelium within fibrous septa, and sometimes may contain cystic components; (2) fetal adenocarcinoma with glandular elements with tubules resembling fetal lung tubules; and (3) enteric adenocarcinoma which resembles colon cancer and can have morphology similar to lung adenocarcinoma with lepidic growth. They are positive for CDX-2, CK20 or MUC2 and CK7 and/or TTF-1.[17]

Question 2: **A. Cardiac risk assessment and pulmonary function test**

From surgical databases, approximately 30% to 35% of patients diagnosed with lung cancer are >70 years of age.[18] It has been advocated that age is not an exclusion criteria for patients who are candidates for curative surgical resection (Grade 1C).[18] Other factors such as stage, comorbidities, and performance status must be considered in the decision on whether to proceed with surgery. Low risk is <1% for mortality. High risk is >10% morbidity and mortality risk.

**

Initial preoperative evaluation should include history, physical examination, ECG, thoracic-revised cardiac risk index (ThRCRI), which is a modified version of the revised cardiac risk index (RCRI), and pulmonary function test, particularly FEV_1 and DLco. Cardiac consultation should be advised if ThRCRI >1.5, new cardiac medication, or limited exercise tolerance. As per ACCP guidelines, the caveat to aggressive cardiac optimization via cardiac interventions does not necessarily decrease mortality risk.[18] Antiplatelet therapy places the patient at high risk for bleeding, and preoperative administration of beta-blocker places the patient at risk for bradycardia and hypotension. If a cardiac intervention such as catheterization is planned, surgery would have to be postponed for at least 6 weeks.

**

Respiratory morbidity and mortality have correlated with FEV_1, PPO FEV_1, DLco, and PPO DLco. Using FEV_1 as a marker, a value of >60% has been determined as a cutoff with lower values associated with higher morbidity and mortality.[19-21] This statement is not always applicable to patients with COPD due to lobar volume reduction effect, which might take place right after surgery. As per the new ACCP guidelines, respiratory function might be slightly reduced or improved 3 to 6 months after lobectomy in moderate to severe COPD. Several studies have suggested that DLco is a better marker for operative risk than FEV_1. Ferguson et al. hypothesize that DLco <60% as a cut-off.[20]

**

Because postoperative values are linked with risks, their values are determined on the basis of preoperative post-bronchodilator FEV_1 and DLco.[18] For pneumonectomy, the calculation for PPO FEV_1 (and PPO DLco) is:

PPO FEV_1 = preoperative post-BD FEV_1 ×
(1 − fraction of total perfusion for resected lung)

**

The value for total perfusion for resected lung is determined via quantitative radionuclide perfusion scan. For lobectomy, the calculation is:

PPO FEV_1 = preoperative post-BD FEV_1 × (1 − Y/Z)
Y = number of functional lung segments to be removed
Z = total number of functional lung segments

According to ACCP guidelines, no additional tests are needed for preoperative evaluation for lung cancer surgery if PPO FEV_1 and DLco >60% predicted (Grade 1C).[18] If either value is <60% predicted, low technology test, such as stair climb or shuttle walk test (SWT), is recommended (Grade 1C). If either PPO FEV_1 or PPO DLco is <30%, a formal CPET with VO_2 max is recommended (Grade 1B). VO_2 max <10 mL/kg/min or <35% predicted is a high risk for mortality and cardiopulmonary complications (Grade 1C). Minimally invasive surgery, sublobar resections or nonoperative approaches should be explored.

**

The SWT requires the patient to walk between two marks that are placed 10 m apart. An audio signal dictates the pace. The end point would be when the patient is too breathless to finish. Correlation with VO_2 max varies per study. One correlates that 25 shuttles = VO_2 max <10 mL/kg/min while another suggested 25 shuttles >VO_2 max >15 mL/kg/min. Interpretation of 6-minute walk test is not standardized. Stair climbing has also been used. Three flights (12–14 m) of stairs indicate FEV 1.7 L and five flights indicate >2 L. According to ACCP guidelines, <25 shuttles (<400 m) on SWT or climb <22 m on stair-climbing test, a formal CPET with VO_2 max is recommended (Grade 1C).

Question 3 A. EGFR = erlotinib, gefitinib

The heterogeneous histologic characteristics of lung cancer has prompted a personalized therapeutic approach based on identified mutations in the signal transduction for cancer cell proliferation.[22-24] One of the mutations involves the surface membrane receptor EGFR. Mutations in the tyrosine kinase domain of EGFR, such as exon 19 deletions and point mutation CTG to CGG in exon 21 leading leucine by arginine (L858R), are responsive to EGFR TKI erlotinib, gefitinib, and afatinib. Patient characteristics with this mutation include female, 50 years of age, Asian, adenocarcinoma histology, and nonsmokers.

**

Another mutation is KRAS which has substitutions of amino acids glycine at position 12, 13, or 61. These involve membrane-bound intracellular GTP-ase and mediate multiple pathways such as mitogen-activated protein kinase (MAPK), signal transducer and activator of transcription (STAT), and phosphoinositide 3-Kinase

(PI3 K). KRAS, EGFR, and ALK are mutually exclusive. KRAS is generally associated with adenocarcinomas, smokers, and carries a poor prognosis. Therapeutic treatments are focused on downstream targets, particularly MEK with selumetinib and mTOR with ridaforolimus.

* *

BRAF is a downstream mediator of RAS and involve with MAPK pathway. BRAF mutations are found 1% to 3% NSCLC and associated with adenocarcinoma and smokers, and have been suggested as a resistant mechanism for patients who are EGFR+. Currently, dabrafenib, a BRAF inhibitor, is being studied for efficacy.

* *

Other potential pathways involved in TKI resistance in patients with EGFR mutations are (1) PIK3CA pathway, catalytic unit of PI3 K that mediates cell survival and (2) B-catenin mutation, which in conjunction with APC, regulates epithelial cell growth.

* *

EML4-ALK is a fusion oncogene of echinoderm microtubule-associated protein-4 with anaplastic lymphoma kinase. It is associated with young age, never or light smoker (<10 pack-years), and adenocarcinoma with signet ring or acinar histology. Crizotinib, a tyrosine kinase inhibitor, has been beneficial with that caveat that almost all will develop resistance within a few years. The resistance mutation is L1196M or G1269 A. Transition to ceritinib, another TKI, is recommended. Complications of ALK inhibitors include nausea, vomiting, diarrhea, hepatotoxicity, pneumonitis, bradycardia, visual changes, and QT prolongation.

* *

Crizotinib is not only restricted to EML4-ALK. ROS1, a tyrosine kinase of insulin, is a driver oncogene via a genetic translocation and found in 1% to 2% NSCLC. Crizotinib has been shown to improve progression—free survival in patients with this mutation. Crizotinib is being tested for patients with MET, a tyrosine kinase receptor for hepatocyte growth factor.

* *

HER2 (ERBB2) is an EGFR mutation involving inframe insertion mutations in exon 20 in 1% to 2% NCSLC. They are found to respond to trastuzumab, afatinib, neratinib, and temsirolimus.

* *

Other potential gene targets include RET translocation, DDR2 mutation, and MEK1 mutation.

CASE 10

Question 1: A. Sarcomatoid carcinoma

Sarcomatoid carcinoma of the lung is a heterogeneous group of NSCLC that generally carries a poor prognosis.[17,25–27] There are five subtypes: Pleomorphic carcinoma is a poorly differentiated nonsmall cell carcinoma mixed with at least 10% malignant spindle cells and/or giant cells. Spindle cells are epithelioid or spindle arranged in haphazard fascicles or storiform pattern. Spindle cell carcinoma is composed only of spindle-shaped tumor cells. Giant cell carcinoma is composed only of giant cells. Carcinosarcoma is a nonsmall cell carcinoma, usually squamous cell carcinoma, with malignant bone, cartilage, or skeletal muscle. These four subtypes generally are associated with smokers, older age (>65 years old), and men. The fifth subtype, pulmonary blastoma, which is composed of cells of fetal adenocarcinoma and primitive stroma that may contain rhabdomyosarcoma, osteosarcoma, or chondrosarcoma, generally occur at a younger age and has better prognosis. Spindle cells have CD34, keratin, and vimentin.

* *

Adenosquamous carcinoma consists of NSCLC which contain at least 10% of each subtype. They tend to be positive for both TTF-1 and P63 and carry a worse prognosis than either pure subtype alone. Frequency of EGFR in adenosquamous carcinoma is comparable to pure adenocarcinoma alone but KRAS appears to have less of a role.[28,29]

* *

Mucoepidermoid carcinoma is derived from submucosal glands from the tracheobronchial tree, 0.2% of all lung cancers.[30] Treatment is primarily surgery with curative intent. This can be successful in patients with low grade more so than high grade which is defined with cellular atypia, necrosis, increased mitotic activity. High-grade MEC may be difficult to distinguish from adenosquamous carcinoma but lack of keratinization and absence of TTF-1 and surfactant can help discern the two.

Question 2: D. Stage IIIB

Refer to the TNM table found in Case 1 *Question 3* for further discussion on staging.

CASE 11

Question 1: E. CD20—Melanoma

Refer to the table in the answer for Case 1 *Question 2* for further explanation.

Question 2: B. Breast cancer

Metastases to the lung are generally asymptomatic because of their peripheral location but can be symptomatic once they approach the central airways. Symptoms would include cough, hemoptysis, fever, and paraneoplastic syndromes. Radiographically, metastases are usually solitary, well-circumscribed lesions that might be cavitary although this is not always the case. The type of initial cancer raises the probability that a new nodule is a metastasis. Sarcoma, melanoma, genitourinary, and colorectal cancer history raises the probability that the new nodule is a metastasis. Head and neck cancer, solitary nodule, and >2 years since resection of first cancer raises the probability that the cancer is a second primary.[31] Elevated-tumor markers such as human chorionic gonadotropin (hCG), carcinoembryonic antigen, and a fetoprotein may lead to further investigation for pulmonary metastases.

* *

There are no randomized trials regarding pulmonary metastasectomy. Data is derived from registry and surgical follow-up studies.[32,34] The indications for pulmonary metastasectomy is usually reserved for chemo-insensitive tumors where complete resection and control can be achieved, absence of extrathoracic tumors, and absence of alternative therapy. Except for rare exceptions, chemosensitive tumors like breast cancer and germ cell tumors generally do not undergo metastasectomy. Additional indications for germ cell tumors include reoccurrence after chemotherapy and to determine if residual viable tumor exists. Recurrence is not uncommon particularly with sarcoma and melanoma. Five-year survival can be up to 44% with repeat metastasectomy and type of malignancy. Regardless, the fewer metastases with long disease free interval indicate longer survival after metastasectomy.

* *

Ten to 20% of colorectal cancer will have pulmonary metastases with 38% to 67% 5-year survival with pulmonary metastasectomy. Hepatic metastases are also not uncommon and can be treated with surgical resection as well. Twenty-five to 30% of renal cell carcinoma will have pulmonary metastases with 5-year survival between 31% and 53% after R0 metastasectomy. Malignant melanoma is an aggressive tumor with 5-year survival of <5% if disseminated. With R0 metastasectomy 5-year survival is between 22% and 33%. Seventy percent of osteosarcoma will develop pulmonary metastases with a 5-year survival of 29% to 43% with R0 metastasectomy. Twenty percent of soft tissue sarcoma will develop pulmonary metastases with 5-year survival 25% to 43% with R0 metastasectomy.

Question 3: E. All of the above

All of these presentations can benefit from surgical resection after a thorough evaluation for the extent of the metastatic disease, via CT and/or MRI with the intent for complete resection (Grade B and Grade C).[35]

* *

Multifocal lung cancer (MFLC) are multiple ground-glass opacities that might develop solid components. They are more common in women, nonsmokers, and are more likely to develop additional pulmonary foci rather than systemic or nodal disease.[35] Hundred percent survival and low recurrence after surgery have been suggested.[35]

* *

Ten percent Stage IV NSCLC have solitary brain metastases. Given the dismal outcomes with just steroids, 2 months, or whole brain radiation therapy, 3 to 6 months, surgical resection of solitary brain metastatic disease and the primary lung cancer have improved survival, with median survival of 6 to 12 months and 5-year survival of 15%.[35] Patients are subsequently followed with whole brain radiation therapy and chemotherapy.

* *

In patients with known cancer and found to have another pulmonary nodule that is suspicious or proven to be malignant, surgical resection is advised provided that the patient has good pulmonary reserve.[35] This applies to patients with two pulmonary nodules in the same lobe, two nodules in different but ipsilateral lobes, and two nodules, one in the contralateral lobe.[35]

* *

Pancoast tumor is cancer that arises in the apex and involves the apical chest wall at the level of the first rib, and can invade the brachial plexus, subclavian vessels, and spine.[35] It is designated as T3 if involves T1–T2 nerve roots and T4 if C8 or higher nerve roots, subclavian vessels, and vertebral bodies or lamina.[4,35] Patients may present with shoulder pain, radiculopathy, and Horner's syndrome. Preoperative chemoradiation followed by surgical resection has improved medial survival from 16 to 22 months and 5-year survival from 20% to 27%.[35]

* *

Other presentations that might benefit from surgical resection include solitary adrenal metastatic disease and chest wall invasion.

CASE 12

Question 1: B. CT at 6 months
For NSCLC who had surgery with curative intent, surveillance CT should take place 6 months for the first 2 years and then yearly afterward (Grade 2C).[36] Surveillance bronchoscopy is advised for patients with central airway squamous cell carcinoma treated with photodynamic therapy at 1, 2, and 3 months.[36] Afterward, every 3 months for the first year and every 6 months for 5 years.[36] Surveillance bronchoscopy is also recommended for intraluminal bronchial carcinoid treated with Nd:YAG or electrocautery at 6 weeks, every 6 months for 2 years and then annually (Grade 2C).[36]

* *

There is no role for surveillance biomarkers or somatostatin receptor scintigraphy.

CASE 13

Question 1: A. Straight-line effect on radiograph is typically seen in conformal radiation therapy, stereotactic body radiation therapy, and gamma knife therapy
The radiation induced lung injury consists of radiation pneumonitis, which occurs 1 to 3 months after completion of radiation therapy, and radiation fibrosis, which takes place from 6 to 24 months.[37] There is also a "hypersensitivity pneumonitis-like reaction" next to lung tissue outside of the radiation port. Risk factors include dose of radiation (>20 Gy), volume of lung, time-dose, concurrent chemotherapy, underlying lung disease, female sex, young age, withdrawal of glucocorticoid therapy, smoking history, and poor performance status.[37] There is also genetic susceptibility via single nucleotide polymorphism in methylene tetrahydrofolate reductase gene (MTHFR) and polymorphisms in ataxia telangiectasia

mutated gene (ATM).[38] Overexpression of manganese superoxide dismutase appears to have protective effects in animal models. Symptoms may precede radiographic findings and consist of cough, dyspnea, low-grade fever, chest pain, and malaise. Diagnosis is in part via imaging studies. The straight-line effect in chest radiographs which typically demarcates the radiation port is not seen in the conformal radiation therapy, stereotactic body radiation therapy, and gamma knife therapy. A focal area with poorly defined margins is seen instead. Pleural effusions may occur but lymphadenopathy is rare. Bronchoscopy is used to rule out other diseases and may have a predominance of CD4[+] in BAL. Treatment is corticosteroids. Symptomatic improvement is possible but after 18 months, it plateaus.

REFERENCES

1. Pelosof LC, Gerber DE. Paraneoplastic syndromes: An approach to diagnosis and treatment. *Mayo Clin Proc.* 2010;85(9):838–854.
2. Jett JR, Schild SE, Kesler KA, et al. Treatment of small cell lung cancer: Diagnosis and management of lung cancer, 3rd ed: American College of Chest Physicians evidence-based clinical practice guidelines. *Chest.* 2013;143(5 Suppl): e400S–e419S.
3. Gould MK, Donington J, Lynch WR, et al. Diagnosis and management of lung cancer 3rd edition: ACCP guidelines: Evaluation of individual with pulmonary nodules: When Is it lung cancer? *Chest.* 2013;143(5 Suppl):e93S–e120S.
4. Detterbeck FC, Mazzone PJ, Naidich DP, et al. Screening for lung cancer: Diagnosis and management of lung cancer, 3rd edition: ACCP evidence-based clinical practice guidelines. *Chest.* 2013;143(5 Suppl):e78S–e92S.
5. National Lung Screening Trial Research Team, Aberle DR, Adams AM, et al. Reduced lung cancer mortality with low dose computed tomographic screening. *N Engl J Med.* 2011;365:395–409.
6. Szabo E, Mao JT, Lam S, et al. Chemoprevention of lung cancer: Diagnosis and management of lung cancer, 3rd edition: ACCP evidence-based clinical practice guidelines. *Chest.* 2013;143(5 Suppl):e40S–e60S.
7. Wisnivesky JP, Yung RCW, Mathur PN, et al. Diagnosis and treatment of bronchial intraepithelial neoplasia and early lung cancer of the central airways: Diagnosis and management of lung cacner, 3rd ed. American College of Chest Physicians evidence-based clinical practice guidelines. *Chest.* 2013;143(5 Suppl):e263s–e277s.
8. Fisseler-Eckhoff A, Demes M. Neuroendocrine tumors of the lung. *Cancers (Basel).* 2012;4:777–798.
9. Travis WD. Advances in neuroendocrine lung tumors. *Ann Oncol.* 2010;21(Suppl 7):Vii65–vi71.
10. Ramnath N, Dilling TJ, Harris LJ, et al. Treatment of stage III non-small cell lung cancer: Diagnosis and management of lung cancer, 3rd edition: ACCP evidence-based clinical practice guidelines. *Chest.* 2013;143(5 Suppl):e314S–e340S.

11. Franquet T, Gimenez A, Prats R, et al. Thrombotic micro-angiopathy of pulmonary tumors: A vascular cause of tree in bud pattern on CT. *AJR Am J Roentgenol.* 2002;179:897–899.

12. Miyoshi S, Hamada H, Chang AC, et al. Pulmonary tumor thrombotic microangiopathy associated with lung cancer. *J Cardiol Cases.* 2010;1(2):e120–e123.

13. Howington JA, Blum MG, Chang AC, et al. Treatment of stage I and II non-small cell lung cancer: Diagnosis and management of lung cancer, 3rd edition: ACCP evidence-based clinical practice guidelines. *Chest.* 2013;143 (5 Suppl):e278S–e313S.

14. Socinski MA, Evans T, Gettinger S, et al. Treatment of stage IV non-small cell lung cancer: Diagnosis and management of lung cancer, 3rd edition: ACCP evidence-based clinical practice guidelines. *Chest.* 2013;143(5 Suppl):e341S–e368S.

15. Schwaiblamir M, Behr W, Haeckel T, et al. Drug induced interstitial lung disease. *Open Respir Med J.* 2012;6:63–74.

16. Limper AH. Chemotherapy-induced lung disease. *Clin Chest Med.* 2004;25:53–64.

17. Travis WD, Brambilla E, Noguchi M, et al. International Association for the Study of Lung Cancer/American Thoracic Society/European Respiratory Society international multidisciplinary classification of lung adenocarcinoma. *J Thorac Oncol.* 2011;6(2):244–285.

18. Brunelli A, Kim AW, Berger KI, et al. Physiologic evaluation of the patient with lung cancer being considered for lung resectional surgery: Diagnosis and management of lung cancer, 3rd edition: ACCP evidence-based clinical practice guidelines. *Chest.* 2013;143(5 Suppl):e166s–e190s.

19. Berrry MF, Vllamizar-Ortiz NR, Tong BC, et al. Pulmonary function tests do not predict pulmonary complications after thoracoscopic lobectomy. *Ann Thoracic Surg.* 2010;89(4):1044–1051.

20. Ferguson MK, Siddique J, Karrison T. Modeling major lung resection outcomes using classification trees and multiple imputation techniques. *Eur J Cardiothorac Surg.* 2008;34(5):1085–1089.

21. Licker MJ, Widikker I, Robert J, et al. Operative mortality and respiratory complications after lung resection for cancer: Impact of chronic obstructive pulmonary disease and time trends. *Ann Thorac Surg.* 2006;81(5):1830–1837.

22. Nana-Sinkam SP, Powell CA. Molecular biology of lung cancer: Diagnosis and management of lung cancer, 3rd edition: ACCP evidence based clinical practice guidelines. *Chest.* 2013;143(5 Suppl):e30s–e39s.

23. Moreira AL, Eng J. Personalized therapy for lung cancer. *Chest.* 2014;146(6):1649–1657.

24. Lee HJ, Lee CH, Jeong YJ, et al. IASCLC/ATS/ERS International Multidisciplinary classification of lung adenocarcinoma: novel concepts and radiologic implications. *J Thorac Imaging.* 2012;27:340–353.

25. Martin LW, Correa AM, Ordonez NG, et al. Sarcomatoid carcinoma of the lung: A predictor of poor prognosis. *Ann Thorac Surg.* 2007;84:973–981.

26. Franks TJ, Galvin JR. Sarcomatoid Carcinoma. *Arch Pathol Lab Med.* 2010;134:49–54.

27. Huan SY, Shen SJ, Li XY. Pulmonary sarcomatoid carcinoma: A clinicopathologic study and prognostic analysis of 51 cases. *World J Surg Oncol.* 2013;11:252.

28. Tochigi N, Dacic S, Nikiforova M, et al. Adenosquamous carcinoma of the lung: A microdissection study of KRAS and EGFR mutational and amplification status in a western patient population. *Am J Clin Pathol.* 2011;135:783–789.

29. Maeda H, Matsumura A, Kawabata T, et al. Adenosquamous carcinoma of the lung: Surgical results as compared with squamous cell and adenocarcinoma cases. *Eur J Cardiothorac Surg.* 2012;357–361.

30. Xi J, Wei J, Lu SH, et al. Primary pulmonary mucoepidermoid carcinoma: an analysis of 21 cases. *World J Surg Oncol.* 2012;10:232.

31. Oien KA, Dennis JL. Diagnostic work-up of carcinoma of unknown primary: from immunohistochemistry to molecular profiling. *Ann Oncol.* 2012;23:271–277.

32. Rusch VW. Pulmonary matastasectomy. *Chest.* 1995;107:322S–332S.

33. Hronbech K, Ravn J, Steinbrüchel DA. Current status of pulmonary metastasectomy. *Eur J Cardio-thorac Surg.* 2011;39:955–962.

34. Treasure T, Milosevic M, Fiorentino F, et al. Pulmonary Metastasectomy: What is the practice and where is the evidence for effectiveness? *Thorax.* 2014;69(10):946–949.

35. Kozower BD, Larner JM, Detterbeck FC, et al. Special treatment issues in non-small cell lung cancer. Diagnosis and management of lung cancer, 3rd ed: American College of Chest Physicians evidence-based clinical practice guidelines. *Chest.* 2013;143(5):e369s–399s.

36. Colt HG, Murgu S, Korst RJ, et al. Follow-up and surveillance of patient with lung cancer after curative-intent therapy. Diagnosis and management of lung cancer, 3rd ed: American College of Chest Physicians evidence–based clinical practice guidelines. *Chest.* 2013;143(5):e437s–454s.

37. Movsas B, Raffin TA, Epstein AH, et al. Pulmonary radiation injury. *Chest.* 1997;111:1061–1076.

38. Williams JP, Johnston CJ, Finkelstein JN. Treatment for radiation-induced pulmonary late effects: Spoiled for choice or looking in the wrong direction? *Curr Drug Targets* 2010;11(11):1386–1394.

14

Occupational Lung Diseases

Brian M. Walsh DO and Paul Simonelli MD, PHD

CASE 1

A 50-year-old man presents to the pulmonary clinic with complaint of progressive dyspnea and dry cough over the past 6 months. He also reports an unintentional weight loss of 10 lbs over the last 6 months. He is given a trial of inhaled albuterol and fluticasone by his PCP without any improvement. He smokes a pack of cigarettes per day since age 15. He has worked in construction most of his life, primarily road construction but reports he is a "jack of all trades." About 1 year ago he took a job of sandblasting metal parts.

**

A chest x-ray is shown from 1 year prior to presentation (left) and current (right).

Question 1: This patient's presentation is most consistent with:

A. Chronic silicosis
B. Accelerated silicosis
C. Acute silicosis
D. Progressive massive fibrosis
E. None of the above

Question 2: Which of the following is an appropriate measure for patients with silicosis?

A. Counseling to avoid any further exposure to silica dust
B. Smoking cessation counseling
C. Placement of tuberculin skin test
D. Influenza and pneumococcal vaccination
E. All of the above

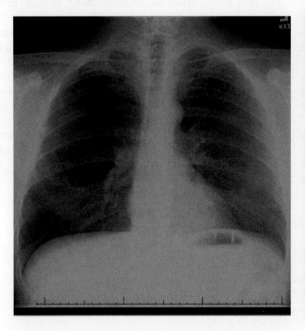 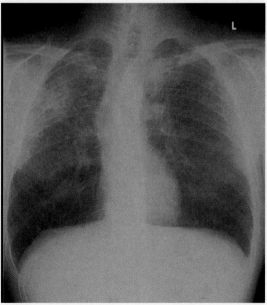

CASE 2

A 78-year-old man presented to the pulmonary clinic for evaluation of chronic cough. He reported a dry cough which had been present for the past 10 years but has been getting progressively worse. Initially he was told the cough was due to acid reflux. He reported this cough to his PCP and a chest x-ray was obtained, followed by a high-resolution chest CT. Old imaging was obtained from his initial complaint 10 years ago which showed increased interstitial markings were present at that time. The patient had never smoked. He worked for 37 years in a foundry making metal alloys used to build machines. He denied any history of asbestos exposure. He denied any symptoms to suggest connective tissue disease. After his initial pulmonary clinic visit the patient explored his prior occupational exposures further and determined that he had significant exposure to Beryllium and his prior supervisor and two coworkers were diagnosed with chronic berylliosis. A beryllium lymphocyte proliferation test and bronchoscopy with transbronchial biopsies were performed.

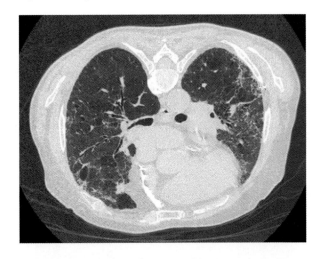

Question 1: Which of the following is true regarding treatment?

A. There is no effective therapy, treatment is supportive including avoidance of further exposure

B. All patients with evidence of beryllium sensitization should receive therapy with glucocorticoids

C. Glucocorticoid therapy has been shown to improve symptoms, pulmonary function tests, and radiographic findings

D. Efficacy of glucocorticoid therapy is not dependent on time from onset of symptoms

E. None of the above

Question 2: Choose the pneumoconiosis with the correct exposure or occupation at risk

A. Siderosis—Aluminum welders

B. Baritosis—Tin miners

C. Stannosis—Iron welders

D. Talcosis—Auto mechanic

E. Flock worker's lung—Nylon workers

CASE 3

A 31-year-old man presents to the pulmonary clinic with complaint of dyspnea. He reports dyspnea which has been slowly progressive over the past 7 months. Two weeks prior to presenting he has had a severe episode of dyspnea which required an emergency department visit. He is started on albuterol as needed and montelukast. Since the ED visit he has been using the albuterol 1 to 2 times per day and does note some improvement. He has no prior personal or family history of asthma, allergic rhinitis, or atopy. He has never smoked but is exposed to second-hand smoke in the workplace. He has worked on the same job for past 8 years, welding stainless steel and aluminum parts for large tanks. About 2 years ago, the company has changes in leadership and instead of leaving large hangar doors open to provide ventilation, the work area is partitioned leading to noticeably worse air quality.

* *

As part of his initial workup, a chest x-ray is obtained which is normal. He underwent spirometry which is shown.

—SPIROMETRY—	Pre-Bronch					Post Bronch		
	Actual	Pred	%Pred	SD	LLN	Actual	%Pred	%Chng
FVC (L)	4.25	5.74	73	0.59	4.77	4.63	80	+8
FEVI (L)	3.30	4.66	70	0.50	3.84	3.65	78	+10
FEVI/TVC (%)	78	82	94	6	72	79	96	+1
FEF 25% (L/sec)	6.53					7.42		+13
FEF 75% (L/sec)	1.27					1.99		+57
FEF 25–75% (L/sec)	2.80	4.58	61	1.02	2.90	3.83	83	+36
FEF Max (L/sec)	7.75	10.63	72	1.48	8.19	9.61	90	+24
FIVC (L)	4.27					3.74		−12
FIF Max (L/sec)	5.95					6.52		+9
FEV6 (L)	4.25	5.66	75	0.58	4.70	4.63	81	+8
Time To FETmex (sec)	0.093					0.071		−23

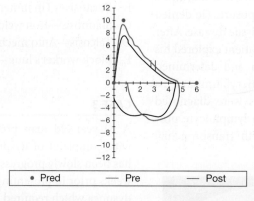

• Pred   — Pre   — Post

Question 1: Which of the following metals have been considered to cause occupational asthma?

A. Aluminum

B. Nickel

C. Cobalt

D. Steel

E. All of the above

CASE 4

A 79-year-old man presents to his primary care office for evaluation of central chest pain which has been present for the past week. He also notes increased fatigue over the past several weeks. He denies any dyspnea, cough, or hemoptysis. He also denies any fevers, chills, sweats.

* *

He has worked for a pharmaceutical company doing general maintenance including "pipe work" for 13 years, followed by 30 years at a sewage and water treatment plant. He does not know of any specific exposures related to his work. He has never smoked.

* *

A chest x-ray is obtained, followed by a CT scan of the chest. A baseline chest x-ray from 7 years prior is also available for review. There is no evidence of calcified pleural plaques on the CT scan. A bronchoscopy with transbronchial biopsies and an EBUS with lymph node sampling are performed. The transbronchial biopsies are nondiagnostic and the lymph node sampling show only a benign mixed population of lymphocytes.

* *

Chest x-ray from 7 years prior to presentation

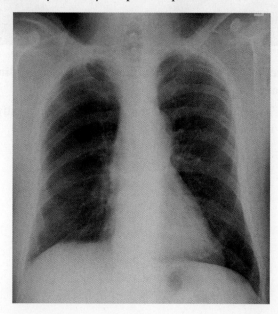

* *

Current PA and lateral chest x-ray

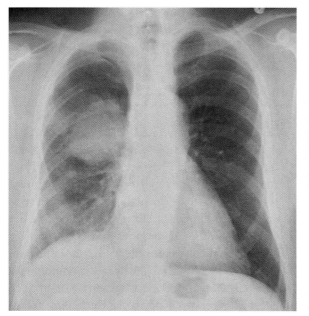 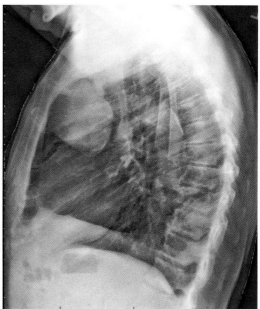

* *

Current chest CT scan

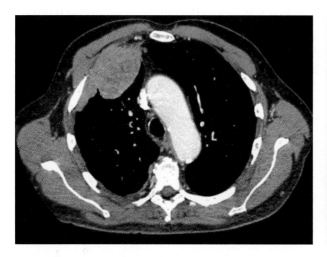 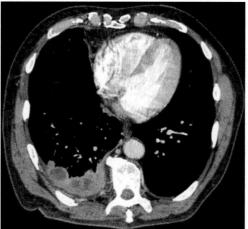

Question 1: **What is the most likely diagnosis?**

A. Asbestosis
B. Rounded atelectasis
C. Benign asbestos-related pleural effusion
D. Diffuse pleural thickening
E. Malignant mesothelioma

CASE 5

A 49-year-old man complains for chronic cough for at least 6 months with dyspnea on exertion. He denies fevers, chills, weight loss. His coworkers have the same symptoms. A chest x-ray is obtained followed by a CT scan which is shown on the next page. Bronchoscopy and biopsy which reveals a collection of pigmented dust and dust-laden macrophages with surrounding focal emphysema.

* *

Patient smoke one pack per day for about 20 years, quit 1 year ago. He has worked as a miner and foreman in an underground coal mine for 19 years mining bituminous coal.

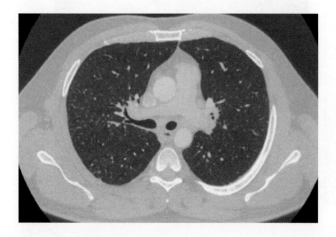

Question 1: **Which of these features is associated with increased risk of coal worker's pneumoconiosis?**

A. Surface mining compared to underground mining
B. Anthracite coal compared to bituminous coal
C. Lower carbon content of coal
D. Working as roof bolter
E. None of the above

Question 2: **Which of the following statements is true regarding coal worker's pneumoconiosis?**

A. Patients are at increased risk of mycobacterial infection.
B. Patients are at increased risk of lung cancer.
C. Patients are at increased risk of chronic obstructive pulmonary disease.
D. Treatment consists of glucocorticoids and cessation of exposure.
E. None of the above.

CASE 6

A 54-year-old man presents for evaluation of intermittent dyspnea which has been progressively worse over the past 2 years. He reports initially having intermittent symptoms while at work which would resolve at night and when on holidays. However over the past 6 months he notes continuous dyspnea and can no longer tolerate his usual daily half mile walk. He is a lifelong non-smoker. He has worked for the past 8 years as a diamond polisher. He has a chest x-ray followed by CT of the chest which showed interstitial thickening and ground-glass opacities predominately in the lower lobes. He has and a surgical lung biopsy which shows interstitial fibrosis with multinucleated giant cells accumulating in the alveolar spaces.

Question 1: **Which of the following exposures is linked to this patient's condition?**

A. Aluminum
B. Carbon
C. Cobalt
D. Heavy metals
E. Iron

Answers

CASE 1

Question 1: C. Acute silicosis

Silicosis results from inhalation of crystalline silica, which can be in the form of quartz, cristobalite, or tridymite. Silica makes up the majority of the Earth's crust so exposure is common in many industries and, although the risk of exposure to silica is well known, new cases of silicosis continue to present in the United States and internationally.[1] Some of the affected occupations include mining, quarrying, foundry work, drilling, and sandblasting.

* *

Silicosis is divided into four primary categories based on clinical and pathological presentation. These categories are chronic silicosis, accelerated silicosis, acute silicosis, and progressive massive fibrosis. Chronic silicosis or classic silicosis presents as multiple small (<1 cm) nodules in a symmetrical and predominately upper lobe distribution. Egg-shell calcification of hilar lymph nodes may also be seen. Usually the time from initial exposure to presentation in chronic silicosis is over 15 years. Accelerated silicosis appears radiographically and pathologically similar to chronic silicosis but occurs after a shorter time period (5 to 10 years) and heavier exposure. Progressive massive fibrosis, sometimes called complicated silicosis, describes the coalescence of multiple small nodules to form larger nodules (>1 cm) which remain predominately in the upper lobes. This condition is often associated with significant restrictive ventilatory defects on lung function testing and exertional hypoxemia. Disease often continues to progress despite complete cessation of silica exposure. Acute silicosis, sometimes called silicoproteinosis, develops following short-term (few months to 2 years), very intense exposure to fine silica particles and has been described with sandblasting. Acute silicosis appears radiographically and pathologically distinct from the other forms of silicosis. Radiographically acute silicosis usually presents as airspace or interstitial opacities rather than nodules and has a tendency for mid- and lower-lung fields. Pathologically acute silicosis has the features of pulmonary alveolar proteinosis.

Question 2: E. All of the above

All patients with silica exposure, even without silicosis, are at increased risk for tuberculosis. Patients with acute and accelerated silicosis are at especially high risk. Patients with newly diagnosed silicosis should have a tuberculin skin test or interferon γ release assay, and if positive without signs of active tuberculosis it should be treated for latent TB. Symptoms of weight loss, fevers, or enlargement and cavitation of nodules should prompt a search for active TB. Although disease may continue to progress despite cessation of exposure, patients should still be advised to avoid further exposure to silica and especially in cases of acute or accelerated silicosis an investigation into the workplace should be performed to protect additional exposed workers. Smoking cessation is always advisable and given the worsening of obstructive airways disease in smokers with silicosis and the possible increased risk of lung cancer in patients with silicosis this should be emphasized.

CASE 2

Question 1: C. Glucocorticoid therapy has been shown to improve symptoms, pulmonary function tests, and radiographic findings

Beryllium is a rare metal with properties that make it useful in many industries: it is lighter than aluminum and six times stronger than steel, and can be alloyed with other metals, most commonly copper. It is used in the aerospace, electronics, and nuclear industries and exposure can occur in workers involved in the manufacture of alloys, ceramics, radiographic equipment, and extraction and smelting.

* *

Chronic beryllium disease (CBD), also referred to as berylliosis, shares many features with sarcoidosis. The primary histologic finding is noncaseating granulomas which can be found throughout the body but occur primarily in the lung, as well as a lymphocytic alveolitis. The granulomas are indistinguishable from those of sarcoidosis. Clinical features include cough, chest pain, dyspnea, weight loss, irregular or nodular opacities on chest x-ray, and bibasilar crackles on examination.

* *

A spectrum of beryllium related disease can be determined by the combination of blood or BAL testing for lymphocyte proliferation, biopsy results, and clinical or radiographic features. A positive blood or BAL beryllium lymphocyte proliferation test (BeLPT) in the absence of clinical or biopsy findings is consistent with beryllium sensitization.[2-6] A positive BeLPT and biopsy evidence of granulomas in the absence of clinical or radiographic findings is defined as subclinical beryllium disease. Positive BeLPT, granulomas on biopsy, and clinical or radiographic features are consistent with chronic beryllium disease or berylliosis. There is a false-negative biopsy rate of up to 10% in patients with chronic berylliosis, a negative biopsy should be confirmed by repeat transbronchial biopsy or surgical lung biopsy when suspicion is high, especially when BAL lymphocytosis is present.

* *

Treatment for chronic beryllium disease includes avoidance of further exposure, supportive care, and glucocorticoids.[2-6] All patients with chronic beryllium disease, and even those with evidence of beryllium sensitization should be counseled to avoid any further exposure to beryllium. Supportive care includes vaccinations (influenza and pneumococcal), supplemental oxygen as indicated, and smoking cessation.

Question 2: E. Flock worker's lung – Nylon workers

There are several mineral dust pneumoconioses which fall into the category of large level dust exposure with minimal lung reaction. These include siderosis (exposure to iron dust from arc welding or iron mining), stannosis (exposure to tin dust), and baritosis (exposure to barium by barium miners or workers). Talcosis (exposure to talc used in many industries including ceramics, cosmetics, paper, paint, plastics) causes a non-necrotizing granulomatous inflammation which can cause progressive fibrosis. Flock worker's lung refers to an interstitial lung disease characterized by lymphocytic bronchiolitis in workers involved in making nylon flock.

CASE 3

Question 1: E. All of the above

Work-related asthma includes both occupational asthma and work-exacerbated asthma (pre-existing asthma which is worsened by exposures present in the workplace). Occupational asthma is triggered by an antigen found at work and can be further divided into categories based on the particular causative agent.[7] Sensitizer-induced asthma requires sensitization to an agent which is capable of producing an immunologic response. These can be classified as high–molecular-weight agents (>10 kD) and low–molecular-weight agents.[7-9] High–molecular-weight agents act as a sensitizing antigen and cause production of specific IgE antibodies and a typical allergic response. Once sensitization occurs, very low level exposures can trigger a response. Some common examples include animal or seafood proteins (farmers, lab workers, veterinarians, seafood processors), grains (mill workers, bakers), plants, and plant products (greenhouse workers, makers, and users of latex products). Low–molecular-weight antigens can also cause sensitization and asthma however the mechanism is not as well understood. Some common examples of low–molecular-weight agents include diisocyanates (polyurethane foam, spray painting), metal salts (welders, metal refinery workers), cleaning agents (domestic and commercial cleaners).

* *

Irritant-induced asthma is a term used to describe asthma symptoms which occur in response to inhaled irritants which do not act as a sensitizing agent. These episodes are typically associated with one or multiple high level exposures rather than long-term low-level exposures. Reactive airways dysfunction syndrome is considered a severe form of irritant-induced asthma. A recent example of irritant-induced asthma was workers in the area of the collapse of the World Trade Center who were exposed to high levels of dusts and later developed new-onset asthma.

* *

The diagnosis of occupational asthma is dependent on a high level of suspicion. Estimates of frequency of work-related asthma vary from 5% to 20% of new-onset asthma in adults. A detailed history of occupational exposures should be obtained in all patients with new-onset asthma as an adult or recurrence of childhood asthma. A latency period of weeks to several years may be present between first exposure and onset of symptoms but generally low–molecular-weight antigens have a shorter latency period than high–molecular-weight antigen. Symptoms and findings on pulmonary function testing and bronchial hyperresponsiveness testing are similar to nonoccupational asthma. Symptom pattern correlates with work exposures: occur early in a work shift, toward the end of a shift, or even after returning home. Often patients can identify a remission during vacations or holiday periods when they are not working. Specific IgE testing is not widely available but does exist for certain antigens and may be helpful in select patients when a specific agent is suspected. Specific IgE testing for common allergens outside the workplace may also identify an alternate trigger.

* *

The cornerstone of management of occupational asthma is complete cessation of exposure, although this is often a difficult decision for patients with socioeconomic consequences. Pharmacologic therapy is the same as for nonoccupational asthma. Asthma symptoms can persist for several years even after complete cessation of exposure.

CASE 4

Question 1: E. Malignant mesothelioma

This patient was found to have malignant mesothelioma confirmed on CT-guided transthoracic needle biopsy. Malignant mesothelioma is an aggressive tumor involving serosal surfaces most commonly the pleura, but also affecting the peritoneum, pericardium, and tunica vaginalis. The primary risk factor for mesothelioma is asbestos exposure. Asbestos refers to a group of six silicate minerals which contain long chains of silicone and oxygen which give them a thin fibrous shape. These fibers are stronger than steel and are fireproof leading to extensive use in industry. Asbestos use increased throughout the 1900s until a peak in 1973 due to increasing evidence of lung toxicity.[10–17] As of 1997, it was estimated that 20% of the US buildings still contain asbestos in the form of shingles, cement pipes, and insulation. Mesothelioma is more common in men with a 5:1 ratio, probably because of differences in rates of occupational exposure. There has been a shift in exposure history from primary asbestos exposure related to the mining of raw materials to users of asbestos containing products in industries like construction, plumbing, heating, auto mechanics, and ship builders. The median lag time between asbestos exposure and development of mesothelioma is 32 years with 99% of cases occurring after a lag time of at least 15 years. Other risk factors for mesothelioma include radiation (i.e., therapy for lymphoma), and simian virus 40 (SV40). Although tobacco smoke increases the risk of other lung cancers synergistically with asbestos exposure, tobacco smoke does not increase risk for mesothelioma. Patients with mesothelioma are usually symptomatic at the time of presentation with chest pain, dyspnea, and pleural effusions being common initial manifestations. Weight loss and fatigue can be present in more advanced disease.

* *

There are several benign pleural manifestations of asbestos exposure: pleural plaques, benign asbestos-related pleural effusions, diffuse pleural thickening, and rounded atelectasis. Pleural plaques are the most common manifestation of asbestos exposure and typically appear 20 to 30 years after exposure. They are most commonly found on the parietal pleura along the posterolateral chest wall, mediastinal pleura, and diaphragm. Half contain calcifications by CT. Pleural plaques can be found in about 50% of exposed workers. Benign asbestos-related pleural effusions (BAPE) tend to be early manifestations of asbestos exposure and can occur within 10 years of exposure. Effusions are usually small and unilateral, are exudative and can be blood tinged. Most patients are asymptomatic but they can have chest pain or fever. BAPE is a diagnosis of exclusion and differentiation from mesothelioma can be difficult. Diffuse pleural thickening is fibrosis primarily of the visceral pleural with involvement of the parietal pleura, adhesions, and obliteration of the pleural space. Diffuse pleural thickening can follow BAPE. Unlike pleural plaques, diffuse pleural thickening often involves the costophrenic angle, apices, and fissures. Patients are often symptomatic with dyspnea and chest pain, and can have significant restrictive lung disease. Rounded atelectasis occurs when visceral pleural fibrosis causes a rolling collapse of lung tissue. It presents as a subpleural mass with a whirling appearance and bands of lung tissue radiating out causing a "comet tail" appearance. It is usually associated with pleural plaques or thickening and is related to asbestos exposure in 70% of cases.

* *

Asbestosis refers to the interstitial lung disease or pneumoconiosis which results from inhalation of asbestos fibers. The diagnosis requires interstitial fibrosis in the setting of an appropriate exposure and latency period (usually over 20 years). Patients often present with insidious onset of dyspnea and have basilar crackles on examination. Imaging classically shows lower lobe predominate fibrotic changes. Imaging can also provide additional evidence to support clinically important asbestos exposure such as pleural plaques. Asbestos fibers are too small to be identified on light microscopy, however asbestos bodies can be seen. Asbestos bodies are fibers which have been coated with a mixture of iron and protein and stain with iron stains (sometimes called ferruginous bodies). Presence of asbestos bodies alone indicates exposure but is not diagnostic of asbestosis. Management is generally supportive and includes patient notification that work exposure related disease is present and compensation may be available. Patients should avoid further exposure, smoking cessation, and immunizations (influenza and pneumococcal vaccines). The ATS consensus guidelines recommend a chest film and PFTs be performed every 3 to 5 years.[12]

CASE 5

Question 1: B. Anthracite coal compared to bituminous coal

Coal workers are susceptible to several respiratory diseases related to exposures including coal worker's pneumoconiosis (CWP), silicosis, and chronic obstructive pulmonary disease.[17-19] Coal worker's pneumoconiosis can be classified as simple or complicated, also called progressive massive fibrosis. Simple CWP is characterized by coal macules and coal nodules. Coal macules are nonpalpable collections of coal dust and dust-laden macrophages usually 1 to 6 mm in diameter, typically with focal emphysema surrounding the macule. Coal nodules develop with ongoing exposure, possibly in combination with silica. In addition to the collection of dust-laden macrophages, coal nodules also contain a haphazard arrangement of collagen fibers making them palpable. Coal nodules can be <7 mm (micronodules) or 7 mm to 2 cm (macronodules). Nodules greater than 2 cm in diameter are the definition of progressive massive fibrosis (PMF). These nodules may cavitate due to ischemic necrosis. Risk factors for progression from CWP to PMF include younger age, total dust burden, rapidly progressive CWP, and increased silica content. PMF is associated with impaired lung function and increased mortality. Patients who develop PMF tend to have progression of disease despite complete cessation of exposure.

**

The risk of developing CWP is dependent on several factors including intensity and duration of exposure, coal type, mine type, and the specific job of the miner. Different types of coal are classified by rank which is based on the percent composition of carbon. The types in order of increasing rank are lignite, subbituminous, bituminous, and anthracite. The higher rank coals are associated with increased risk of developing CWP, with anthracite miners having the highest risk. Underground miners are at increased risk of CWP compared to surface miners. However, surface miners have higher exposure to silica due to the rock drilling involved. In addition to mining, workers involved in coal trimming (loading and storing coal) are at risk of developing CWP. The level of silica exposure in coal miners is dependent on the silica content of the ore being mined, the type of mine (surface higher than underground), the type of coal (anthracite higher than bituminous), and the specific job (increased exposure from tunnel drilling, roof bolting).

Question 2: C. Patients are at increased risk of chronic obstructive pulmonary disease

Coal workers are at increased risk of chronic obstructive pulmonary disease with an effect similar in magnitude to cigarette smoking. They also have an increased rate of mucous hypersecretion and chronic bronchitis, although this tends to improve or resolve after cessation of exposure. Unlike silicosis, coal worker's pneumoconiosis is not associated with increased risk of mycobacterial infection. Coal workers have not been shown to have an increased risk of lung cancer, however they do have increased rates of gastric cancer. Management of patients with CWP includes cessation of dust exposure and smoking cessation counseling.

CASE 6

Question 1: C. Cobalt

Giant cell interstitial pneumonitis (also called hard metal lung disease) is an occupational lung disease found in both hard metal workers and workers exposed to cobalt dust. Hard metal (different from heavy metal) is produced by the combination of tungsten carbide and cobalt along with other metals in a process called sintering.[20,21] As the name suggests, this is used in industries such as drilling, cutting, and grinding due to its hardness, which is close to diamond.[20,21] However the same pathology has been found in diamond polishers who were exposed to cobalt dust without any hard metal suggesting that cobalt is the inciting factor.

* *

The clinical symptoms from exposure can range from occupational asthma with intermittent symptoms upon exposure to progressive fibrosis. Pathology shows accumulation of unusual appearing multinucleated giant cells in the alveolar spaces. There is evidence of a hypersensitivity pneumonitis process. Elemental analysis often shows presence of tungsten in the areas of fibrosis. Cobalt is rarely identified, probably because of its solubility in tissue.

* *

Treatment consists of early recognition so that patients can avoid further exposure. If recognized early symptoms can resolve with avoidance, and there have been reports of improvement with corticosteroids.

REFERENCES

1. Parker J, Wagner GR. 10. Respiratory system, David A, Wagner GR, eds. *Encyclopedia of Occupational Health and Safety*. Jeanne Mager Stellman, Editor-in-Chief. Geneva: International Labor Organization; 2011.
2. Taylor TP, Ding M, Ehler DS, et al. Beryllium in the environment: a review. *J Environ Sci Health A Tox Hazard Subst Environ Eng*. 2003;38(2):439–469.
3. Kreiss K, Mroz MM, Zhen B, et al. Risks of beryllium disease related to work processes at a metal, alloy, and oxide production plant. *Occup Environ Med*. 1997;54(8):605–612.
4. Marchand-Adam S, El Khatib A, Guillon F, et al. Short- and long-term response to corticosteroid therapy in chronic beryllium disease. *Eur Respir J*. 2008;32(3):687–693.
5. Newman LS, Mroz MM, Balkissoon R, et al. Beryllium sensitization progresses to chronic beryllium disease: a longitudinal study of disease risk. *Am J Respir Crit Care Med*. 2005;171(1):54–60.
6. Sood A, Beckett WS, Cullen MR. Variable response to long-term corticosteroid therapy in chronic beryllium disease. *Chest*. 2004;126(6):2000–2007.
7. Tarlo SM, Balmes J, Balkissoon R, et al. Diagnosis and management of work-related asthma: American College Of Chest Physicians Consensus Statement. *Chest*. 2008: 134(3 Suppl):1S–41S.
8. Mapp CE, Boschetto P, Maestrelli P, et al. Occupational asthma. *Am J Respir Crit Care Med*. 2005;172:280–305.
9. Tarlo SM, Lemiere C. Occupational asthma. *N Engl J Med*. 2014;370:640–649.
10. Alleman JE, Mossman BT. Asbestos revisited. *Scientific Am*. 1997;277(1):54–57.
11. Chapman SJ, Cookson WO, Musk AW, et al. Benign asbestos pleural diseases. *Curr Opin Pulm Med*. 2003;9(4): 266–271.
12. Ghio AJ, Roggli VL. Diagnosis and initial management of nonmalignant diseases related to asbestos. *Am J Respir Crit Care Med*. 2005;171(5):527–527.
13. Lanphear BP, Buncher CR. Latent period for malignant mesothelioma of occupational origin. *J Occup Med*.1992; 34(7):718–721.
14. Lee YC, Light RW, Musk AW. Management of malignant pleural mesothelioma: a critical review. *Curr Opin Pulm Med*. 2000;6(4):267–274.
15. Robinson BW, Lake RA. Advances in malignant mesothelioma. *N Engl J Med*. 2005;353(15):1591–1603.
16. Scherpereel A, Astoul P, Baas P, et al. Guidelines of the European Respiratory Society and the European Society of Thoracic Surgeons for the management of malignant pleural mesothelioma. *Eur Resp J*. 2010;35(3):479–495.
17. Tsao AS, Wistuba I, Roth JA, et al. Malignant pleural mesothelioma. *J Clin Oncol*. 2009;27(12):2081–2090.
18. Petsonk EL, Rose C, Cohen R. Coal mine dust lung disease. New lessons from an old exposure. *Am J Respir Crit Care Med*. 2013;187(11):1178–1185.
19. Attfield MD, Morring K. An investigation into the relationship between coal worker's pneumoconiosis and dust exposure in US coal miners. *Am Ind Hyg Assoc J*. 1992; 53(5):486–492.
20. Moriyama H, Kobayashi M, Takada T, et al. Two-dimensional analysis of elements and mononuclear cells in hard metal lung disease. *Am J Respir Crit Care Med*. 2007;176(1): 70–77.
21. Nemery B, Abraham JL. Hard metal lung disease: still hard to understand. *Am J Respir Crit Care Med*. 2007;176(1): 2–3.

15

Sleep Medicine

**Michael Marino MD, Ronaldo Collo Go MD,
Evelyn Mai MD, and Alfred Astua MD**

CASE 1

A 50-year-old morbidly obese man with history of diabetes mellitus and hypertension complains of excessive daytime sleepiness. He complains of morning headaches, lightheadedness, and fatigue. His wife has witnessed that he chokes at night and snores. He says his symptoms improve when he sleeps on his side. On physical examination his vital signs were unremarkable and he is noted to have a Mallampati IV.

Question 1: **What type of sleep study would you prescribe?**

A. Type I
B. Type II

C. Type III
D. Type IV
E. Out of center testing

Question 2: **During the sleep study, this wave form is observed. What sleep stage is this?**

A. Stage wake
B. Stage N1
C. Stage N2
D. Stage N3
E. REM

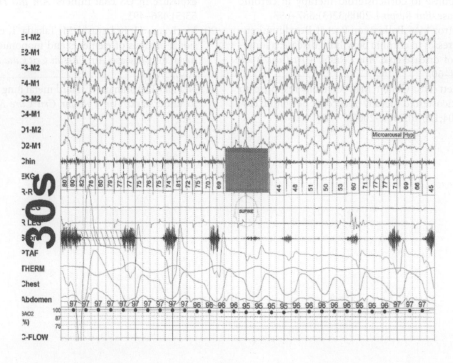

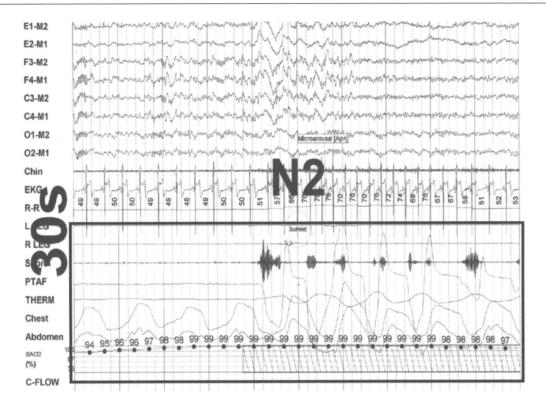

Question 3: After reviewing the sleep study, the diagnosis of the patient is:

A. Malingering
B. Obstructive sleep apnea
C. Central sleep apnea
D. Mixed sleep apnea
E. Obesity hypoventilation syndrome

CASE 2

A 55-year-old woman with severe obstructive sleep apnea returns to you with her compliance chip and this is what it shows:

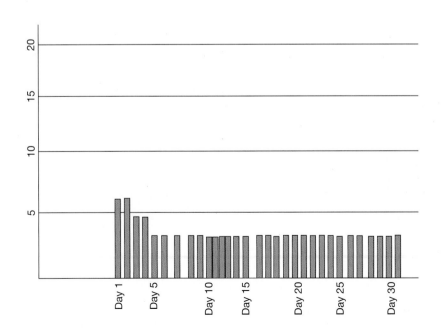

Question 1: **What is the next step?**

A. None
B. Uvuloplasty
C. Mouth guard
D. Tracheostomy
E. Eszopiclone

CASE 3

A 50-year-old man with history of atrial fibrillation and CHF complains of daytime sleepiness and fatigue. He has a polysomnograph and the results are below:

Question 1: **He did not tolerate CPAP. What would be the next best option for him?**

A. Adaptive servo ventilation
B. BPAP
C. Theophylline
D. Acetazolamide
E. Oxygen supplementation

CASE 4

A 41-year-old woman with a history of depression and anemia presents with increasing fatigue for the last 3 months. She has noticed that upon awakening in the morning she is now chronically unrefreshed. Once she gets ready for the day, fatigue tends to abate and she is able to function adequately. She clearly states that she experiences physical fatigue and not daytime sleepiness. After work she may rest in front of the television for a few minutes, but then finds that she cannot get comfortable. She will then get up and walk to the kitchen. She also experiences similar difficulty when going to bed.

* *

She admits to recent increased work-related stress. In response to increased depressive symptoms, her primary care physician placed her on Sertraline 50 mg daily.

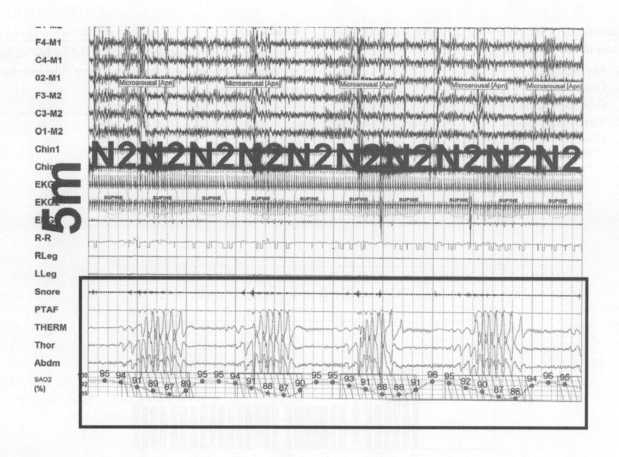

After a dose increase to Sertraline 100 mg daily, depression resolved but fatigue worsened.

* *

During screening for obstructive sleep apnea, she states that neither she nor her husband is aware of snoring, choking, gasping, or witnessed apneas. On examination, her BMI is 23 kg/m² and her neck circumference is 13.5 in. No mandibular abnormalities are noted. Tonsils and adenoids are not present; she has a history of surgical removal at age 5. Family history is negative for sleep apnea. Epworth sleepiness scale score is 5.

Question 1: **What further information would you want to elicit?**

A. Additional symptoms of sleep apnea
B. Symptoms of restless legs syndrome
C. Split night polysomnogram
D. Multiple sleep latency test (MSLT)
E. Maintenance of wakefulness test (MWT)

Question 2: **What factor(s) may have exacerbated the patient's condition?**

A. Worsening depression
B. Age of onset
C. Use of a serotonergic agent
D. B and C
E. Body habitus, including BMI, and neck circumference

Question 3: **What medication changes can be considered to help alleviate her symptoms?**

A. Discontinuation of Sertraline
B. Initiation of Bupropion
C. Initiation of Venlafaxine
D. A and B
E. A and C

Question 4: **What are some predisposing factors that are associated with this disorder?**

A. Iron deficiency
B. Chronic renal disease
C. Pregnancy
D. A and C
E. A, B, and C

CASE 5

A 55-year-old man with a history of obstructive sleep apnea currently treated with CPAP 10 cm H_2O, hyper-tension, obesity, and cardiovascular disease has been complaining of increased fatigue during the day. Subjective reporting and objective data confirm adherence to CPAP therapy. Cessation of snoring and witnessed apneas is present as long as he uses CPAP. A recent CPAP titration study confirmed that patient is on the optimal CPAP pressure setting: his Apnea Hypopnea Index (AHI) was 1/hour and supine REM sleep is recorded at the final pressure. His weight has been stable and he denies any changes to his medical history in the interim period since the study was completed. His epworth sleepiness scale score is 12, an improvement from the pre-CPAP score of 18.

Question 1: **What would be an appropriate treatment consideration in this patient?**

A. Split night polysomnogram
B. Initiation of methylphenidate
C. Initiation of Modafinil
D. A and C
E. A and B

Question 2: **On the CPAP titration study, it is noted that the patient's periodic limb movement index is 28/hour. Periodic limb movements (PLMS) are commonly seen in which of the following disorders?**

A. Obstructive sleep apnea (OSA)
B. Narcolepsy
C. REM sleep behavior disorder (RBD)
D. Delayed sleep–wake phase disorder
E. A, B, and C

CASE 6

A 19-year-old man with a history of anxiety presents with a 3-year history of escalating excessive daytime sleepiness (EDS). His symptoms has started in high school when he received repeated reprimands and after school detention for tardiness. He has experienced significant difficulty getting up in the morning to get to school on time. In screening for sleep disorders he mentions that when he tells jokes to his friends he occasionally experiences weakness in his face; he does not lose consciousness during these episodes. Otherwise he denies feeling like he is paralyzed or hearing/seeing things that are not actually present during the sleep–wake transition.

* *

On examination about 3 hours after his usual wake time he appears mildly sleepy and yawns repeatedly. His BMI is 21 kg/m^2 and his neck circumference is 16 in. His oropharynx is normal. His Epworth Sleepiness Scale score is 21/24. Family history is negative for OSA, but he does note that his father has been known to fall asleep at family gatherings very easily. The diagnostic polysomnogram is notable for AHI 2/hour of sleep, a total sleep time of 8 hours, and REM latency of 90 minutes.

Question 1: Assuming appropriate diagnostic studies were performed in the patient to help confirm the diagnosis, what changes might you expect if a lumbar puncture was performed?

A. Decreased hypocretin-1 level
B. Decreased glucose level and elevated cell count
C. Elevated glutamine level
D. Elevated lactate dehydrogenase level
E. Elevated chloride level

Question 2: Which of the following results is associated with this diagnosis?

A. Mean sleep latency of <11 minutes on multiple sleep latency test (MSLT)
B. Mean sleep latency of £8 minutes on MSLT
C. 3 sleep onset REM periods (SOREMPs) on MSLT
D. 1 SOREM on MSLT
E. B and C

Question 3: Which medication can be used to treat the episodes of facial weakness?

A. Venlafaxine
B. Methylphenidate
C. Carbamazepine
D. Modafinil
E. Bupropion

Question 4: This diagnosis has been associated with which of the following infectious agents?

A. *Pseudomonas*
B. *Staphylococcus*
C. H1N1
D. Adenovirus
E. *Escherichia*

CASE 7

A 25-year-old woman with no significant medical history presents with a complaint of difficulty falling and staying asleep, even as an infant. Due to poor sleep, she sometime reports fatigue during the day. She does not notice any change in her sleep quality when sleeping in a new environment nor does she deny any excessive anxiety around sleep.

* *

She estimates her total sleep time at 6 hours. A 2-week sleep diary and actigraphy confirms this sleep estimate.

* *

She has tried different medications, including Zolpidem, Trazodone, and most recently Clonazepam. She has tried to modify her lifestyle to exclude caffeine, nicotine, or alcohol as well as exercise or heavy meals close to bedtime. She does not watch television or use her computer or phone in the bedroom.

* *

On examination her BMI is 19 kg/m^2 and her neck circumference is 12.5 in. Her oropharynx is normal. Her Epworth Sleepiness Scale score is 5/24.

Question 1: What diagnosis best fits this patient?

A. Inadequate sleep hygiene
B. Idiopathic insomnia
C. Paradoxical insomnia
D. Psychophysiological insomnia
E. Behavioral insomnia of childhood, mixed type

Question 2: A previous polysomnograph has shown sleep spindles. What does this imply?

A. Decreased N3 sleep
B. Increased REM sleep
C. Decreased N2 sleep
D. Increased N1 sleep
E. Increased sleep fragmentation

Question 3: Which of the following findings has been associated with insomnia?

A. Decreased cortisol
B. Decreased brain metabolism
C. Hypocretin/orexin agonism
D. Increased norepinephrine
E. Increased sodium

CASE 8

A 75-year-old man with a history of hypertension presents with a 1-year history of difficulty falling asleep at night, worsening in the last 6 months. Previously he could fall asleep within 15 minutes of getting into bed and sleep until his usual morning wake time.

* *

He denies changes to his medical history or medication list. He denies symptoms suggestive of RLS, parasomnia, or hypersomnia. He does not have a bed partner that could confirm snoring, choking, or witnessed apneas. He states that he has been waking up earlier than he would like.

* *

On examination he is alert appearing slightly younger than his stated age. His BMI is 24 kg/m^2 and his neck circumference is 16 in. His oropharynx is unremarkable.

* *

A diagnostic polysomnogram is performed. No evidence of significant sleep apnea or other sleep disorder is found. He is noted to awaken around 4:30 AM after falling asleep at 8 PM. Sleep latency is abbreviated at 10 minutes. He states the bed time and wake time noted on the polysomnogram are consistent with his sleep schedule at home.

Question 1: Which disorder best describes the patient's presentation?

A. Delayed sleep–wake phase disorder
B. Irregular sleep–wake rhythm disorder
C. Non-24-hour sleep–wake rhythm disorder
D. Advanced sleep–wake phase disorder
E. B and C

Question 2: Which treatment options could be considered in this patient?

A. Zolpidem CR 12.5 mg at bed time, nightly
B. Diphenhydramine 50 mg at bed time, nightly
C. Chronotherapy in the evening, nightly
D. Clonazepam 1 mg at bedtime, nightly
E. Weight loss

Question 3: In elderly patients, what polysomnographic findings may be present?

A. Increased N1 sleep, decreased N3 sleep
B. Decreased N2 sleep, increased REM sleep
C. Increased N3 sleep, decreased REM sleep
D. Decreased sleep efficiency, no change in N1 sleep
E. B and D

CASE 9

A 57-year-old man is referred to you for observed behaviors during sleep. His wife has commented that he will punch and kick during sleep. She describes it as if he were fighting someone. On occasion this has caused her injury. He does not snore or have had witnessed apnea. On further review she remarks that he also talks and yells out partial sentences during his sleep. She has noted these episodes up to four times a week over the past 6 months. His wife has woken him up right after these episodes and he denies any awareness of the events. He appears oriented to place and time. There is no change in his personality, incontinence, daytime sleepiness, snoring, recurrent headaches, or head injury. There are no complaints of neurologic issues during waking hours. He denies marital discord. His past medical history is significant for hypertension and has been on lisinopril. His blood pressure has been under good control by review of his chart.

Question 1: These sleep observations are most likely explained by which of the following?

A. Temporal lobe seizure
B. REM sleep behavior disorder
C. Medication side effect
D. Psychiatric illness
E. Advance sleep phase disorder

Question 2: You have made your evaluation and made a clinical treatment plan that includes:

A. MRI of the brain followed by neurosurgical consultation
B. Use of clonazepam 30 minutes prior to bedtime
C. EEG followed by prophylactic treatment with phenytoin
D. Change his antihypertensive regimen to HCTZ
E. Use of zolpidem 5 mg at bedtime

CASE 10

A 45-year-old man with a history of obesity, hypertension, and dyslipidemia presents to clinic for continued fatigue. The patient recently switched jobs. He has been working as a mechanic during the day, but in the last 3 months has started to drive a truck for local deliveries. His work schedule has changed from 8 am to 6 pm 5 days a week to 11 pm to 7 am. While he enjoys the change in his work, he has found that he is now more sleepy. His Epworth Sleepiness Scale score is 15/24.

* *

On examination, his BMI is noted to be 35. Oropharynx showed Mallampati 4 with 2+ tonsillar tissue. A polysomnogram is ordered; results show severe obstructive sleep apnea with an Apnea-Hypopnea Index of 48. CPAP is initiated at 10-cm H2O per recommendation from polysomnogram.

* *

At first, the patient admits to difficulty using CPAP. He complains of air leaking from his mask, claustrophobia with mask, some skin breakdown over bridge of nose, as well as a severe dry mouth.

* *

After working with the patient to acclimate to CPAP therapy, documented adherence to CPAP is noted. The CPAP download shows resolution of breathing disturbances. Epworth Sleepiness Scale score showed improvement at 11/24.

* *

A maintenance of wakefulness test (MWT) is requested by his company before the patient continue driving.

Question 1: **Which of the following choices is true about the MWT?**

A. MWT is used to objectively measure daytime sleepiness.
B. MWT recording montage includes oronasal airflow and oxygen saturation recordings.
C. MWT is performed in an active, brightly lit environment to simulate daytime conditions.
D. MWT protocol follows three 20-minute trials.
E. MWT trials are concluded after 40 minutes of no sleep or after unequivocal sleep (three consecutive epochs of N1 or 1 epoch of any other sleep stage).

Question 2: **Which of the following options may be considered to aid in CPAP use?**

A. Heated humidifier use on CPAP
B. Proper mask fitting with possible change to different mask interfaces
C. Avoidance of overtightening mask
D. Desensitization protocol
E. All of the above

Question 3: **Given the patient's history of night time shift work with continued fatigue related to shift change, aside from general education about shift work disorder, what other treatment options can be considered?**

A. Light exposure on the commute home to aid in sleep quality

B. Scheduled nap prior to beginning of night shift to aid in alertness
C. Use of Melatonin prior to beginning of night shift
D. Use of Modafinil at end of night shift to aid in alertness on commute home
E. A and D

CASE 11

A 64-year-old woman is referred to the sleep clinic due to snoring. Her husband notes that her snoring was mild for many years and he hardly noticed it. He has observed that her snoring has worsened over the past 2 years. It is associated with a weight gain of 25 lb over this period. She denies history of sinus disease, allergic rhinitis or recurrent URIs. There is no witnessed apneas, although she does wake herself up snoring if she falls asleep sitting in a chair watching a movie at night. She typically wakes once a night secondary to nocturia. No history of parasomnias. She feels refreshed on awakening after 8 hours of sleep and has no daytime naps. The snoring has caused her husband to sleep in a different bedroom from his wife. Her past medical history is significant for Type 2 DM, well controlled with metformin 1,000 mg bid. The physical examination is significant for a BMI of 34.8. A home sleep study is interpreted as inconclusive and she was underwent an in lab PSG. That study reveals an AHI of 0.3/hour and RDI of 1/hour. No positional effect present on review of the data. No significant hypoxemia is noted. She wakes up from the study stating it was a typical night sleep. The sleep tech notes loud snoring throughout the night. She presents one week later to review the results.

Question 1: **After reviewing the data you suggest the following as first-line treatment:**

A. CPAP titration study
B. Referral for UPPP
C. Diet and exercise with the goal of weight loss
D. Referral to surgery for palatal implants
E. No intervention

CASE 12

A 27-year-old man presents for a PAP titration study. He has had a PSG 1 week earlier secondary to a history of witnessed apnea, loud snoring, and hypersomnia. He denies medical problems and is not on any medications. His examination is unremarkable except for a BMI of

38.6. The PSG shows moderate OSA. The overall AHI is 26.2/hour. All episodes are obstructive in etiology. The AHI during Stage R is 52/hour. After placement of appropriate leads the study is started at a CPAP of 4 cwp. Zolpidem 5 mg is provided prior to the study secondary to prolonged SOL of 55 minutes. During the course of the titration the obstructive events persists as the CPAP was increased up to 6 cwp. Noted on this study is the appearance of central apneic events that appeared at an increasing frequency during the course of the titration. These central events are noted in Stages N1, N2, N3, and R. The obstructive apneas/hypopneas are suppressed at a CPAP of 10 cwp but the central events persist and compromise more than 50% of sleep disordered breathing encountered on this study.

Question 1: The appearance of central sleep apnea on this titration study is indicative of:

A. Primary central sleep apnea not noted on the PSG
B. Complex sleep apnea related to introduction of CPAP

C. First night effect related to the sleep environment
D. Medication-related central events
E. None of the above

CASE 13

An 8-year-old boy wakes up from his sleep and runs to his parents complaining of dreams regarding monsters chasing him. He had a similar dream last week.

Question 1: What is his diagnosis?

A. Night terrors
B. Nightmares
C. Confusional arousals
D. Sleepwalking
E. None of the above

Answers

CASE 1

Question 1: A. Type I

There are four types of polysomnography. Type I is performed at a sleep laboratory with an attendant and at least seven physiologic markers being evaluated which includes: EEG, EOG, Chin, ECG, airflow, respiratory effort, and oxygen saturation. Type II is portable monitoring which includes the parameters of Type I. Type III is also a portable monitoring which is limited to sleep apnea. Type IV is also portable monitoring which measures only two markers such as oxygen saturation and flow.

**

Portable monitoring (PM) or out of center sleep testing (OCST) is recommended for (1) diagnosis of obstructive sleep apnea with a high pretest probability and no associated comorbidities or other sleep disorders; (2) evaluation of effectiveness of oral appliance or surgery for OSA; (3) and guide titration of CPAP and auto-titration.

**

Protocols include split night and daytime sleep studies. Split night studies diagnose OSA during the first half and titration of positive-airway pressure on the second half. It is recommended for: AHI >40 events per hour during >2 hours of sleep or positive-airway pressure titration >3 hours and elimination of obstructive events are noted with positive-airway pressure.

**

Daytime sleep studies are recommended for night workers.

Question 2: D. Stage N3

The PSG below depict the stages of sleep (Figs. 15–1 to 15–5).

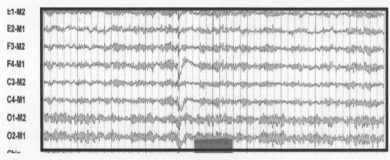

Figure 15–1   Stage Wake: Alpha waves, Beta 15–30 Hz.

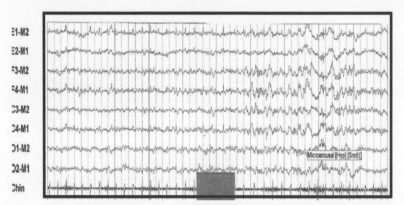

Figure 15–2   Stage N1: 5% of sleep cycle; Theta 4–8 Hz for 50% of epoch.

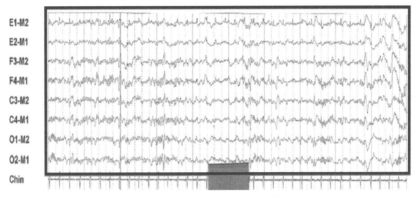

Figure 15–3   Stage N2: 45% of sleep cycle; Sleep Spindles and K Complexes.

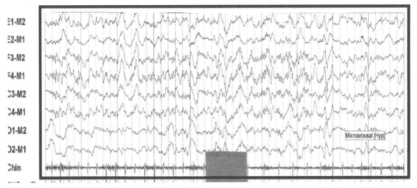

Figure 15–4   Stage N3: 25% of sleep cycle Delta 1–3 Hz.

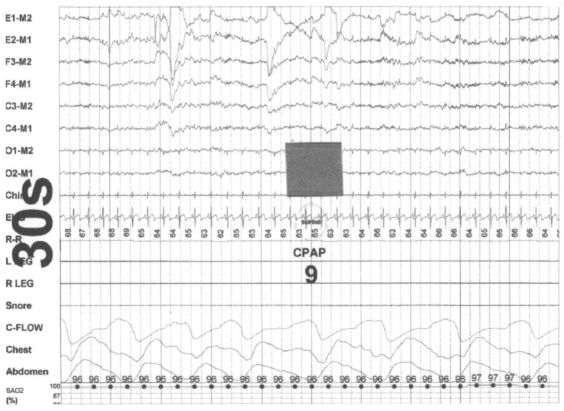

Figure 15–5   REM: 25% of sleep cycle. It consists of sharp, conjugate, irregular movements with the EOG (E1-M2 and E2-M1), muscle atonia, and EEG shows low voltage fast pattern reminiscent of awake stage.

Question 3: **B. Obstructive sleep apnea**

There are two types of sensors for respiratory events: oronasal thermal sensor (TFLOW or THERM) and nasal pressure transducer (PFLOW or PTAF). Apneas are measured via reduced TFLOW. Apnea is when there is reduced or cessation of flow to less than 10% of baseline for >10 seconds (Fig. 15–6). Hypopneas are reduced flow in PTAF, >30% from baseline for at least 10 seconds with a >4% desaturation while there is sustained or reduced flow in THERM (Fig. 15–7). Respiratory effort related arousals (RERA) are increased respiratory effort or flattening of nasal pressure for at least 10 seconds followed by arousal (Fig. 15–8). Obstructive pattern of apnea is noted when there is cessation of flow but ventilatory effort is present. Central pattern of apnea is when there is cessation of flow and ventilator effort. Mixed apnea usually involves central apnea followed by obstructive pattern apnea.

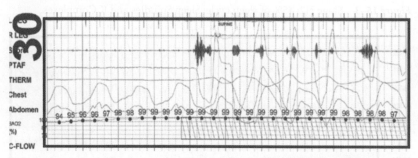

Figure 15–6   Apnea pattern: Notice the ventilatory effort (Chest and Abdomen) is maintained.

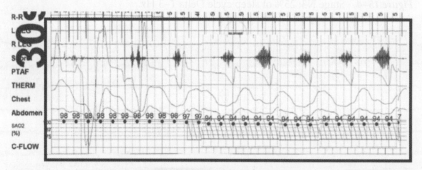

Figure 15–7   Hypopnea: Notice the reduced flow in PTAF >30% and 4% desaturation for at least 10 seconds.

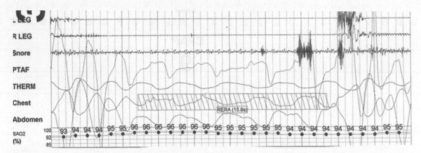

Figure 15–8   RERA: Notice flattening on nasal pressure followed by arousal.

**

Obstructive sleep apnea (OSA) secondary to recurrent collapse of pharyngeal airway and is diagnosed via two indexes: AHI (Apnea and hypopnea index) which is used by American Academy of Sleep Medicine and the RDI (respiratory disturbance index which measures apnea, hypopnea, and respiratory related arousals) which is used by Centers of Medicare and Medicaid Services.[1-3] OSA is diagnosed when there are >5 obstructive respiratory events (hypopneas, apneas, or RERA) per hour in PSG with symptoms.[1-3] These symptoms include daytime sleepiness, fatigue, arousals with choking sensation, snoring, breathing interruptions, and/or associated disease such as hypertension, coronary artery disease, atrial fibrillation, diabetes mellitus, mood disorder, and cognitive dysfunction. OSA can also be diagnosed if there are >15 obstructive respiratory events without symptoms and associated diseases.

**

There are three levels of severity: mild AHI 5–15 where sleep cycle is preserved and no cardiovascular complications, moderate AHI 15–30 where daytime sleepiness is more apparent, and severe AHI >30.

**

Central sleep apnea (CSA) is diagnosed when there are >5 central respiratory events for at least >50% of the total respiratory events, symptoms which include fatigue, snoring, witnessed apneas, and insomnia, absence of hypoventilation, and absence of other possible cause. Risk factor is age >65, men, CVA, and heart failure.[1,4] There are three subtypes. CSA with Cheyne–Stokes with >3 consecutive central hypopneas or apneas separated by 40 seconds of cresendo–decresendo pattern and is associated with atrial fibrillation, CHF, or neurologic disease (Fig. 15-9).[1,4] The other two subtypes include CSA secondary to high altitudes (>2,500 m) and CSA secondary to medications.[1,4]

**

Obesity hypoventilation syndrome (OHS) is found in patients with BMI >30 kg/m^2 and awake hypoventilation ($PaCO_2$ >45 mm Hg). Pulmonary hypertension is common and it is usually associated with OSA. Chest radiograph, sleep study, pulmonary function tests, and cardiac imaging are utilized to exclude other causes of symptoms or identify concommitant diseases.

CASE 2

Question 1: E. Eszopiclone

Nonadherence to positive-airway pressure therapy is defined by use £4 hours per night. Although mean use of positive-airway pressure therapy is >5 hours per night, the beneficial effects are generally seen >6 hours per night. Predictors of adherence include use within the first week, moderate to severe OSA with increased awareness of daytime sleepiness, desaturation, large nasal passages, CPAP titration with attended PSG, and motivated and optimistic.

**

Nonpharmacologic methods to help with adherence include patient's choice of mask and interface, chin strap, humidification, and behavioral therapy. Although a weak recommendation, the use of sedatives and hypnotics such as eszopiclone 3 mg have been shown to improve duration of use per night and the number of nights compared to placebo.[5-8]

**

Oral appliances are alternatives for mild to moderate OSA who have failed positive-airway pressure therapy. Surgery is generally deferred until a 3-month trial of oral appliances and positive-airway pressure therapy. Tracheostomy is preferred when everything else fails.

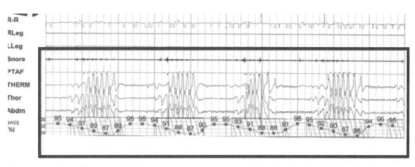

Figure 15-9   Cheyne–Stokes.

CASE 3

Question 1: A. Adaptive servo ventilation

The patient has central sleep apnea with Cheynne's stokes. Positive-airway pressure therapies for patients with CSA include: continuous positive-airway pressure (CPAP), adaptive servo-ventilation (ASV) and Bilevel positive-airway pressure (BPAP). The first modality preferred is CPAP which keeps the pharynx open and prevents the generation of higher negative pressures to initiate a breath. If that modality fails, ASV is preferred which has a variable amount of inspiratory pressure on a fixed level of CPAP with a backup respiratory rate. For patients that have failed both CPAP and ASV, BPAP with a backup rate is preferred, particularly in patients who have CSA with hyperventilation. BPAP is the first modality preferred if CSA is with hypoventilation. BPAP has two different pressures during inspiration and expiration and the tidal volume is the difference between the two pressures. Oxygen supplementation is an adjunct treatment for patients who are hypoxic during sleep. Pharmacologic interventions such as acetazolamide and theophylline are respiratory stimulants and used for patients who have failed positive-airway pressure therapies.

CASE 4

Question 1: B. Symptoms of restless legs syndrome

Restless leg syndrome (RLS) is a clinical diagnosis and may manifest as other symptoms, including insomnia and fatigue. Therefore, direct questioning about RLS is necessary to establish the diagnosis. Otherwise the diagnosis may be missed. In this case, fatigue may be secondary to sleep-onset insomnia from RLS as well as possible continued leg movements during sleep.

* *

The patient's description of discomfort when relaxing, that is sitting quietly, while watching TV and then again while trying to go to bed is suggestive of RLS. The temporal relationship of her symptoms, i.e. increased in the evening, is also consistent with the diagnosis. Finally her description of "walk(ing) to the kitchen" may indicate some relief of leg symptoms with movement.

* *

The cardinal features of RLS are:[9–10]

(1) An urge to move the legs, usually an uncomfortable sensation, which worsens with inactivity/lack of movement, improves with/during movement, and occurs primarily at night;
AND

(2) Symptoms are not solely due to another underlying condition such as neuropathy, arthritis, or myalgia;
AND

(3) Symptoms lead to distress or concern, sleep disturbance, and impairment of functioning.

* *

Her risk for sleep apnea based on clinical and physical presentation as well as lack of family history is low. While a sleep study can useful to look for underlying sleep apnea, OSA is less likely in her case. Polysomnogram may detect increased arousal from sleep and periodic limb movements. A MSLT is used to evaluate hypersomnia. Her Epworth Sleepiness Scale score is normal and she specifically denies daytime sleepiness. A MWT is used to objectively assess alertness; she reports normal functioning during the daytime.

Question 2: C. Use of a serotonergic agent

Certain medications can worsen RLS. Primary offending agents include serotonergic medications such as Sertraline, antihistamines, and dopamine receptor antagonists. The patient's depression actually improved with Sertraline. Fatigue and insomnia are therefore not likely to be secondary to worsening depression.

* *

The patient's age of onset, early 40s, places her in the early onset category (<age 45). Patients in this category may also have a family history of RLS. Progression of the disease is thought to be more gradual. In comparison, later age of onset is associated with more rapid progression and other associated disorders. The patient's body habitus is not an exacerbating factor for RLS.

Question 3: D. A and B

If concern for depression remains and antidepressant medication is required, cross-tapering of Sertraline and Bupropion could be considered. As a dopaminergic agent, Bupropion is one antidepressant that is thought to be "RLS-neutral," i.e., does not worsen RLS symptoms. Another treatment that could be considered if Sertraline was discontinued is psychotherapy.

* *

Venlafaxine is an SNRI (serotonin norepinephrine reuptake inhibitor) and can worsen RLS.

Question 4: E. A, B, and C

All patients with suspected RLS should be screened for iron deficiency by checking a ferritin level. If ferritin <50 µg/dL, iron supplementation should be considered. Symptoms of RLS may improve once the ferritin level is >50 mg/dL. A posited connection between low iron stores in the central nervous system and RLS may help to explain this symptomatic improvement. Iron is used in dopamine production. Therefore, supplementation of iron when necessary and use of dopaminergic agents such as Pramipexole and Ropinirole can alleviate symptoms.

CASE 5

Question 1: C. Initiation of Modafinil

Assuming the patient is optimized on CPAP treatment for OSA, reports that he believes he is doing well on CPAP, and has documented adherence to CPAP. Modafinil can be used to treat residual daytime sleepiness that has not responded to CPAP.[11] The other indications for Modafinil are excessive daytime sleepiness associated with either narcolepsy or shift work disorder.

* *

Methylphenidate is not recommended as a first-line treatment in a patient with pre-existing hypertension and cardiovascular disease as it could potentially exacerbate these underlying conditions.

* *

A polysomnogram is not indicated in a patient with a recent CPAP titration and lack of change to weight and medical history.

Question 2: E. A, B, and C

Periodic limb movements of sleep (PLMS) are repetitive movements of the extremities that can involve flexion of leg at the knee, ankle, or hip and extension of the big toe. Less commonly, the upper extremities may be involved as well. PLMS have been associated with RLS, untreated OSA, narcolepsy, and RBD.[12,13]

* *

Periodic limb movement disorder (PLMD) is an uncommon disorder in which the periodic limb movement index is >15/hour and PLMS causes a sleep disturbance, such as difficulty falling or staying asleep or unrefreshing sleep quality, and/or impairment in functioning. PLMD is not diagnosed in the setting of a concurrent sleep or medical disorder that could contribute to the presence of the leg movements, such as undertreated OSA, RLS, etc. If PLMS are present in a patient with RLS, the diagnosis would be RLS with notation given to the presence of PLMS rather than a diagnosis of PLMD.

* *

Delayed sleep–wake phase disorder, in which the patient's preference for a later bed and wake time is out of sync with the demands of his/her daily schedule, has not been linked to increased PLMs. Sleep–wake phase disorders are diagnosed based on history obtained during clinic visit. Use of actigraphy may provide objective information to correlate with sleep logs.

CASE 6

Question 1: A. Decreased hypocretin-1 level

Narcolepsy is a disorder characterized by repetitive episodes of daytime sleepiness that have occurred for at least 3 months, sleep paralysis (sensation of muscle paralysis during sleep–wake transition), hypnagogic or hypnopompic hallucinations (awareness of auditory, visual, or tactile sensations during wake–sleep or sleep–wake transition), and cataplexy (brief, bilateral loss of muscle tone with preserved consciousness).[14-16] Cataplexy is usually triggered by a strong emotion such as laughter. There is a usual bimodal distribution of narcolepsy onset: first peak in adolescence and second peak in mid-30s.

* *

Narcolepsy can be associated with a decreased level of hypocretin-1 or orexin level, decreased <110 pg/mL or <1/3 mean values for normal subjects.[14] A patient with a low level of hypocretin-1/orexin is now classified as Narcolepsy Type 1 regardless of whether cataplexy is present. The former nomenclature for these patients was Narcolepsy with Cataplexy. Therefore, his formal diagnosis would be Narcolepsy Type 1.

Question 2: E. B and C

To diagnose Narcolepsy Type 1, in addition to complaints of hypersomnia the patient must have an abnormal MSLT result (defined as mean sleep latency of ≤8 minutes and >2 sleep-onset REM periods) and/or low CSF hypocretin-1/orexin levels.[17] A change in the SOREMP definition now allows a REM latency <15 minutes on preceding diagnostic polysomnogram to count as a SOREMP on MSLT.

* *

The MLST should be preceded by a polysomnogram the previous night to ensure adequate total sleep time. If evidence of sleep apnea is found on the polysomnogram, sleep apnea should be adequately treated first in case breathing disturbances contribute to poor sleep quality. A sleep diary filled out in the weeks prior to the MSLT as well as a urine toxicology screen on the day of MSLT can also help to rule out insufficient sleep syndrome and hypersomnia secondary to substance effects respectively.

Question 3: A. Venlafaxine

The patient is likely describing cataplexy, a brief loss of muscle tone in the setting of strong emotion. Patients with cataplexy may benefit from REM-suppressing serotonergic agents such as Venlafaxine (75–150 mg in the morning) or Fluoxetine. In this patient, a serotonergic agent could be used to treat both cataplexy and underlying anxiety disorder.

* *

Of note, another medication to consider would be sodium oxybate. Sodium oxybate is considered to be a first-line medication in the in treatment of narcolepsy with cataplexy. It has been shown to help both with hypersomnia and disrupted sleep quality, a common complaint in narcoleptics.

* *

Methylphenidate and Modafinil can be used in narcoleptic patients to treat hypersomnia, but improvement in cataplexy would not be expected.

Question 4: C. H1N1

It is thought that narcolepsy may be related to an autoimmune process. A connection between H1N1 infection and H1N1 vaccination (as seen in an increased incidence of the diagnosis in 2010 following use of the vaccination in Europe) as triggers for narcolepsy has been posited.[16]

CASE 7

Question 1: B. Idiopathic insomnia

Insomnia is defined as difficulty falling asleep, staying asleep, and/or waking up too early at least three times per week. An additional symptom include fatigue, difficulty with concentration or memory, functional impairment, sleepiness, concern about sleep, accident proneness, and decreased motivation.[18–20] Short-Term Insomnia occurs for less than 3 months, while Chronic Insomnia is present for 3 months or more.

* *

Idiopathic Insomnia is associated with a lifelong onset and duration of insomnia symptoms. Symptoms tend to start in childhood and persist through the life span without significant remission.

* *

Inadequate sleep hygiene refers to daily practices that are not compatible with good sleep quality, such as use of substances like nicotine or caffeine close to bedtime, napping late in the day, and overtly stimulating activities or exercise close to bedtime. These suboptimal sleep practices were not observed in this patient.

* *

Paradoxical insomnia refers to a subjective description of insomnia that does not correlate with objective data. A patient may state that he/she sleeps only 3 hours, but objective testing, such as with polysomnogram or actigraphy, may indicate a total sleep time on the same night of 7 hours. In this patient, this mismatch between actual and perceived sleep times was not observed with actigraphy.

* *

Psychophysiological insomnia refers to conditioned arousal that makes good quality sleep difficult. Patients may excessively dwell on their poor sleep quality, and how lack of sleep may effect their physical and emotional well-being.

* *

Behavioral insomnia of childhood refers to difficulty with insomnia in children, specifically related to a need for a certain situation at sleep onset, such as being rocked to sleep, or lack of firm limits around bed time, such as allowing a child to delay bedtime.

Question 2: A. Decreased N3 sleep

The polysomnograph sample shows evidence of pseudo-spindles, likely related to use of the benzodiazepine clonazepam.

* *

Benzodiazepines, which work by nonselectively binding to inhibitory GABAA receptor subunits in the central nervous system, are known to suppress N3 (slow wave) sleep. N2 sleep can be increased.[21] During N2 sleep, the presence of pseudo-spindles may be noted. REM sleep may either remain unchanged or be decreased slightly.

Other noted effects of benzodiazepines include decreased sleep latency and decreased awakenings.

Question 3: D. Increased norepinephrine

Insomnia is thought to be a disorder of hyperarousal, both day and night.[18-20] Increased norepinephrine, cortisol and brain metabolism have been noted. Orexin/hypocretin is one the major neurotransmitters involved in wake-promotion; Suvorexant, an orexin receptor antagonist, has been approved to treat insomnia. Abnormal sodium levels have not been linked to insomnia.

CASE 8

Question 1: D. Advanced sleep–wake phase disorder

Circadian rhythm disorders refer to a group of disorders in which the timing of sleep is misaligned with the external environment.[22-24] In this case, the patient is most closely describing an advanced sleep–wake phase disorder. In this disorder, there is an advancement in the timing of sleep compared to the patient's desired sleep time. Therefore, a patient may complain of falling asleep and waking up earlier than he or she would prefer for at least 3 months. If allowed to sleep without external pressures from work, school, or other societal cues, the patient will naturally fall into an advanced pattern of sleep.

* *

A risk factor for this disorder is increased age.[23,24] While a clinical diagnosis, advanced sleep–wake phase disorder can be clarified by use of a sleep log in conjunction with actigraphy for a 2-week period; results could show an advanced sleep phase.

* *

Delayed sleep–wake phase disorder shows the opposite: a delay in the sleep period and a consequent delay in wake up time which is not aligned with the patient's preferred sleep/wake schedule. This disorder is more common in adolescents.

* *

Irregular sleep–wake rhythm disorder demonstrate a pattern of irregular sleep–wake schedules through a 24-hour period. Thus, they may present with a combination of both insomnia (during normal sleep period at night) and daytime sleepiness (during normal wake period during the day). This condition may be associated with neurodegenerative disorders such as dementia as well as in patients with developmental disorders.

* *

Non–24-hour-sleep–wake rhythm disorder refers to patients with insomnia, daytime sleepiness, or a combination that occurs because of misalignment to a normal 24-hour sleep–wake cycle. This disorder may be seen in blind patients who do not undergo proper entrainment to the sleep–wake cycle due to lack of photic stimulation.

Question 2: C. Chronotherapy in the evening, nightly

While therapy has not been standardized for advanced sleep–wake phase disorder, use of light therapy in the evening can be considered. In addition, timed use of melatonin could also prove beneficial.

* *

In an elderly patient, use of high dose Zolpidem CR, Diphenhydramine, and Clonazepam could lead to CNS depression and/or significant grogginess the next day that could impair daily activities. The patient's BMI falls within the normal range; therefore weight loss is not required.

Question 3: A. Increased N1 sleep, decreased N3 sleep

With aging, changes to sleep architecture can be noted, including a marked decline in N3 sleep (particularly when compared to young children) and an increase in N1 sleep. REM sleep may be stable in a healthy older adult or may decrease mildly. Additional changes to sleep may include decreased total sleep time, decreased sleep efficiency, and increased N2 sleep.

CASE 9

Question 1: B. REM sleep behavior disorder

REM sleep behavior disorder is characterized by dream-enacting activity.[25,26] REM sleep is normally accompanied by relative atonia of the peripheral muscles. A REM sleep disorder represents a lack of suppression of these movements. Patients may be unaware of the events and the history is often obtained from the bed partner. Historically it may present as laughing, talking, crying, running or fighting during sleep. PSG may reveal sustained muscle activity on chin EMG during REM sleep. >50% of REM sleep epochs will contain bursts of skeletal muscle activity. Partial seizures need to be considered in the differential diagnosis of parasomnias. Temporal lobe seizures typically present with daytime symptoms. Nocturnal symptoms of temporal lobe seizures may include automatisms such as lip smacking and chewing. Many medications can have an effect on sleep. Use of ACE inhibitors can be associated with both insomnia and nightmares.

* *

REM sleep behavior disorders affect 30% to 90% of patients with synucleopathies.[26] The physician should consider that a REM sleep behavior disorder may precede the clinical appearance of Parkinson's disease, Lewy body dementia, and multiple system atrophy by several years.[25]

Question 2: B. Use of clonazepam 30 minutes prior to bedtime

Use of clonazepam 0.5 to 2.0 mg use 30 minutes prior to bedtime has been shown to decrease REM sleep disorder frequency and severity.[27,28] Melatonin in doses of between 3 and 12 mg has been shown to be helpful in decreasing the number of epochs of Stage R sleep without atonia. There is no indication for MRI at this point. The lack of daytime symptoms does not rule out seizure disorder but empiric use of phenytoin is not indicated at this point.

CASE 10

Question 1: E. MWT trials are concluded after 40 minutes of no sleep or after unequivocal sleep (3 consecutive epochs of N1 or 1 epoch of any other sleep stage)

The maintenance of wakefulness test (MWT) is a study used to objectively measure the ability of a person to stay awake. The MWT may be useful in situations when a person's ability to keep awake may compromise safety, such as in the driving or piloting professions. In this case, the patient's continued sleepiness despite treatment of OSA in combination with his work as a truck driver do argue that a MWT may provide helpful information in the assessment of wakefulness.

* *

While there is no one MWT protocol that has been universally applied, American Academy of Sleep Medicine guidelines recommend that the test be performed as four 40-minute trials spaced apart at 2-hour intervals. The patient is asked to stay awake while seating in bed in a room not exposed to excess ambient light. Recording montage for the MWT includes central and occipital EEG derivations, right and left electrooculograms, chin electromyogram, and EKG. It is important that the patient have adequate sleep time and adequate sleep quality on the night prior to the MWT. A polysomno-

gram can be performed on the previous night per the ordering practitioner's discretion.

Question 2: E. All of the above

While changes in mask type and PAP pressures are not necessarily associated with improved PAP adherence, interventions to make the patient more comfortable with PAP are still commonly employed.

* *

To this effect, a proper mask fit with avoidance of overtightening (to avoid skin breakdown) can help with patient comfort. For dry mouth, heated humidifier use can be considered. For claustrophobia, change to nasal pillow interface and/or PAP desensitization protocol can be implemented.

Question 3: B. Scheduled nap prior to beginning of night shift to aid in alertness

Shift work disorder, defined as excessive daytime sleepiness and/or insomnia with decreased total sleep time for at least 3 months, can be treated in a variety of ways. In this case, the patient complained of sleepiness that started with a change to a night time work schedule. While sleepiness improved with CPAP initiation, some residual sleepiness was still present.

* *

In this case, scheduled naps prior to beginning of the night shift may be helpful with respect to alertness on the job. Use of melatonin on arrival home from the morning commute may aid in sleep quality. Use of sunglasses on the commute home to block excess light exposure may also help with sleep quality during the day. Modafinil can be considered for treatment of sleepiness associated with shift work disorder; it is usually used on awakening at night or at the beginning of the shift.

CASE 11

Question 1: C. Diet and exercise with the goal of weight loss

Snoring is one of the most common symptoms encountered in the sleep medicine clinic. It is a result of soft tissue vibration in the upper airway. In this instance a PSG was done as part of her assessment. No significant sleep disordered breathing was noted in a patient with minimal complaints. Options for treatment include weight loss, consideration for an oral appliance that would be fashioned by a dentist, surgical interventions including nasal, radio frequency ablation, UPPP and palatal implants. Surgical options often help with snoring however are not consistent in result. Without finding an obvious abnormality of the upper airway this should not be considered amongst first-line treatment. Use of an oral appliance offers a noninvasive option; it should be considered in patients with mild OSA (AHI 5–15/hour without evidence of significant hypoxemia) and in patients with primary snoring. In this patient's history however weight gain was specifically noted as occurring, and most likely leading, to the loud snore. Discussion of life style modification that would include exercise and dietary adjustments would be most appropriate and may lead to improvement in both the snoring and DM. Referral to a nutritionist could be considered if not previously done. Use of CPAP could be considered. It would resolve the snoring by working as a pneumatic splint. Most insurance companies would not cover this intervention however given the absence of OSA/UARS. The most appropriate intervention in this patient would be diet and exercise with follow up in the office in 3 months to assess progress and look for symptom improvement.

CASE 12

Question 1: B. Complex sleep apnea related to introduction of CPAP

The patient has moderate severity OSA based on his baseline PSG. All events were obstructive in etiology. The presence of central apneic events may occur with the introduction of CPAP. Complex sleep apnea refers to the presence of central apneic events that comprise more than 50% of the episodes of sleep disordered breathing during a titration for OSA. These central events may be transient and extinguish with CPAP. Interventions would include switching to other types of positive-airway pressure therapy such as adaptive servo-ventilation or biPAP or continuation of CPAP for another 2 to 3 months.

* *

In cases where there are significant central events interfering with oxygenation, a backup rate may be required. Medications can contribute to the appearance of central apneic events. Opiate analgesics classically can induce this phenomenon. It is not associated with the use of sedative hypnotics/benzodiazepines such as zolpidem. Auto PAP is a useful modality that should be considered in patients with OSA if an optimal treatment pressure

was not achieved and there is absence of complex sleep apnea. The use of acetazolamide – a carbonic anhydrase inhibitor – may lead to a shift in the $PaCO_2$ threshold to a lower value. It has the potential to offer some improvement in idiopathic central sleep apnea where hypersomnia is the predominant symptom presentation. There is a paucity of studies however evaluating its therapeutic benefit in central sleep apnea. It is not indicated for the treatment of complex sleep apnea.

CASE 13

Question 1: B. Nightmares

Parasomnias are involuntary movements or experiences that occur before, during, or after arousals from sleep. They occur predominantly in children and occur during NREM or REM stages. The NREM parasomnias generally occurring during N3 stage and include: confusional arousals, sleep terrors, and sleep walking. Confusional arousals generally occur in children <5 years of age and are characterized by 5- to 30-minute episode where the child will sit up from bed and appears to be distressed with no sweating, flushing of face, or stereotypic movement. The child has no recollection of the event. Sleep terrors occur between ages 4 and 12 years and patient is agitated and scream and may have sweating, flushing of face, and tachycardia. The child will have no recollection of the event. Sleep walking occurs between 8 and 12 years of age and the child might walk up to parents bedroom and will have autonomic dysfunction.

* *

Nightmares are REM parasomnias that generally occur during the early morning hours and are disturbing dreams that awaken the child. Body movements are rare since muscle activity is inhibited during REM sleep. Treatments for recurrent nightmares predominantly are behavioral techniques such as reassurance, rescripting, desensitization, hypnotherapy, and cognitive behavioral therapy.

REFERENCES

1. Michael S, ed. *International Classification of Sleep Disorders.* 3rd ed. Darien, IL: American Academy of Sleep Medicine; 2014.
2. Strohl KP, Brown DB, Collop N, et al; ATS Ad Hoc Committee on Sleep Apnea, Sleepiness, and Driving Risk in Noncommercial Drivers. An Official American Thoracic Society Clinical Practice Guideline: Sleep apnea, sleepiness, and driving risk in noncommercial drivers. An

update of a 1994 statement. *Am J Respir Crit Care Med.* 2013;187(11):1259–1266.

3. Hiestand D, Philips B. Obstructive sleep apnea syndrome: Assessing and managing risk in motor vehicle operators. *Curr Opin Pulm Med.* 2011;17(6):412–418.

4. Garcia-Touchard A, Somers VK, Olson LJ, et al. Central sleep apnea: Implications for congestive heart failure. *Chest.* 2008;133:1495–1504.

5. Lettieri CJ, Collen JF, Eliasson AH, et al. Sedative use during continuous positive airway pressure titration improves subsequent compliance: A randomized, double-blinded, placebo-controlled trial. *Chest.* 2009;136(5):1263–1268.

6. Park JG, Olsen EJ, Morgenthaler TL. Impact of zaleplon on continuous positive airway pressure therapy compliance. *J Clin Sleep Med.* 2013;9(5):439–444.

7. Bradshaw DA, Ruff GA, Murphy DP. An oral hypnotic medication does not improve continuous positive airway pressure compliance in men with obstructive sleep apnea. *Chest.* 2006;130(5):1369–1376.

8. Lettieri CJ, Shah AA, Holley AB, et al. CPAP promotion and prognosis--The Army Sleep Apnea Program Trial. *Ann Intern Med.* 2009;151(10)L696.

9. Hubner A, Krafft A, Gadient S, et al. Characteristics and determinants of restless legs syndrome in pregnancy: A prospective study. *Neurology.* 2013;80(8):738–742.

10. Gigli GL, Adorati M, Dolso P, et al. Restless legs syndrome in end-stage renal disease. *Sleep Med.* 2004;5(3):309–315.

11. Schwartz JR, Hirshkowitz M, Erman MK, et al. Modafinil as adjunct therapy for daytime sleepiness in obstructive sleep apnea: A 12 week, open-label study. *Chest.* 2003;124(6):2192–2199.

12. Hening W, Allen R, Earley C, et al. The treatment of restless legs syndrome and periodic limb movement disorder. An American Academy of Sleep Medicine Review. *Sleep.* 1999;22(7):970–999.

13. Aurora RN, Kristo DA, Bista SR, et al. Practice parameters for the treatment of restless legs syndrome and periodic limb movement disorder in adults–An update for 2012. *Sleep.* 2012;35(8):1039–1062.

14. Andlauer O, Moore H, Jouhier L, et al. Nocturnal rapid eye movement latency for identifying patients with narcolepsy/hypocretin deficiency. *JAMA Neurol.* 2013;70(7):891–902.

15. Guilleminault C, Tao, MT . Narcolepsy: Diagnosis and management. In: Kryger, Meir H., et al. *Principles and Practice of Sleep Medicine.* 5th ed. St. Louis, MO: Elsevier; 2011:957–968.

16. Partinen M, Kornum BR, Plazzi G, et al. Narcolepsy as an autoimmune disease: The role of H1N1 infection and vaccination. *Lancet Neurol.* 2014;13(6):600–613.

17. Littner MR, Kushida C, Wise M, et al; Standards of Practice Committee of the American Academy of Sleep Medicine. Practice parameters for the clinical use of the multiple sleep latency test and the maintenance of wakefulness test. *Sleep.* 2005;28:113–121.

18. McClure T, Drake C, Roth T, et al. Sleep and endocrine responses to psychological stress in primary insomnia. *Sleep.* 2003;26:A311.

19. Herring WJ, Snyder E, Budd K, et al. Orexin receptor antagonism for the treatment of insomnia: A randomized clinical trial of suvorexant. *Neurology.* 2012;79(23):2265–2274.

20. Nofzinger EA, Buysse DJ, Germain A, et al. Functional neuroimaging evidence for hyperarousal of insomnia. *Am J Psychiatry.* 2004; 161(11):2126–2128.

21. Nowell PD, Mzaumdar S, Buysse DJ, et al. Benzodiazepines and zolpidem for chronic insomnia: A meta-analysis of treatment efficacy. *JAMA.* 1997;278(24):2170–2177.

22. Morganthaler TI, Lee-Chiong T, Alessi C, et al. Practice parameters for the clinical evaluation and treatment of circadian rhythm sleep disorders. *Sleep.* 2007;30(11):1445–1459.

23. Floyd JA, Janisse JJ, Jenuwine ES, et al. Change in REM-sleep percentage over the adult lifespan. *Sleep.* 2007;30(7):829–836.

24. Moraes W, Piovezan R, Poyares D, et al. Effects of aging on sleep structure throughout adulthood: A population-based study. *Sleep Med.* 2014;15(4):401–409.

25. Plazzi G, Corsini R, Provia F, et al. REM sleep behavior disorders in multiple system atrophy. *Neurology.* 1997;48:1094–1097.

26. Boeve B, Siber MH, Ferman TJ, et al. Association of REM sleep behavior disorder and neurodegenerative disease may reflect an underlying synucleopathy. *Mov Disord.* 2001;16:622–630.

27. Roux FJ, Kryger MH. Medication effects on sleep. *Clin Chest Med.* 2010;31:397–405.

28. Seda G, Tsai S, Lee-Chiong T. Medication effects on sleep and breathing. *Clin Chest Med.* 2014;35(3):557–569.

16

Interventional Pulmonology

Amit Mahajan MD and Adnan Majid MD

CASE 1

A 73-year-old woman presents with persistent cough and weight loss. She describes the cough as productive of yellow sputum for as long as she can remember, but recently she has noted occasional streaks of blood in her sputum. Her appetite has been poor recently, and she has had an unintentional weight loss of 15 lb over the past 4 months. Her past medical history includes chronic obstructive pulmonary disease (COPD), diabetes, HTN, and CHF. She has a 50 pack-year smoking history, and she does not describe any occupational exposures.

* *

Her primary care physician orders a chest x-ray that reveals a right-sided lung nodule. A follow-up CT scan of the chest shows a right-lower lobe, spiculated lung nodule along with enlarged subcarinal and station 11 L lymph nodes. The patient's primary care provider is concerned that the speculated nodule is malignant. A whole body PET scan is performed that shows the right-sided nodule and the subcarinal lymph node to be FDG-avid with only mild FDG-avidity of the 11 L lymph node.

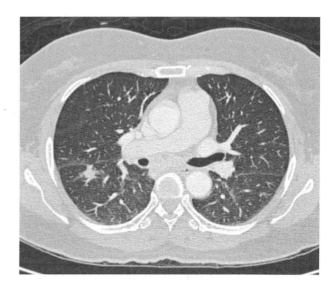

Question 1: **What is the appropriate next step in diagnosis?**

A. Surgical resection of the nodule
B. Convex probe endobronchial ultrasound (CP-EBUS) bronchoscopy with transbronchial needle aspiration of the mediastinal, hilar, and interlobar lymph nodes
C. CT-guided needle biopsy of the lung nodule
D. Flexible bronchoscopy with transbronchial biopsies
E. Mediastinoscopy

Question 2: **The patient undergoes flexible bronchoscopy and CP-EBUS bronchoscopy for diagnosis and staging. Which abnormality should be sampled first?**

A. Right lower lobe nodule
B. Subcarinal lymph node
C. Right hilar lymph node

D. Left hilar lymph node

E. Left interlobar lymph node

Question 3: **Which of the following lymph node stations is not accessible by CP-EBUS TBNA?**

A. 2R

B. 4L

C. 7

D. 8

E. 11R

Question 4: **Cytology results from the patients CP-EBUS bronchoscopy reveal the presence of malignant cells in the subcarinal node. What stage could classify this patient according to the TNM staging system?**

A. Stage I

B. Stage II

C. Stage IIIa

D. Stage IIIb

E. Stage IV

CASE 2

A 66-year-old man with an extensive smoking history is referred to a pulmonologist for an abnormal chest x-ray which reveals complete atelectasis of the right lung. A bronchoscopy is performed and an image of the findings is featured below. The patient is referred to interventional pulmonology for further treatment options. The patient endorses progressive shortness of breath and a new cough over the past few months. He does not report chest pain, fevers, chills, or weight loss. His past medical history includes COPD on 4 L of home oxygen, DM, and HTN. His physical exam is normal except for decreased breath sounds over the right chest and a slight right-sided expiratory wheeze.

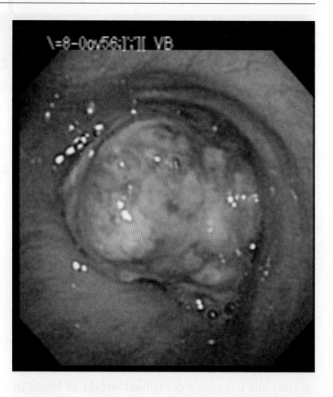

Question 1: **What type of lung cancer is most commonly associated with endobronchial involvement?**

A. Squamous cell carcinoma

B. Adenocarcinoma

C. Small cell lung cancer

D. Large cell cancer

E. Mucoepidermoid carcinoma

Question 2: **What percentage of patients with lung cancer will develop complications associated with airway obstruction?**

A. 0–10%

B. 20–30%

C. 40–50%

D. 60–70%

E. 90–100%

Question 3: **Which of the following bronchoscopic interventions is contraindicated in the management of this patient?**

A. ND-YAG laser

B. Cryodebridement

C. Brachytherapy

D. Endobronchial electrocautery

E. Airway stenting

Question 4: Which of the following comorbidities would preclude the patient from undergoing rigid bronchoscopy?

A. Obesity

B. Vocal cord paralysis

C. Thrombocytopenia (platelet count 50,000)

D. Rheumatoid arthritis with involvement of the cervical vertebral bodies

E. Micrognathia

CASE 3

A 61-year-old female cross-country runner presents to the emergency room with progressive dyspnea on exertion and orthopnea. She endorses right upper quadrant pain, fatigue, and malaise 3 weeks prior to admission along with low-grade fevers. She also endorses a 10-lb weight loss over the past 3 months. A right upper quadrant ultrasound shows a normal liver and gall bladder, but a moderate right pleural effusion is noted. A chest x-ray is performed which confirms the presence of the moderate right pleural effusion. The patient's past medical history includes rheumatoid arthritis for which she is currently being treated with Infliximab and prednisone. The patient has emigrated from Cape Verde 7 years prior. A recent PPD prior to starting biologic therapy was negative. Based on the patient's presentation, a chest tube is placed with drainage of the fluid and the fluid is sent for analysis.

* *

Fluid Analysis: pH – 7.46

WBC – 4325

RBC – 6525

Neutrophils – 6%

Lymphocytes – 79%

Mesothelial cells – 3%

Total protein – 6.0 g/dL

Glucose – 122

LDH – 298

Cholesterol – 91

Albumin – 3.1

Triglycerides – 50

Gram stain – Negative

Cultures – Pending

Cytology – Negative for malignancy

Question 1: Which best describes the pleural fluid analysis?

A. Transudative with lymphocyte predominance

B. Bacterial empyema

C. Chylothorax

D. Exudative with lymphocyte predominance

E. Pseudo-chylothorax

Question 2: What is the appropriate next diagnostic step for this patient?

A. Repeat thoracentesis

B. Await culture results

C. Closed Abram's needle biopsy

D. Induced sputum with AFB cultures

E. None of the above

Question 3: Which of the following is the most likely diagnosis in this patient?

A. *S. Pneumoniae* empyema

B. Extrapulmonary tuberculosis

C. Malignant pleural effusion

D. Chylothorax

E. Pseudo-chylothorax

Question 4: Which of the following pleural fluid studies has high sensitivity for pleural tuberculosis?

A. Fluid beta natriuretic peptide

B. Fluid galactomannan

C. Fluid adenosine deaminase

D. Fluid triglycerides

E. Fluid cholesterol-triglyceride ratio

CASE 4

A 59-year-old man presents with a nonresolving cough following a viral illness. He states that the cough has been persistent for 3 months and is nonproductive until this past week when he coughs up a small amount of bright red blood. The patient is a lifetime nonsmoker without any occupational exposures. He states that he ran a 5-km race 2 weeks ago without any difficulty. The hemoptysis has prompted his doctor to order a CT scan of the chest, which reveals a spiculated, left upper lobe mass continuous with the major fissure with enlarged left hilar and subcarinal lymph nodes. The patient has had bronchoscopy with endobronchial ultrasound (EBUS) and is diagnosed with adenocarcinoma of the lung. Eight weeks later, the patient presents to the interventional pulmonary clinic with shortness of breath. A chest x-ray revealed a large left-sided pleural effusion. The patient has had diagnostic and therapeutic thoracentesis with removal of 1 L of serosanguinous fluid. Pleural manometry performed during the thoracentesis reveals a change in pleural pressure of 30 mm Hg and the postprocedure chest x-ray does not reveal full re-expansion of the lung. He states that his shortness of breath significantly has improved following drainage. Cytology from the pleural fluid reveals presence of malignant cells.

Question 1: What is the diagnostic yield for an initial thoracentesis for malignant pleural cells?

A. 100%
B. 80%
C. 55%
D. 25%
E. 5%

Question 2: The presence of a malignant pleural effusion would classify the patient as what TNM stage?

A. Stage Ia
B. Stage IIa
C. Stage IIIa
D. Stage IIIb
E. Stage IV

Question 3: Which of the following interventions would be the best treatment option of this patient's malignant pleural effusion?

A. Serial thoracenteses
B. Starting the patients on a low dose diuretic
C. Referral to hospice
D. Tunneled pleural catheter placement
E. Talc pleurodesis

Question 4: Which of the following mechanisms is responsible for this improvement in the patient's dyspnea?

A. Improvement in V/Q mismatch
B. Improvement in alveolar hypoventilation
C. Improvement in diffusion capacity
D. Improvement in chest wall and diaphragm mechanics
E. Improvement in alveolar oxygenation

Question 5: The patient's tunneled pleural catheter is draining less than 50 mL after three consecutive drainages. Which of the following interventions is NOT indicated?

A. Chest x-ray
B. Instillation of t-PA/DNAse into the catheter
C. Flushing the catheter with sterile saline
D. Chest ultrasound
E. None of the above

CASE 5

A 49-year-old man with a history of hypertension, peptic ulcer disease, emphysema, atrial fibrillation, and recurrent left lower lobe pneumonia presented with fevers, chills, night sweats, and a cough productive of green sputum. He endorsed some blood-tinged sputum the day prior to presentation. A CT scan was performed that was concerning for an endobronchial lesion in the distal left mainstem bronchus. The patient was on Coumadin 5 mg for history of atrial fibrillation and has an INR of 2.3. Later that afternoon, the patient had a coughing fit and then began coughing up copious amounts of bright red blood. The patient became tachycardic and had a drop in oxygen saturations to 80% on room air and increased respiratory distress. A portable chest x-ray was performed revealing increased haziness of the left lung. He continued to cough up approximately 200 mL of bright red blood with increased shortness of breath.

Question 1: What is the next appropriate intervention for this patient?

A. Repeat CT scan of the chest
B. Turning the patient onto his right side followed by transfer to the ICU
C. Emergent intubation with preferential advancement of the endotracheal tube into the right mainstem bronchus
D. Bilevel positive pressure ventilation
E. Increase FiO$_2$ and cough suppression with IV codeine

Question 2: The patient is deemed unstable and bright red blood continues to be suctioned from the endotracheal tube. Flexible bronchoscopy is performed at bedside with the presence of clotted blood obstructing the distal trachea. The clot is unable to be cleared with flexible suction. What is the next step in care?

A. Rigid bronchoscopy with aspiration of clot and possible electrocautery to the airway lesion
B. Continue supportive care with adjustment of ventilator settings
C. Plan for repeat flexible bronchoscopy through the endotracheal tube the following day
D. Allow INR to trend down to sub-therapeutic ranges followed by repeat flexible bronchoscopy
E. Allow INR to trend down to sub-therapeutic range followed by rigid bronchoscopy and possible electrocautery to airway lesion

CASE 6

A 77-year-old woman with severe aortic regurgitation, diabetes, and hypertension presents to the emergency department with progressive dyspnea on exertion. The patient endorses neck fullness along with difficulty swallowing over the past 3 weeks. She is using accessory muscles and complains of difficulty taking in air. Harsh stridor is heard during physical examination. She quickly deteriorates requiring intubation. The anesthesiologist has difficulty passing a 7-mm endotracheal tube due to resistance past the vocal cords and is only able to pass a 6-mm endotracheal tube. CT scan of the chest is seen above. Over the next several days, the patient is awake and alert, but continuously fails spontaneous breathing trials due to increased work of breathing. After 3 weeks of intubation, the ear, nose, and throat service is consulted and considers surgery, but is concerned about the patient's inability to be weaned from the ventilator.

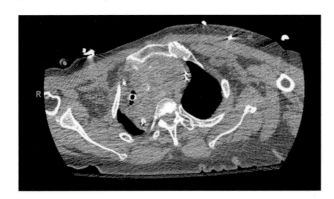

Question 1: **What is the most effective therapeutic option for improving the patient's chances for liberation from the ventilator?**

A. Increase level of positive end-expiratory pressure during spontaneous breathing trial
B. Laying the patient on her left side during spontaneous breathing trial
C. Tracheal stent placement prior to spontaneous breathing trial
D. Tracheostomy placement
E. Surgical resection of the goiter

CASE 7

A 48-year-old man with a history of emphysema and coronary artery disease presents to the emergency room with new onset chest pain and shortness of breath. Chest x-ray reveals a left-sided pneumothorax and oxygen saturation in the mid-70s with right-sided tracheal shift.

An electrocardiogram reveals ST-segment depressions. A chest tube is emergently placed with re-expansion of the left lung and resolution of ST-segment depressions. A large air leak is noted on tidal inspiration and exhalation. Extensive subcutaneous emphysema develops over the next 6 hours. The patient remains hospitalized requiring suction to prevent recurrence of lung collapse for 2 weeks without improvement in the air leak.

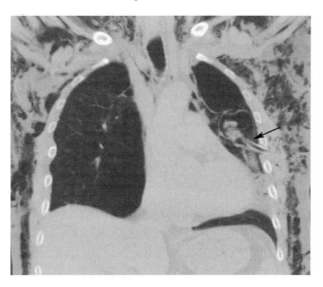

Question 1: **What therapeutic intervention is appropriate for the treatment of the patient's alveolopleural fistula?**

A. Video assisted thoracoscopic surgery (VATS) with muscle flap
B. Open surgical muscle flap
C. Intrabronchial valve placement
D. Observation on wall suction
E. Discharge with heimlich valve

Question 2: **How many weeks are recommended for intrabronchial valves to remain within the airways following successful resolution of a persistent air leak?**

A. 2 weeks
B. 4 weeks
C. 6 weeks
D. 8 weeks
E. 10 weeks

CASE 8

A 74-year-old man with a history of stroke presents with fevers, shortness of breath, and right-sided chest pain. A chest x-ray reveals complete white out of the right lung and shift of the trachea to the right. The patient's wife states that while taking his morning potassium pill yesterday, he began coughing incessantly and has been feeling unwell since. He is hemodynamically stable and his oxygen saturation is 93% on 2 L nasal cannula.

Question 1: **Which therapeutic approach should be utilized for the treatment of the patient's underlying medical problem?**

A. Flexible bronchoscopy
B. Rigid bronchoscopy
C. Whole lung lavage
D. Chest percussion
E. 7% saline nebulization

CASE 9

A 67-year-old male with a history of heavy smoking, severe COPD on home oxygen, coronary artery disease, hypertension, diabetes, and renal insufficiency was incidentally found to have a left lower lobe spiculated lung nodule an a screening low dose chest CT scan. He endorsed daily cough, and dyspnea on exertion class III, but denies weight loss. A PET scan revealed FDG avid nodule (SUV 7.0).

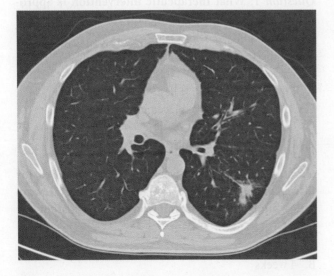

Question 1: **If the nodule represents cancer, which of the following bronchoscopic approaches will provide the best chance for both diagnosis and staging for the patient?**

A. Flexible bronchoscopy with fluoroscopy-guided transbronchial biopsy(TBBX), brush, and transbronchial needle aspirate (TBNA)
B. Linear EBUS-TBNA
C. Flexible bronchoscopy with radial EBUS-guided transbronchial biopsy(TBBX), brush and transbronchial needle aspirate (TBNA)
D. Navigation bronchoscopy–guided transbronchial biopsy(TBBX), brush and transbronchial needle aspirate (TBNA)
E. Linear EBUS-TBNA, navigation bronchoscopy and radial EBUS-guided transbronchial biopsy (TBBX), brush and transbronchial needle aspirate (TBNA)

Question 2: **Compared to CT-guided needle biopsy, navigation bronchoscopy has a lower incidence of which of the following?**

A. Alveolar hemorrhage
B. Respiratory failure
C. Pneumonia
D. Pneumothorax
E. Post-procedural stridor

Answers

CASE 1

Question 1: B. Convex probe endobronchial ultrasound (CP-EBUS) bronchoscopy with transbronchial needle aspiration of the mediastinal, hilar, and interlobar lymph nodes

As the incidence of lung cancer continues to increase, the ability to diagnose and stage malignancy remains a pillar of effective therapy. Convex probe endobronchial ultrasound (CP-EBUS) bronchoscopy is a relatively new procedure that provides real-time ultrasound imaging of airway walls, blood vessels, and lymph nodes in the thoracic cavity. This technology is considered minimally invasive and is currently utilized for staging and diagnosing lung cancer. According to the *Diagnosis and Management of Lung Cancer, 3rd ed. American College of Chest Physicians Evidence-Based Clinical Practice Guidelines* patients with high suspicion of N2,3 involvement, either by discrete mediastinal lymph node enlargement or PET uptake (and no distant metastases), a needle technique (convex probe endobronchial ultrasound [CP-EBUS]-needle aspiration, EUS-NA or combined EBUS/EUS-NA) is recommended over surgical staging as a best first test (Grade 1B).[1]

* *

Choice A is incorrect because the stage of the cancer has not been determined based on advanced imaging modalities. ACCP guidelines recommend surgery only in clinical stage I or II nonsmall cell lung cancer (NSCLC) with no medical contraindications (Grade 1B).[1] Choice C, CT-guided needle biopsy of the lung nodule, does not provide information regarding the stage of the cancer. Choice D is incorrect, since this procedure has a low yield for the diagnosis of lung cancer, with lesions </ = 2 cm had a diagnostic yield of 14% when located in the peripheral third versus 31% when located in the inner two thirds of the lung.[2] In addition, it does not provide information regarding the stage of the cancer. ACCP guidelines recommend performing mediastinoscopy in patients with suspected lung cancer if the pretest probability of malignancy is high and minimally invasive testing (EBUS-TBNA or EUS-NA) are deemed nondiagnostic or negative.[1]

Question 2: E. Left interlobar lymph node
Station 11 L corresponds to the interlobar lymph nodes. Staging of the mediastinum in patients with lung cancer requires a methodical and disciplined approach. While the largest and most easily accessible lymph nodes may be closest to a suspicion primary lesion, determining the appropriate stage of the patient allows clinicians to adequately determine if a tumor is resectable. When appropriately staging the mediastinum, EBUS-TBNA should start with the N3 nodal station followed by N2 followed by N1 depending on size and accessibility.[3,4] This avoids upstaging patients and allows for appropriate management based on degree of metastasis. In settings where rapid on site cytology examination (ROSE) is available, positive sampling an N3 node may justify completion of CP-EBUS-TBNA. Yet, in patients with suspected or confirmed NSCLC, further specimen collection may be necessary to test for specific molecular markers.

Question 3: D. 8
Anatomic mapping of the mediastinum provides guidance as to which nodal stations are accessible by various sampling modalities. Sampling of stations 1, 2, 4, 7, 10, 11, and 12 can be reliably sampled with endobronchial ultrasound–guided transbronchial needle aspiration (EBUS-TBNA). Stations 4, 5, 7, 8, and 9 can be reliably sampled by esophageal endoscopic ultrasound-guided fine-needle aspiration (EUS) with a sensitivity of 84% and a specificity of 99.5%.[4,5]

Question 4: C. Stage IIIa
Lung cancer mortality is high since it is often detected after development of late stage disease and stage at diagnosis is a strong predictor of lung cancer mortality. The majority (67.6%) of patients diagnosed with lung cancer between 2003 and 2006 present at stage III or stage IV.[6]

This patient would be characterized as stage IIIa according to the seventh TNM staging system due to involvement on the mediastinal lymph nodes without spread to the contralateral lymph nodes (stage IIIb).[7]

CASE 2

Question 1: **A. Squamous cell carcinoma**

The most common cause of central airway obstruction is due to direct extension into the airway lumen by extrinsic tumors, most commonly bronchogenic carcinomas. Squamous cell carcinomas or adenoid cystic carcinomas make up 70% to 80% central airway obstructions.[8] Unlike adenoid cystic carcinomas, squamous cell carcinomas occur typically later in older men with a history of smoking. Symptoms of malignant airway obstructions depend on size and location. Late findings associated with central airway obstructions include dyspnea, cough, wheezing, and stridor. In addition, post obstructive pneumonia may be present. While small cell carcinoma and adenocarcinoma may cause extrinsic airway obstruction, they are rarely derived from the endobronchial lining and do not typically invade the large airways.

Question 2: **B. 20–30%**

Various types of central airway obstructions may stem from both malignant and nonmalignant processes. The most common cause of malignant central airway obstruction is direct extension from an adjacent tumor, most commonly bronchogenic carcinoma. Esophageal carcinoma and thyroid carcinoma are also commonly associated with malignant airway obstruction. An estimated 20% to 30% of patients with lung cancer will develop complications associated with airway obstruction (atelectasis, pneumonia, dyspnea, etc.).[9,10] In addition, up to 40% of lung cancer deaths may be attributed to locoregional disease. Complications such as distal airway collapse or pneumonia may be insidious in progression or may develop suddenly when a critical airway diameter is reached. Dyspnea on exertion is typically present when the trachea is narrowed to less than 8 mm and symptoms at rest may be present when the trachea is narrowed to less than 5 mm. Benign central airway obstructions continue to be more commonly recognized with the increased use of artificial airways and an aging population.

Question 3: **C. Brachytherapy**

The evaluation and treatment of central airway obstruction requires understanding of airway anatomy and careful planning. Bronchoscopy, preferably rigid bronchoscopy, is necessary to assess the extent of obstruction and to determine intraluminal or extraluminal involvement.[8,11,12] While flexible bronchoscopy can be used to assess airway obstruction, this modality may be dangerous as it allows for further obstruction of the remaining lumen and securing the airway may be difficult. In addition, the use of conscious sedation may also pose danger as respiratory muscles may relax and ventilation may be depressed. Rigid bronchoscopy allows the airway to be secured in addition to controlling of oxygenation and ventilation. Various instruments can be safely passed through the rigid bronchoscope, making debridement more expeditious and effective. Silicone stent placement generally requires rigid bronchoscopy and if excessive bleeding occurs, the barrel of the rigid bronchoscope can be used to tamponade bleeding. Finally, the rigid bronchoscope itself can be used to core out lesions in the trachea and proximal mainstem bronchi. Cryodebridment relies on utilizing extreme cold temperature (below −40°C). The cryotherapy probe is used to make direct contact and freeze obstructing tissue. During the freezing process, the probe is withdrawn pulling the obstructing tissue from the lumen in large chunks. Maximal cellular damage can result from the rapid cooling and slow thawing of tissues. Freezing tissue results in the formation of intracellular ice crystals and cell death. In addition, vasoconstriction of arterioles and venules helps reduce bleeding and activate clotting. Cryodebridement is a safe modality without risk of perforation or residual stenosis. Importantly, no FiO_2 ceiling is required for the use of cryodebridement, unlike hot therapies like electrocautery, argon-plasma coagulation, and laser. Balloon bronchoplasty is an integral part of the treatment of central airway obstruction. Balloon dilation is used to improve the lumen size in symptomatic airway stenosis. Various balloons can be used for balloon dilation including the compliant Fogarty balloon or the controlled radial expansion balloon, which is more rigid and is commonly used for tight areas of stenosis. Balloon bronchoplasty results in less trauma than rigid-barrel dilation and is immediately effective in intrinsic and extrinsic compression. Complications of balloon bronchoplasty are rare, but include airway rupture, pneumothorax, and bleeding. Airway stenting is a therapeutic option that has gained significant favor since the first endoluminal stent was introduced by Jean-Francois Dumon in 1990. Stents are typically made from silicone or metal and are used to maintain patency in airways which are narrowed from either endoluminal or extraluminal disease. The ideal stent would be easy to insert and remove without migration, sufficient strength to support the airway, yet flexible enough to mimic normal airway physiology and promote secretion clearance, biologically inert to minimize the formation of granulation tissue, and available in a variety of sizes. Stents may be placed via flexible bronchoscopy or rigid bronchoscopy depending on the operator's comfort. Stents are an important device for maintaining airway patency in patients with malignant endobronchial disease. While metallic stents are considered a therapeutic option for patients with malignant disease, the Food and Drug Administration (FDA) has issued a black box warning against using metallic stents in benign airway disease.

* *

Brachytherapy is contraindicated in the setting of obstructing endobronchial tumors that cannot be traversed.[8,12] This treatment option involves the placement of radioactive source in or around a malignant lesion in order to provide local radiation therapy. This treatment modality delivers high dose radiation to the tumor, which may be more effective than external beam radiation. While the tumor can either be extrinsic or intrinsic to the airway, the radiation catheter must be able to pass distal to the obstruction. Due to the extent of the obstruction, the catheter would not be able to pass the tumor in this patient.

Question 4: D. Rheumatoid arthritis with involvement of the cervical vertebral bodies

Rigid bronchoscopy is a procedure typically used to manage patients with central airway obstructions involving the trachea or proximal bronchi. This form of bronchoscopy provides operators with a secure airway along with the ability to utilize suctioning, tissue removal, and stent placement. The barrel of the rigid bronchoscope can vary between 2 and 14 mm along with various tube lengths. While the procedure is very safe in trained hands, the few complications that may arise from rigid bronchoscopy include tooth damage and vocal cord injury during insertion. Absolute contraindications for rigid bronchoscopy include an unstable cervical spine, severe maxillofacial trauma or deformity, or obstructing oral or laryngeal disease.

CASE 3

Question 1: D. Exudative with lymphocyte predominance

Pleural effusions results from increased pulmonary capillary pressure, decreased oncotic pressure, increased

pleural membrane permeability, or obstruction of lymphatic flow. Pleural effusions can be classified as exudative or transudative. Transudative effusions result from a decrease in colloid osmotic pressure (decreased protein synthesis, e.g., liver disease; increased protein loss, e.g. kidney disease) or increased hydrostatic pressure (venous outflow obstruction, e.g. congestive heart failure). Exudative pleural effusion result from fluid and protein leakage due to an inflammatory process resulting in vasodilation and increased interendothelial spaces. According to Light's criteria, pleural fluid can be defined as an exudate if the pleural fluid protein divided by serum protein is >0.5 g/dL, pleural fluid LDH divided by serum LDH >0.6, or pleural fluid LDH is more than two-thirds the upper limit of normal serum LDH.[13] More recently, modified Light's criteria have been validated to have the same sensitivity as the original Light's criteria without the need of serum studies. Modified Light's criteria suggest an exudate if the pleural fluid protein is >2.9 g/dL, pleural fluid LDH is >0.45 upper limit of normal, or fluid cholesterol is >45 mg/dL.[13,14] Pleural fluid differential cell counts further classify pleural fluid, but are rarely diagnostic alone. Parapneumonic effusions or empyema is typically a neutrophilic exudate with empyemas having >50,000 WBCs. Exudates with lymphocytic predominance can be seen in malignancy, tuberculosis, lymphoma, sarcoidosis, chylothoraces, or rheumatoid effusions. In addition, mesothelial cells >5% of total cells would essentially rule out tuberculosis.

* *

Choice A is incorrect as the effusion would not be defined as transudative based on Light's criteria. Choice B is incorrect as bacterial empyema would be unlikely as the fluid does not feature a neutrophil predominance, the Gram stain is negative, and the fluid pH is not significantly decreased. Choice C is incorrect as a chylothorax is defined as a pleural fluid triglyceride level greater than 110 mg/dL. Choice E is incorrect as a pseudochylothorax or a cholesterol effusion is defined as a pleural fluid cholesterol greater than 200 mg/dL and cholesterol to triglyceride ratio >1.

Question 2: C. Closed Abram's needle biopsy

The Abram's pleural needle consists of three parts, with two concentric tubes and a stylet. The needle biopsy performed using the Abram's needle is a blind biopsy yielding an excellent yield in cases of pleural tuberculosis due to the diffuse nature of the infection. In fact, the initial biopsy via blind pleural biopsy may demonstrate granulomas in

50% to 80% of patient's samples. The addition of tissue culture, pleural fluid smear culture, ADA, and lymphocyte/neutrophil ratio further improves the sensitivity to 93% and specificity to 100%. While pleural tuberculosis is a diffuse pleural process, malignant implant may be randomly distributed throughout the pleura. In such cases, biopsies using a modality utilizing direct visualization of the pleura, such as thoracoscopy, would be the desired approach.

* *

While repeat thoracentesis may be reasonable in the setting of malignancy prior to thoracoscopic biopsy, the suspicion for malignancy is low in this patient. Waiting for cultures to grow in such a patient may take up to 6 weeks in patients with tuberculosis. Treatment should be started as soon as a diagnosis is determined in patients with suspected pleural tuberculosis, therefore choice B is incorrect. Finally, although analysis of induced sputum may provide a diagnosis of pulmonary tuberculosis, sputum smears tend to be positive in less than 2% of cases of pleural tuberculosis cases.

Question 3: B. Extrapulmonary tuberculosis
The case described features a patient with pleural tuberculosis. She is an immigrant from an endemic region found to have low-grade fevers, fatigue, and weight loss combined with findings of a lymphocyte predominant pleural effusion. Thoracoscopic images of the patient's pleura are featured below.

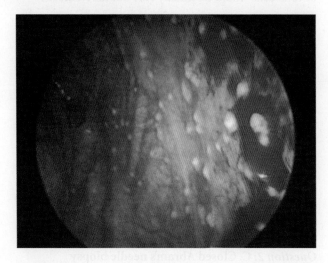

* *

Pleural tuberculosis should be entertained in patients with lymphocytic pleural effusions. Tuberculosis involving the pleural fluid is the most common extrapulmonary site following lymph node involvement. Unfortunately, the precise number of pleural tuberculosis cases yearly is difficult to determine since it is not routinely distinguished from other forms of pulmonary tuberculosis. Pleural tuberculosis is postulated to arise as the sequela of primary pulmonary tuberculosis infection or through reactivation of latent tuberculosis. The effusion resulting from the infection is thought to result from the rupture of subpleural foci into the pleural space resulting in a delayed hypersensitivity reaction to the tuberculus antigen. Symptoms related to pleural tuberculosis include recurrent pleuritic chest pain, low-grade fevers, fatigue, and weight loss. Foreign-born patients comprise a large proportion of both pleural and pulmonary tuberculous cases. Antimicrobial therapy for pleural tuberculosis is the same as that for pulmonary tuberculosis, comprising of four-drug therapy for 2 months followed by 4 months of two-drug therapy. Treatment with steroids has not proven to show significant benefit.[15]

Question 4: C. Fluid adenosine deaminase
Adenosine deaminase (ADA) is an enzyme in the purine salvage pathway considered important in differentiation of lymphoid cells and is found to have increased activity as lymphocyte activity increases. The sensitivity of ADA in tuberculosis is high (90–100%). Galactomannan is typically tested from bronchoalveolar lavage specimens for the diagnosis of aspergillus infections, while beta-natriuretic peptide is typically elevated in cases of pleural effusions caused by fluid overload states such as congestive heart failure. The diagnosis of chylothorax is established by measuring triglyceride levels to be greater than 110 mg/dL. When the triglyceride levels are between 50 and 110 mg/dL, lipoprotein analysis should be performed.[16] Chylomicrons in the fluid establish the diagnosis of chylothorax. Pseudo-chylothorax in any condition associated with a chronic pleural effusion with or without thickened pleural membranes. In the past, one of the more common causes was induced pneumothorax therapy for pulmonary tuberculosis. At present, the two most common etiologies are tuberculous and chronic rheumatoid pleural effusions. The diagnosis is made with pleural fluid cholesterol level >200 mg/dL and a cholesterol to triglyceride ratio >1.[16]

CASE 4

Question 1: C. 55%
Approximately 200,000 pleural effusions secondary to malignant disease occur every year in the United States.

The presence of pleural effusions in patients with diagnosed or undiagnosed cancer can often present as a diagnostic dilemma. A pleural effusion represents a readily accessible source of tissue for either diagnosis or staging of cancer. Unfortunately, the diagnostic yield of malignant cells from pleural fluid in patients with cancer is much lower than would be expected. While pleural implants may be present in metastatic disease, cancerous cells are not always shed into pleural fluid. In fact, pleural fluid cytology is positive for malignant cells after the first thoracentesis in patients with malignancy from various primary sources only 50% to 60% of the time.[13,17] Further thoracenteses typically result in diminishing returns, as the yield from a second thoracentesis is only 27% and the third only 5%.[13,17] Patients deemed to have a high pretest probability for malignant involvement of the pleura typically undergo more invasive diagnostic and therapeutic interventions, such as thoracoscopy with pleural biopsies and possible pleurodesis, after two thoracenteses with negative cytology.

Question 2: E. Stage IV

In the case of lung cancer patients, over 50% will develop effusions during their illness and the presence of a malignant pleural effusion would characterize the disease as stage IV according to the seventh TNM staging system. Patients with malignant pleural effusions have a median survival of 3 to 12 months.[13,18,19] The shortest survival is seen in patients with lung cancer, while the longest survival is seen in patients with ovarian cancer.[19]

Question 3: D. Tunneled pleural catheter placement

Malignant pleural effusions manifest as dyspnea close to 60% of the time. Over 50% of patients with lung cancer will develop pleural effusions during their illness.[18] The majority of malignant pleural effusions are symptomatic and over 90% are exudative. There are a number of therapeutic options available for managing pleural effusions involving drainage. The etiology of malignant pleural effusions involves obstruction of stoma situated between pleural mesothelial cells due to tumor infiltration. This obstruction decreases fluid reabsorption resulting in pleural effusion formation. The recurrence rate of malignant effusions after drainage is close to 100%. The tunneled pleural catheter is a management option that has greatly improved the care of patients with malignant pleural effusions. These catheters are tunneled under the skin and inserted into the pleural space for home drainage and can be placed on an outpatient basis with a low rate of complications. The catheter is typically hidden under clothing and is only exposed from its dressing when drainage is being performed. Either visiting nurses or family members can perform drainage. Tunneled pleural catheters offer the freedom to drain fluid on an as needed basis based on day-to-day symptoms. Serial thoracenteses, choice A, had previously been recommended for patients with poor functional ability and extremely short-life expectancy, on the order of days. More recently, even patients with short-life expectancies benefit from tunneled pleural catheter placement rather than repeated trips to the outpatient setting for drainage. Choice B, low-dose diuretic, is unlikely to be beneficial, as pleural effusions from malignancy do not result from changes in hydrostatic pressure. Finally, while hospice referral, choice C, may be appropriate in the future, the patient is highly functional and is unlikely near end of life. Choice E is unlikely to be beneficial in a patient who shows a nonexpandable lung on chest radiograph and pleural manometry.

Question 4: D. Improvement in chest wall and diaphragm mechanics

Patient with pleural effusions suffer from considerable dyspnea. Despite the presence of dyspnea, hypoxia is rarely present and is only a concern when significant bilateral atelectasis is present. The presence of pleural fluid results in changes in the chest wall mechanics, namely in the shape of the ipsilateral diaphragm. Diaphragm contour is changed from a curved to flat. This prevents the necessary diaphragm contraction and descent to generate negative intrapleural pressure to facilitate ventilation. When patients are unable to contract their diaphragms to generate appropriate negative intrathoracic pressure, accessory muscles are utilized to generate the necessary negative pressure. Drainage of pleural fluid through thoracentesis or tunneled pleural catheter results in correction of the mechanical disadvantage, efficient diaphragmatic contraction, and improved shortness of breath.[20]

Question 5: B. Instillation of t-PA/DNAse into the catheter

Patients with minimal drainage of pleural fluid following tunneled pleural catheter placement should be evaluated for the development of autopleurodesis or catheter obstruction. Evaluation for absence of pleural fluid or obstruction of the catheter with the subsequent build-up of pleural fluid can be assessed with chest radiography or chest ultrasound. The absence of pleural fluid on three consecutive drainages without the presence of pleural fluid likely represents the achievement of autopleurodesis warranting removal of the tunneled catheter. Presence of pleural fluid without significant drainage may indicate obstruction of the catheter or poor placement.[21] Catheter obstruction may benefit from intrapleural fibrinolytics with follow-up drainage.[22] The incorrect therapeutic option for this patient would be use of recombinant tissue plasminogen activator (t-PA) and dornase-alpha (DNAse), choice B.[23–25] These medications are utilized in patients with pleural infections. The mortality rate from pleural infections ranges between 10% and 20% in both children and adults. Standard therapy for pleural infections includes systemic antibiotic therapy and tube drainage. While surgery was the standard of care for patients with poorly controlled pleural infections, the use of intrapleural administration of tPA and DNAse reduces the frequency of failed drainage and the need for surgical intervention. The belief that pleural septations can be released with use of fibrinolytic agents will result in improved pleural drainage that has gained increasing favor. In addition, the presence of extracellular DNA and other bacterial components in the pleural space may increase viscosity and permit biofilm formation. The use of t-PA/DNAse is becoming increasingly popular in patients with infected pleural spaces was associated with a reduction in hospital stays compared to placebo.[25]

CASE 5

Question 1: C. Emergent intubation with preferential advancement of the endotracheal tube into the right mainstem bronchus

Patients with hemoptysis require close monitoring and detailed action plans. While diagnosing the source of bleeding is essential, patient positioning and establishing a secure airway are the primary objective. Identification of the bleeding etiology can be performed following stabilization of the patient. While massive hemoptysis is typically described as expectoration of large amounts of blood and/or rapid rate of bleeding, the quantity of blood needed to deem hemoptysis as "massive" is poorly defined.[26,27,28] Quantities of blood anywhere between 100 mL and 1000 mL over 24 hours have been described as "massive."[26,27,28] Because the amount of blood and characteristic of blood, bright or dark, are often difficult to describe by patients, some physicians choose to consider hemoptysis to be significant if gas exchange is affected. The initial management of massive hemoptysis includes turning the patient onto the side of the likely bleeding lung to prevent soiling of the contralateral lung

and intubation to secure the airway with preferential intubation into the mainstem bronchus of the nonbleeding lung versus use of an endobronchial blocker. Following establishment of a secure airway, flexible bronchoscopy or rigid bronchoscopy can be performed to identify the source of bleeding with possible therapeutic intervention. Choice A would offer no therapeutic option for the patient and may worsen respiratory status by laying flat. Choice B is incorrect as the patient should be turned onto the side of suspected bleeding, the left side, to avoid soiling the contralateral lung. Choice D is incorrect as bi-level positive pressure ventilation (BIPAP) would not provide a stable airway for the patient. Choice E is incorrect as this patient has life-threatening hemoptysis and cough suppression in patients with nonmassive hemoptysis remains to be controversial.

Question 2: A. Rigid bronchoscopy with aspiration of clot and possible electrocautery to the airway lesion

Flexible bronchoscopy is the preferred procedure for patients with massive hemoptysis following intubation. The goal of bedside flexible bronchoscopy is to localize the site of bleeding and to develop a plan for further intervention. In specialized centers, rigid bronchoscopy can be performed in the operating room and is valuable in situations where greater suction capacity is necessary. In addition, therapeutic interventions can be performed more readily with rigid bronchoscopy such as electrocautery, argon plasma coagulation, and laser ablation. Choices B, C, and D are inadequate for therapeutic intervention on this patient with a worsening respiratory status and would not be effective in removing the obstructing blood clots. Choice E is inadequate as patient is unstable and requires emergent treatment.

CASE 6

Question 1: C. Tracheal stent placement prior to spontaneous breathing trial

The patient in the above case was diagnosed with a massive goiter of the thyroid gland. Unfortunately, attempts at liberation from the ventilator posed a challenge due to the resistive forces associated with the severe airway narrowing. Stenting of the airway allows for relief of significant extrinsic compression. This patient underwent placement of a covered self-expanding stent in the proximal trachea with subsequent successful extubation. Unfortunately, increased PEEP during spontaneous breathing trial (Choice A) or positioning the patient on her left side (Choice B) may improve success of the SBT, but will not equate to avoiding reintubation. In addition, tracheostomy (Choice D) placement would be extremely difficulty considering the position of the mass. Finally, taking the patient to the operating room for goiter removal would be deemed high risk due to the inability to secure her airway and her other comorbidities.

CASE 7

Question 1: C. Intrabronchial valve placement

Intrabronchial valves are umbrella-shaped devices utilized for the treatment of persistent air leaks. These valves are placed bronchoscopically and allow secretions to drain proximally while preventing air to travel distally.[29] The resulting atelectasis results in a decreased air leak and allows for reduced healing time. Intrabronchial valves are placed using balloon localization in order to identify the segment responsible for the air leak and remain in place for approximately 6 weeks until they are taken out, again bronchoscopically. While intrabronchial valves harbor an FDA humanitarian device exemption for persistent air leaks following thoracic surgical resection, they are often used in the off label use for traumatic or spontaneous pneumothoraces.

Question 2: C. 6 weeks

Intrabronchial valves typically remain in for 6 weeks following placement. After 6 weeks, the valves are removed endoscopically after the persistent air leak has healed.

CASE 8

Question 1: B. Rigid bronchoscopy

Pill aspiration is a common cause of airway obstruction, especially in individuals with a history of stroke. Potassium pills are large pills often considered difficulty to swallow. Patients may see an airway obstruction, typically seen in the right-sided airways due to the angle at which the right mainstem projects from the trachea.

* *

Rigid bronchoscopy remains the gold standard for treatment of foreign-body aspiration. Insertion of the rigid bronchoscopy provides a conduit to ventilate the patient in addition to utilize powerful suction along with rigid forceps. In addition, foreign bodies with substantial water content can be easily removed using cryotherapy. The foreign body can be easily withdrawn using the cryotherapy probe without suffering from fragmentation.

CASE 9

Question 1: E. Linear EBUS-TBNA, navigation bronchoscopy and radial EBUS-guided transbronchial biopsy (TBBX), brush and transbronchial needle aspirate (TBNA)

Navigation bronchoscopy utilizes three-dimensional reconstructions of axial CT imaging to create a virtual airway map. Electromagnetic navigation bronchoscopy (ENB) is an image-guided localization procedure that allows the operator to steer a bronchoscope to peripheral lung lesions.[4] The ENB system consists of steerable navigation catheters used in concert with navigation software to create virtual three-dimensional reconstructions of bronchial anatomy. Operators utilize localization software to maneuver small airways in real-time using a virtual bronchoscopic map outlined prior to the procedure. The objective of this study was to evaluate the diagnostic yield of peripheral pulmonary nodules using ENB in high-risk patients and the rate of complications associated with the procedure. A study by Eberhardt et al. showed that the diagnostic yield when using ENB and radial EBUS in combination was higher (88%) compared to radial EBUS alone (69%) and ENB alone (59%) ($p = 0.02$).[36] In addition, linear endobronchial ultrasound (EBUS) bronchoscopy allows for real-time imaging of mediastinal lymph nodes and transbronchial needle aspiration. Thus, combining linear EBUS, ENB, and radial EBUS provides staging and diagnosis of patients with lung cancer.

Question 2: D. Pneumothorax

Transthoracic fine-needle biopsy of pulmonary lesions can be associated with a risk of pneumothorax up to 64%.[30-35] The benefit of navigation bronchoscopy stands in the minimally invasive nature of the procedure combined with the lower pneumothorax rate. The incidence of pneumothorax with ENB is 2% to 3%.[36]

REFERENCES

1. Detterbeck FC, Lewis SZ, Diekemper R, et al. Executive summary: Diagnosis and management of lung cancer. 3rd ed. American College of Chest Physicians evidence-based clinical practice guidelines. *Chest*. 2013;143:7S–37S.

2. Baaklini WA, Reinoso MA, Gorin AB, et al. Diagnostic yield of fiberoptic bronchoscopy in evaluating solitary pulmonary nodules. *Chest.* 2000;117:1049–1054.

3. Vincent BD, El-Bayoumi E, Hoffman B, et al. Real-time endobronchial ultrasound-guided transbronchial lymph node aspiration. *Ann Thorac Surg.* 2008;85:224–230.

4. Folch E, Yamaguchi N, VanderLaan PA, et al. Adequacy of lymph node transbronchial needle aspirates using convex probe endobronchial ultrasound for multiple tumor genotyping techniques in non-small-cell lung cancer. *J Thorac Oncol.* 2013;8(11):1438–1444.

5. Gomez M, Silvestri GA. Endobronchial ultrasound for the diagnosis and staging of lung cancer. *Proc Am Thorac Soc.* 2009;6:180–186.

6. Horner MJ, Ries LAG, Krapcho M, eds, et al. *SEER Cancer Statistics Review.* 1975–2006; National Cancer Institute. Bethesda, MD.

7. Detterbeck FC, Boffa DJ, Tanoue LT. The new lung cancer staging system. *Chest.* 2009;136(1):260–271.

8. Ernst A, Feller-Kopman D, Becker HD, et al. Central airway obstruction. *Am J Respir Crit Care Med.* 2004;169(12):1278–1297.

9. Ayers ML, Beamis JF Jr. Rigid bronchoscopy in the twenty-first century. *Clin Chest Med.* 2001;22:355–364.

10. Ginsberg RJ, Vokes EE, Ruben A. Non-small cell lung cancer. In: DeVita VT, Hellman S, Rosenberg SA, eds. *Cancer: Principles and Practice of Oncology.* 5th ed. Philadelphia, PA: Lippincott-Raven; 1997:858–911.

11. Dumon JF. A dedicated tracheobronchial stent. *Chest.* 1990;97:328–332.

12. Hilaris BS, Mastoras DA. Contemporary brachytherapy approaches in non-small cell lung cancer. *J Surg Oncol.* 1998;69:258–264.

13. Light RW. *Pleural diseases.* 3rd ed. Baltimore, MD: Williams and Wilkins; 1995.

14. Heffner JE, Brown LK, Barbieri CA. Diagnostic value of tests that discriminate between exudative and transudative pleural effusions. Primary Study Investigators. *Chest.* 1997; 111:970–980.

15. Wyser C, Walzl G, Smedema IP, et al. Corticosteroids in the treatment of tuberculous pleurisy. A double-blind, placebo-controlled, randomized study. *Chest.* 1996;110(2):333–338.

16. Staats BA, Ellefson RD, Budhan LL, et al. The lipoprotein profile of chylous and nonchylous pleural effusions. *Mayo Clin Proc.* 1980;55:700–704.

17. Starr RL, Sherman ME. The value of multiple preparations in the diagnosis of malignant pleural effusion: a cost-benefit analysis. *Acta Cytol.* 1991;35:533–537.

18. Chernow B, Sahn SA. Carcinomatous involvement of the pleura. *Am J Med.* 1977;63:695–702.

19. van de Molengraft FJ, Vooijs GP. Survival of patients with malignancy-associated effusions. *Acta Cytol.* 1989;33: 911–916.

20. Klecka M, Maldonado F. Symptom relief after large volume thoracentesis in the absence of lung perfusion. *Chest.* 2014;145(5):1141–1143.

21. Nasim F, Folch E, Majid A. Tunneled pleural catheter malfunction: Case report and review of complications. *J Bronchology.* 2012;19(2):149–152.

22. Davies RJ, Traill ZC, Gleeson FV. Randomised controlled trial of intrapleural streptokinase in community acquired pleural infection. *Thorax.* 1997;52:416–421.

23. Heffner JE. Multicenter trials of treatment for empyema – after all these years. *N Engl J Med.* 2005;352:926–928.

24. Hall-Stoodley L, Nistico L, Sambanthamoorthy K, et al. Characterization of biofilm matrix, degradation by DNase treatment and evidence of capsule downregulation in Streptococcus pneumoniae clinical isolates. *BMC Microbiol.* 2008;8:173–173.

25. Rahman NM, Maskell NA, West A, et al. Intrapleural use of tissue plasminogen activator and DNase in pleural infection. *N Engl J Med.* 2011;365:518–526.

26. Jean-Baptiste E. Clinical assessment and management of massive hemoptysis. *Crit Care Med.* 2000;28:1642–1647.

27. Ibrahim WH. Massive haemoptysis: the definition should be revised. *Eur Respir J.* 2008;32:1131–1132.

28. Cahill BC, Ingbar DH. Massive hemoptysis. Assessment and management. *Clin Chest Med.* 1994;15:147–167.

29. Mahajan AK, Doeing CD, Hogarth DK. Isolation of persistent airleaks and placement of intrabronchial valves (IBV). *J Thorac and Cardiovasc Surg.* 2013;135(3):626–630.

30. Cox JE, Chiles C, McManus CM, et al. Transthoracic needle aspiration biopsy: variables that affect risk of pneumothorax. *Radiology.* 1999;212:165–168.

31. Li H, Boiselle PM, Shepard JO, et al. Diagnostic accuracy and safety of CT-guided percutaneous needle aspiration biopsy of the lung: comparison of small and large pulmonary nodules. *AJR Am J Roentgenol.* 1996;167: 105–109.

32. Westcott JL. Percutaneous transthoracic needle biopsy. *Radiology* 1988;169:593–601.

33. Khouri NF, Stitik FP, Erozan YS, et al. Transthoracic needle aspiration biopsy of benign and malignant lung lesions. *AJR Am J Roentgenol* 1985;144:281–288.

34. Kazerooni EA, Lim FT, Mikhail A, et al. Risk of pneumothorax in CT-guided transthoracic needle aspiration biopsy of the lung. *Radiology.* 1996;198:371–375.

35. Laurent F, Michel P, Latrabe V, et al. Pneumothoraces and chest tube placement after CT-guided transthoracic lung biopsy using a coaxial technique: incidence and risk factors. *AJR Am J Roentgenol.* 1999;172:1049–1053.

36. Eberhardt R, Anantham D, Herth F, et al. Electromagnetic navigation diagnostic bronchoscopy in peripheral lung lesions. *Chest* 2007;131:1800–1805.

17

Lung Transplantation

Irene Louh MD, Hilary Robbins MD, and Lori Shah MD

CASE 1

A 34-year-old woman had bilateral lung transplantation for severe pulmonary arterial hypertension. Postoperatively she developed acute renal failure requiring hemodialysis and subsequently, a reduction in her tacrolimus level. Two months later, she complained of shortness of breath and chest tightness. Her physical examination was otherwise unremarkable. Her pulmonary function testing showed a forced expiratory volume (FEV_1) of 3.3 L, a 12% decrease from prior. She had a bronchoscopy that showed minimal exudate at the anastomosis but no secretions. The transbronchial biopsies showed perivascular infiltrates with focal endothelialitis. Cultures were negative.

Question 1: The appropriate next therapy is:

A. Levofloxacin 500 mg daily for 14 days
B. Methylprednisolone 1,000 mg IV daily for 3 days, followed by an oral prednisone taper
C. Voriconazole 200 mg twice daily for 6 months
D. Antithymocyte globulin 1.5 mg/kg/day IV daily for 5 days
E. Rituximab 375 mg/m² IV weekly for 4 weeks

Question 2: Over the next 2 years, her FEV_1 continued to decline to 0.7 L (17% predicted) despite aggressive therapy. All of the above were considered potential contributors to this clinical syndrome EXCEPT:

A. Acute cellular rejection
B. Cytomegalovirus infection
C. Native lung disease
D. Gastroesophageal reflux
E. Severe primary graft dysfunction

Question 3: A serum luminex assay revealed the presence of high titer circulating donor-specific antibodies (DSA). Which of the following is NOT true regarding DSA?

A. The risk of chronic allograft dysfunction and mortality following lung transplant is increased in patients with circulating DSA.
B. The development of DSA leads to complement activation which in turn causes allograft injury.
C. The antigens recognized by DSA are human leukocyte antigen class I and class II antigens.
D. DSA may have specificity for type V collagen and K-a1 tubulin.
E. Treatment for DSA includes intravenous immunoglobulin (IVIG) and/or rituximab.

CASE 2

A 69-year-old woman with history of hypertension and hypothyroidism presents to your office with complaints of dyspnea with dry cough for 3 years. Vital signs in your office show BP 125/78, HR 78, RR20, and POx of 93% on room air. Physical examination is significant for crackles on lung examination, no murmurs, and no peripheral edema. Her chest CT demonstrates diffuse fibrotic changes, basilar and peripheral predominance. Rheumatological serologies and all other laboratory findings are normal. PFTs performed demonstrate FEV_1 1.32 (56%), FVC 1.41 L (46%), ratio91%, TLC 2.22 (44%), and DLco of 7.3 (31%). Patient's 6 MWT was 820 ft on 2 LPM O_2 via nasal cannula.

Question 1: At what point should this patient be referred for evaluation for lung transplantation?

A. At time of diagnosis

B. BODE index >5

C. Presence of pulmonary hypertension

D. 30% decrease in 6-minute walk test

E. When oxygen therapy is prescribed

Question 2: Which of the following would prevent this patient's candidacy for lung transplantation?

A. Age >65

B. BMI >30

C. Tobacco use 5 months prior to current evaluation

D. History of basal cell carcinoma of the skin

E. Coronary artery disease with preserved LVEF

Question 3: What findings would suggest this patient should be listed for transplantation?

A. 5% decrease in FEV_1 in past 2 months

B. Chronic hypercapnea

C. DLco 35%

D. 6MWT of <1,000 ft

E. Progression of disease on HRCT

CASE 3

A 44-year-old man with a past medical history significant for cystic fibrosis-related diabetes and chronic sinusitis underwent double lung transplantation for cystic fibrosis 14 years ago. He now presented with 1 month of enlarging and painful skin nodules on his left thigh and bilateral forearms. He was seen by his local dermatologist and was diagnosed with molluscum contagiosum. He was given topical therapy, with no beneficial effect. In addition, he had a 10-lb unintentional weight loss, intermittent headaches, nausea, and vomiting for the last 8 weeks. He had new onset of mild dyspnea upon strenuous exertion. He was found to have a creatinine of 3.3, which was above his baseline of 1.9. He was noted to have an RML infiltrate on CXR upon admission. A skin biopsy yielded "yeast-like forms with surrounding halos" consistent with *Cryptococcus Neoformans*.

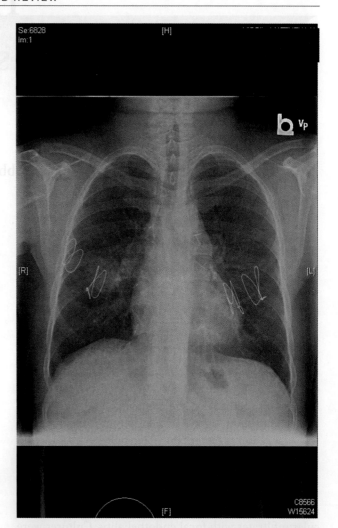

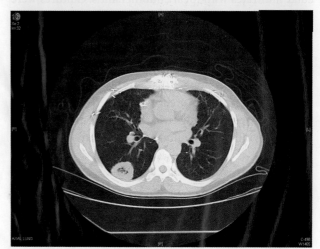

He was initially started on intravenous fluconazole therapy at a dose of 12 mg/kg.

Question 1: Which lung transplant-related immunosuppressant medication must be adjusted due to the addition of fluconazole to this patient's medication regimen?

A. Mycophenolate mofetil
B. Tacrolimus
C. Prednisone
D. Trimethoprim-sulfamethoxazole
E. None of the above

Question 2: A serum cryptococcal antigen is positive at a titer of 1:2,048. A lumbar puncture is performed which is positive for cryptococcus with a CSF cryptococcal antigen titer of 1:1,024. What is the best course of therapy at this time?

A. Continue fluconazole at current dose of 12 mg/kg
B. Discontinue fluconazole and start liposomal amphotericin B and flucytosine (5FU)
C. Continue fluconazole and start intrathecal amphotericin
D. Change fluconazole to voriconazole (VFEND) at a dose of 200 mg BID
E. None of the above

Question 3: The appropriate dose reduction for flucytosine in a patient with renal dysfunction is:

A. No dose reduction is required.
B. The dose should not be reduced, if the patient's disease is severe.
C. The dose should be reduced on the basis of the patient's creatinine clearance.
D. The dose should be reduced when the patients' clinical status improves.
E. None of the above.

CASE 4

A 31-year-old woman with cystic fibrosis underwent bilateral lung transplant 9 years ago. Her other history includes cystic fibrosis related diabetes, pancreatic insufficiency, Crohn's disease, nephrolithiasis, hyperlipidemia, and depression. She presented with epigastric pain radiating to her back for 3 weeks, unrelieved with oral narcotic therapy. She had no fevers, nausea, or vomiting. She had regular bowel movements. She denied urinary symptoms. Her CT of the abdomen and pelvis showed a 4.8 × 2.4 cm mass between the liver and the pancreas.

Surgical biopsy of the mass revealed sheets of large monomorphic CD 20+ B cells, with an increased mitotic rate, apoptotic debris, and increased proliferation index. In situ hybridization for the Epstein–Barr virus (EBV) is positive.

Question 1: The incidence of posttransplant lymphoproliferative disorder (PTLD) following lung transplant is:

A. 0.5%
B. 3.7%
C. 12.5%
D. 20%
E. 35%

Question 2: The following statements are true regarding PTLD in lung transplant EXCEPT:

A. Fifty percent of patients who develop PTLD do so within the first year after transplant.
B. PTLD developing within the first year occurs most commonly in the allograft.
C. PTLD that develops after the first posttransplant year often develops in extrathoracic sites and may be EBV-negative.
D. Approximately 15% of PTLDs are of B cells in origin.
E. EBV is associated with the development of PTLD in about 80% of samples.

Question 3: Therapy for PLTD may include all of the following EXCEPT:

A. Cessation of mycophenolate or azathioprine
B. Rituximab 375 mg/m² IV weekly × 4 weeks
C. Antithymocyte globulin 1.5 mg/kg/day IV daily for 5 days
D. Cyclophosphamide, doxorubicin, vincristine, and prednisolone
E. Dose reduction of tacrolimus or cyclosporine

CASE 5

A 36-year-old woman who underwent double-lung transplant for cystic fibrosis 2 years ago, presents with fatigue and malaise for about 2 weeks duration. At the time of her transplant, she was a cytomegalovirus (CMV) mismatch (donor CMV IGG positive/recipient CMV IGG negative) and received a 3-month course of intravenous ganciclovir followed by an additional 9 months of therapy with oral valganciclovir. At 1 year, her oral valganciclovir therapy was discontinued and her CMV PCR was negative thereafter. Upon admission, her CMV PCR was 12,100 IU/mL. Her creatinine was in normal range. She is started on intravenous ganciclovir therapy at a dose of 5 mg/kg twice daily. Her subsequent CMV PCR was 14,000 IU/mL. She continued to have fatigue, but was otherwise asymptomatic. There was no change made to her therapeutic regimen. After 2 weeks of therapy, her CMV PCR was 23,000 IU/mL. A CMV resistance panel was shown below:

CMV Antiviral Resistance Assay	
Ganciclovir UL97 gene target	Resistant at site H520Q
Cidofovir UL54 gene target	Resistant at site A987G
Foscarnet UL54 gene target	None detected
Ganciclovir UL54 gene target	Resistant at site A987G

Question 1: **What is the incidence of ganciclovir-resistant CMV in the post-lung transplant population?**

A. 0%
B. Up to 15%
C. 50%
D. 100%
E. Resistance is based on the CMV status of donor and recipient and cannot be quantified.

Question 2: **Based on this patients resistance assay, IV Foscarnet is initiated. What is the greatest toxicity concern about the use of IV Foscarnet?**

A. Hepatotoxicity
B. Cardiac toxicity
C. Interaction with tacrolimus
D. Nephrotoxicity
E. Ocular toxicity

The patient developed a cough and mild dyspnea on exertion. Her oxygen saturations were now in the 90% to 92% range, lower than her prior range of 98% to 100%. Fiberoptic bronchoscopy and transbronchial biopsy were performed revealing "owls eye" inclusions. There was no evidence of acute cellular rejection.

Question 3: **Based on the patient's clinical course so far, which factor increases her risk of bronchiolitis obliterans syndrome (chronic rejection)?**

A. Presence of CMV viremia
B. Degree of CMV viremia
C. Presence of CMV pneumonitis
D. Cystic fibrosis
E. None of the above

Answers

CASE 1

Question 1: B. Methylprednisolone 1,000 mg IV daily for 3 days, followed by an oral prednisone taper

The patient had acute cellular rejection. This is most common within the first year after transplant and can be asymptomatic or characterized by symptoms such as cough, dyspnea, fever, hypoxemia, infiltrates on chest imaging, or decline in pulmonary function testing. The gold standard for diagnosis of acute cellular rejection is bronchoscopy with transbronchial biopsy, which allows for determination of infection as well as rejection. Rejection is characterized pathologically as the presence of perivascular mononuclear infiltrates. The presence of endothelialitis suggests grade A2 rejection.

* *

The pathologic grading of rejection is described in Table 17-1.[1] Acute rejection is graded by the presence and degree of perivascular and interstitial mononuclear cell infiltrates (A grade) and the presence and degree of lymphocytic bronchiolitis (B grade). Chronic rejection (C grade) indicates the presence of obliterative bronchiolitis, the pathologic correlate of bronchiolitis obliterans syndrome (BOS).

* *

The treatment of acute cellular rejection is with high dose steroids. Although varying protocols exist, we typically use 10 to 15 mg/kg of solumedrol for 3 days with an oral prednisone taper starting at 60 mg daily for 3 days and decreasing by 10 mg every 3 days.

Table 17-1 PATHOLOGIC GRADING OF REJECTION

A. Acute Rejection	
Grade 0	None
Grade 1	Minimal
Grade 2	Mild
Grade 3	Moderate
Grade 4	Severe
B. Airway inflammation	
Grade 0	None
Grade 1R	Low grade
Grade 2R	High grade
C. Chronic airway rejection—obliterative bronchiolitis	
0	Absent
1	Present

Question 2: C. Native lung disease

The patient has bronchiolitis obliterans syndrome (BOS), which is the most common form of chronic allograft dysfunction following lung transplant.[1-3] It is characterized by persistent airflow obstruction on pulmonary function testing, with the exclusion of other etiologies (e.g., infection, acute rejection, airway complications). It is graded by the degree of decline in pulmonary function compared to baseline (Table 17-2). This patient has BOS stage 3.

Table 17-2 STAGES OF BOS

BOS 0	FEV_1 >90% of baseline
BOS 0p	FEV_1 81–90% of baseline and/or FEF 25–75 ≤75% of baseline
BOS 1	FEV_1 66–80% of baseline
BOS 2	FEV_1 51–65% of baseline
BOS 3	FEV_1 <50% of baseline

* *

The most important currently identified risk factor for BOS is acute cellular rejection and lymphocytic bronchiolitis, particularly repeated episodes. Infections, including cytomegalovirus and other respiratory viral infections, severe primary graft dysfunction, and gastroesophageal reflux and aspiration have all been associated with BOS. Native lung disease (i.e., indication for transplant) does not appear to be a risk factor.

Question 3: D. DSA may have specificity for type V collagen and K-a1 tubulin

The luminex assay is one of several means of determining the presence of circulating antibodies to human leukocyte antigens (HLA). The assay uses a bead array in which each different bead is bound with a single HLA antigen; donor specificity is determined by comparing recipient serum HLA antibodies to the donor HLA panel. In contrast, type V collagen and K-a1 tubulin are self-antigens located on airway epithelium and other sites.

* *

In transplant recipients who develop antibodies to donor HLA, these circulating antibodies may initiate the complement cascade and cause injury to the allograft. This process is known as antibody mediated rejection (AMR), and is well recognized in kidney and heart transplant, although the pathologic correlate in lung transplant has proven difficult to establish. As a surrogate marker for AMR, the presence of DSA has been shown to increase the risk of chronic rejection and death after lung transplant.[2,3] Evaluation for AMR is important as therapy differs from that of acute cellular rejection, and includes the use of IVIG and rituximab or plasmapheresis in select cases.

CASE 2

Question 1: A. At time of diagnosis

The most updated guidelines from IHLBT recommend referral of patients for evaluation at time of diagnosis of UIP, as median survival from time of diagnosis for these patients is 2.5 to 3.5 years, and these patients have the highest mortality on the waiting list for transplant.[4] BODE index is only utilized for referral of patients with COPD. Pulmonary hypertension is not the criteria for interstitial lung disease, though it is used as criteria for referral in cystic fibrosis. Six-minute walk distance is not used as referral criteria for IPF. While oxygen therapy indicates worsening pulmonary function, it has not used as criteria for lung transplant referral. It is, however, a guideline for transplantation in patients with cystic fibrosis.

Question 2: C. Tobacco use 5 months prior to current evaluation

Any tobacco use or substance use within 6 months is an absolute contraindication to transplant. Other absolute contraindications include malignancy in last 2 years except squamous or basal cell tumors of the skin, untreatable advanced dysfunction of another organ, noncurable extrapulmonary infection, such as chronic hepatitis B, hepatitis C, and HIV, documented nonadherence or inability to follow through with medical therapy, and absence of reliable or consistent social support system.[4,5] Age, BMI, and current CAD or history of CAD are only relative contraindications to transplant referral. Other relative contraindications to lung transplantation include critical/ unstable clinical condition, severely limited functional status with poor rehabilitation potential, colonization with highly resistant organisms, severe obesity, severe osteoporosis, and mechanical ventilation.

Question 3: C. DLco 35%

Guidelines for transplantation in IPF are based on multiple studies suggesting an increased mortality in patients that have significant decreases in physiologic variables over time. Guidelines for transplantation of IPF require histologic or radiographic evidence of UIP and any of the following: a DLco of less than 39% predicted, 10% or greater decrement in FVC during 6 months of follow-up, decrease in pulse oximetry below 88% during a 6MWT, or honeycombing on HRCT (fibrosis score >2).[4,6,7] Length of 6MWT is not used as criteria for lung transplantation. Chronic hypercapnea is not used as an indication for lung transplantation in IPF, however it is used as a guideline for transplantation in patients with cystic fibrosis.

CASE 3

Question 1: B. Tacrolimus

Tacrolimus (previously known as FK506) is a calcineurin inhibitor. It binds to a family of cytoplasmic proteins present in most cells known as FK binding proteins. The drug-receptor complex binds and inhibits calcineurin, a calcium- and calmodulin-dependent phosphatase. This process leads to reduced transcriptional activation of interleukin (IL)-2 and several other cytokines, mainly in T helper lymphocytes. Ultimately, lymphocyte activity is reduced.

* *

Oral tacrolimus is only partially absorbed due to fractional metabolism by enzymes in the bowel mucosa and first-pass hepatic metabolism. Tacrolimus is metabolized by the cytochrome P450 family of enzymes in the liver and excreted into the bile. Since tacrolimus is metabolized by hepatic cytochrome P450 enzymes, a variety of important drug interactions with drugs that either affect or are metabolized by these enzymes can occur. As a result, the tacrolimus dosing in patients treated with fluconazole must be reduced.

Question 2: B. Discontinue fluconazole and start liposomal amphotericin B and flucytosine (5FU)

The primary antifungal agents used for the treatment of cryptococcal meningoencephalitis include intravenous amphotericin B deoxycholate or its lipid formulations, flucytosine and fluconazole.[8-10] Combination therapy with amphotericin B and flucytosine is fungicidal, while fluconazole alone is only fungistatic. Clinical data suggests that a combination treatment regimen with fungicidal activity such as amphotericin B and flucytosine rapidly sterilizes the cerebrospinal fluid during induction therapy.[8-10] During the initial phase of therapy, this has been associated with better clinical outcomes.

Question 3: C. The dose should be reduced on the basis of the patient's creatinine clearance

Flucytosine dosage modification is required in any patient with renal dysfunction. Empiric dose adjustments can be based on measured or estimated creatinine clearance.

CASE 4

Question 1: B. 3.7%

The incidence of posttransplant lymphoproliferative disease (PTLD) following lung transplant has varied widely in single center reports, although is clearly higher than in liver and kidney transplant where immunosuppression rates are lower. An analysis of the Scientific Registry of the United Network of Organ Sharing from 1988 to 1999 showed an overall incidence of PTLD in 2,365 (1.2%) recipients, with 3.7% occurring in patients receiving lung transplants.[11]

Question 2: D. Approximately 15% of PTLDs are of B cells in origin

The majority (>80%) of all cases of PTLD are B cells in origin and associated with EBV infection.[11-14] EBV infection results in latent B cell infection with the viral genome and is controlled in the immunocompetent host by EBV-specific cytotoxic T cells. Transplant immunosuppression leads to an acquired T-cell immunodeficiency which can result in uncontrolled proliferation of EBV-infected B cells.

* *

Presentation of PTLD in lung transplant is often divided into early and late stage disease. Early stage disease occurs within the first year after transplant and encompasses approximately 50% of cases; typically these tumors occur in the allograft. Late stage disease, that is, after the first posttransplant year, typically is extrapulmonary in presentation and may be EBV negative.

Question 3: C. Antithymocyte globulin 1.5 mg/kg/day IV daily for 5 days

PTLD is associated with the presence and degree of immunosuppression, and lympholytic therapy with antithymocyte globulin or OKT3 appears to be a risk factor for the development of disease. The initial therapy for PTLD is reduction in immunosuppression (RI). RI typically consists of cessation of cell-cycle inhibitor therapy (azathioprine and mycophenolate) and a 25% to 50% reduction in dose of calcineurin inhibitor therapy.[13,14] Therapeutic response to RI varies widely in reported studies. Frequently, more aggressive chemotherapy is required and typically consists of rituximab (anti-CD20 monoclonal antibody) with or without CHOP (cyclophosphamide, doxorubicin, vincristine, and prednisolone).[13,14]

CASE 5

Question 1: B. Up to 15%

Ganciclovir-resistant CMV has been reported in up to 15% of lung transplant recipients who develop active infections.[15-18] Genotypic resistance arises from mutations at hot spots in the UL97 gene, which encodes the viral DNA phosphotransferase that monophosphorylates ganciclovir, and/or the UL54 gene, which encodes viral DNA polymerase. UL54 mutations are less common and may confer cross-resistance to cidofovir or foscarnet.

* *

Occasionally, viral loads may rise following initiation of therapy in some patients but this does not necessarily signify ganciclovir resistance. Ganciclovir resistance should be considered in patients who fail to improve after 2 weeks of adequate doses of antiviral therapy, have frequent relapses, or breakthrough CMV viremia/disease while on prophylaxis.

Question 2: **D. Nephrotoxicity**

Due to foscarnet's poor oral bioavailability, it must be administered intravenously. Foscarnet is excreted solely by the kidneys, mainly via glomerular filtration and tubular secretion. It appears to be directly toxic to the renal tubular cells. Tubular damage is likely the principal factor underlying foscarnet-induced renal dysfunction.

Question 3: **C. Presence of CMV pneumonitis**

Multiple retrospective studies of posttransplant patients have shown that presence of tissue invasive CMV pneumonitis may a risk factor for bronchiolitis obliterans syndrome.[19-20] CMV viremia has not been shown to be correlated to BOS. The presence of a pretransplant diagnosis of cystic fibrosis has not been associated with BOS.

REFERENCES

1. Stewart, S, Fishbein MC, Snell GI, et al. Revision of the 1996 working formulation for the standardization of nomenclature in the diagnosis of lung rejection. *J Heart Lung Transplant.* 2007;26:1229–1242.

2. Martinu T, Chen D, Palmer S. Acute rejection and humoral sensitization in lung transplant recipients. *Proc Am Thorac Soc.* 2009;6:54–65.

3. Belperio J, Weigt SS, Fishbein MC, et al. Chronic lung allograft rejection. *Proc Am Thorac Soc.* 2009;6:108–121.

4. Orens, JB, Estenne M, Arcasoy S, et al. Pulmonary Scientific Council of the International Society for Heart and Lung Transplantation. International guidelines for the selection of lung transplant candidates: 2006 update—a consensus report from the pulmonary scientific council of the international society for heart and lung transplantation. *J Heart Lung Transplant.* 2006;25(7):745–755.

5. Yusen, RD, Christie JD, Edwards LB, et al; International Society for Heart and Lung Transplantation. The Registry of the International Society for Heart and Lung Transplantation: Thirtieth Adult Lung and Heart-Lung Transplant Report—2013; Focus Theme: Age. *J Heart Lung Transplant.* 2013;32(10):965–978.

6. Collard HR, King TE Jr, Bartelson BB, et al. Changes in clinical and physiologic variables predict survival in idiopathic pulmonary fibrosis. *Am J Respir Crit Care Med.* 2003;168:538–542.

7. Flaherty KR, Mumford JA, Murray S, et al. Prognostic implications of physiologic and radiographic changes in idiopathic interstitial pneumonia. *Am J Respir Crit Care Med.* 2003;168:543–548.

8. Yao AQ, Lu X, Shen C, et al. Comparison of flucytosine and fluconazole combined with amphotericin B for the treatment of HIV-associated cryptococcal meningitis: a systematic review and meta-analysis. *Eur J Clin Microbiol Infect Dis.* 2014;33(8):1339–1344.

9. Saag MS, Powderly WG, Cloud GA, et al. Comparison of amphotericin B with fluconazole in the treatment of acute AIDS-associated cryptococcal meningitis. The NIAID Mycoses Study Group and the AIDS Clinical Trials Group. *N Engl J Med.* 1992;326(2):83–89.

10. Perfect JR, Dismukes WE, Dromer F, et al. Clinical practice guidelines for the management of cryptococcal disease: 2010 update by the Infectious Diseases Society of America. *Clin Infect Dis.* 2010;50(3):291–322.

11. Dharnidharka VR, Tejani AH, Ho PL, et al. Post-transplant lymphoproliferative disorder in the United States: young Caucasian males are at highest risk. *Am J Transplant.* 2002;2(10) 993–998.

12. Kremer, BE, Reshef R, Misleh JG, et al. Post-transplant lymphoproliferative disorder after lung transplantation: A review of 35 cases. *J Heart Lung Transplant.* 2012;31(2):296–304.

13. Trappe R, Oertel S, Leblond V, et al. German PTLD Study Group; European PTLD Network. Sequential treatment with rituximab followed by CHOP chemotherapy in adult B-cell post-transplant lymphoproliferative disorder (PTLD): the prospective international multicenter phase 2 PTLD-1 trial. *Lancet Oncology.* 2012;13(2):196–206.

14. Al-Mansoure, A, Nelson BP, Evens AM, et al. Post-transplant lymphoproliferative disease (PTLD): risk factors, diagnosis and current treatment strategies. *Curr Hematol Malig Rep.* 2013;8(3):173–183.

15. Limaye AP, Raghu G, Koelle DM, et al. High incidence of ganciclovir-resistant cytomegalovirus infection among lung transplant recipients receiving preemptive therapy. *J Infect Dis.* 2002;185(1):20–27.

16. Kotton CN, Kumar D, Caliendo AM, et al. Updated international consensus guidelines on the management of cytomegalovirus in solid-organ transplantation. *Transplantation.* 2013;96(4):333–360.

17. Razonable RR, Humar A. Cytomegalovirus in solid organ transplantation. *Am J Transplant.* 2013;13 (Suppl 4):93–106.

18. Ahmad S, Shlobin OA, Nathan SD, et al. Pulmonary complications of lung transplantation. *Chest.* 2011;139(2):402–411.

19. Snyder LD, Finlen-Copeland CA, Turbyfill WJ, et al. Cytomegalovirus pneumonitis is a risk for bronchiolitis obliterans syndrome in lung transplantation. *Am J Respir Crit Care Med.* 2010;181(12):1391–1396.

20. Minces LR, Nguyen MH, Mitsani D, et al. Ganciclovir-resistant cytomegalovirus infections among lung transplant recipients are associated with poor outcomes despite treatment with foscarnet-containing regimens. *Antimicrob Agents Chemother.* 2014;58(1):128–135.

18

Bacterial and Viral Diseases

Navitha Ramesh MD, Aloke Chakravarti MD, and Ronaldo Collo Go MD

CASE 1

A 21-year-old woman with no known medical history or prior hospitalization presents to the emergency department with complaints of shortness of breath, cough, and fever for 3 days. On physical examination, her vital signs show blood pressure of 120/80 mm Hg, heart rate of 110/min, respiratory rate of 18/min, temperature of 38.1°C, and oxygen saturation 95% on room air. She has rhonchi in the left lower lung field and chest radiography reveals left lower lobe consolidation. Laboratory evaluation shows white blood cell count of 14,000/m/μL with a left shift, hemoglobin 14 g/dL, platelets 300,000/μL, sodium 145 mEq/L, potassium 4 mEq/L, chloride 101 mEq/L, bicarbonate 28 mEq/L, blood urea nitrogen 16 mg/dL, creatinine 0.6 mg/dL, glucose 100 mg/dL. She receives a dose of ceftriaxone and azithromycin in the emergency department.

Question 1: What level of care should this patient receive?

A. Outpatient management
B. Medical/surgical floor
C. Telemetry floor
D. Intensive care unit
E. One dose of antibiotics in the emergency department

Question 2: Which of the following is the best treatment choice?

A. Ceftriaxone 1 g intramuscularly once a day
B. Azithromycin and ceftriaxone for at least 3 days and then continue to de-escalate if patient improves
C. Vancomycin and cefepime for at least 3 days and then continue to de-escalate if patient improves
D. Hold antibiotics until further testing such as Legionella urine antigen and strep urine antigen
E. Azithromycin 500 mg PO daily followed by 250 mg PO daily for 4 additional days

Question 3: What is the accurate association between antibiotic and cause of resistance?

A. Vancomycin–gyrase
B. Moxifloxacin–topoisomerase IV
C. Levofloxacin–topoisomerase IV and gyrase
D. Azithromycin–gyrase
E. Cefepime–oxacillin mediated

CASE 2

A 60-year-old man with history of insulin dependent diabetes mellitus, hypertension, chronic obstructive pulmonary disease, current everyday smoking history (one pack per day), and recent bout of influenza is admitted to the hospital for acute respiratory failure secondary to community-acquired pneumonia. Sputum and blood cultures show methicillin sensitive staphylococcus aureus. He is given 7 days of nafcillin but fails to improve. He is persistently febrile and his leukocytosis does not improve. Repeat cultures show *Staphylococcus aureus* in sputum and blood. Below are his sequential chest CT scans, 1 week apart.

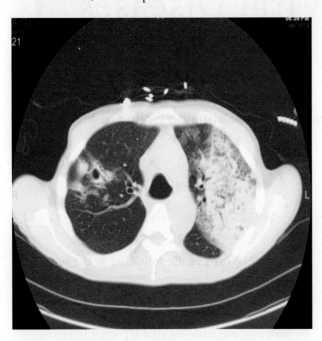

* *

CT chest 1 week later:

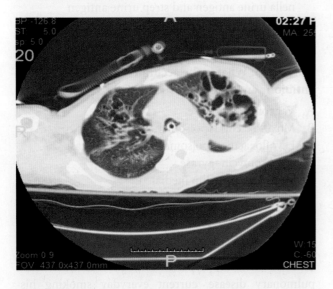

Question 1: Which of the following antibiotics would need to be initiated?

A. Cefepime
B. Linezolid
C. Vancomycin
D. Meropenem
E. Ceftazidime

Question 2: What other organism is closely related with this disease?

A. Adenovirus
B. Influenza
C. Cryptococcus
D. Pseudomonas
E. Klebsiella

Question 3: What risk factor is associated with this disease in this patient?

A. Diabetes mellitus
B. Smoking history
C. Hypertension
D. Influenza
E. Age

CASE 3

A 51-year-old obese man is admitted for delirium tremens. During his hospital stay he develops shortness of breath and is noted to have a right lower lobe opacity on chest radiograph. He is started on metronidazole 500 mg IV every 6 hours.

Question 1: Monotherapy for aspiration pneumonia with metronidazole is generally not advised because of resistance to which organism?

A. *Microaerophilic streptococcus*
B. *Enterococcus*
C. *Acinobacter*
D. *Candida*
E. *Klebsiella*

Question 2: What would be the appropriate antibiotic?

A. Clindamycin
B. Meropenem
C. Tobramycin
D. Vancomycin
E. Ampicillin

Question 3: After 1 day of antibiotics, the infiltrate on chest radiograph has disappeared. What would be the next best step?

A. Change IV antibiotics to PO
B. Discontinue all antibiotics
C. CT chest
D. Chest physiotherapy
E. Continue the same antibiotics for a total of 7 days

CASE 4

A 67-year-old man with history of COPD has been residing in a long-term acute care facility for 3 months, following a traumatic brain injury. He has required mechanical ventilation via tracheostomy, and has had four previous episodes of pneumonia that have been attributed to aspiration. He now presents with a 7-day history of temperatures up to 38.5°C, decreased responsiveness, and a white blood cell count of 9,100/μL. Tracheal secretions are unchanged, though FiO_2 requirements have increased to 50%, with a PaO_2 of 100. A portable chest x-ray shows chronic-appearing, bilateral hazy opacities. A procalcitonin level is obtained.

Question 1: Which of the following is true regarding the use of procalcitonin in this patient?

A. An elevated procalcitonin may be secondary to traumatic brain injury and not infection
B. TNF-alpha, IL-6, IL-1, and interferon gamma increase the level of procalcitonin
C. A procalcitonin level >0.5 ng/mL suggests bacterial infection
D. A procalcitonin level <0.25 ng/mL suggests bacterial infection
E. Procalcitonin can only be used inpatient

CASE 5

A 45-year-old man had a bone marrow transplantation 3 months ago.

Question 1: When would you consider varicella zoster virus infection?

A. Day 0
B. Day 15
C. Day 45
D. Day 100
E. Day 365

CASE 6

A 62-year-old woman with a history of hypertension and diabetes, and a nonhealing ulcer on the ankle for which she receives daily dressing changes from a visiting nurse at her home, is brought to the emergency department with a 3-day history of fevers, chills, lethargy, and difficulty breathing. She is arousable, but slow to respond. Her blood pressure is 104/66 mm Hg, pulse rate is 97/min and regular. Respiratory rate is 22/min, associated with rattling sound of secretions in the upper airway.

A complete blood count shows a leukocyte count of 14,800/μL, with 8% band forms. A chemistry panel discloses normal renal function. A chest radiograph shows a dense opacity in the right middle lobe. The patient is started on empiric therapy for health care associated pneumonia with vancomycin, cefepime, and levofloxacin, after blood and sputum cultures are obtained. Three days later, the sputum culture grows *pseudomonas aeruginosa*.

Question 1: What is the most appropriate next step?

A. Continue the same antibiotic regimen
B. Add tobramycin 1 mg/kg IV every 8 hours
C. Discontinue levofloxacin.
D. Continue cefepime at 2 g IV every 8 hours
E. Add polymixin

Question 2: Which option best describes the pharmacodynamic profile of cefepime?

A. Concentration-dependent
B. Time-dependent
C. AUC/MIC
D. Bacteriostatic
E. Bactericidal

CASE 7

A 30-year-old man with no known medical history presents to the pulmonary clinic with complaints of nonproductive cough, rhinorrhea, and fever for 12 days duration. His primary care doctor has treated him with anti-inflammatory agents, intranasal fluticasone, and oral antihistamines. He initially felt better for 2 days but after that he felt generalized weakness, cough, and purulent nasal secretions. Examination reveals temperature of 100°F, blood pressure of 120/90 mm Hg, heart rate of 90/min, saturating 98% on room air. He has tenderness over the left maxillary sinus on percussion and he has a yellowish mucoid secretion on the posterior pharyngeal wall. His lungs are clear to auscultation and cardiac examination is within normal limits.

Question 1: Which of the following helps in identifying patients with acute bacterial rhino sinusitis from acute viral rhino sinusitis?

A. Presence of postnasal drip
B. Temperature of 100°F
C. Duration of symptoms more than 5 days
D. New onset fever after initial improvement
E. All of the above

Question 2: What should you do next?

A. Obtain nasopharyngeal swab for culture and sensitivity
B. Obtain cultures from direct sinus aspiration
C. Start empiric amoxicillin-clavulanic acid
D. Start azithromycin
E. Obtain CT of the para-nasal sinuses

Question 3: What is the duration of the antimicrobial therapy?

A. 3 days of azithromycin
B. 5 days of trimethoprim-sulfamthoxazole
C. 7 days of amoxicillin-clavulanic acid
D. 10 days of cephalexin
E. 5 days of levofloxacin

Question 4: The adjunctive therapy for acute rhinosinusitis includes all EXCEPT:

A. Analgesics
B. Nasal irrigation with physiologic saline
C. Nasal irrigation with hypertonic saline
D. Oral decongestants
E. Intranasal corticosteroids

CASE 8

A 71-year-old man is transferred to the hospital from a nursing home for cough and fevers. He is in his usual state of health until 4 days ago when he started having a cough and difficulty breathing. He endorses worsening malaise, productive cough, nasal congestion, and dyspnea. He also complains of mild abdominal pain and anorexia. On physical examination, you note that he is a frail man, who appears tired and generally unwell. He has a low-grade fever, tachypnea, and tachycardia. Mucous membranes are dry and skin turgor is poor. Lung examination discloses biphasic wheezes bilaterally. A chest radiograph reveals faint bibasilar opacities. A rapid influenza screen is negative.

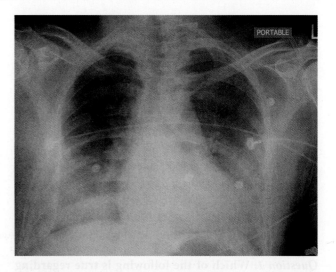

Question 1: The most likely etiology of his symptoms is:

A. Influenza B virus
B. Respiratory syncytial virus
C. Coronavirus
D. Rhinovirus
E. Parainfluenza virus

Question 2: Generally, Influenza A produces a more severe disease than RSV. In which of the following populations does RSV have a comparable morbidity and mortality?

A. 15 to 25 years of age
B. 25 to 40 years of age
C. 40 to 55 years of age
D. Greater than 55 years of age
E. Patients who have had the influenza vaccine

CASE 9

A 58-year-old woman is being evaluated in the emergency department for cough, fevers, and malaise. She complains of a cough, which is productive of yellow sputum for the past 4 days. Her symptoms began with subjective fevers, and now include the productive cough, chills, difficulty breathing, and pleuritic pain on the right side. In the ED, she has a temperature of 101.2°F, RR of 22, HR of 104, and BP of 132/76. A chest radiograph demonstrates a dense opacity in the right lower lobe. She is started on broad-spectrum antibiotics after a sputum sample is obtained for microbiological analysis, and transferred to the medical floor. On the following day the gram stain of the sputum sample discloses 8 squamous epithelial cells, and 32 PMNs, in addition to many gram-positive diplococci.

Question 1: **Which of the following is true about sputum analysis in the setting of respiratory infections?**

A. Given the number of squamous epithelial cells, specimen is likely contaminated by saliva, and cannot be interpreted

B. Given the number of host cells, this sample is highly sensitive and specific for the infective organism

C. Sputum cultures have a low sensitivity and specificity, and their use is not recommended by the IDSA

D. Sputum samples often yield more than one organism, and rarely change management

E. Sputum cultures are equally sensitive in typical and atypical pneumonias

Question 2: **A second sputum sample, which is obtained at the same time, reveals gram-positive cocci in chains. What is the most likely explanation for the differing results?**

A. Contamination of the specimen

B. A second infective organism

C. Mislabeling of specimens by hospital staff

D. Laboratory error

E. Antibiotic administration prior to obtaining samples

CASE 10

A 32-year-old man is seen at the pulmonary clinic with complaints of episodic hemoptysis, cough with yellowish sputum, fever, and poor appetite of 1-week duration. He has just returned from a business trip to Taiwan. Review of systems is negative for history of positive PPD positivity, recent incarceration, or sick contacts. He does not have any known chronic medical conditions and does not take any medications. He is afebrile with a blood pressure of 100/90, heart rate of 110 beats per minute, saturating 98% on 2-L nasal cannula. Laboratory examination is notable for white count of 12,000 with 35% eosinophils. The remainder of the liver and kidney panel appears normal. Chest radiograph shows multiple nodules and cavitations in both lungs especially in the lower lobes. Smears of the sputum are negative for acid-fast bacilli, fungi, pyogenic organisms, and malignant cells. Cultures of the sputum are also negative for *Mycobacterium tuberculosis*. Microscopic examination of the BAL shows eggs from the lung fluke.

Question 1: **What is the treatment of choice?**

A. Praziquantel

B. Rifampin, isoniazid, pyranamide, ethambutol

C. Vancomycin and cefepime

D. Albendazole

E. Ceftriaxone and azithromycin

Answers

CASE 1

Question 1: A. Outpatient management

For community-acquired pneumonia, the decision to avoid unnecessary hospital admissions is based on: (1) cost, where inpatient treatment is 25 times more expensive than outpatient treatment; (2) faster recovery times with outpatient treatments; (3) patient preference; (4) less risk of thromboembolic events; and (5) avoid super-infection from hospital-acquired bacteria.[1] Severity of illness scores such as CURB-65 (Confusion, Uremia with BUN >7, Respiratory rate >30, Blood pressure <90/60, Age >65) with a score >2 warrants ICU admission and prognostic scores such as PORT have been devised.[1] This patient has a CURB-65 score of 0 and PORT class 1, which warrants outpatient treatment.

**

Decision to admit risk class 1 to 3 would be based on a complication from pneumonia, exacerbation of disease, inability to take medications, or multiple risk factors close to threshold score. Because PSI is based on history of disease whereas CURB 65 does not, utilization of one type of validation tool might underestimate or overestimate the need for appropriate level of care.

**

For ICU admission, prognostication from CURB-65 (>2), PSI severity (IV or V), or severe CAP (any major or three minor) can be used.

Severe Community-Acquired Pneumonia Criteria
Major: (1) Invasive mechanical ventilation (1) Septic shock
Minor: (1) Respiratory rate $\geq$30 bpm (2) PaO$_2$/FiO$_2$ $\leq$250 (3) Multilobar infiltrates (4) Confusion (5) Uremia (BUN $\geq$20 mg/dL) (6) Platelets <100,000 cells/mm^3 (7) WBC <400 cells/mm^3 (8) Temp <36°C (9) Hypotension requiring fluid resuscitation

Question 2: E. Azithromycin 500 mg PO daily followed by 250 mg PO daily for 4 additional days

Routine microbiological studies should not delay administrating appropriate antibiotics on patients on outpatient CAP treatment although it is appropriate in the event of nonresponding pneumonia. The only randomized comparing empirical antibiotics versus microbial targeted antibiotics show no difference in survival.[1] Urine antigen of streptococcus and legionella can remain positive for a few weeks despite antibiotic treatment. Rapid testing for influenza should be performed in the appropriate clinical testing.

**

Antibiotic treatment is usually continued for minimum of 5 days, longer duration in pseudomonal infections. In the outpatient setting, the most commonly encountered pathogens are *Streptococcus pneumoniae, Mycoplasma pneumoniae, Haemophilus influenzae, Chlamydophila pneumoniae*, and respiratory viruses. In the inpatient setting, the same outpatient pathogens with *Legionella* and aspiration are considerations. In the ICU setting, *S. pneumoniae, Staphylococcus aureus, Legionella*, gram-negative bacilli and *H. Influenzae* are included.

COMMUNITY ACQUIRED PNEUMONIA OUTPATIENT AND INPATIENT ANTIBIOTICS

Outpatient treatment:	
Healthy and risk factors for drug resistant *S. pneumoniae*	Macrolide or doxycycline
Comorbids such as chronic heart, lung, live, renal disease, DM, alcoholism, malignancies, asplenia, immunosuppressant conditions, antimicrobials within 3 months, or high rates of macrolide resistant *S. pneumoniae*	Fluoroquinolone or beta-lactam and macrolide
Inpatient treatment:	Beta-lactam (cefotaxime, ceftriaxone, or ampicillin-sulbactam) plus azithromycin or doxycycline; ertapenem in certain patients; or fluoroquinolone. Transition to PO antibiotics after 72 hours and can be discharge on that day if there no other associated diseases or complications.
ICU treatment: For Pseudomonas	Beta-lactam plus azithromycin or fluoroquinolone; for pseudomonal coverage antipneumococcal, antipseudomonal beta-lactam (piperacillin-tazobactam, cefepime, imipenem or meropenem) plus quinolone (750-mg dose) Antipneumococcal and antipseudomonal beta-lactam plus quinolone (ciprofloxacin or levofloxacin at 750-mg dose) duration usually for 14 days or beta-lactam plus aminoglycoside plus azithromycin or beta-lactam plus aminoglycoside and antipneumococcal fluoroquinolone or aztreonam for penicillin allergy
For MRSA	Add vancomycin or linezolid

Question 3: C. Levofloxacin–topoisomerase IV and gyrase

Antibiotic resistance can lead to infection progression. For macrolides, low-level resistance ($MIC_{90} = 0.5–8$ ug/mL) is secondary to bacterial efflux pump mechanisms via mefE gene and M phenotypes. High-level resistance ($MIC_{90} \geq 16$ ug/mL) is secondary to macrolide binding site (ermAMgene MLSB phenotype). In fluoroquinolones, resistance is secondary to mutations in quinolone resistance-deforming regions (QRDR), topoisomerase IV, or DNA gyrase. One gene target leads to low-level resistance whereas multigene leads to high-level resistance. Ciprofloxacin resistance is secondary to topoisomerase mutation; moxifloxacin resistance is secondary to gyrase mutation; and levofloxacin resistance is secondary to topoisomerase and gyrase mutations.

CASE 2

Question 1: B. Linezolid

The patient has necrotizing pneumonia from methicillin sensitive staphylococcus aureus producing panton-valentine leukocidin (PVL) endotoxin. Previously thought to be restricted to MRSA, PVL forms pores in membranes of infected cells. Monotherapy might eradicate the bacteria but has no effect on the endotoxin. Linezolid can eradicate the bacteria and the endotoxin. Other options include dual regimen of penicillin or vancomycin with clindamycin or rifampin. Antibiotic duration is from 4 to 8 weeks. If improperly treated, mortality is 70%.[2,3]

Question 2: E. Klebsiella

Other causes of necrotizing pneumonia include *streptococcus*, *enterococcus*, *tuberculosis*, certain fungal infections, and *acinobacter*. *Klebsiella* has been documented in literature to cause the more severe form of necrotizing pneumonia called pulmonary gangrene.[4,5] Necrosis of the alveoli leads to air seeping outside of the airspaces, leading to cavitary-like appearance. Patients generally have copious respiratory secretions which in part have elements of sloughed off pulmonary parenchyma.

Question 3: D. Influenza

For MSSA-associated necrotizing pneumonia, a recent bout of influenza is an important risk factor. The other answer choices do not necessarily predispose patients to necrotizing pneumonia.

CASE 3

Question 1: A. *Microaerophilic streptococcus*

Pathogens in an aspiration pneumonia can include *bacteroides*, *prevotella*, *fusobacterium*, and *peptostreptococcus*.

Question 2: A. Clindamycin

The other antibiotics will not be able to cover the oral flora, particularly in this patient with alcohol abuse history.

Question 3: **B. Discontinue all antibiotics**

The patient most likely has aspiration pneumonitis and it would appropriate to discontinue antibiotics on a patient that is hemodynamically stable. Despite clinical improvement, pneumonia can take at least 2 weeks to improve radiographically. Although repeat chest radiograph is advised, it is still debatable whether pneumonic consolidation can evolve after hydration since this has not been in shown in animal models and in theory.

CASE 4

Question 1: **C. A procalcitonin level >0.5 ng/mL suggests bacterial infection**

Procalcitonin (PCT) is a precursor to calcitonin and serum levels increase after inflammatory states. They have been used to help discriminate bacterial causes of SIRS, bacterial superinfections in patients with known viral disease, gauge patients who would benefit from antibiotics and their duration, and have prognostic implications.[6-10] It is believed that IL-1B, TNF-alpha, and IL-6 increase PCT as a response to bacterial infections and interferon gamma, which is excreted after viral infections, suppress it.[8] It has an interesting kinetic profile in that it is not affected by corticosteroids and the levels increase 6 to 12 hours after stimulation and decreased daily by 50% with effective antibiotic treatment.[8] It has become a desirable option because of the limitations of cultures via duration, contamination, and colonization and risks of *Clostridium difficile* with excessive use of antibiotics.[8]

* *

In general, PCT levels <0.1 ng/mL exclude the diagnosis of bacterial infection. PCT levels of 0.1 to 0.25 warrant the withholding of antibiotic therapy, except for at-risk populations. PCT >0.5 rule in the diagnosis of bacterial infection and warrant antibiotics. Levels should be repeated 6 to 24 hours and/or daily. If PCT levels

decrease to <0.25, it might indicate de-escalation of antibiotic therapy.

* *

Another important factor to PCT is the presence of false-positives, such as in hepatitis C, severe trauma, burns, thoracic or abdominal surgery, and multiorgan failure. The PCT levels begin to fall within 24 to 48 hours.

* *

Prognostication is possible with the PCT level—in CAP, HCAP, as well as in the setting of ventilator-associated pneumonia (though the data suggests that the PCT elevations are generally lower in VAP). Higher initial levels, as well as levels above 0.5 ng/mL at day 7, even in the setting of appropriate medical management, are associated with increased mortality. In the appropriate clinical context, procalcitonin provides useful supportive data. PCT levels have also been shown to increase the sensitivity and specificity of clinical assessment scales such as the Pneumonia Severity Index and the Clinical Pulmonary Infection Score. Multiple validated prognostic scales, including the APACHE-2 Score, and the SOFA Score have directly correlated with PCT levels.

CASE 5

Question 1: **D. Day 100**

Infection is the most common cause of pulmonary complication after bone marrow transplantation. During the period before engraftment (0–30 days), profound neutropenia and mucosal damage occur. This makes patients vulnerable to fungal, bacterial, and RSV pneumonias. During the period after engraftment (31–100 days), there is impairment of both cellular and humoral immunity that predisposes the patient to mainly CMV and RSV infections.[11] During the late posttransplantation period (>100 days), infection in the absence of graft-versus-host disease is uncommon because of the relative normal immunologic function at this phase.[11]

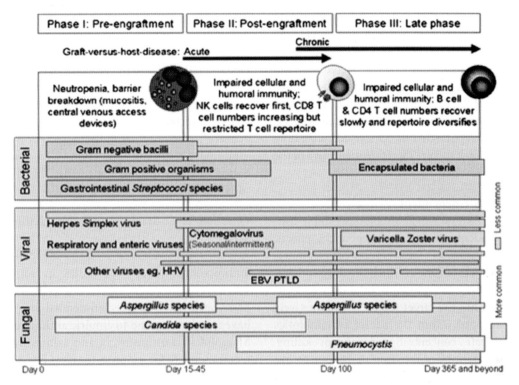

Figure 18-1   Phases of opportunistic infections among allogeneic HCT recipients Abbreviations: EBV, Epstein-Barr virus; HHV6, human herpesvirus 6; PTLD, posttransplant lymphoproliferative disease. (Reproduced with permission from Tomblyn M, Chiller T, Einsele H, et al. Guidelines for preventing infectious complications among hematopoietic cell transplantation recipients: A global perspective. *Biol Blood Marrow Transplant.* 2009;15(10):1143–1238.)

CASE 6

Question 1: D. Continue cefepime at 2 g IV every 8 hours

Given the history of wound care at home, this patient meets criteria for healthcare-associated pneumonia (HCAP).

* *

HCAP is defined by one of the following:
- Acute hospitalization for 2 days within the last 90 days
- Having resided in a nursing home or LTAC facility within 30 days
- Receipt of IV infusion therapy within the last 30 days
- Wound care at home within 30 days
- Treatment in a dialysis clinic within 30 days
- Close contact with a known multidrug-resistant infection[12]

* *

Subsets of HCAP include ventilator-associated pneumonia (VAP), which is one that presents on or after ventilator day 3, and hospital-acquired pneumonia (HAP), which presents >48 hours after admission. VAP can be prevented with the implementation of "ventilator bundles." These consist of measures such as head-of-bed elevation and chlorhexidine decontamination of the oropharynx. Antibiotic decontamination of the GI tract has also shown efficacy. The classification of pneumonia aids in the predicted pathogens, and the most likely efficacious treatment. While community-acquired pneumonia is most often due to gram-positive organisms, HCAP is associated with a higher prevalence of gram-negative and anaerobic organisms, as well as drug-resistant organisms.

* *

Recommended therapy for HCAP includes two antimicrobial agents with activity against *Pseudomonas aeruginosa* such as both levofloxacin and cefepime. Both of these drugs should be continued, given the presence of pseudomonas in the sputum culture. Tobramycin does not need to be added, as levofloxacin would provide the adequate coverage. As with all antibiotics, the penetration into the target tissue must be considered. In cases of pseudomonal pneumonia, cefepime must be administered at a dose of 2 g every 8 hours in order to achieve the necessary concentration within the lung parenchyma. Doses of 1 g of cefepime do not achieve adequate lung tissue concentrations, and are therefore ineffective in the treatment of pneumonia.

Question 2: B. Time-dependent

It is important to know which antibiotics exhibit concentration-dependent effects, time-dependent effects, and postantibiotic effects.[13,14] The efficacy of cefepime is related to proportion of time at which the drug concentration remains above the minimum inhibitory concentration (MIC) within the target tissue.[13,14] Alternatively fluoroquinolones are within the subset of antibiotics which demonstrate concentration-dependent killing, requiring concentrations of the drug up to four to five times higher than the MIC within the target tissue.[13,14] A third subset of antibiotics (which includes macrolides) demonstrates a sustained postantibiotic effect, which can be measured by observing the AUC/MIC rather than the peak concentration itself.[13,14]

* *

In the case of cefepime in pseudomonal pneumonia, it becomes crucial to ensure that the drug penetrates the lung parenchyma with a concentration above the MIC of pseudomonas, as well as for an effective duration. As a result, the concentration of 2 g per dose, with an 8-hour dosing interval (rather than 12 hours) is advised. Pharmacokinetic and pharmacodynamic studies not only suggest outcome benefits with the more frequent dosing interval, but also extend the infusion time of the dose from 30 minutes to 4 hours.

CASE 7

Question 1: D. New onset fever after initial improvement

Acute rhinosinusitis usually lasts for less than 4 weeks and the most common cause is a virus.[15] Viral rhinosinusitis typically resolves in less than 10 days.

* *

The pointers toward a bacterial rhinosinusitis include: (A) Persistent symptoms or signs compatible with

acute rhinosinusitis, lasting for more than 10 days without any evidence of clinical improvement; (B) Onset with severe symptoms or signs of high fever (>39°C [102°F]) and purulent nasal discharge or facial pain lasting for at least 3 to 4 consecutive days at the beginning of illness; and (C) worsening symptoms or signs characterized by the new onset of fever, headache, or increase in nasal discharge following a typical viral upper respiratory infection (URI) that lasted 5 to 6 days and were initially improving. This is described as "double sickening."[15]

Question 2: C. Start empiric amoxicillin-clavulanic acid

Amoxicillin-clavulanate is recommended as empiric antimicrobial therapy for ABRS in adults. Cultures obtained by direct sinus aspiration rather than by nasopharyngeal swab are recommended in patients who have failed to respond to empiric antimicrobial therapy. Macrolides (clarithromycin and azithromycin) are not recommended for empiric therapy due to high rates of resistance among *S. pneumoniae* (>30%). Trimethoprim-sulfamethoxazole (TMP/SMX) is not recommended for empiric therapy because of high rates of resistance among both *S. pneumoniae* and *H. influenzae* (>30–40%).

* *

Routine antimicrobial coverage for *S. aureus* or MRSA during initial empiric therapy is not recommended.

Question 3: C. 7 days of amoxicillin-clavulanic acid

The recommended duration of therapy for uncomplicated acute bacterial rhinosinusitis in adults is 5 to 7 days.

Question 4: D. Oral decongestants

According to the current guidelines, oral or nasal decongestants and antihistaminics are not recommended as adjunctive therapy for acute bacterial rhinosinusitis.[15]

CASE 8

Question 1: B. Respiratory syncytial virus

RSV is the second most common cause of community-acquired viral pneumonia in the adult population, and is attributable to approximately 10,000 deaths annually.[16,17] In contrast to *Influenza* virus, which is the most common, RSV has a more gradual onset of symptoms.[17] In addition, nasal congestion, wheezing, and gastrointestinal symptoms are common. As with influenza, radiographic evidence of RSV pneumonia is neither sensitive, nor specific. Initial diagnosis is mainly clinical, with laboratory analysis as a confirmatory test. Rapid screens for RSV are insensitive, and RT-PCR of the nucleic acid, though sensitive and specific, is not widely available. A fourfold increase in RSV-specific IgG supports the diagnosis. There is no specific antiviral therapy for RSV, and treatment is mainly supportive.

* *

Influenza virus is the most common cause of community-acquired viral pneumonia, and has been implicated in pandemics over the past century. The frequent antigenic drifts of the hemagglutinin and neuraminidase are responsible for the seasonal epidemics of the disease. Diagnosis is supported by a rapid influenza antigen test, which is only 50% to 60% sensitive for the antigen but 90% specific. Therefore, in the appropriate clinical presentation – rapid onset of fevers, cough, and myalgias – appropriate therapy should be instituted.[16-20] If the patient presents within 48 hours of onset, antiviral therapy with zanamivir, or oseltamivir should be initiated. Zanamivir should be avoided in patients with underlying COPD or asthma, as the parainfluenza virus is known to cause croup and epiglottitis in the pediatric population. However, the virus is also detected in as many as 14% of patients with viral pneumonia, notably in cases of fatality, where it was perhaps a precursor to a more serious pulmonary infection. Coronavirus and rhinovirus are the most common causes of the common cold. In the elderly and immunocompromised population they have been shown to cause pneumonia. Treatment of these types of community-acquired viral pneumonia is supportive.

Question 2: D. Greater than 55 years of age

Cohorts of patients more than 55 years of age have been shown to have a high incidence of viral pneumonia due to RSV.[17] Particularly in patients who have cardiac disease and are functional at NYHA class 2 or higher, or have pulmonary disease with secondary activity restriction or long-term medication use, the burden of RSV infection is higher. In this population, in comparison to Influenza A, the hospital length of stay, admission to the ICU, and need for mechanical ventilation is similar. Notably, in patients admitted from a long-term care facility, or in the years when the Influenza vaccine is particularly efficacious, the mortality is higher than that of Influenza A.

CASE 9

Question 1: B. Given the number of host cells, this sample is highly sensitive and specific for the infective organism

A sputum culture with less than 10 squamous epithelial cells and more than 25 PMNs is considered an adequate sample, and as such is highly sensitive and specific for the causative organism. The IDSA recommends the use of sputum gram stain and culture, while the ATS does not.[1] For several decades, there has been controversy surrounding the clinical utility of this diagnostic test. Indeed, it is difficult to obtain an adequate sample—one showing minimal contamination with saliva, and an appropriate immune response. A majority of the study designs evaluating sputum analysis have used a statistical protocol wherein an inadequate sample is recorded as a false-negative, lowering the sensitivity of the test. Typical pneumonias are associated with productive cough, whereas atypical pneumonias are classically associated with a dry cough, which is corroborated in studies, which show that the latter are cultured less often. A recent study, which adjusted for the actual collection of a sputum sample, and then adjust for its adequacy and clinical utility, found this disparity in 30% to 50% of patients with atypical pneumonia. However, recent data suggests that when an adequate sample is obtained, a single pathogen can be identified in <u>83% of cases</u>. A majority of these are *S. pneumoniae* and *H. influenzae*, yielding a positive-predictive value for typical pathogens at above 90%. In combination with tests for specific antigens in body fluids, an adequate and uncontaminated sputum specimen is of high clinical utility.

Question 2: D. Laboratory error

Although not explicitly studied, a not insignificant degree of inter-observer variability exists in the interpretation of gram stains. A sensitivity and specificity as low as 15% and 11% respectively has been reported in gram stain interpretation when compared to reference standard (i.e., final cultures).[21] Pretest probability and clinical correlation remain essential in the interpretation of sputum gram stains.

CASE 10

Question 1: A. Praziquantel

Pulmonary paragonimiasis is a food-borne parasitic disease caused by the lung fluke (trematode) especially *Paragonimus westermani*.[22,24] Humans, through consumption of undercooked freshwater crabs or crayfish, acquire *Paragonimus*. Immature forms migrate through the duodenal wall, peritoneal cavity, and diaphragm to become encapsulated and mature within the pulmonary parenchyma. When the encapsulated cyst bursts, eggs are extruded into the bronchioles and subsequently are coughed up and swallowed, passing back into the environment with the stool.

* *

The initial illness is characterized by diarrhea, abdominal pain, urticaria, fever, malaise, and eosinophilia that last from days to weeks, when the immature flukes are migrating. As larvae penetrate the diaphragm and migrate within the pleural cavity, pleuritic chest pain may develop, occasionally associated with pleural effusion and pneumothorax. Pulmonary manifestations include dyspnea, cough, and hemoptysis. Leukocytosis with prominent eosinophilia and transient pulmonary infiltrate occurs during this time. Signs and symptoms due to the involvement of ectopic locations can also be seen at this stage.

* *

Praziquantel (75 mg/kg/day in three divided doses, for 3 days) is generally considered the treatment of choice for all species of paragonimiasis.

REFERENCES

1. Mandell LA, Wunderink RG, Anzueto A, et al. Infectious Diseases Society of America/American Thoracic Society consensus guidelines on the management of community-acquired pneumonia in adults. *Clin Infect Dis.* 2007;44: S27–S72.
2. Noah MA, Dawrant M, Faulkner GM, et al. Panton-valentine leukocidin expressing staphylococcus aureus pneumonia managed with extracorporeal membrane oxygenation: experience and outcome. *Crit Care Med.* 2010;38(11): 2250–2253.
3. Tsai YF, Ku YH. Necrotizing pneumonia: A rare complication of pneumonia requiring special consideration. *Curr Opin Pulm Med.* 2012;18(3):246–252.
4. Hammond JMJ, Lyddell C, Potgieter PD, et al. Severe pneumococcal pneumonia complicated by massive pulmonary gangrene. *Chest.* 1993;104:1610–1612.
5. Chen CH, Huang WC, Chen TY, et al. Massive necrotizing pneumonia with pulmonary gangrene. *Ann Thorac Surg.* 2009;87(1):310–311.
6. Schuetz P, Briel M, Mueller B. Algorithms to guide antibiotic therapy in respiratory tract infections. *JAMA.* 2013;309(7):717–718.
7. Schuetz P, Raad I, Amin DN. Using procalcitonin-guided algorithms to improve antimicrobial therapy in ICU patients with respiratory infections and sepsis. *Curr Opin Crit Care.* 2013;19(5):453–460.
8. Schuetz P, Amin DN, Greenwald JL. Role of procalcitonin in managing adult patients with respiratory tract infections. *Chest.* 2012;141(4):1063–1073.
9. Bloos F, Marshall JC, Dellinger RP, et al. Multinational, observational study of procalcitonin in ICU patients with pneumonia requiring mechanical ventilation: A multicenter observational study. *Crit Care.* 2011;15(2):R88.
10. Charles PE, Kus E, Aho S. Serum procalcitonin for the early recognition of nosocomial infection in the critically Ill patients: A preliminary report. *BMC Infect Dis.*2009;9:49.
11. Tomblyn M, Chiller T, Einsele H, et al. Guidelines for preventing infectious complications among hematopoietic cell transplant recipients. *Biol Blood Marrow Transplant.* 2009;15:1143–1238.
12. Infectious Diseases Society of America/American Thoracic Society. Guidelines for the management of adults with hospital-acquired, ventilator-associated, and healthcare-associated pneumonia. *Am J Respir Crit Care Med.* 2005;171(4):388–416.
13. Bauer KA, West JE, O'brien JM, et al. Extended-infusion cefepime reduces mortality in patients with pseudomonas aeruginosa infections. *Antimicrob Agents and Chemother.* 2013;57(7):2907–2912.
14. Levison ME. Pharmacodynamics of antimicrobial drugs. *Infect Dis Clin North Am.* 2004;18(3):451–465.
15. Chow AW, Benninger MS, Brook I, et al. IDSA clinical practice guidelines for acute bacterial rhinosinusitis in children and adults. *Clin Infec Dis.* 2012;54(8):1–41.
16. Falsey AR. Community-acquired viral pneumonia. *Clin Geriatr Med.* 2007;23(3):535–552.
17. Falsey AR, Hennessey PA, Formica MA, et al. Respiratory syncytial virus infection in elderly and high-risk adults. *N Engl J Med.* 2005;352(17):1749–1759.
18. Mitchell MD, Mikkelsen ME, Umscheid CA, et al. A systematic review to inform institutional decisions about the use of extracorporeal membrane oxygenation during the H1N1 influenza pandemic. *Crit Care Med.* 2010;38(6): 1398–1404.
19. Myles P, Nguyen-Van-Tam JS, Semple MG, et al. Differences between asthmatics and nonasthmatics hospitalised with influenza a infection. *Eur Respir J.* 2013;41(4): 824–831.
20. Polakowski LL, Sandhu SK, Martin DB, et al. Chart-confirmed Guillain-Barre Syndrome after 2009 H1N1 influenza vaccination among the medicare population, 2009–2010. *Am J Epidemiol.* 2013;178(6):962–973.
21. Rosón B, Carratalà J, Verdaguer R, et al. Prospective study of the usefulness of sputum gram stain in the initial approach to community acquired pneumonia requiring hospitalization. *Clin Infect Dis.* 2000;31(4):869–867.
22. Haswell-Elkins MR, Elkins DB. Lung and liver flukes. In: Leslie C, Albert B, Max S, eds. *Topley and Wilson's Microbiology and Microbial Infections.* 9th ed. Vol. V. New York, NY: Oxford University Press; 1998:507–520.
23. Johnson RJ, Jong EC, Dunning SB, et al. Paragonimiasis: Diagnosis and the use of praziquantel in treatment. *Rev Infect Dis.* 1985;7:200–206.
24. Toscano C, Hai YS. Paragonimiasis and tuberculosis: Diagnostic confusion: A review of the literature. *Trop Dis Bull.* 1995;92:R1–R27.

19

Mycobacterial Diseases

Michael Bergman MD and Ronaldo Collo Go MD

CASE 1

A 30-year-old man from Kentucky recently moved to New York City for work. He had a history of asthma on albuterol as needed and 2 weeks ago finished oral prednisone 10 mg PO for 7 days as prescribed by his primary care physician. For hospital preemployment, he had a TST and an unremarkable chest radiograph. His PCP read the TST as 4 mm induration and 15 mm erythema and referred the patient to you.

Question 1: What would be the next step?

A. Start isoniazid 5 mg/kg/d to max of 300 g or 15 g/kg biweekly to max of 900 g for 6 to 9 months
B. Start rifampin, isoniazid, pyrazinamide, ethambutol
C. Order sputum AFB
D. Order interferon-gamma release assay
E. Do nothing

Question 2: Upon further inquiry, you found out he is HIV positive and you decide to evaluate his TST which shows a 4-mm induration and 15-mm erythema. What would be your interpretation of his PCP's findings?

A. He still has a negative TST
B. He has a positive TST but should be referred for IGRA
C. Repeat TST in 4 weeks
D. Rifampin 10 mg/kg for 4 months or rifampin with pyrazinamide daily for 2 months
E. Tuberculosis genotype

Question 3: Which of the following is NOT a preferred treatment regimen for latent tuberculosis?

A. Rifampin 900 mg twice weekly for 6 to 9 months
B. Rifampin plus pyrazinamide daily for 2 months
C. Rifampin 300 mg daily for 9 months
D. Rifampin 600 mg daily for 4 months
E. Rifampin 900 mg plus rifapentine 900 mg once weekly for 12 weeks

CASE 2

A 30-year-old man is referred to you for right sided pleural effusion. He has recently immigrated from China and has been complaining of fevers, night sweats, and cough with blood-streaked sputum. His CXR shows right-sided pleural effusion. A thoracentesis is performed and almost all of the fluid is removed.

Question 1: Based on his clinical symptoms and radiograph, what can you infer?

A. He probably has primary tuberculosis
B. He can either have primary or postprimary tuberculosis
C. He has influenza
D. A TST will help determine whether he has an infection from a mycobacterium
E. He has community acquired pneumonia and should be treated with ceftriaxone and azithromycin or levoquin for 5 days

Question 2: **Sputum smears have been negative for AFB. In addition to a thoracentesis, what would aide in the diagnosis?**

A. Sputum for bacterial and viral cultures

B. Pleural culture

C. Pleural biopsy

D. Adenosine deaminase

E. PCR

Question 3: **He informs you that he recently took levofloxacin for 7 days for his symptoms. What would be the next best step?**

A. Rifampin, isoniazid, pyrazinamide, ethambutol, levofloxacin

B. Rifampin, isoniazid, pyrazinamide, ethambutol

C. Start rifampin, isoniazid, pyrazinamide

D. Surgery

E. None of the above

CASE 3

A 39-year-old man from the United States presented to the hospital with fever to 102.1°F, cough with yellow-green sputum, and scant hemoptysis mixed with sputum. He was recently incarcerated for the past 5 years and was released 2 months ago. One week ago, he saw his primary care physician who gave him a 5-day course of azithromycin which did not provide relief. A TST done at that time produced a 12-mm area of induration. On admission, he was placed in respiratory isolation after chest imaging revealed a left upper lobe cavitary lesion. Serial daily sputum samples for AFB were negative. A subsequent bronchoscopy with BAL for AFB and culture were also negative. Eight days into the hospitalization, this patient remains with fevers to 101.5°F, persistent cough with intermittent scant hemoptysis, and vague left-sided anterior chest pain. All AFB smears and cultures remain negative.

Question 1: **What is the best next step in treatment for this patient?**

A. Repeat bronchoscopy with transbronchial biopsies

B. Start broad spectrum antimicrobial treatment to cover gram-negative, gram-positive, and anaerobic organisms

C. Start treatment with rifampin, isoniazid, pyrazinamide, and ethambutol

D. Await culture results prior to initiation of antituberculous treatment

E. Observe off treatment

Question 2: **After initiation of rifampin, isoniazid, pyrazinamide, and ethambutol, which of the following is FALSE regarding monitoring during treatment?**

A. Drug-induced hepatitis is common and liver-function tests should be monitored throughout the course of therapy

B. Mild gastrointestinal symptoms are common in patients taking this standard four-drug regimen

C. New or persistent fever while on this four-drug regimen could represent a drug fever

D. Drug–drug interactions involving rifampin are rare and dose adjustments are rarely necessary

E. All four drugs may cause a drug rash

Question 3: **Which of the following is a true statement regarding the role of surgery for active tuberculosis?**

A. Surgical biopsy of the lung or pleura may be useful in the diagnosis of active tuberculosis

B. Mediastinoscopy is useful in the diagnosis of thoracic lymph node involvement by *Mycobacterium tuberculosis*

C. Surgery plays an important role in the management of tuberculosis with bone and joint involvement

D. Surgery may play an important role in the treatment of MDR and XDR strains of M. tuberculosis

E. All of the above

CASE 4

A 71-year-old woman with a past medical history of essential hypertension, hyperlipidemia, and breast cancer status post bilateral mastectomy with breast reconstruction presents to the outpatient pulmonary clinic with cough productive of yellow sputum for 4 months. She denies chest pain or hemoptysis but has noticed a 10-lb unintentional weight loss since the onset of symptoms. She also reports intermittent low-grade fevers without chills or rigors and denies other constitutional symptoms and night sweats. She has had no sick contacts and has not had recent travel outside the United States. Her internist has given her one course of azithromycin 2 months ago and another course of levofloxacin 1 month ago with minimal relief of symptoms. She never receive neoadjuvant or adjuvant radiotherapy for her previous breast cancer. Temperature is 100.9°F, respiratory rate 18, heart rate 88 bpm, and SaO$_2$ 95% on room air. On examination, she is generally well appearing and in no distress. Notable is thin stature and moderate kyphoscoliosis. Her heart exam is normal and lung exam reveals bilateral inspiratory wet rhonchi with bronchial breath sounds anteriorly. There is no peripheral edema or jugular venous distension. Laboratory studies are significant for a hemoglobin of 10.2 g/dL and white blood cell count of 12,300/μL.

* *

A chest CT is shown:

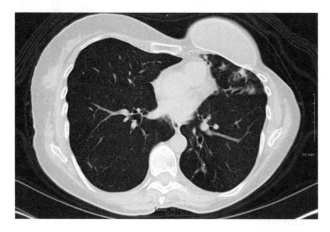

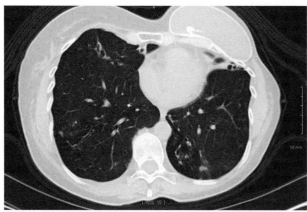

Question 1: Which of the following is adequate in making the diagnosis of mycobacterium avium-intracellulare complex (MAC) in this patient?

A. One induced sputum specimen with confirmed acid-fast bacilli smear and cultures confirming MAC
B. Two expectorated sputum specimens with confirmed acid-fast bacilli smear and cultures confirming MAC
C. One bronchial wash or lavage specimen with confirmed acid-fast bacilli smear and culture confirming MAC
D. One transbronchial biopsy demonstrating granulomatous inflammation and positive MAC culture and one bronchial lavage or sputum specimen with a positive MAC culture
E. B, C, and D

Question 2: Which of the following presentations is NOT typical for a primary infection with MAC?

A. A 74-year-old thin postmenopausal Caucasian woman with essential hypertension and pectus excavatum who presents with right middle lobe and lingular bronchiectasis, chronic cough, and low-grade fevers
B. A 38-year-old man with HIV and a CD4+ T-lymphocyte number of 22/μL who presents with low-grade fevers, weight loss, hepatosplenomegaly, anemia, and diffuse lymphadenopathy
C. A 44-year-old man who is a heavy smoker and history of ethanol abuse presents with high fevers, cough with mild hemoptysis, a 15-lb weight loss, and a left upper lobe cavity
D. A 68-year-old heavy smoker with moderate COPD who is admitted with frequent COPD exacerbations and a chronic cough productive of yellow-green sputum
E. A 32-year-old woman with no medical history who frequently uses hot tubs who presents with 4 months of chronic cough and 2 weeks of chest discomfort and worsening dyspnea on exertion

Question 3: Which of the following is an appropriate treatment regimen for MAC?

A. A patient with nodular MAC disease treated with clarithromycin, ethambutol, rifampin, and pyrazinamide
B. A patient with fibrocavitary MAC disease treated with azithromycin, rifampin, ethambutol, and amikacin
C. A patient with Lady Windermere's disease treated with clarithromycin, azithromycin, ethambutol, and rifampin
D. An HIV+ patient with disseminated MAC infection treated with azithromycin, ethambutol, and streptomycin
E. A patient with hypersensitivity pneumonitis secondary to MAC exposure treated with prednisone 10 mg daily for 1 week

CASE 5

A 49-year-old African American man presents to the hospital with 3 weeks of intermittent fevers, chills, and cough productive of green sputum. He endorses dull anterior chest discomfort with cough and a diminished appetite associated with an unintentional 8-lb weight loss. He denies night sweats or rash. On admission, his temperature is 101.4°F, heart rate 111, and oxygen saturation 93% on 4 liters supplemental oxygen. Examination is significant for right-sided rhonchi without wheezing.

A chest CT is shown:

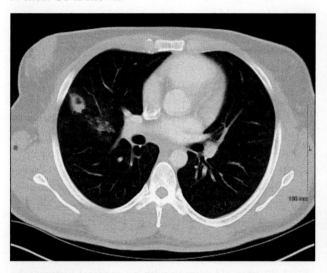
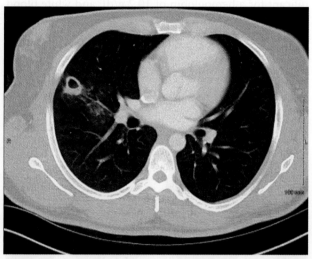

The patient is admitted to the hospital and placed on respiratory isolation in a negative pressure room.

Question 1: Which of the following is the best way of distinguishing tuberculosis from other causes of cavitary lung disease?

A. PCR

B. Sputum induction with AFB staining with inhaled hypertonic saline

C. Bronchoscopy with transbronchial biopsy of the lesion and BAL for cell count, acid-fast staining, and cultures

D. TST

E. Quantiferon gold assay

CASE 6

A 65-year-old man with a previous history of reactivation tuberculosis 30 years ago after being incarcerated, diet controlled type 2 diabetes mellitus, and history of tongue cancer 15 years ago status-post glossectomy, radiotherapy, and tracheostomy without disease recurrence now presents to the hospital with a 6-day history of intermittent fevers and chills. He also reports 3 days of night sweats and poor appetite, although denies significant weight loss. He has had yellow-green sputum production with scant mixed fresh blood without clots. He denies chest pain or pleurisy. He has not had recent travel outside the United States and does not report sick contacts. His examination is significant for warm and flushed skin, tachycardia without audible cardiac murmurs, and

bilateral rhonchi and right upper posterior bronchial breath sounds.

**

A chest x-ray is shown:

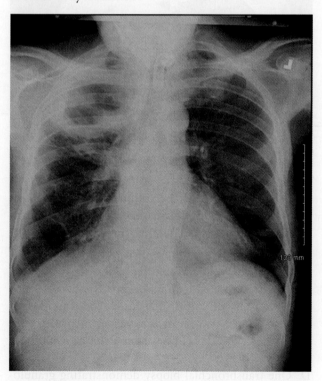

A subsequent chest CT reveals scattered tree-in-bud opacities and a right upper lobe cavity without an air fluid level.

* *

His white blood cell count is 18,900/μL with a differential count of 82% neutrophils, 16% lymphocytes, 2% monocytes, and no bands. Blood cultures are negative and two expectorated sputum samples grow *Mycobacterium kansasii.*

Question 1: What is the next step?

A. Proceed with bronchoscopy for BAL and transbronchial biopsy

B. Begin treatment with rifampin, ethambutol, and isoniazid to complete a 9-month total course of treatment

C. Begin treatment with rifampin, ethambutol, and isoniazid to complete a minimum of an 18-month total course of treatment and with a minimum of 12 months of negative expectorated sputum samples

D. Begin treatment with rifampin, ethambutol, and isoniazid for 6 months

E. Repeat chest CT

CASE 7

A 36-year-old man with a history of cystic fibrosis presents to the emergency department with a chief complaint of hemoptysis. He has previously been diagnosed with cystic fibrosis 5 years prior to his current presentation after referral from his PMD for recurrent sinopulmonary infections. Since diagnosis, he has had two episodes of hemoptysis caused by bronchial artery bleeding status-post embolization on both occasions. He has been compliant to his outpatient treatment regiment, which includes inhaled dornase alfa, inhaled tobramycin, and airway clearance treatments. He has not been hospitalized in the past 1 year, has not had recent travel, and has not been exposed to new sick contacts. For the past 1 month he has noticed intermittent fevers, some reported as high as 102°F, associated with increased yellow-green sputum production that has not responded to his current treatment regimen. He has noticed unspecified weight loss and generalized malaise. Over the past 2 days he has noticed occasional teaspoon-sized hemoptysis when he vigorously coughs. After conferring with his outpatient CF physician, he was referred to the ED for further evaluation. In the ED, his respiratory rate was 22, SaO$_2$ 96% on room air, and temperature 101.2°F. He is generally ill appearing but not toxic. Lung examination is significant for scattered wet rhonchi with a focus of bronchial breath sounds and squeaks over the posterior right upper lung field. His leukocyte count is 16,900/μL with a differential count of 92% neutrophils.

* *

Selected chest CT images are shown:

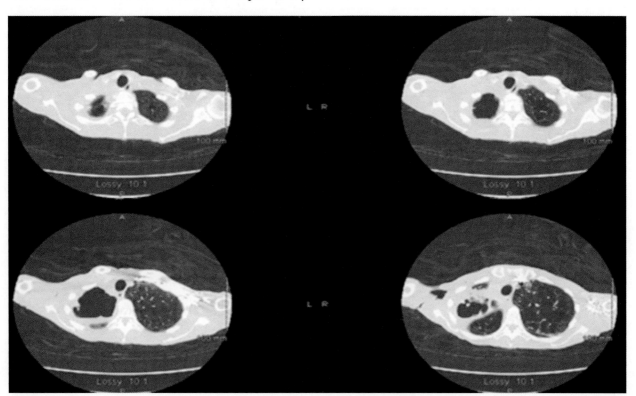

Blood cultures are negative and two separate sputum cultures grow *Mycobacterium abscessus*.

Question 1: **Which of the following statements is true about mycobacterium abscessus?**

A. Mycobacterium abscessus infection rarely affects patients in their fourth and fifth decade of life

B. Patients with bronchiectasis are at increased risk of Mycobacterium abscessus lung disease

C. Mycobacterium abscessus does not cause cutaneous abscess formation

D. Mycobacterium abscessus is the most common non-tuberculous mycobacterium isolate from cystic fibrosis patients

E. None of the above

Answers

Question 1: E. Do nothing

Tuberculin skin test (TST) or PPD is primarily used to determine exposure to tuberculosis. It is based on delayed hypersensitivity reaction to certain mycobacterial antigens. 0.1 mL of 5 tuberculin units is injected subcutaneously on the arm and the induration is read after 48 to 72 hours. Based on the patient's current description from his PCP, he appears to have a negative TST result.

TST positive if Induration Size	Patient Population
≥5 mm	Close contacts to other people with tuberculosis, HIV, organ transplants, TNF-alpha blocker users such as RA or IBD, or patients on prednisone ≥15 mg of >1 month
≥10 mm	Recent immigrants (<5 years) from endemic areas, employees of high risk areas
≥15 mm	Low risk patients

* *

Isoniazid 5 mg/kg/d to max of 300 g or 15 g/kg biweekly to max of 900 g for 6 to 9 months would be the starting medication for latent tuberculosis. Rifampin, isoniazid, pyrazinamide, and ethambutol is the initial drug regimen for active tuberculosis.

Question 2: A. He still has a negative TST

The risk factors for progression of latent tuberculosis to active tuberculosis include HIV, DM, latent TB during infancy or early childhood, apical fibrosis on chest radiograph, and use of TNF-alpha blockers such as in Crohn's disease and rheumatoid arthritis. The demographic distribution of tuberculosis includes male adults from 15 to 64 years of age, foreign born with Asians > Blacks > Hispanics > American Indian > White and lower socioeconomic class.

* *

Latent tuberculosis can be identified with the use of tuberculin skin test, which uses a delayed hypersensitivity reaction, or interferon-gamma release assay (IGRA), which measures a component of cell mediated immune response. Advantages to IGRA include no effect from BCG vaccination, results within a few hours, and they are usually negative in NTM. However, newer IGRA can cross react with other NTM such as *M. marinium* and *M. kansasii*. Other drawbacks include lack of definition in the young and immunocompromised and the need to have it assessed within 12 hours.

* *

Repeating the tuberculosis skin test 4 to 8 weeks after the initial test is indicated if the initial test is negative and the patient has close contacts with individuals with active tuberculosis, ongoing occupational exposure, or in individuals with prior mycobacterial antigen exposure in the form of BCG, NTM, or prior TB exposure. The second TST is considered positive if the induration is >10 mm and has increased by >6 mm from the prior study. This suggests a booster effect, which is the awakening response to prior BCG, NTM, or remote TB exposure. It can also suggest conversion, which might suggest a new tuberculosis infection.

* *

Tuberculosis genotyping is considered to determine transmission relationships between tuberculosis patients, distinguish recent new infections from old infections, and detect laboratory cross contamination.

* *

If he did have latent TB, Rifampin 10 mg/kg for 4 months or rifampin with pyrazinamide daily for 2 months is an alternative chemoprophylaxis for HIV patients.

Question 3: B. Rifampin plus pyrazinamide daily for 2 months

Once the diagnosis of latent tuberculosis is attained, either by PPD or IGRA, treatment should be initiated.

The CDC guidelines for treatment of latent tuberculosis specify multiple acceptable treatment regimens.[1]

Treatment Regimens for Latent Tuberculosis

Regimen	Duration
Isoniazid 300 mg daily	9 months
Isoniazid 900 mg twice weekly	9 months (administered as DOT)
Isoniazid 300 mg daily or 900 mg twice weekly	6 months (not for HIV-infected patients, children, or fibrotic lung disease)
Rifampin 600 mg daily	4 months
Rifapentine 900 mg plus isoniazid 900 mg daily	12 weeks

**

Isoniazid monotherapy is the most studied and widely used regimens for the treatment of latent tuberculosis. However, a regimen consisting of rifampin is a viable alternative for those patients who develop side effects to or are intolerant of isoniazid. More recently, a regimen of rifapentine plus isoniazid as a daily regimen for 3 months was studied in the PREVENT TB trial and was found to be a noninferior regimen when compared to isoniazid in prevention of progression to active tuberculosis.[2] Rifampin plus pyrazinamide is no longer a preferred regimen for the treatment of latent tuberculosis as an excess number of adverse events, mainly hepatotoxicity, were attributed to this regimen.

CASE 2

Question 1: B. He can either have primary or postprimary tuberculosis

Pleural effusion can be found in both primary and postprimary tuberculosis.[1,3] Tuberculosis is transmitted through their air in 1 to 5 um droplet nuclei which can contain 1 to 400 organisms. The smallest organisms make it to the alveoli where they are phagocytized by alveolar macrophages; marking the primary infection. Within 2 weeks they are transported into the lymphatics to establish secondary sites. Delayed type hypersensitivity develops within 4 weeks leading to granuloma formation with decreased number of bacilli, which is detected by TST. Radiographic manifestations of primary tuberculosis include: parenchymal disease in lower and middle lobes with lymphadenopathy that fails to improve

with antibiotics; lymphadenopathy, usually unilateral and right paratracheal >2 cm, and considered active if with necrosis; miliary disease which is a complication of erosion of parenchymal focus into blood or lymphatics, manifests initially as hyperinflation with 2 to 3 mm nodules lower lobe predominance and resolves with 2 to 5 months; and unilateral pleural effusion.[3,4] Radiographic manifestations of postprimary tuberculosis are marked by upper lobe cavitary lesions, usually apical or posterior right upper lobe, no lymphadenopathy, parenchymal disease, airway disease, and pleural effusions. Postprimary tuberculosis is usually from reinfection or reactivation of tuberculosis.[3,4]

Question 2: D. Adenosine deaminase

The paucity of organisms and the nonspecific presentation of a pleural effusion secondary to tuberculosis can make diagnosis difficult. Tuberculous effusions are secondary to a ruptured subpleural focus followed by cell mediated immune response. Ninety percent of the effusions are exudative with lymphocytic predominance, although neutrophilic predominance can occur.[1] These effusions generally have glucose values between 60 and 100 with pH 7.30. If low glucose and low pH, consider chronic tuberculosis empyema.

**

Although usually positive, PPD can be negative if circulating mononuclear cells suppress sensitive T lymphocytes but not in pleural space or sequestration of PPD reactive lymphocytes in pleural space. Sputum AFB stains and cultures are usually negative because has it requires 10,000 to 100,000 organisms in 1 ml. Five to ten milliliters of sputum are needed for a good study. Sputum cultures can require 8 weeks of incubation. Nuclei acid amplification can detect tuberculosis with a few strands and have >90% sensitivity and 99% specificity in smear-positive cases. Sensitivity decreases up to 60% in smear negative cases.[1]

**

Several studies have shown that adenosine deaminase (ADA) >45 U/L have been found to be 100% sensitivity and 85% to 100% specificity for tuberculosis.[1,5-7] ADA <40 U/L does not occur in tuberculosis. The lower specificity can be due to that other conditions, such as rheumatoid arthritis, empyema, and malignancies can have elevated ADA. This is in part due to that most kits test for total ADA despite the existence of two types of ADA: ADA-I n empyemas and ADA-2 is in tuberculosis.

* *

Pleural fluid lysozymes of >15 mg/dL and/or ratio 1.2 pleural to serum lysozyme ratio has 100% sensitivity and 95% specificity for tuberculosis although others have argued it cannot discern from bacterial empyema or malignancy.[5–8] Other markers, such as IFN-gamma < 140pg/mL has a sensitivity 94 and specificity of 92%.[9,10]

* *

Pleural biopsies can have a diagnostic yield between 60% and 95% of cases and medications can be tailored to the appropriate antimicrobial sensitivities.[1,10] However, it requires a certain amount of pleural fluid to remain to perform the procedure. In this case, almost all of the fluid was removed after the thoracentesis.

Question 3: B. Rifampin, isoniazid, pyrazinamide, ethambutol

Fluoroquinolones are considered monotherapy for tuberculosis. Repeated administration of these antibiotics on a patient with an undiagnosed tuberculosis can lead to multidrug resistance variants; therefore are generally avoided. However, one course of fluoroquinolones is generally tolerable.

CASE 3

Question 1: C. Start treatment with rifampin, isoniazid, pyrazinamide, and ethambutol

A high index of suspicion is necessary to rapidly diagnose and treat pulmonary tuberculosis. In high-risk patients, pulmonary tuberculosis should be promptly identified by acid-fast staining of respiratory sputum samples, and subsequently confirmed by AFB culture. *M. tuberculosis* is a slow-growing organism; therefore, culture results may take up to 8 weeks. This should not delay initiation of antituberculous treatment in symptomatic patients in whom the suspicion of active tuberculosis is high. Repeat bronchoscopy with transbronchial biopsies may reveal the presence of caseating granulomas and provide further evidence of active infection; however, given the already high suspicion of active tuberculosis, this is not required prior to initiation of antitubuculous treatment. Initiation of broad-spectrum antimicrobial treatment to cover gram-negative, gram-positive, and anaerobic organisms is a reasonable treatment option in patients who are acutely ill and hospitalized with pneumonia. However, this patient's presentation is highly suggestive of active tuberculosis and treatment with broad-spectrum antimicrobials in this case would

lead to an unnecessary delay in appropriate antituberculous treatment. After initiation of treatment in patients with AFB-negative sputum smears, culture results and repeat imaging should be monitored during the course of treatment. If, after 2 months of antituberculous treatment there is clinical and radiographic improvement and no other diagnosis has been established, the diagnosis of culture-negative tuberculosis is made. In these cases, the total duration of antimicrobial treatment is generally less than culture-positive cases. After an initial 2-month course of rifampin, INH, pyrazinamide, and ethambutol, an additional 2 months of INH plus rifampin is required to complete a total of 4 months of therapy.[1] Note that if TB cultures remain negative but there is no clinical or radiographic improvement, then the diagnosis of culture-negative TB cannot be established, and further testing to establish an alternative diagnosis must be pursued. Further observation would not be appropriate as this patient is already acutely ill and has not improved despite prolonged observation.

Question 2: D. Drug–drug interactions involving rifampin are rare and dose adjustments are rarely necessary

Monitoring during therapy for tuberculosis is necessary as adverse reactions are common and can occur with all antituberculous antimicrobials.[1] Many patients have mild GI symptoms and may include nausea, vomiting, abdominal pain, and poor appetite. When these symptoms occur, this should prompt the evaluation of underlying hepatotoxicity related to these medications. In most cases, changing the dosing schedule or administration of one or more of these drugs with food is an adequate solution. In the absence of significant hepatotoxicity, these GI side effects are generally manageable with conservative management. Significant elevation in liver enzymes is common in patients treated with the standard four-drug regimen and an asymptomatic elevation of AST is found in up to 20% of patients.[1] INH, rifampin, and pyrazinamide are most often implicated. Elevation in AST may be characterized as mild, defined as <5× the upper limit of normal, moderate, defined as 5 to 10× the upper limit of normal, and severe, defined as >10× the upper limit of normal. Mild elevations in AST in asymptomatic patients should be monitored on regular basis, but should not cause a change in regimen. More significant rises in AST, either 3× the upper limit of normal in symptomatic patients or 5× the upper limit of normal in asymptomatic patients, should prompt the discontinuation of antituberculous treatment.[1] When treatment is halted, the initiation of three non-hepatotoxic drugs should occur until the time that the liver enzymes return to normal. Once normal, rifampin should be restarted as it is the least likely to cause hepatotoxicity; thereafter, INH and pyrazinamide may be restarted once weekly while monitoring for recurrent elevation in liver enzymes. If recurrent hepatotoxicity occurs upon reinitiation of these drugs, then an alternative regimen should be started.

* *

Fever that persists despite initiation of this four-drug regimen could indicate the presence of a multidrug resistant strain of tuberculosis; however, persistent fever may also be a sign of drug fever. The consideration of drug fever should especially be prompted by the recurrence of fever after several weeks of treatment, especially in those patients who initially had a clinical and/or radiographic improvement on therapy. Classically, a drug fever in this context occurs in a patient who otherwise is clinically well. The initial consideration when a new fever arises is to assess whether the tuberculosis infection has worsened or a new superinfection has occurred. If no new or worsened infection is identified, then all drugs should be stopped and restarted one at a time every 2 to 3 days once the fever has dissipated. Rash during treatment is also relatively common and may be seen with any of the antituberculous drugs. Minor drug rashes should be treated symptomatically with antipruritic medications and antihistamines, as needed. More severe rashes, generalized drug eruptions, or rashes with mucous membrane involvement should prompt discontinuation of all drugs. Rechallenging one drug at a time every 2 to 3 days once the rash subsides is recommended, and if the rash recurs, then switching to an alternative regimen is required. Other well-described drug-related adverse effects are peripheral neuropathy attributed to INH use, bone marrow suppression and hyperuricemia attributed to pyrazinamide use, and optic neuritis attributed to ethambutol use.

* *

It is important to consider drug–drug interactions when prescribing this four-drug regimen. Antituberculous drugs affect the concentrations of other drugs. The most common drug–drug interactions involve rifampin. Rifampin is metabolized via the cytochrome CYP3 A P450 pathway, and drugs also metabolized by this pathway will have their metabolism altered. Common drug interactions include HIV medications, including protease inhibitors and nonnucleoside reverse transcriptase inhibitors; macrolide antibiotics; levothyroxine;

theophylline; hormone replacement therapy; and multiple cardiovascular medications.[11] While not prohibitive to use rifampin and these drugs together, it is important to consider these drug–drug interactions and make appropriate dose adjustments.

Question 3: E. All of the above

Current noninvasive or minimally invasive techniques for the diagnosis of active tuberculosis are highly specific, but are not 100% sensitive. This includes sputum samples, bronchoscopic BAL samples and transbronchial biopsy samples, pleural fluid analysis, and closed pleural biopsies. While limitations in sampling and diagnosis should not delay treatment in a symptomatic patient with a strongly suggestive history supporting tuberculosis, more invasive surgical biopsies may be of benefit in many patients. Pleuroscopy can provide for direct sampling of the affected pleura. VATS techniques have improved and is generally a safe and effective method for obtaining tissue for diagnosis from the affected lung. Mediastinoscopy is a well-tolerated method for the diagnosis of intrathoracic lymph node involvement by tuberculosis. The identification of granulomas and obtain positive culture results from these lymph nodes may help in guiding treatment in these patients. The more widespread use of EBUS-TBNA may obviate the need for a more invasive mediastinoscopic approach. The overall rate of significant complications from mediastinoscopy is <1%. No randomized trials have compared EBUS-TBNA and mediastinoscopy in this setting, and therefore mediastinoscopy remains a useful method for lymph node sampling in these patients. Patients with bone and joint involvement may respond to medical treatment with combination chemotherapy. However, when spinal disease is present (Pott's disease), especially with extension into the spinal canal and epidural space, surgery remains a mainstay of treatment. Laminectomy, fusion, and other surgical techniques have good success in stabilizing the spine and also in the acute setting when nerve structures are compromised, especially with cord compression. Extra-spinal joint involvement, especially involving large joints, may require serial surgical washouts in addition to antituberculous chemotherapy. Synovitis, if present, may require synovectomy if medical management fails. One realm where surgery may play an especially important role in the treatment of tuberculosis is in the treatment of MDR or XDR strains. The failure rate with medical management in these strains is reported to be as high as 40%.[1,12,13] In these cases, careful surgical resection of the affected area may provide a significant benefit. Multiple studies have evaluated the surgical resection of either cavities or destroyed lung in these patients, and the results of these studies is mixed. However, there exists potential to benefit these patients, as many of them fail medical therapy. In addition, patients with persistently positive sputum despite prolonged medical treatment and those with persistent hemoptysis may also benefit from surgical resection. VATS may be an effective approach in many patients; however, complicated cases and those with multiple adhesions may require open thoracotomy.

CASE 4

Question 1: E. B, C, and D

This patient is presenting with a subacute to chronic cough productive of sputum, weight loss, and low-grade fevers that did not respond to two separate courses of treatment for community-acquired pneumonia. Chest imaging demonstrates bronchiectasis preferentially affecting the lingula and right middle lobe. This presentation is consistent with chronic infection with *Mycobacterium avium*-intracellulare *complex* (MAC). The diagnosis requires compatible clinical, radiographic, and microbiologic criteria to be met. A patient must have pulmonary symptoms, which most often is chronic productive cough, and often accompanied by low-grade fevers and weight loss over time. A plain chest x-ray is adequate if cavitary MAC disease is demonstrated; otherwise an HRCT is required to demonstrate nodular opacities with multifocal bronchiectasis. Tree-in-bud opacities are often present and contiguous local spread of disease is common.[14,15] Susceptible patients with underlying structural lung disease in whom MAC is present, radiographic disease originates at or near sites of bronchiectasis, fibrosis, or emphysema. Specific microbiologic evidence of MAC must also be present. One sputum sample demonstrating MAC is not adequate. Two separate sputum samples, one bronchial wash or BAL specimen, or one lung biopsy specimen demonstrating granulomatous inflammation and one BAL or bronchial wash or expectorated sputum sample culturing MAC are required for diagnosis.[14,15]

Question 2: D. A 68-year-old heavy smoker with moderate COPD who is admitted with frequent COPD exacerbations and a chronic cough productive of yellow-green sputum

The majority of patients exposed to MAC in the environment will not develop clinically significant pulmonary disease. However, skin testing to lipoarabinomannan, a mycobacterial antigen seen in nontuberculous mycobacteria, has revealed rising prevalence throughout childhood and is common in previously healthy patients who later develop clinically significant MAC disease.[14,15] Different phenotypes develop depending on host-mycobacterial interaction and local and systemic immune deficiency. One form of disease is upper lobe cavitary MAC disease that mimics reactivation TB in clinical course and radiographic appearance. Fevers, rigors, productive cough, and hemoptysis may be seen with a progressive clinical course. This is most common among elderly man with COPD, although local and systemic immune deficiency seen in middle aged men who are heavy smokers and alcoholics may also lead to cavitary lung disease. Second, patients with underlying structural lung disease, such as those with preexistent bronchiectasis, may develop new radiographic opacities and MAC disease at sites of old structural lung disease. Third, MAC may affect patients without preexistent underlying lung disease and who are generally healthy. This preferentially affects thin elderly patients and causes the subacute presentation of cough with sputum production, low-grade fevers, and weight loss. This phenotype has the unique radiographic distribution of the lingula and right-middle lobe, thought to be anatomic straightening and narrowing of these lung segments with resultant poor clearance of mucus. Ongoing infection leads to bronchiectasis and the clinical syndrome of Lady Windermere's disease. Fourth, advanced HIV/AIDS and other states of severe immunodeficiency lead to disseminated MAC disease. The source of infection in disseminated MAC is likely oral ingestion of the organism since much of the disease begins in the GI tract. This is also true for MAC-associated lymphadenitis seen mostly in the pediatric population. From the GI tract, a MAC bacteremia allows for systemic disease to occur, which accounts for persistent low-grade fevers, diffuse lymphadenopathy, hepatosplenomegaly, and bone marrow involvement, causing anemia which is often out of proportion to the degree expected with HIV disease alone. Finally, exposure to MAC antigens found in standing water, such as that in spas or hot tubs, may lead to a hypersensitivity-like pneumonitis called "hot-tub lung."[16] MAC is often resistant to disinfectants and may survive in a wide range of temperatures, promoting its ability to sustain growth in environments such as hot tubs. Patients often present with cough, dyspnea on exertion, and interstitial and alveolar infiltrates on imaging. While COPD is a risk factor for superimposed MAC disease, this is not the most common cause of COPD exacerbations in this population.

Question 3: **B. A patient with fibrocavitary MAC disease treated with azithromycin, rifampin, ethambutol, and amikacin**

Once the diagnosis is made, the treatment is dictated by the severity of disease, immune competence or incompetence, and disease phenotype. Below is a summary of the treatment recommendations from the ATS Guidelines.[14]

Treatment Recommendations for MAC	
Disease phenotype	Medications
Lady Windermere's disease/nodular or bronchiectatic diseases	Macrolide (Azithromycin or Clarithromycin) + Ethambutol + Rifampin
Fibrocavitary disease	Macrolide (Azithromycin or Clarithromycin) + Ethambutol + Rifampin +/– Aminoglycoside (Streptomycin or Amikacin)
Severe or previously treated disease	Macrolide (Azithromycin or Clarithromycin) + Ethambutol + Rifabutin + Aminoglycoside (Streptomycin or Amikacin)
Disseminated disease	Clarithromycin + Ethambutol +/– Rifabutin

* *

Pyrazinamide is not routinely used to treat MAC infection. Pyrazinamide and other antituberculous medications have been shown to be ineffective in treating MAC disease, with poor in vitro and in vivo effects. Furthermore, the side effect profile of antituberculosis medications is poor, especially in the setting of sporadic success in treating MAC. Two macrolides (azithromycin and clarithromycin) are not required in the treatment of Lady Windermere's disease. Acceptable treatment regimens include ethambutol, rifampin, and one macrolide, not two. Treatment regimen for disseminated MAC does not include an aminoglycoside. The initial regimen is a macrolide plus ethambutol, with or without rifabutin. Clarithromycin has been shown to more rapidly resolve MAC bacteremia, and therefore is the preferred macrolide over azithromycin. Overall, treatment is for prolonged periods, frequently longer than

1 year. The recommendation for termination of antibiotics is at least 12 months of sputum samples which are negative for MAC while on treatment. The exception to this rule is in disseminated MAC, where treatment is life-long unless immune reconstitution is obtained and sustained while on HAART. Therefore, MAC treatment should be combined with HAART whenever possible. Patients with hypersensitivity pneumonitis secondary to MAC, also termed "hot-tub lung" (generally improve to normal within weeks to months following abstinence from exposure to the reservoir of infection. For those patients with severe lung disease or respiratory failure, prednisone should be given at higher doses (1–2 mg/kg daily) and tapered over 1 to 2 months.

CASE 5

Question 1: **C. Bronchoscopy with transbronchial biopsy of the lesion and BAL for cell count, acid-fast staining, and cultures**

This patient is presenting with the subacute onset of fever, productive cough, and constitutional symptoms associated with cavitary lung disease. This patient was admitted and placed on respiratory isolation due to the need to rule out tuberculosis. However, there is significant overlap between reactivation pulmonary tuberculosis and other infections, malignancies, rheumatologic diseases, and inflammatory disorders. Symptoms of reactivation tuberculosis are not specific. Ongoing infection and inflammation result in clinical symptoms of fever, chest pain, and productive cough; necrosis may ensue which results in cavity formation. The type of necrosis is variable and includes suppurative necrosis seen in lung abscesses, ischemia-induced necrosis in pulmonary infarctions, necrosis secondary to tumor growth and abnormal local vasculature, and caseous necrosis seen in tuberculosis. Likewise, there is a broad differential diagnosis for cavitary lung disease. Clues from the patient's history, physical examination, and radiographic appearance of the cavity and surrounding parenchyma may aid in narrowing the diagnosis. However, there is no one sign or symptom that may definitively obviate the need for further testing to confirm the diagnosis. See following table for selected diseases that most commonly cause cavitary lung disease.

CAUSES OF CAVITARY LUNG DISEASE

Category	Types	Features
Bacterial Infections	*Streptococcus pneumoniae*	Infrequently cavitates; when cavities occur tends to be associated with bacteremia
	Staphylococcus aureus	Sequelae of viral infection; 1/4–1/3 cavitate
	Klebsiella pneumoniae	Most common bacterial infection causing cavities; risk factors include alcoholism, chronic renal disease, and steroid use
	Actinomyces	May mimic *M. tuberculosis* Male predominance; poor dentition
	Nocardia	Seen in COPD, malignancy, and steroid use
Fungal Infections	Invasive Aspergillosis	Immunocompromised; air-crescent sign; halo sign
	Histoplasma capsulatum	Ohio and Mississippi River Valleys; spelunkers, heavy machine operators and poultry breeders; chronic infection may cavitate
Other infections	*Mycobacterium tuberculosis* NTMs (*M. abscessus, M. kansasii, MAC*)	Extensive caseous necrosis, upper lobe predominance
Inflammatory diseases	Sarcoidosis	7% cavitate; peribronchovascular and fissural nodule distribution; fibrosis; hilar/mediastinal LN
Malignancy	Primary lung cancer	22% cavitate; squamous cell most common
	Metastatic cancers	Cavitate less commonly than primary lung malignancies
Rheumatologic diseases	Granulomatosis with polyangiitis	35–50% of nodules cavitate
Other	Pulmonary embolism	Look for feeding vessel
	Langerhan's cell histiocytosis	Afflicts 20–40-year-old smokers

**

When *M. tuberculosis* infection is suspected, respiratory isolation and collection of three sputum samples is appropriate. Reported sensitivity of induced sputum for culture is up to 80%, with the caveat that many of these samples may stain acid-fast negative with a resultant 2- to 8-week delay in diagnosis due to the slow growth of the organism.[1,17] In addition, expectorated sputum is generally inadequate to diagnose other diseases such as sarcoidosis, fungal infections, atypical infections such as *Nocardia* and *Actinomyces*, and malignancies. When a patient is unable to produce adequate expectorated sputum or when stained sputum samples are AFB negative, adjunctive testing is required.

**

The purified protein derivative (PPD) test or tuberculosis skin test (TST) may be useful to rule out infection with tuberculosis, but is not an adequately sensitive or specific test.[17] False negatives occur when a patient has energy and fails to develop the adequate delayed-type hypersensitivity response required for a positive skin test. Even when positive tests occur, tuberculosis cannot be definitively diagnosed as false positives may occur when infected with other nontuberculous mycobacteria.

**

Quantiferon Gold, an interferon-gamma release assay (IGRA), is a test that is highly sensitive and specific for latent tuberculosis.[1,17,18] Quantiferon Gold assay is both sensitive and specific for latent tuberculosis. With the newer IGRA, they contain antigens which have genetic sequences that are found in two NTM, *M. marinum* and *M. kansasii*. Therefore, they will be positive in patients exposed to these NTM. IGRA may not be positive acute infection and will not be able to distinguish active from latent tuberculosis.

**

Nucleic acid amplification (NAA) assays have several advantages over routine culture of sputum samples. NAA allows for a more rapid and reliable way of identifying tuberculosis in sputum than awaiting mycobacterial cultures, especially in those patients with negative acid-fast sputum stains. The reported sensitivity of NAA in identifying *M. tuberculosis* for acid-fast positive sputum samples is >95%, while the sensitivity drops to 75% to 80% for sputum-negative patients. Limitations to NAA testing do exist.[19,20] Sensitivity for sputum-negative cases is only 75% which is only as good and may be slightly less sensitive than awaiting culture results in these patients. False-negative results also exist, which may be due to inhibitors that reduce or inhibit the DNA amplification process. Finally, the cost of NAA is much greater than culture. Given these limitations, NAA is recommended as an adjunctive test rather than a replacement for AFB staining and culture. While a positive NAA test will definitively diagnose *M. tuberculosis*, a negative test has the limitation of failing to diagnose an alternative disease such as sarcoidosis, malignancy, or other infections.

**

Flexible bronchoscopy is reserved for those patients in whom a high suspicion of tuberculosis exists and whose sputum samples fail to demonstrate AFB.[22] It is also reserved for those patients in whom the diagnosis of tuberculosis is in question and biopsy specimens will help delineate one disease process from another. Certain BAL features may point toward an alternative diagnosis; for example, the demonstration of sputum lymphocytosis, activated macrophages, and high CD4:CD8 ratio may assist in diagnosing sarcoidosis rather than tuberculosis. The sensitivity of routine sputum cultures for atypical infections such as *Nocardia* and *Actinomyces* is low, and bronchial washing and BAL cultures are more sensitive for these organisms. Transbronchial biopsy in these patients is also useful in identifying characteristics of other diseases such as noncaseating granulomas in sarcoidosis, fungal elements in invasive fungal infections, and cancer cells in malignant cavities. The combination of high resolution computed tomography and flexible bronchoscopy in this group of patients is highly sensitive in patients in whom tuberculosis is highly likely and will be of most use in definitively diagnosing tuberculosis and distinguishing it from other disease states.

CASE 6

Question 1: **C. Begin treatment with rifampin, ethambutol, and isoniazid to complete a minimum of an 18-month total course of treatment and with a minimum of 12 months of negative expectorated sputum samples**

Mycobacterium kansasii is a slow growing nontuberculous mycobacterium (NTM) that mainly causes lung disease in humans. Unlike many other nontuberculous mycobacteria, *M. kansasii* has not been found in

the soil or outdoor water sources. It is ubiquitous in municipal tap water, which is the major reservoir for human infection. It is most common in urban environments and concentrated to the South and Central portions of the United States.[15,22–24] Diagnosis of disease is similar to other NTM, requiring clinical disease, radiographic abnormalities consistent with *M. kansasii* infection, and isolation of *M. kansasii* in two separate expectorated sputum cultures, one BAL or bronchial wash specimen, or one lung biopsy culture plus an additional BAL or sputum culture. Epidemiologically, *M. kansasii* preferentially inflicts middle aged Caucasian males and is the second most common NTM isolated after MAC in the United States.[22–24] Risk factors include prior lung disease including tuberculosis, bronchiectasis, COPD, pneumoconiosis, immunocompromised states such as transplantation or HIV and ethanol abuse. The most common form of lung disease caused by *M. kansasii* infection in fibrocavitary disease similar in appearance to that seen with reactivation *M. tuberculosis*.

**

He has clinical symptoms, radiographic fibrocavitary lung disease, and two expectorated sputum isolates confirming growth of *M. kansasii*. Therefore, treatment should be initiated in this patient without awaiting sensitivity results for *M. kansasii*. It is recommended that sensitivity results to only rifampin be obtained because resistance to isoniazid and ethambutol are very rare. The preferred antimicrobial regimen for treatment of *M. kansasii* is isoniazid 300 mg daily, rifampin 600 mg daily, and ethambutol 25 mg/kg for the first 2 months followed by 15 mg/kg for the remainder of the course of treatment. Guidelines dictate that at lease 12 months of negative expectorated sputum are required while on treatment prior to the termination of antibiotics, which translates usually to at least an 18-month course of treatment. Shorter courses of treatment have been tried and have good initial success in sputum clearance. However, these shorter courses resulted in higher rates of disease relapse and are therefore not recommended When rifampin-resistant isolates are cultured, this should trigger testing for other antimicrobial sensitivities. The preferred regimen for treatment of rifampin-resistant isolates is daily high-dose isoniazid 900 mg, ethambutol 25 mg/kg, and sulfamethoxazole 1 g along with either streptomycin or amikacin for the first 6 months.

CASE 7

Question 1: **B. Patients with bronchiectasis are at increased risk of Mycobacterium abscessus lung disease**

Mycobacterium abscessus is a nontuberculous mycobacterium (NTM) found in environmental sources such as soil, water, and dusts.[14,25-27] It is classified as a rapidly growing mycobacteria (RPM), along with *M. chelonae* and *M. fortuitum*, due to its ability to form colonies when incubated within seven days, as opposed to the typically very slow growth of other mycobacterium species.[27] *M. abscessus* will generally grow well in routine culture media; therefore, specialized mycobacterial media are not required. *M. abscessus* may cause lung disease that typically occurs at sites of previous lung destruction such as bronchiectasis or prior tuberculosis. While nodular-bronchiectatic disease may occur and mimic the disease course of MAC, especially in female nonsmokers over 60 years of age, cavitary lung disease and abscess formation with surrounding continuous spread of disease is more common. In fact, it is not uncommon to isolate more than one species of NTM in the same patient with lung disease. It is the third most common NTM and typically affects younger populations of patients, typically in the fourth to fifth decade of life. Extra-pulmonary disease including penetrating traumatic wound infections (especially when contaminated with soil), iatrogenic skin and soft-tissue infections at sites of transdermal needle injection causing purple nodules and small abcesses, and rarely disseminated cutaneous lesions in severely immunocompromised individuals. Cutaneous lesions may spontaneously resolve within weeks to months, although antibiotic treatment and drainage of abscesses may be required.

* *

Because *M. abscessus* isolates are very frequently resistant to multiple antimicrobial agents, such as isoniazid, rifamycins, ethambutol, and aminoglycosides. Only macrolides have a reasonably reliable efficacy against *M. abscessus*, although macrolide-resistant isolates have been identified. Either clarithromycin 1 g/day or azithromycin 250 mg/day, plus one or more parenteral antibiotics. Amikacin is also used, although cefoxitin and imipenem are reasonable alternatives. The likelihood of cure is greater than that seen with pulmonary *M. abscessus* disease. For those patients with localized *M. abscessus* lung disease, the combination of antibiotic treatment to reduce bacterial burden followed by surgical resection is suggested as a means of maximizing the chance for cure. Due to low cure rates and high rates of disease relapse, in many patients the goal is not cure but instead control of disease.

REFERENCES

1. American Thoracic Society; Centers for Disease Control and Prevention; Infectious Diseases Society of America. Treatment of tuberculosis. *Am J Respir Crit Care Med.* 2003;167:603–662.
2. Sterling TR, Villarino ME, Borisov AS, et al. Three months of rifapentine and isoniazid for latent tuberculosis infection. *NEJM.* 2011;365:2155–2166.
3. Burrill J, Williams CJ, Bain G, et al. Tuberculosis: A radiologic review. *Radiographics.* 2007;27:1255–1273.
4. McAdams HP, Erasmus J, Winter JA. Radiologic manifestations of pulmonary tuberculosis. *Radiol Clin North Am.* 1995;33(4):655–678.
5. Burgess LJ, Maritz FJ, Le Roux I, et al. Combined use of pleural adenosine deaminase with lymphocyte/neutrophil ratio: Increased specificity for the diagnosis of tuberculous pleuritis. *Chest.*1996;109(2):414–419.
6. Valdes L, San Jose E, Alvarez D, et al. Diagnosis of tuberculous pleurisy using the biologic parameters adenosine deaminase, lysozyme and interferon gamma. *Chest.* 1993;103:458–465.
7. Valees L, Alvarez D, San Jose E, et al. Value of adenosine deaminase in the diagnosis of tuberculous pleural effusinos in young patients in a region of high prevalence of tuberculosis. *Thorax.* 1995;50:600–603.
8. Near KA, Lefford MJ. Use of serum antibody and lysozyme levels for diagnosis of leprosy and tuberculosis. *J Clin Microbiol.* 1992;30(5):1105–1110.
9. Villegas MV, Lbrada LA, Saravia NG. Evaluation of polymerase chain reaction, adenosine deaminase, and interferon-gamma in pleural fluid for the differential diagnosis of pleural tuberculosis. *Chest.* Nov 2000;118(5):1355–1364.
10. Gopi A, Madhavan SM, Sharma SK, et al. Diagnosis and treatment of tuberculous pleural effusion in 2006.*Chest.* 2007;131:880–889.
11. Centers for Disease Control and Prevention. Updated guidelines for the use of rifabutin or rifampin for the treatment and prevention of tuberculosis among HIV-infected patients taking protease inhibitors or nonnucleoside reverse transcriptase inhibitors. *Morb Mortal Wkly Rep.* 2000;49:185–189.
12. Chan ED, Laurel V, Strand MJ, et al. Treatment and outcome analysis of 205 patients with multidrug-resistant tuberculosis. *AJRCCM.* 2004;169:1103–1109.
13. Mukherjee JS, Rich ML, Socci AR, et al. Programmes and principles in treatment of multidrug-resistant tuberculosis. *Lancet.* 2004;363(9407):474—481.
14. Griffith DE, Aksamit T, Brown-Elliott BA, et al. An official ATS/IDSA statement: Diagnosis, treatment, and prevention of nontuberculous mycobacterial diseases. *Am J Respir Crit Care Med.* 2007;175(4):367–416.

15. Kasperbauer SH, Daley CL. Diagnosis and treatment of infections due to mycobacterium avium complex. *Semin Respir Crit Care Med.* 2008;29(5):569–576.

16. Aksamit TR. Hot tub lung: Infection, inflammation, or both? *Semin Respir Infect.* 2003;18:33–39.

17. ATS Statement: Targeted Tuberculin Testing and Treatment of Latent Tuberculosis Infection. *AJRCCM.* Aug 2000;161:S221-S247.

18. Diel R, Loddenkemper R, Meywald-Walter K, et al. Comparative performance of tuberculin skin test, Quantiferon-TB-Gold In Tube Assay, and T-Spot. TB test in Contact Investigations for Tuberculosis. *Chest.* 2009;135(4):1010–1018.

19. Larque f, Griggs A, SlopenM, Munsiff S. Performance of nucleic acid amplification tests for diagnosis of tuberculosis in a large urban setting. *Clin Infect Dis.* 2009;49(1): 46–54.

20. Report of An Expert Consultation on the Sues of Nucleic Acid Amplification Tests for the Diagnosis of Tuberculosis. http://www.cdc.gov/tb/publications/guidelines/amplification_tests/reccomendations.htm. Accessed Dec 2014.

21. de Gracia J, Curull V, Vidal R, et al. Diagnostic value of bronchoalveolar lavage in suspected pulmonary tuberculosis. *Chest.* 1988;93(2):329–332.

22. Ahn CH, McLarty IW, Ahn SS, et al. Diagnostic criteria for pulmonary disease caused by *Mycobacterium kansasii* and *Mycobacterium intracellulare. Am Rev Respir Dis.* 1982;125: 388–391.

23. Bert LP, Steadham JE. Improved technique for isolation of *Mycobacterium kansasii* from water. *J Clin Microbiol.* 1981; 13:969–975.

24. Block KC, Zwerling L, Pletcher MJ, et al. Incidence and clinical implications of isolation of *Mycobacterium kansasii. Ann Intern Med.* 1998;129:698–704.

25. Brown BA, Wallace RJ Jr, Onyi GO, et al. Activities of four macrolides, including clarithromycin, against *Mycobacterium fortuitum, Mycobacterium chelonae,* and *Mycobacterium chelonae* like organisms. *Antimicrob Agents Chemother.* 1992;36:180–184.

26. Cullen AR, Cannon CL, Mark EJ, et al. *Mycobacterium abscessus* infection in cystic fibrosis: Colonization or infection? *Am J Respir Crit Care Med.* 2000;161:641–645.

27. Daley CL, Griffith DE. Pulmonary disease caused by rapidly growing mycobacteria. *Clin Chest Med.* 2002;23:623–632.

20

Fungal Diseases

Jimmy Johannes MD, Tessy Paul MD, and Tisha Wang MD

CASE 1

A 61-year-old morbidly obese woman with diabetes, a 35 pack-year smoking history, and coronary artery disease with chronic stable angina is referred to your clinic for an abnormal chest CT shown below. She denies any new systemic or respiratory complaints including wheezing, fevers, night sweats, or cough.

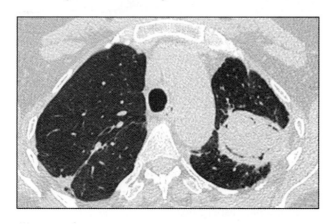

Question 1: What is the most likely diagnosis?

A. *Mycobacterium tuberculosis*
B. Nonsmall cell lung cancer
C. Aspergilloma
D. Nocardiosis
E. Lung abscess

Question 2: Which factor(s) can predispose patients to this condition?

A. Bullous emphysema
B. Bronchiectasis
C. Tuberculosis
D. All of the above
E. None of the above

Question 3: Six months after her initial visit, she presents to the ER with acute hemoptysis with two cups of frank blood. Chest CT with contrast shows an increased opacity surrounding the previous lesion. What is the next step in management after securing her airway?

A. Bronchial artery embolization
B. Chest tube placement
C. Surgical resection
D. Diagnostic bronchoscopy
E. Observation

CASE 2

A 48-year-old woman is referred to your clinic for uncontrolled asthma with a prior FEV1 of 58% and FEV1/FVC ratio of 62%. She is currently on high-dose salmeterol-fluticasone, Singulair, an oral antihistamine, and as-needed short-acting bronchodilators. She has also tried theophylline and zileuton in the past without any benefit. She continues to have nightly wheezing and shortness of breath. Further evaluation shows complete blood count (CBC) with eosinophilia and IgE level of 1,600 IU/mL. CT findings are seen on the following page.

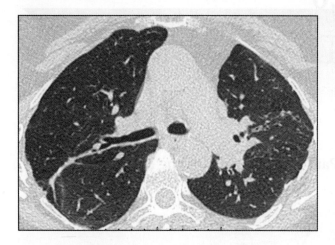

Question 1: **What additional testing can support the suspected diagnosis?**

A. Sputum acid-fast cultures
B. Open lung biopsy
C. Skin-test reactivity to *Aspergillus* antigen
D. Serum ACE levels
E. Methacholine challenge

Question 2: **What is the next step in controlling the patient's respiratory symptoms?**

A. Add theophylline
B. Systemic glucocorticoids
C. Bronchial thermoplasty
D. Add inhaled budesonide
E. Add tiotropium

Question 3: **What is the most common complication that develops in these patients?**

A. Bronchiectasis
B. Hemoptysis
C. Pulmonary fibrosis
D. Chronic pulmonary aspergillosis (CPA)
E. Lung cancer

CASE 3

A 30-year-old woman with a history of poorly controlled diabetes developed productive cough, wheezing, and shortness of breath. She was initially treated as an outpatient with multiple courses of antibiotics for presumed bacterial pneumonia based on chest x-ray findings. She subsequently was evaluated with a chest CT scan which revealed >10 pulmonary nodules and right-mainstem obstruction along with sinusitis seen on head CT. She underwent bronchoscopy with endobronchial biopsy of the mass. Pathology findings are shown at upper right.

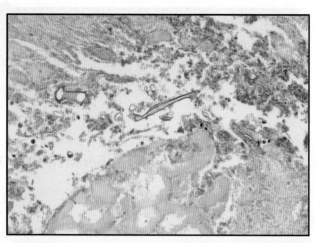

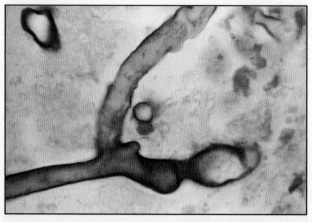

Top image used with permission of W. Dean Wallace, MD, Department of Pathology and Laboratory Medicine, David Geffen School of Medicine, UCLA

Bottom image reproduced with permission from Centers for Disease Control and Prevention (CDC). Public Health Image Library (PHIL)

Question 1: **What is the most likely diagnosis?**

A. Nocardiosis
B. Pulmonary aspergillosis
C. Mucormycosis
D. Fusarium
E. Mycobacterium tuberculosis

Question 2: **Which of the following is a risk factor for this diagnosis?**

A. Diabetes
B. Hematologic malignancy
C. Solid organ transplant
D. High-dose glucocorticoids
E. All of the above

Question 3: **What is the treatment approach in addition to surgical debridement?**

A. Voriconazole
B. Amphotericin B
C. Caspofungin
D. Itraconazole
E. Trimethoprim/sulfamethoxazole

CASE 4

A 57-year-old man with a history of lupus with associated interstitial lung disease on chronic steroids and multiple immunomodulating agents, most recently mycophenolate mofetil, is referred to your clinic for persistent cough, fevers, dyspnea, and an abnormal chest CT scan below.

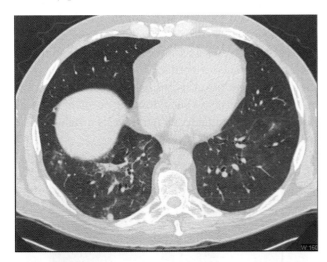

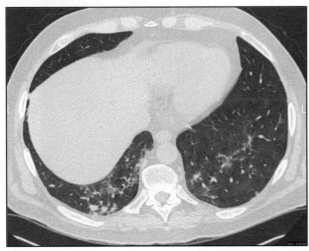

Used with permission of Yasir Tarabichi, MD and Ariss Derhovanessian, MD, Division of Pulmonary and Critical Care Medicine, David Geffen School of Medicine, UCLA.

Question 1: **What is the most appropriate next step in the management of this patient?**

A. Bronchoscopy with bronchoalveolar lavage (BAL)
B. VATS lung biopsy
C. Empiric antibiotic therapy with azithromycin
D. Increase dose of mycophenolate
E. Increase dose of steroids

Question 2: **The patient is evaluated with a bronchoscopy with BAL. Culture of BAL fluid grows the organism shown below. What is the most likely diagnosis?**

A. Histoplasmosis
B. Cryptococcosis
C. Rhizopus
D. Coccidioidomycosis
E. Blastomycosis

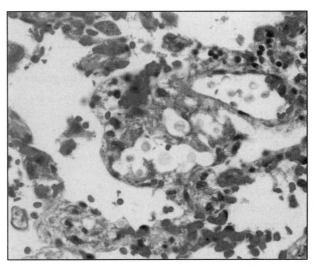

Used with permission of W. Dean Wallace, MD, Department of Pathology and Laboratory Medicine, David Geffen School of Medicine, UCLA.

Question 3: **What is the best treatment plan for this patient?**

A. Monitor clinically
B. Fluconazole
C. Amphotericin B
D. Caspofungin
E. Flucytosine

CASE 5

A 56-year-old man with a history of HIV, who recently immigrated from Central America, presents with low-grade fevers and weight loss. He denies any TB exposures and has a recent negative skin purified protein derivative

(PPD) test. He previously worked as a construction worker and a gardener. Physical examination reveals cervical and axillary lymphadenopathy and oral ulcers. His chest imaging shows infiltrates in his upper lung fields and his sputum culture shows the following organism:

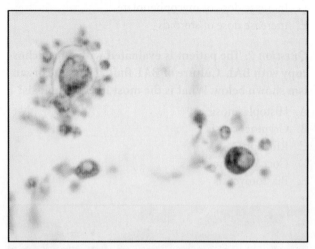

Reproduced with permission from Centers for Disease Control and Prevention (CDC). Public Health Image Library (PHIL).

Question 1: What is the most likely diagnosis?

A. Histoplasmosis
B. Paracoccidioidomycosis
C. Blastomycosis
D. Coccidioidomycosis
E. Cryptococcosis

Question 2: Which of these agents have activity against this mycosis?

A. Itraconazole
B. Cotrimoxazole
C. Amphotericin B
D. Terbinafine
E. All of the above

CASE 6

A 36-year-old woman with a recent diagnosis of acute lymphocytic leukemia is admitted to the medical intensive care unit with septic shock, pneumonia and respiratory failure. You send labs for infectious work-up including those for fungal etiologies.

Question 1: Which of the following is true regarding biochemical diagnostics for fungal infections?

A. Galactomannan is a polysaccharide component of Aspergillus cell wall that can be measured in the serum
B. (1–3)-β-D-glucan can be useful in identifying Candida and Pneumocystis
C. Galactomannan has variable sensitivity and specificity in different populations
D. Results of galactomannan can be altered in patients taking amoxicillin-clavulanic acid
E. All of the above

CASE 7

A 42-year-old man nonsmoker with no significant past medical history presents with cough, weight loss, and night sweats. He is an avid camper and recently spent a week camping in Mississippi. Physical examination reveals subcutaneous nodules and verrucous lesions in his lower extremities as shown below. He notes that some of his skin lesions have been draining purulent material. A chest x-ray is obtained which reveals a right-middle lobe lung mass.

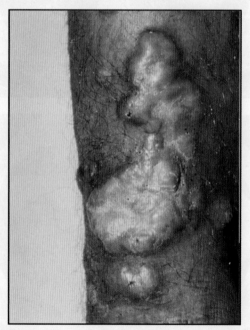

Reproduced with permission from Centers for Disease Control and Prevention (CDC). Public Health Image Library (PHIL).

Question 1. What is the most appropriate next step?

A. PET-CT of the chest
B. Transbronchial biopsy of lung mass
C. Examination of skin lesion and drainage with KOH preparation
D. VATS with wedge resection of lung mass
E. CT-guided biopsy of lung mass

Question 2. What is the best therapeutic regimen in this patient?

A. Amphotericin B
B. Itraconazole
C. Caspofungin
D. Anidulafungin
E. No therapy since the disease is self-limited

CASE 8

A 54-year-old man status post renal transplant presents with a 2-week history of progressive fatigue and dyspnea without cough or fever. His immunosuppressive regimen consists of tacrolimus, mycophenolate mofetil, and prednisone. Three months ago, he is diagnosed with cryptogenic organizing pneumonia responsive to a prolonged steroid course and is currently on prednisone at 40 mg daily. Vital signs reveal a low-grade fever (100.1°F), mild tachycardia, a respiratory rate of 26, and oxygen saturation of 87% on room air. On examination, he appears fatigued, tachypneic, and cushingoid and lung examination reveals diminished breath sounds and scattered bilateral rhonchi.

**

A chest x-ray reveals multifocal consolidation and he is treated empirically with vancomycin, piperacillin-tazobactam, and ciprofloxacin along with stress dose steroids. A chest CT is obtained (see bottom of page):

**

Bronchoscopy with bronchoalveolar lavage is performed and cultures grow *Aspergillus fumigatus*. Serum *Aspergillus* galactomannan enzyme-linked immunosorbent assay (EIA) returns positive.

Question 1: Which of the following is the most appropriate therapeutic change?

A. Add itraconazole
B. Add lipid formulation amphotericin B
C. Add voriconazole
D. Add posaconazole
E. Add recombinant interferon-gamma

Question 2: Which of the following medications is most likely to cause a false-positive galactomannan EIA?

A. Tacrolimus
B. Mycophenolate mofetil
C. Piperacillin-tazobactam
D. Vancomycin
E. Ciprofloxacin

Question 3: Which of the following is most likely to be resistant to amphotericin B?

A. *Aspergillus flavus*
B. *Aspergillus terreus*
C. *Aspergillus niger*
D. *Aspergillus claidoustus*
E. *Aspergillus fumigatus*

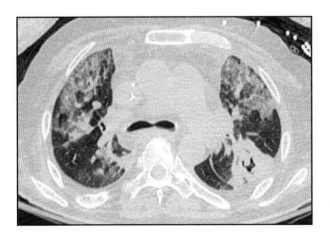
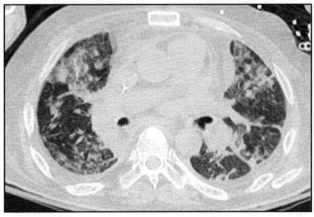

Question 4: The histopathologic features of *Aspergillus* with septate branching hyphae are often indistinguishable from which other potentially invasive opportunistic mold?

A. Scedosporium
B. Mucorales
C. Curvularia
D. Wangiella
E. Alternaria

CASE 9

A 51-year-old man with severe COPD and bullous emphysema presents with intermittent fevers and progressively worsening dyspnea, cough, hypoxia, and a 10-pound weight loss over the past 4 months. Six months prior, he underwent lung volume reduction surgery without complications with initially improved exertional dyspnea. He is currently on an inhaler regimen of fluticasone with salmeterol, tiotropium, and as needed albuterol. Vital signs are unremarkable, and on examination he is thin with scattered mild expiratory wheezing.

* *

Because of some concern for malignancy, a chest CT is obtained:

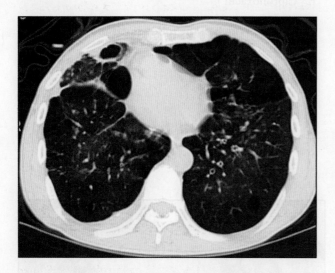

* *

Sputum culture is positive for *Aspergillus fumigatus*. Serum *Aspergillus* antigen EIA is negative, but serum precipitating *Aspergillus* IgG is positive.

Question 1: Which of the following is the LEAST appropriate alternative to voriconazole to treat this condition?

A. Fluconazole
B. Caspofungin
C. Lipid formulation amphotericin B
D. Posaconazole
E. Itraconazole

Question 2: Which of the following tests is most consistently positive for this condition?

A. *Aspergillus* IgG precipitins
B. Galactomannan EIA
C. *Aspergillus*-specific IgE
D. Bronchoalveolar lavage culture for *Aspergillus*
E. Histopathology from transbronchial biopsy

Question 3: Despite an initial response with voriconazole, after several months of therapy there is evidence of disease progression. Which of the following is the most appropriate next step?

A. Continue therapy and reevaluate in 1 month
B. Change antifungal therapy to itraconazole
C. Start interferon-gamma therapy
D. Surgical resection of affected lung
E. Check serum voriconazole level

CASE 10

A 53-year-old man with no past medical history presents with fevers, chills, and cough for 3 weeks. He lives in Missouri and works as a construction worker. Prior to presentation, he is given a course of amoxicillin and ciprofloxacin without improvement. On examination he is febrile to 102°F but otherwise his examination is unremarkable. Labs reveal pancytopenia with WBC 1.2 (ANC 400), Hb 7.1, and Plt 10,000. A chest CT obtained after an abnormal chest x-ray shows bulky mediastinal and hilar lymphadenopathy and a lingular mass as below, along with splenomegaly. Mediastinoscopy is performed with lymph node biopsies revealing fungal organisms consistent with *Histoplasma capsulatum*. A bone-marrow biopsy reveals hypocellularity consistent with myelodysplastic syndrome. Urine and serum *Histoplasma* antigen return positive.

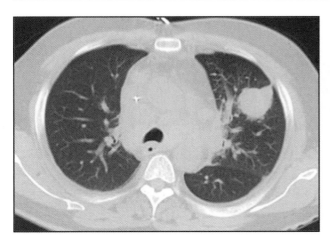
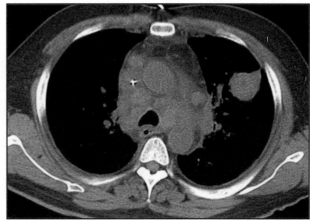

Question 1: **Which of the following is the most appropriate treatment?**

A. Itraconazole
B. Lipid formulation amphotericin B
C. Voriconazole
D. Caspofungin
E. No antifungal treatment

Question 2: **The patient presents 6 months later with worsening cough and dyspnea despite continuous antifungal therapy. A chest CT is repeated and reveals the following:**

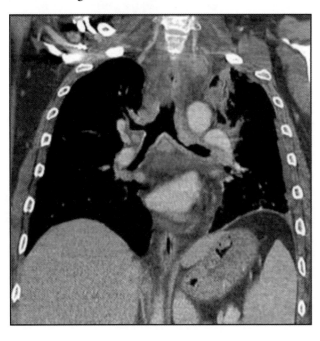

What is the most likely cause for the bronchial obstruction and stenosis?

A. Mediastinal lymphadenitis
B. Extrinsic compression from a mediastinal granuloma
C. Endobronchial fistula from a mediastinal granuloma
D. Fibrosing mediastinitis
E. Broncholithiasis

Question 3: **Antifungal therapy is most indicated for which of the following pulmonary histoplasmosis-related complications?**

A. Histoplasmoma
B. Symptomatic fibrosing mediastinitis
C. Broncholithiasis
D. *Histoplasma* pneumonia with mild symptoms lasting 2 weeks
E. Symptomatic mediastinal granuloma

CASE 11

A 60-year-old Filipino man develops 8 days of fevers, chills, nonproductive cough, and bilateral pleuritic chest pain. He lives in Southern California, works in construction, and denies any sick contacts. On examination, he has a low-grade fever with bilateral rhonchi on lung examination. Labs reveal a WBC of 11 with an absolute eosinophil count of 550 (normal <500). His chest imaging reveals the following:

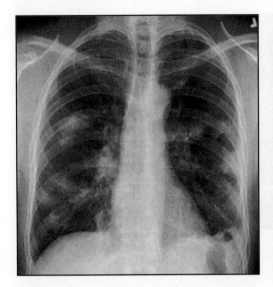

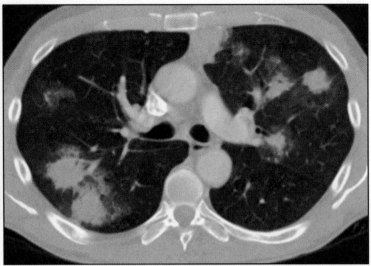

* *

Coccidioides IgG and IgM enzyme-linked immunosorbent assay (EIA) return positive.

Question 1: Which of the following can be used to evaluate response to treatment?

A. Peripheral eosinophil count
B. *Coccidioides* antibody EIA
C. *Coccidioides* antibody immunodiffusion
D. *Coccidioides* antibody complement fixation
E. None of the above

Question 2: Which of the following in confirmed Coccidioidomycosis is the LEAST likely to require antifungal treatment?

A. Pulmonary cavitary lesions
B. Weight loss of 20%
C. Night sweats persistent for 4 weeks
D. *Coccidioides* antibody complement fixation titer 1:32
E. Comorbid HIV with CD4 count of 180 cells/μL

Question 3: He is treated with Fluconazole for 3 months with symptomatic and radiographic improvement. He is subsequently lost to follow-up but presents 2 years later with several months of fevers, chills, night sweats, weight loss, cough, fatigue, and persistent low back pain. He is found to have an L5 spinal abscess as well as

mediastinal, hilar, and supraclavicular lymphadenopathy. *Coccidioides* antibody complement fixation titer is elevated at 1:1,024, and a biopsy of a supraclavicular lymph node shows the following:

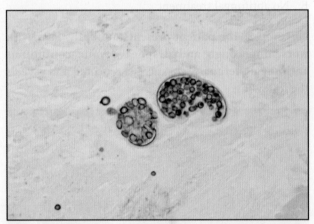

Used with permission of Gregory Fishbein, MD, David Geffen School of Medicine, UCLA.

Which of the following is the LEAST appropriate option for initial treatment?

A. Caspofungin
B. Fluconazole
C. Itraconazole
D. Posaconazole
E. Lipid formulation amphotericin B

CASE 12

A 28-year-old woman with a history of allergic rhinitis and severe persistent asthma for the past several years with frequent exacerbations requiring corticosteroids presents with an asthma exacerbation with associated cough productive of mucus plugs. She has been on high-dose inhaled corticosteroids, a long-acting beta agonist, and montelukast. CBC reveals an eosinophil count of 1,250 (normal <500) and serum IgE of 2,320. Skin prick test and IgE to *Aspergillus fumigatus* are negative. Sputum cultures grow *Curvularia lunata.*

Question 1: **Aside from initiating oral corticosteroid therapy, which of the following is the most appropriate next step in management?**

A. Start omalizumab
B. Start itraconazole
C. Start inhaled amphotericin B
D. Start immunotherapy for *Curvularia*
E. Skin pinprick testing for *Curvularia*

Answers

CASE 1

Question 1: C. Aspergilloma

The patient's radiographic finding is consistent with an aspergilloma, defined as the presence of a fungus ball, fungal hyphae mixed with inflammatory cells, fibrin and mucus, inside a cavity or dilated airway. A fungus ball is usually from aspergillus but can be seen with other fungal species such as *Zygomycetes* and *Fusarium*. The aspergilloma mass can be seen moving within the cavity if the patient is rotated and reimaged. In general, patients are asymptomatic and are diagnosed based on incidental findings on chest radiographs. Others may develop hemoptysis and chronic cough.[1,2]

* *

Although *Nocardia*, mycobacterial infections, and non-small cell lung cancer can present with cavitary lung masses, the presence of a mass within a cavity is unlikely. Lung abscesses often present with systemic symptoms including fevers, cough, and night sweats, and air-fluid levels are typically seen on imaging.

Question 2: D. All of the above

Aspergillomas develop when preexisting pulmonary cavities become colonized with *Aspergillus* species. Aspergillomas are most commonly associated with pulmonary tuberculosis but they have also been associated with nontuberculous mycobacterial infections, allergic bronchopulmonary aspergillosis (ABPA), COPD, fibrocavitary sarcoidosis, lung cancer following treatment, and pneumothorax with bullae formation.[1,2] This patient's risk factor is likely undiagnosed COPD given her significant smoking history.

Question 3: A. Bronchial artery embolization

Observation may be appropriate in asymptomatic, immunocompetent patients. Conservative measures with humidified oxygen, cough suppressants, and postural drainage may be sufficient with mild hemoptysis. Aggressive treatment is recommended if there is disease progression or if patients develop significant hemoptysis.

* *

Immunocompromised patients may progress to chronic or invasive pulmonary aspergillosis and can be treated with voriconazole or itraconazole. Surgery is the first-line treatment for patients with hemoptysis related to aspergilloma. However, bronchial artery embolization is the option in high-risk patients who have moderate to massive hemoptysis or are not good surgical candidates, as is the case in this patient with coronary artery disease and angina. Diagnostic bronchoscopy may assist in localizing the source of bleeding but this was already confirmed on CT angiogram and definitive management should be the next step. Chest tube placement has no role in hemoptysis management. Mortality associated with hemoptysis from aspergilloma has been reported to be between 2% and 14% and observation alone is not appropriate.[1,2]

CASE 2

Question 1: C. Skin-test reactivity to *Aspergillus* antigen

Allergic bronchopulmonary aspergillosis (ABPA) should be considered in patients with poorly controlled asthma despite appropriate therapy. ABPA is a hypersensitivity reaction usually caused by *Aspergillus fumigatus*. It typically occurs in patients with asthma or cystic fibrosis (CF). Asthmatics often present with frequent exacerbations requiring corticosteroids, fevers, malaise, and cough with copious sputum production. ABPA is difficult to differentiate from an exacerbation in the CF population and should be considered when a CF flare fails to respond to antimicrobials.

* *

The diagnosis of ABPA in asthma is based on a combination of clinical, radiographic and laboratory findings (see Table 20–1). Although a variety of diagnostic

Table 20-1 MAJOR AND MINOR CRITERIA FOR THE DIAGNOSIS OF ABPA

Major	Minor
• Asthma • Peripheral blood eosinophilia • IgE >1,000 IU/mL • Positive immediate (type I) skin reaction to *Aspergillus* • Serum *Aspergillus* –specific IgE • Serum precipitating or IgG antibodies to *A. fumigatus* • Chest x-ray or CT with central bronchiectasis and fleeting infiltrates	• *Aspergillus* in sputum on repeated studies • History of brown mucous plugs • Late (type III) skin reaction to *Aspergillus*

criteria have been proposed, the most commonly used includes major and minor criteria. However, the necessary findings required to come to a definitive diagnosis have yet to be established. In the above patient with uncontrolled asthma and elevated IgE levels, a positive immediate cutaneous reaction to *Aspergillus* would add to the major criteria.[3]

* *

Lung biopsies are rarely performed in the diagnostic evaluation of ABPA. Serum ACE levels and sputum acid-fast cultures can aid in the evaluation and diagnosis of sarcoidosis and mycobacterial infections respectively, but have no utility in the diagnosis of ABPA. This patient has known asthma with obstruction on prior pulmonary function tests; therefore a methacholine challenge is unnecessary.

Question 2: B. Systemic glucocorticoids

The goal of treatment in ABPA is to both prevent and control exacerbations as well as to limit disease progression to fibrosis. Corticosteroids are the mainstay of treatment although there is limited data on duration and dose of therapy. In general, the recommendation is prednisone 0.5 mg/kg/day for 2 weeks with a gradual taper, individualized to each patient's clinical status. Most will require prolonged low-dose corticosteroid therapy to control symptoms and to prevent relapse. Response to therapy can be monitored with reduction in IgE levels, peripheral eosinophilia, and symptoms along with resolution or improvement in radiographic infiltrates.

* *

Several trials have also shown utility of antifungal agents with resultant reduction in steroid dose, pulmonary infiltrates, IgE levels, and symptoms with the use of itraconazole. Voriconazole also has excellent activity against *Aspergillus* and has been shown to have a good response in some trials in ABPA. The duration of antifungal therapy is not established although 4 to 8 months has been suggested with itraconazole and up to a 12-month course with voriconazole.[3,4]

* *

The patient is already on high-dose inhaled steroids and although theophylline (failed therapy in the past) and tiotropium can be utilized in asthma, they will not target the patient's underlying ABPA. Bronchial thermoplasty has no utility in ABPA and its role in uncontrolled asthma remains unclear.

Question 3: A. Bronchiectasis

The most common complication of ABPA is bronchiectasis, which is often already present at the time of diagnosis. In its most severe forms, bronchiectasis can lead to pulmonary hypertension and respiratory failure. Hemoptysis is not commonly reported with ABPA. Patients with ABPA have also been documented to develop chronic cavitary pulmonary aspergillosis (CCPA) as well as upper lobe fibrosis without cavitation, but less commonly than bronchiectasis. CCPA is characterized by multiple cavities with or without mycetomas that can further progress to extensive fibrosis, resulting in chronic fibrosing pulmonary aspergillosis (CFPA). CFPA falls under the umbrella term chronic pulmonary aspergillosis (CPA). There is no data on the utility of antifungals or corticosteroids in preventing bronchiectasis, cavitation or fibrosis. However, long-term antifungal therapy is currently recommended in all patients who transform from ABPA to CPA with cavitation.[3] Finally, lung cancer is not a known complication of ABPA.

CASE 3

Question 1: C. Mucormycosis

Mucormycosis commonly presents with sinopulmonary involvement. Clinical symptoms are often indistinguishable from that of *Aspergillus*. Mucormycosis manifests as nonproductive cough, progressive dyspnea, pleuritic chest pain, and fevers refractory to broad-spectrum antibiotics. Infection can be angioinvasive resulting in fatal hemoptysis and has a propensity to traverse tissue planes in the chest including the bronchi, chest wall, diaphragm, and pleura. The presence of severe sinusitis, rhinoorbital extension, and necrotic palatal lesions can be clues to mucormycosis rather than *Aspergillus* infection.

**

Chest imaging can show numerous abnormalities including cavities, masses, nodules, and consolidation. The presence of multiple nodules (>10) can favor mucormycosis over aspergillosis.

**

Diagnosis relies on histopathology and cultures of sterile tissue. Pathology shows characteristic broad nonseptate hyphae with 90° angle branching, unlike the septate hyphae with 45° angle branching seen with *Aspergillus* or *Fusarium*. Sputum cultures and bronchoalveolar lavage fluid are often nondiagnostic, and blood cultures rarely are positive despite the angioinvasive nature of the disease.[5] *Nocardia* and mycobacterium tuberculosis (MTB) have rarely been shown to cause sinusitis. On histology, *Nocardia* appears as weakly acid-fast positive filamentous organisms while MTB appears as strongly acid-fast positive bacilli.

Question 2: E. All of the above

Patients with hematological malignancies, those with prolonged and severe neutropenia, those on high-dose glucocorticoid therapy, and recipients of hematopoietic stem cell and solid organ transplant are all at increased risk for infections from *Mucorales*. Patients with uncontrolled diabetes mellitus are also at increased risk, and they tend to develop endobronchial lesions more often as seen in this patient.

**

Different host immune deficiencies can predispose patients to different forms of mucormycosis. Patients with diabetic ketoacidosis for example develop the rhinocerebral form more frequently while those with severe immunocompromise (organ transplant recipients and patients with hematologic malignancies) tend to develop pulmonary disease. Recent studies have identified mucormycosis as a breakthrough infection in the setting of antifungal prophylaxis or treatments that are effective against aspergillosis (voriconazole and echinocandins) but not mucormycosis.[5]

Question 3: B. Amphotericin B

Given the rarity of the disease, there are no prospective randomized trials evaluating the treatment of mucormycosis. Early administration of an effective antifungal agent is crucial as delayed treatment is associated with increased mortality. Based on small studies, the current recommendation includes antifungal therapy with the lipid formulation of amphotericin B or amphotericin B deoxycholate. There are case reports using alternate routes for amphotericin administration such as inhaled drug for pulmonary disease as well as instillation into abscess/pleural cavities, but the efficacy of these methods remains unclear.

**

An alternate regimen is posaconazole, which is the only oral agent in its class that has activity against *Mucorales*, with success rates of 60% to 70% in open label and retrospective trials with refractory cases. However this drug is currently not FDA-approved for mucormycosis given the need for additional studies. Echinocandins lack in vitro activity against *Mucorales*. However, caspofungin has been studied in animal models and there are case reports with some success. Combination therapy with amphotericin and caspofungin was shown to have success in a study with biopsy proven rhinoorbital cerebral mucormycosis. However, since there have been cases of breakthrough mucormycosis in the setting of echinocandin use, additional studies are needed. Mucormycosis is often angioinvasive with resultant tissue necrosis and thrombosis that impedes antifungal penetration at the site of infection. Thus, surgical debridement of infected tissue should be performed urgently and has been shown to improve survival compared to those who were treated only with antifungals.[5-9]

**

Trimethoprim/sulfamethoxazole is used in the treatment of infections caused by organisms such as *Nocardia*, *Stenotrophomonas* and *Pneumocystis jirovecii* but has no role in the treatment of mucormycosis.

CASE 4

Question 1: A. Bronchoscopy with BAL

An immunosuppressed patient with new respiratory symptoms with nodular and ground glass changes on chest CT is concerning for atypical or fungal infection. Further infectious work-up is warranted and augmenting immunosuppression is inappropriate at this time. Although an atypical pneumonia is possible, treatment with azithromycin alone without additional evaluation is not appropriate. An invasive procedure such as a VATS lung biopsy is not indicated in this patient before less invasive procedures are attempted. This patient was further evaluated with a bronchoscopy with bronchoalveolar lavage.

Question 2: B. Cryptococcosis

Cryptococcal pneumonia is most often associated with HIV but other conditions that predispose patients to this infection include solid organ transplant, hematologic malignancies, chronic corticosteroid treatment, sarcoidosis, and dysfunction of cell-mediated immunity as with anti-tumor necrosis factor-alpha (TNF-alpha) therapy. Infection can also occur in immunocompetent patients although the incidence in the normal population is not well characterized. *C. neoformans* is the most common cause of cryptococcosis and typically occurs in immunocompromised patients. *C. gattii*, on the other hand, is an emerging pathogen causing disease in the immunocompetent host, typically in the Pacific Northwest, Canada, and the tropics. Meningitis is the most common manifestation of cryptococcosis in both normal and immunocompromised hosts. Other secondary sites of infection include the skin, bone, prostate, and eye.

* *

The clinical presentation of cryptococcal pneumonia varies and commonly includes cough, fever, dyspnea, and chest pain. Disease in immunocompetent patients may be asymptomatic with isolated pulmonary nodules that may self-resolve. Radiographic findings include solitary or multiple pulmonary nodules, segmental or lobar consolidation, a diffuse interstitial pattern, and cavitary lesions.

* *

Diagnosis relies on the isolation of *Cryptococcus* species from a lung specimen in the appropriate clinical setting. Cryptococcal antigen testing in sputum and BAL fluid are unreliable. Serum antigen testing is highly sensitive and specific for disseminated infection and cryptococcal meningitis but has a more limited role in patients with only pulmonary involvement. A lumbar puncture is recommended in patients with cryptococcal pneumonia with any concern for dissemination, neurologic symptoms or positive serum cryptococcal antigen titers.[6,10]

* *

The patient is not known to have traveled to areas that would place him at risk for endemic mycoses and BAL fluid findings show *Cryptococcus neoformans* on H&E stain as shown previously, with the classic halo from the polysaccharide capsule.

Question 3: B. Fluconazole

Choice and regimen of antifungal therapy for Cryptococcosis depend on disease severity and immune status. See Table 20-2 for specific recommended regimens based on American Thoracic Society Guidelines. Fluconazole 400 mg/day for 6 to 12 months followed by a maintenance dose of 200 mg/day would be appropriate for this immunocompromised patient with disease limited to the lungs.[6]

Table 20-2 TREATMENT OF CRYPTOCOCCOSIS

Immunocompetent Patients	
Disease Severity	**Treatment**
Colonization	No antifungal therapy
Localized pulmonary disease	Fluconazole or itraconazole × 6 months[a]
Central nervous system (CNS) or disseminated disease	Amphotericin B ± flucytosine × 2 weeks, then fluconazole or itraconazole × 10 weeks[a] OR Amphotericin B ± flucytosine × 6–10 weeks[a]

Immunocompromised Patients	
Disease Severity	**Treatment**
Pulmonary disease, asymptomatic or mild	Fluconazole or itraconazole × 6 months, followed by secondary prophylaxis
CNS or disseminated disease	Amphotericin B + flucytosine × 2 weeks then fluconazole or itraconazole × 8 weeks, followed by maintenance OR Lipid formulation of amphotericin B × 6–10 weeks followed by maintenance
Maintenance (secondary prophylaxis)	Fluconazole

[a]Can extend therapy if incomplete response.

CASE 5

Question 1: B. Paracoccidioidomycosis

Paracoccidioidomycosis (PCM) is an endemic mycosis caused by *Paracoccidioides brasiliensis*, a dimorphic soil fungus, found mainly in rural workers in Latin America. Most primary pulmonary infections are subclinical and individuals may remain infected throughout their life without ever progressing to have clinical signs of infection. The respiratory system is the most common site of primary infection.

**

A small fraction of individuals can develop clinical disease in two patterns, acute or subacute (juvenile type) form, or chronic (adult type) form. Lung involvement is frequent in the chronic form but not the acute form. The acute and chronic form can progress to disseminated disease with secondary lesions affecting mucous membranes, lymph nodes, adrenal glands, the CNS, and the skin. Most PCM cases in HIV patients present as disseminated disease with fevers, lung involvement, generalized lymphadenopathy, weight loss, rash, and hepatosplenomegaly.

**

The diagnosis is made in patients with appropriate clinical symptoms from endemic areas, with microbiological isolation from clinical specimens. The characteristic morphology is that of large fungal cells surrounded by multiple budding yeast resembling a "pilot's wheel" or as mother cells only with two budding yeast resembling a "mickey mouse head." These findings are not consistent with the organisms in the other answer choices.[11]

Question 2: E. All of the above

Although PCM has high incidence and mortality in South America, few studies are available to determine optimal treatment. PCM is very sensitive to a large number of drugs including sulfonamides, azoles, amphotericin B, and terbinafine. In general, itraconazole is used to treat mild to moderate disease and amphotericin B is utilized for severe cases of disseminated disease.[11]

CASE 6

Question 1: E. All of the above

Galactomannan is a polysaccharide component of *Aspergillus* cell wall that can be measured in serum and other body fluids allowing for the evaluation of invasive aspergillosis. Based on data from leukemia patients and hematopoietic stem cell transplant recipients, high sensitivity (81%) and specificity (89%) were demonstrated, which were much higher than in the solid organ transplant population (22% and 84% respectively). The sensitivity of galactomannan assay in BAL was much higher than in serum. However, the utility of BAL galactomannan in detecting invasive aspergillosis is complicated by the inability to differentiate it from colonization and chronic forms of Aspergillosis.

**

Results of galactomannan assays can be affected by several factors. False-positives are seen in patients on antimicrobial treatment with certain beta-lactam antibiotics, in patients with respiratory colonization with other molds, and if Plasma-Lyte solutions are used with BAL collection. False-negatives are seen in patients on antifungal therapy with antimold activity.

**

(1–3)-β-D-glucan (BDG) is another fungal cell wall component used to detect invasive fungal infections including *Aspergillus*, *Pneumocystis*, *Fusarium*, *Candida* and *Trichosporon*. It has high sensitivity and specificity, and can be used in conjunction with the galactomannan assay. Unfortunately, BDG is ubiquitous in the environment and similar to the galactomannan assay, several factors can lead to false-positive results, such as poor specimen handling and bacteremia.[12]

CASE 7

Question 1: C. Examination of skin lesion and drainage with KOH preparation

Blastomycosis should be considered in patients presenting with lung masses or alveolar infiltrates with extrapulmonary manifestations such as cutaneous involvement, in the appropriate clinical context. *Blastomyces dermatitidis* is a dimorphous fungus endemic to areas along the Ohio, Mississippi and St. Lawrence River, as well as the areas around the Great Lakes in New York and Canada. Blastomycosis can occur in immunocompetent patients but is typically more severe or disseminated in the immunocompromised population.

**

After exposure through inhalation of *Blastomyces* spores, patients can present acutely with fevers and productive cough similar to a bacterial pneumonia. The course can also be indolent with cough, night sweats, weight loss and hemoptysis, often resembling tuberculosis or histoplasmosis. Radiographic findings can include alveolar infiltrates, lung masses and pleural effusions. Less often, patients can present with diffuse miliary disease or ARDS (acute respiratory distress syndome).

**

Blastomycosis can involve virtually every organ although the most common are bone, skin, the CNS, and the genitourinary system. As in this patient, skin findings include ulcerated or verrucous lesions that can drain purulent material. Subcutaneous nodules and abcesses can be present but are less common.

* *

The most rapid and noninvasive way to diagnose blastomycosis is examination of clinical specimens such as scrapings from skin lesions or cutaneous drainage under KOH (potassium hydroxide) preparation. Sputum samples and BAL fluid can be examined similarly. Visualization of the characteristic broad-based budding yeast (shown below) can lead to the correct diagnosis, although this needs to be confirmed with culture of the specimen, which is the gold standard. Blastomyces urine antigen detection is commercially available although it is limited by a high degree of cross-reactivity with histoplasmosis. Invasive procedures such as transbronchial, CT-guided, or VATS biopsies are not indicated in this patient as initial diagnostic steps. Although this patient's lung mass raises suspicion for malignancy, this non-smoker has a low risk for lung cancer and blastomycosis is more likely given the clinical context.

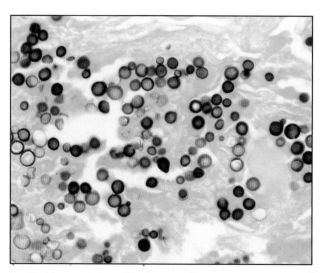

Used with permission of W. Dean Wallace, MD, Department of Pathology and Laboratory Medicine, David Geffen School of Medicine, UCLA.

Question 2: B. Itraconazole

Prompt diagnosis and treatment of blastomycosis is crucial since it can be associated with mortality rates of up to 60%. Although acute pulmonary blastomycosis is self-limited in some immunocompetent patients, current recommendations suggest treating all recognized cases of blastomycosis since it is impossible to predict who will recover and who will develop extrapulmonary disease. The initial mainstay of therapy is itraconazole and amphotericin depending on the disease manifestations and severity (Table 20-3). Itraconazole is appropriate in this patient without life threatening disease or CNS involvement. Echinocandins have variable in vitro activity against *Blastomyces* and there is no human data to support their use in blastomycosis.[6,13]

Table 20-3   TREATMENT OF BLASTOMYCOSIS

Extent of Disease	Antifungal Agent
Skin disease	Itraconazole × 24 weeks
Bone disease	Itraconazole × 24 weeks
Mild to moderately ill with pulmonary and non-meningeal involvement	Itraconazole × 24 weeks
Life-threatening disease including ARDS	Liposomal amphotericin B or amphotericin B until clinical improvement, then itraconazole for 6–12 months
Meningeal disease	Liposomal amphotericin B or amphotericin B until clinical improvement, and concurrent or sequential itraconazole or fluconazole for 6–12 months

CASE 8

Question 1: C. Add voriconazole

Voriconazole is first-line therapy for invasive pulmonary aspergillosis (IPA). IPA is an opportunistic infection typically affecting those with significant immune compromise, such as allogeneic hematopoietic stem cell transplant (HSCT) recipients and solid organ transplant (SOT) patients (see Table 20–4).[4,14–16] The incidence in SOT ranges

Table 20-4   TYPICAL HOST RISK FACTORS FOR INVASIVE ASPERGILLOSIS[4,14,15]

Prolonged neutropenia (<500 neutrophils/mm^3 for >10 days)
HSCT or SOT, particularly lung transplant
Systemic corticosteroid use for >3 weeks at a mean dose of ≥0.3 mg/kg/day of prednisone or equivalent
Hematologic malignancy, particularly leukemias
Chemotherapy
AIDS
Inherited immunodeficiencies

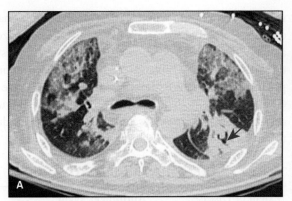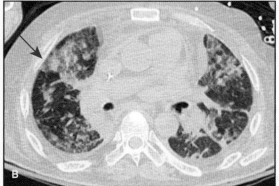

Note the air-crescent sign in panel A and the halo sign in panel B (red arrows).

from 10% to 15% and occurs most commonly in lung transplant recipients. IPA is also becoming increasingly recognized in patients without traditional risk factors, i.e., in COPD patients and critically ill patients in the ICU.

* *

Diagnosing IPA can be challenging. Definitive diagnosis requires histopathologic evidence of *Aspergillus* tissue invasion and destruction, but tissue sampling is often high risk. Alternatively, probable disease requires an immunocompromised host along with clinical evidence of disease and laboratory evidence of *Aspergillus* involvement (Table 20-5).[15] Serum (1–3)-β-D-glucan assay is a useful test to detect invasive mycoses but is not specific to *Aspergillus*. The limited sensitivity and specificity of many of these studies complicates the diagnosis of IPA. Nevertheless, our patient meets criteria for probable IPA.

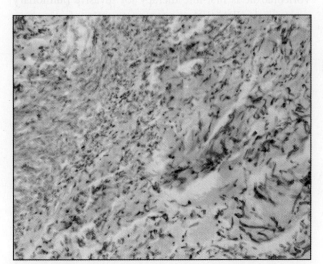

Note the septated hyphae branching at 45-degree angles.
(Used with permission of Gregory Fishbein, MD, David Geffen School of Medicine, UCLA.)

Table 20-5 PROBABLE INVASIVE PULMONARY ASPERGILLOSIS[14,15]

Immunocompromised Host	See Table 20-4
Clinical evidence of disease (≥1 needed)	• Characteristic CT findings: dense, well-circumscribed consolidations with or without halo sign, air-crescent sign, or cavity (see below) • Noncharacteristic CT findings with pleural rub, pleuritis, or hemoptysis • Bronchoscopic evidence of tracheobronchitis (suggestive of invasive tracheobronchial aspergillosis)
Laboratory evidence of disease (≥1 needed)	• *Aspergillus* in cytology or culture from sputum, BAL, or bronchial brushing (see below) • Galactomannan in serum or BAL • Serum (1–3)-β-D-glucan positivity

* *

An alternative therapy to voriconazole in the treatment of IPA is lipid formulation amphotericin B. Itraconazole, caspofungin, and posaconazole can also be used as salvage therapy but voriconazole remains first line. Combination therapy is often used clinically but data supporting this approach is lacking. Cessation of therapy requires clinical and radiographic resolution, fungal eradication, and reversal of immune suppression. Reduction or cessation of immunosuppressive agents should thus be pursued if possible.[4,14–16] Immunomodulation with recombinant interferon-gamma and granulocyte-colony stimulating factor or granulocyte macrophage-colony stimulating factor can be considered as salvage therapy in life-threatening invasive fungal disease refractory to conventional antifungal therapy, though supporting evidence is limited.[17]

Question 2: C. Piperacillin-tazobactam

False-positive galactomannan EIA can be seen in patients who have been treated with semi-synthetic beta-lactams, including piperacillin and amoxicillin. Cross-reactivity with *Histoplasma capsulatum* or *Blastomyces dermatitidis* can also cause false-positive results. The other agents are not known to cause a false-positive galactomannan EIA test.

* *

Galactomannan EIA levels can be followed to assess response to therapy and for prognostication; declining values are associated with improved outcomes.[9,18]

Question 3: B. *Aspergillus terreus*

The most common cause of aspergillosis is *Aspergillus fumigatus*, comprising >50% of cases. This is followed by *A. flavus* and *A. terreus*. Most *Aspergillus* species are sensitive to amphotericin B; however *A. terreus* is generally resistant to amphotericin B and best treated with voriconazole.[16]

Question 4: A. Scedosporium

Aspergillus is often difficult to distinguish from *Scedosporium* and *Fusarium* species on histopathologic examination as they all have septate acute-angle branching hyphae. *Mucorales* on the other hand have broad-based nonseptate or pauciseptate ribbon-like hyphae. *Curvularia*, *Wangiella*, and *Alternaria* have characteristic pigmented hyphae and are easily distinguished from the colorless *Scedosporium*, *Aspergillus*, and *Mucorales*.

* *

While *Aspergillus* is by far the most common cause of invasive pulmonary mold infections in the immuno-compromised population, other molds can also cause similar opportunistic infections. Invasive *Mucorales*, *Fusarium*, and *Scedosporium* infections are becoming more common and often present similarly to *Aspergillus* with similarly poor outcomes.

* *

Culture identification is crucial to distinguish *Aspergillus* from *Scedosporium* and *Fusarium* in order to guide antifungal therapy. *Scedosporium* and *Fusarium* have variable sensitivities to various antifungal agents, including voriconazole.[15,16,19]

CASE 9

Question 1: A. Fluconazole

This patient has chronic pulmonary aspergillosis (CPA), which is characterized by progressive pulmonary cavitations surrounded by consolidation or pleural thickening.[19] The serum *Aspergillus* precipitins (IgG) test is usually positive.[1] Isolation of *Aspergillus* species on culture aids in the diagnosis. CPA typically presents with an indolent course with fever, cough, weight loss, and fatigue lasting months. It usually affects patients with underlying lung disease (i.e., COPD) with either mild or no immune compromise (i.e., low-dose corticosteroids) and with defective pulmonary mucociliary clearance. CPA straddles the spectrum of pulmonary *Aspergillus* disease, between simple aspergilloma on one end and invasive pulmonary aspergillosis on the other. CPA can be further divided into chronic cavitary pulmonary aspergillosis, which is more indolent and progresses over several months, and chronic necrotizing pulmonary aspergillosis, which is more subacute and progresses over weeks to months.

* *

Prolonged antifungal therapy is indicated in CPA. First-line treatment of CPA is voriconazole, although itraconazole, posaconazole, lipid formulation amphotericin B, and caspofungin are options. Fluconazole has no activity against *Aspergillus* species.[21]

Question 2: A. *Aspergillus* IgG precipitins

The serum *Aspergillus* IgG precipitins test is the most useful test for CPA. A positive result along with characteristic radiographic and appropriate clinical presentation is sufficient for the diagnosis for CPA. Its sensitivity is 75% to 90% with a specificity of 85% for CPA. Galactomannan EIA, BAL cultures, and histopathology from transbronchial biopsies all have limited sensitivity in CPA and aspergillus-specific IgE is used in the diagnostic criteria for ABPA rather than CPA.[20,22]

Question 3: E. Check serum voriconazole level

Progression of *Aspergillus* infection despite appropriate voriconazole therapy may indicate inadequate drug levels, and serum levels should be checked. Some experts recommend routine voriconazole level monitoring. If itraconazole or posaconazole is used to treat *Aspergillus* infection, serum levels should be monitored routinely to ensure adequate tissue exposure and avoid toxicity.[15]

* *

Progression of disease despite appropriate antifungal therapy should also raise suspicion for resistance, which is not uncommon in the treatment for chronic pulmonary aspergillosis. Testing for antifungal sensitivity can thus be useful. *Aspergillus* infection refractory to primary antifungal therapy with voriconazole may require transition to lipid formulation amphotericin or caspofungin. Transitioning to itraconazole or posaconazole from voriconazole for suspected resistance is inappropriate because of the high likelihood of cross-resistance.[15]

* *

Adjunctive interferon-gamma may be considered for refractory chronic pulmonary aspergillosis, but supporting evidence is limited. Ensuring adequate antifungal tissue exposure and changing antifungal therapy in cases of resistance are more appropriate initial steps.[1,15] Surgery may be considered for chronic pulmonary aspergillosis in select patients. However because of high rates of postoperative complications, it should be limited to younger patients with limited comorbidities, good pulmonary reserve, and focal disease and those who are either not tolerating or refractory to antifungal therapy. In this case, consideration for surgery would be premature; ensuring appropriate antifungal levels and consideration for changing antifungal therapy in cases of resistant disease should first be considered for refractory chronic pulmonary aspergillosis.[4,20]

CASE 10

Question 1: **B. Lipid formulation amphotericin B**

This patient has severe progressive disseminated histoplasmosis, and lipid formulation amphotericin B is first-line therapy. Amphotericin B is preferred for severe disease, disease affecting the CNS, and in pregnant patients. Itraconazole is preferred monotherapy for mild-to-moderate disease or as step-down therapy from amphotericin B for severe disease but is not the preferred option for initial therapy for severe disseminated disease. While voriconazole has in vitro activity against *Histoplasma*, it has not been well-studied clinically. Echinocandins, including caspofungin, do not have significant activity against *Histoplasma* in vitro and are not considered treatment options for histoplasmosis. Treatment is certainly indicated in severe progressive disseminated histoplasmosis.

* *

Histoplasma capsulatum is endemic to the Ohio and Mississippi River valleys with propensities for humid climates and damp soil. Common niches include river banks, caves contaminated with bat guano, old chicken coops, and construction sites. Inoculation with spores by inhalation results in conversion to yeast form at body temperature. Subsequent dissemination is usually self-limited with 99% of primary infections being asymptomatic in nature (see Table 20–6). Symptomatic disease manifests in a variety of ways. Immunosuppression increases the risk for symptomatic, severe, and disseminated disease.

Table 20-6 MANIFESTATIONS OF HISTOPLASMOSIS[23,24]

Manifestation	Clinical Characteristics	Treatment

Acute Pulmonary Histoplasmosis	Symptomatic pneumonia <1 month	• Mild—no treatment, usually self-limited
		• Severe pneumonia with respiratory failure
		  • Amphotericin B then Itraconazole
		  • Corticosteroids in first 1–2 weeks

Subacute pulmonary histoplasmosis	Symptomatic pneumonia >1 month; associated with focal infiltrate, hilar, and mediastinal lymphadenopathy	• Mild/Moderate—Itraconazole
		• Severe pneumonia with respiratory failure
		  • Amphotericin B then Itraconazole
		  • Corticosteroids in first 1–2 weeks

Chronic pulmonary histoplasmosis	Symptomatic pneumonia >3 months; cavitary apical infiltrates associated with underlying lung disease	• Itraconazole for >1 year (high risk of relapse)
Progressive disseminated histoplasmosis	Multi-organ involvement; can be life-threatening if left untreated	• Mild/Moderate—Itraconazole • Severe—Amphotericin B then Itraconazole • Prolonged or lifelong suppressive Itraconazole for persistent immune compromise

* *

Cytology, histopathology, and culture of infected tissue can show budding yeast (see below). *Histoplasma* antigen detection sensitivity varies based on disease duration and severity. The sensitivity of *Histoplasma* urine antigen and serum antigen are ~60% each but they have a combined sensitivity of >80% to 90% for acute pulmonary histoplasmosis. Urine *Histoplasma* antigen is particularly useful for disseminated disease with a sensitivity of ~90%. Antigen concentrations correlate with severity of disease, particularly in disseminated disease. *Histoplasma* antigen can also be evaluated in bronchoalveolar lavage fluid with a sensitivity of 97% when combined with cytology. There is cross-reactivity for *Histoplasma* antigen testing with other endemic mycoses (i.e., coccidioidomycosis and blastomycosis), which can lead to false-positive results, though overall, specificity is 99%.[23,24]

* *

Serologic testing of *Histoplasma* antibody by immunodiffusion and complement fixation can be used after 1 month of disease, with sensitivities ranging from 40% to 90% depending on disease severity and whether there is pulmonary involvement. It has limited sensitivity prior to 1 month of disease onset and is most sensitive in subacute pulmonary disease (>4 weeks), chronic pulmonary disease (>3 months), and severe pulmonary disease. Sensitivity is more limited in disseminated disease and immunocompromised patients. Serologic testing is the most sensitive test for disease limited to the mediastinum (mediastinal granulomas and fibrosing mediastinitis), with a sensitivity of 67%. Serologic tests can remain positive for years after an episode of histoplasmosis.

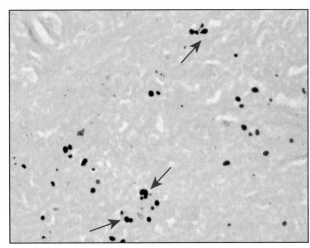

Note the budding yeast (red arrows).
(Used with permission of Gregory Fishbein, MD, David Geffen School of Medicine, UCLA.)

Question 2: D. Fibrosing mediastinitis

This is a rare late complication of pulmonary histoplasmosis caused by a fibrotic reaction to *Histoplasma* antigens in mediastinal and hilar lymph nodes, resulting in occlusion of airways or vessels. Complications of histoplasmosis are described in Table 20-7. The chest

Table 20-7   COMPLICATIONS OF HISTOPLASMOSIS[23,24]

Complication	Characteristics	Treatment
Pericarditis	Due to adjacent inflammation of mediastinal lymph nodes Early manifestation	Mild: NSAIDs Severe: Prednisone with itraconazole
Rheumatologic syndromes	Polyarthritis, erythema nodosum Early manifestation	NSAIDs, rarely corticosteroids
Mediastinal lymphadenitis	Causes chest pain, cough, airway obstruction, and dysphagia Early manifestation	Asymptomatic: No therapy Symptoms of compression: Prednisone with itraconazole
Mediastinal granuloma	Large (3–10 cm) encapsulated matted conglomeration of caseating lymph nodes Usually asymptomatic but compression of adjacent structures and fistulization to bronchus, esophagus, and skin can occur Late manifestation	Asymptomatic: No therapy Symptomatic: itraconazole; surgery if no response to itraconazole
Mediastinal fibrosis	Invasive fibrosis of mediastinal and hilar lymph nodes Can cause obstruction of airway and vessels Late manifestation	No role for antifungal therapy Intravascular stents can be considered for vessel obstruction
Broncholithiasis	Erosion of calcified lymph node into the airway Can cause cough productive of white chalky material, hemoptysis, and obstruction Late manifestation	No role for antifungal therapy Bronchoscopy or surgery to remove stones

CT and chronicity of the lesions are most consistent with fibrosing mediastinitis. There is no apparent compression from surrounding enlarged lymph nodes, as in mediastinal lymphadenitis, or a mediastinal granuloma. The presentation and imaging is not consistent with either endobronchial fistula from a mediastinal granuloma or broncholithiasis.

Question 3: E. Symptomatic mediastinal granuloma

Mediastinal granulomas are large matted conglomerations of caseating mediastinal lymph nodes with a surrounding capsule often affecting the paratracheal and subcarinal lymph nodes. They are a late manifestation of histoplasmosis. Patients are typically asymptomatic and do not require treatment.[23-25]

* *

Mediastinal granulomas however can cause compression of adjacent structures leading to SVC obstruction, pulmonary artery or vein obstruction, bronchial obstruction, and dysphagia. The granulomas can also fistualize into the bronchus, skin, or esophagus and drain its caseous contents. For symptomatic cases, antifungal therapy with 6 to 12 weeks of itraconazole is recommended, though data supporting its efficacy is limited. Surgical drainage or resection can be considered for persistent symptoms despite treatment with itraconazole. Mediastinal granulomas do not appear to progress to mediastinal fibrosis.[25]

* *

Histoplasmomas are residual pulmonary nodules that may persist despite resolution of pulmonary histoplasmosis. They usually have concentric or central calcification and are asymptomatic.

* *

Antifungal therapy is generally not indicated for histoplasmomas, fibrosing mediastinitis, broncholithiasis, and mild pulmonary histoplasmosis lasting <4 weeks in duration.[23-25]

CASE 11

Question 1: D. *Coccidioides* antibody complement fixation

This patient has acute coccidioidomycosis. Coccidioidomycosis is caused by *Coccidioides immitis* or *Coccidioides*

posadasii, which are endemic in the southwest United States and northwest Mexico. Coccidioidomycosis most commonly causes a self-limited acute or subacute pneumonia, typically 1 to 3 weeks after inoculation, and can be indistinguishable from bacterial community acquired pneumonia. Less than 5% develop chronic pulmonary infection or extrapulmonary disease.

* *

Coccidioidomycosis can sometimes present with a mild eosinophilia, though this is neither sensitive nor specific. Evaluation includes obtaining sputum, BAL, fluid, or tissue samples for fungal staining and culture. Identification of spherules with enclosed endospores is pathognomonic. Serum *Coccidioides* IgG and IgM EIA is the most sensitive serologic test and the initial screening test of choice. If positive, it is confirmed using the *Coccidioides* antibody immunodiffusion test and the *Coccidioides* antibody complement fixation (CF) test. The *Coccidioides* antibody CF can be further quantified as a titer, which is associated with disease severity and decreases with reduction in disease burden. As a result, the *Coccidioides* antibody CF titers can be used to follow response to therapy.[26-28] The other tests are not followed to monitor response to therapy.

Question 2: A. Pulmonary cavitary lesions

After a primary *Coccidioides* pneumonia, thin-walled cavitary lesions may develop. Antifungal therapy is usually not indicated unless they are adjacent to the pleura and at risk for causing a bronchopleural fistula.

* *

While most cases of pulmonary coccidioidomycosis are self-limited and do not require antifungal therapy, current guidelines recommend treatment for patients with symptoms >8 weeks, weight loss of >10%, night sweats for >3 weeks, infiltrates involving more than half of one lung or portions of both lungs, prominent or persistent hilar adenopathy, and *Coccidioides* antibody CF titer of >1:16. Immunocompromised patients also warrant therapy. Antifungal therapy is recommended for coccidioidomycosis in all HIV patients with CD4 count <250 cells/μL.

* *

First-line therapy is fluconazole. For refractory disease, severe disease, or skeletal involvement, amphotericin B is preferred. Table 20-8 describes various manifestations of coccidioidomycosis and their treatment.[26,27]

Table 20-8 MANIFESTATIONS OF COCCIDIOIDOMYCOSIS[26–30]

Manifestation	Treatment/Characteristics
Uncomplicated acute pneumonia	Treatment can usually be withheld unless high-risk disease is present. Treatment: Fluconazole first-line. Use amphotericin B in pregnancy (azoles teratogenic)
Diffuse pneumonia	Treat with fluconazole. Consider amphotericin B as initial therapy for rapidly progressive disease or hypoxemia, followed by fluconazole step-down therapy
Pulmonary nodule	No treatment if asymptomatic
Pulmonary cavity	No treatment if asymptomatic. Treat with antifungals for local discomfort/hemoptysis and for lesions abutting the pleura at high risk for formation of bronchopleural fistulas. If cavity ruptures into pleura, treat with antifungal therapy and pleural drainage. Consider resection of ruptured cavity and decortication
Chronic progressive fibrocavitary pneumonia	Multilobar infiltrates and cavities with chronic constitutional symptoms; often associated with poorly controlled diabetes. Treat with antifungals for ≥1 year
Disseminated coccidioidomycosis	Most commonly affects skin, bone, and meninges. Treatment: Fluconazole and itraconazole generally first-line; amphotericin B is alternative therapy; voriconazole and posaconazole can also be considered, usually as salvage therapy

Question 3: A. Caspofungin

The patient has relapsed coccidioidomycosis and now presents with disseminated disease. The risk of relapse after completion of therapy for primary coccidioidomycosis is 15% to 30%. Thus after completion of therapy, continued follow-up and serial *Coccidioides* antibody CF titers every 3 to 6 months are needed to monitor for relapse.[26–28]

* *

Disseminated disease can affect any organ, but it most commonly affects skin, bone, and the CNS.

Immunocompromised patients are at higher risk for disseminated disease, as are those of African American and Filipino descent.

* *

The treatment of choice for disseminated coccidioidomycosis is fluconazole or itraconazole. Itraconazole may be more effective than fluconazole for skeletal involvement.[29] Lipid formulation amphotericin B serves as alternative therapy, though it may be favored as initial therapy in severe disease or disease affecting the spine. Dual therapy with amphotericin B and fluconazole or itraconazole is sometimes utilized for widespread dissemination and refractory disease, but data supporting its efficacy is limited. Antagonism with combination polyene and azole therapy has been reported, potentially limiting the efficacy of this strategy.

* *

Voriconazole and posaconazole can also be used for disseminated coccidioidomycosis, typically as salvage therapy for refractory disease.

* *

In addition to antifungal therapy, skeletal dissemination warrants consideration for surgical debridement, especially in refractory disease.[26,27,30]

* *

Echinocandins, such as caspofungin, have little activity against *Coccidioides* in the mold form, and their effectiveness has been reported only in a limited number of case reports.[31]

CASE 12

Question 1: E. Skin pinprick testing for *Curvularia*

Curvularia is a ubiquitous pigmented mold found in soil and is a rare cause of allergic bronchopulmonary mycosis (ABPM), which resembles allergic bronchopulmonary aspergillosis (ABPA).[32,33] The diagnosis of ABPM includes the presence of asthma, sensitivity to non-*Aspergillus fumigatus* fungus by skin prick test and/or specific IgE, elevated IgE, and peripheral eosinophilia. *Curvularia* also rarely causes allergic rhinosinusitis. In the immunocompromised host, it is a rare cause of invasive sinus, orbital, CNS, and pulmonary disease as well as pulmonary mycetomas.[34]

* *

ABPM is typically less severe compared to ABPA, though severe forms have been described as the syndrome of severe asthma with fungal sensitization (SAFS). Common fungi associated with SAFS include *Candida, Penicillium, Alternaria,* and *Curvularia,* among others.

* *

Treatment of SAFS entails usual treatment for asthma, including omalizumab. In this case, excessively high IgE precludes omalizumab as a treatment option.[35]

* *

Prior to consideration of antifungal therapy or immunotherapy for fungal sensitization, fungal sensitization needs to be verified, which requires either a positive skin prick test or an elevated specific IgE to *Curvularia.* The role of antifungal treatment of SAFS remains controversial with only one small randomized controlled study showing that treatment of SAFS with itraconazole may be beneficial in ~60% of patients. While inhaled amphotericin B is a plausible alternative to azoles for SAFS, there is no evidence for its use in ABPM or SAFS.

* *

Controlled studies support the use of immunotherapy for asthma associated with fungal sensitization, specifically in patients with *Alternaria* and *Cladosporium* sensitization. Nevertheless, immunotherapy is considered high risk and is relatively contraindicated in patients with severe or uncontrolled asthma due to the potential for inducing life-threatening bronchospasm.[36–38]

REFERENCES

1. Riscili BP, Wood, KL. Noninvasive pulmonary Aspergillus infections. *Clin Chest Med.* 2009;30(2):315–335, vii.
2. Lee JK, Lee YJ, Park SS, et al. Clinical course and prognostic factors of pulmonary aspergilloma. *Respirology.* 2014; 19(7):1066–1072.
3. Hogan C, Denning DW. Allergic bronchopulmonary aspergillosis and related allergic syndromes. *Semin Respir Crit Care Med.* 2011;32(6):682–692.
4. Kousha M, Tadi R, Soubani AO. Pulmonary aspergillosis: A clinical review. *Eur Respir Rev.* 2011;20(121):156–174.
5. Hamilos G, Samonis G, Kontoyannis DP. Pulmonary mucormycosis. *Semin Respir Crit Care Med.* 2011;32(6): 693–702.
6. Limper AH, Knox KS, Sarosi GA, et al. An official American Thoracic Society statement: Treatment of fungal infections in adult pulmonary and critical care patients. *Am J Respir Crit Care Med.* 2011;183(1):96–128.
7. Greenberg RN, Mullane K, van Burik JA, et al. Posaconazole as salvage therapy for zygomycosis. *Antimicrob Agents Chemother.* 2006;50(1):126–133.
8. Van Burik JA, Hare RS, Solomon HF, et al. Posaconazole is effective as salvage therapy in zygomycosis: A retrospective summary of 91 cases. *Clin Infect Dis.* 2006;42(7):e61–e65.
9. Reed C, Bryant R, Ibrahim AS, et al. Combination polyene-caspofungin treatment of rhino-orbital-cerebral mucormycosis. *Clin Infect Dis.* 2008;47(3):364–371.
10. Brizendine KD, Baddley JW, Pappas PG. Pulmonary cryptococcosis. *Semin Respir Crit Care Med.* 2011;32(6): 727–734.
11. Queiroz-Telles F, Escuissato DL. Pulmonary paracoccidioidomycosis. *Semin Respir Crit Care Med.* 2011;32(6): 764–774.
12. Lease ED, Alexander BD. Fungal diagnostics in pneumonia. *Semin Respir Crit Care Med.* 2011;32(6):663–672.
13. Bariola JR, Vyas KS. Pulmonary blastomycosis. *Semin Respir Crit Care Med.* 2011;32(6):745–753.
14. De Pauw B, Walsh TJ, Donnely JP, et al. Revised definitions of invasive fungal disease from the EORTC/MSG Consensus Group. *Clin Infect Dis.* 2008;46(12):1813–1821.
15. Walsh TJ, Anaissie EJ, Denning DW, et al. Treatment of aspergillosis: Clinical practice guidelines of the Infectious Diseases Society of America. *Clin Infect Dis.* 2008;46(3): 327–360.
16. Thompson GR 3rd, Patterson TF. Pulmonary aspergillosis: Recent advances. *Semin Respir Crit Care Med.* 2011;32(6): 673–681.
17. Safdar A. Immunotherapy for invasive mold disease in severely immunosuppressed patients. *Clin Infect Dis.* 2013; 57(1):94–100.
18. Pfeiffer CD, Fine JP, Safdar N. Diagnosis of invasive aspergillosis using a galactomannan assay: A meta-analysis. *Clin Infect Dis.* 2006;42(10):1417–1427.
19. Chen SC, Blyth CC, Sorrell TC, et al. Pneumonia and lung infections due to emerging and unusual fungal pathogens. *Semin Respir Crit Care Med.* 2011;32(6):703–716.
20. Godet C, Philippe B, Laurent F, et al. Chronic pulmonary aspergillosis: An update on diagnosis and treatment. *Respiration.* 2014;88(2):162–174.
21. Denning DW, Riniotis K, Dobrashian R, et al. Chronic cavitary and fibrosing pulmonary and pleural aspergillosis: Case series, proposed nomenclature change, and review. *Clin Infect Dis.* 2003;37 (Suppl 3):S256–S280.
22. Kitasato Y, Tao Y, Hoshino T, et al. Comparison of Aspergillus galactomannan antigen testing with a new cut-off index and Aspergillus precipitating antibody testing for the diagnosis of chronic pulmonary aspergillosis. *Respirology.* 2009;14(5):701–708.
23. McKinsey DS, McKinsey JP. Pulmonary histoplasmosis. *Sem Respir Crit Care Med.* 2011;32(6):735–744.
24. Wheat LJ, Freifeld AG, Kleiman MB, et al. Clinical practice guidelines for the management of patients with histoplasmosis: 2007 update by the Infectious Diseases Society of America. *Clin Infect Dis.* 2007;45(7):807–825.
25. Parish JM, Rosenow EC 3rd. Mediastinal granuloma and mediastinal fibrosis. *Semin Respir Crit Care Med.* 2002; 23(2):135–143.

26. Galgiani JN, Ampel NM, Blair JE, et al. Coccidioidomycosis. *Clin Infect Dis.* 2005;41:1217–1223.

27. Thompson GR. Pulmonary coccidioidomycosis. *Semin Respir Crit Care Med.* 2011;32(6):754–763.

28. Nguyen C, Barker BM, Hoover S et al. Recent advances in our understanding of environmental, epidemiological, immunological, and clinical dimensions of coccidioidomycosis. *Clin Microbiol Rev.* 2013;26(3):505–525.

29. Galgiani JN, Catanzaro A, Cloud GA, et al. Comparison of oral fluconazole and itraconazole for progressive, nonmeningeal coccidioidomycosis. A randomized, double-blind trial. *Ann Intern Med.* 2000;133:676–686.

30. Blair JE. State-of-the-art treatment of coccidioidomycosis skeletal infections. *Ann N Y Acad Sci.* 2007;1111:422–433.

31. Dodds Ashley ES, Lewis R, Lewis JS, et al. Pharmacology of systemic antifungal agents. *Clin Infect Dis.* 2006;43:S28–S39.

32. Knutsen AP, Bush RK, Demain JG et al. Fungi and allergic lower respiratory tract diseases. *J Allergy Clin Immunol.* 2012;129(2):280–291.

33. Agarwal R. Severe asthma with fungal sensitization. *Curr Allergy Asthma Rep.* 2011;11:403–413.

34. Rinaldi MG, Phillips P, Schwartz JG, et al. Human curvularia infections. *Diagn Microbiol Infect Dis.* 1987;6(1):27–39.

35. Holgate S, Buhl R, Bousquet J, et al. The use of omalizumab in the treatment of severe allergic asthma: A clinical experience update. *Respir Med.* 2009;103(8):1098–1113.

36. Denning DW, O'Driscoll BR, Powell G, et al. Randomized controlled trial of oral antifungal treatment for severe asthma with fungal sensitization: The fungal asthma sensitization trial (FAST) study. *Am J Respir Crit Care Med.* 2009;179(1):11–18.

37. Moss RB. Treatment options in severe fungal asthma and allergic bronchopulmonary aspergillosis. *Eur Respir J.* 2014;43(5):1487–500.

38. Cox L, Nelson H, Lockey R, et al. Allergen immunotherapy: A practice parameter third update. *J Allergy Clin Immunol.* 2011;127(1):S1–S55.

21

HIV-Associated Pulmonary Diseases

Anthony F. Arredondo MD, Richard H. Huynh MD, and Steven Y. Chang MD

CASE 1

A 48-year-old man from Mexico presents with 2 weeks of progressive shortness of breath, fevers, and night sweats. His CXR shows questionable infiltrates in the right middle and upper lobes and laboratory data reveals lymphopenia. Ceftriaxone and azithromycin are initiated for community-acquired pneumonia. Examination reveals significant cervical lymphadenopathy. His hospital course is significant for a new diagnosis of HIV infection with a CD4+ count of 44/μL and 3 AFB sputum stains are sent and return negative. The patient's hospital course is further complicated by sepsis, including persistent fever and tachycardia, despite 3 days of antibiotics. A chest CT performed on day 4 is shown below. Blood cryptococcal antigen and coccidioidomycosis serologies are undetectable, and he has no evidence of CNS or bone disease.

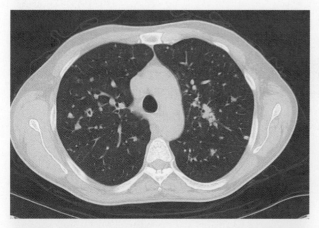
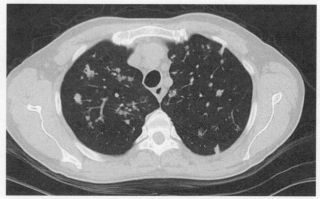
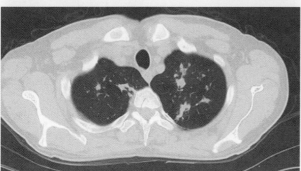

Used with permission of Harbor-UCLA Medical Center Department of Internal Medicine, Division of Infectious Disease and HIV Medicine.

Question 1: This patient has developed worsening sepsis during his hospital course despite appropriate antibiotics for community-acquired pneumonia. What should be the next therapeutic step?

A. Broaden antibiotics to include piperacillin-tazobactam

B. Initiate IV trimethoprim-sulfamethoxazole (TMP-SMX)

C. Initiate RIPE therapy

D. Initiate oseltamivir

E. Initiate antifungal therapy

Question 2: What diagnostic test(s) should be pursued at this time?

A. Continue AFB sputum collection

B. Transcutaneous lung biopsy

C. Repeat CT scan of the chest

D. Bronchoscopy with BAL

E. Lymph node biopsy and AFB blood cultures

Question 3: Biopsy and blood cultures are consistent with disseminated tuberculosis. What is the appropriate RIPE therapy?

A. RIPE therapy for 2 months followed by isoniazid and rifampin for 4 months

B. RIPE therapy for 2 months followed by isoniazid and rifampin for 8 months

C. RIPE therapy for 2 months followed by isoniazid and rifampin for 4 months and prednisone for 11 weeks

D. RIPE therapy for 2 months followed by isoniazid and rifampin for 10 months

E. RIPE therapy for 2 months followed by isoniazid and rifampin for 12 months

Question 4: What is the recommended time for initiation of antiretroviral therapy for this patient?

A. Within 2 weeks of starting RIPE therapy

B. At 2 to 4 weeks during the induction phase of RIPE

C. At 8 to 12 weeks during the continuous phase of isoniazid and rifampin therapy

D. Antiretroviral therapy is not recommended during the treatment of TB

E. After RIPE therapy is completed

CASE 2

A 36-year-old HIV-positive woman presents with persistent cough associated with hemoptysis, fevers, chills, night sweats, and unintentional weight loss for 2 months. CXR and chest CT are shown below. The patient is placed in respiratory isolation for TB, and RIPE is initiated empirically. Patient reports noncompliance with antiretroviral therapy and her CD4+ count is 220/μL.

**

Sputum reveals positive AFB stains and culture is consistent with *Mycobacterium tuberculosis*.

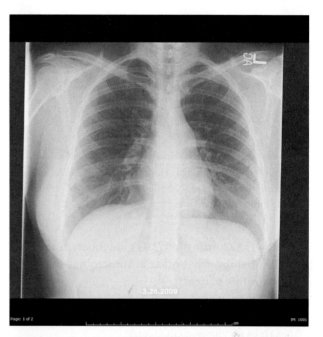

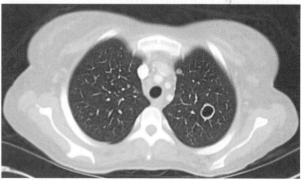

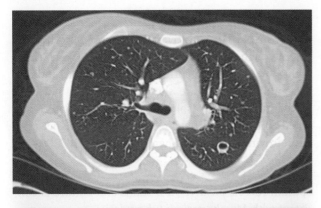

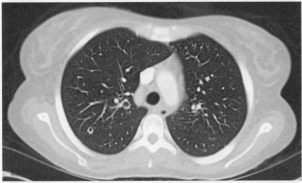

Used with permission of Harbor-UCLA Medical Center Department of Internal Medicine, Division of Infectious Disease and HIV Medicine.

Question 1: According to WHO guidelines, in addition to RIPE therapy, what other antimicrobial should be started for this patient?

A. Amoxicillin
B. Levofloxacin
C. TMP-SMX (PCP prophylaxis)
D. Fluconazole
E. Azithromycin

Question 2: What factor in this patient's presentation most influences radiographic findings in HIV-associated TB?

A. Presence of hemoptysis
B. CD4 cell count
C. AFB stain positivity
D. Weight loss
E. Night sweats

Question 3: After 4 weeks of RIPE therapy, sputum AFB stains remain positive and symptoms have minimally improved. Drug susceptibility testing (DST) reveals resistance to isoniazid, rifampin, levofloxacin, and amikacin. What best characterizes this type of TB infection and its associated mortality?

A. Super MDR-TB, mortality up to 90%
B. MDR-TB, mortality up to 30%
C. XDR-TB, mortality up to 30%
D. MDR-TB, mortality up to 90%
E. XDR-TB, mortality up to 90%

Question 4: Rifampin reduces levels of protease inhibitors and nonnucleoside reverse transcriptase inhibitors by what mechanism?

A. Decreases gut absorption
B. Increases renal clearance
C. Inhibition of cytochrome P450 enzyme
D. Induction of cytochrome P450 enzyme
E. None of the above

CASE 3

A 24-year-old man in South Africa complains of fatigue and is found to have HIV. His CD4+ count is 94/μL. Further evaluation reveals normal physical exam and CXR. Symptoms are not temporally related to the time of day of ART administration. Physical examination now reveals cervical lymphadenopathy and CXR shows right middle lobe infiltrate and effusion.

Question 1: Which of the following is the most likely diagnosis?

A. Adverse reaction to ART
B. Latent tuberculosis infection
C. HIV-associated TB immune reconstitution inflammatory syndrome (IRIS)
D. HIV-associated cryptococcal IRIS
E. HIV-associated pneumocystis

Question 2: Antiretroviral therapy should be discontinued in which of the following scenarios?

A. All cases of IRIS
B. If corticosteroid therapy is initiated
C. Only if IRIS is life threatening
D. If antituberculosis treatment is initiated
E. None of the above

CASE 4

A 32-year-old man diagnosed with HIV 4 months prior presents for evaluation. At the time of diagnosis his CD4+ count was 47 cells/µL. Further workup revealed cryptococcal meningitis and cryptococcemia. Initial lumbar puncture showed an elevated opening pressure of 28 cm H_2O and CSF analysis with WBC 15 cells/µL. He subsequently received therapeutic lumbar punctures and antifungal therapy without complications. His presenting symptoms of headache and nausea eventually resolved. One month after initial presentation ART was initiated concurrently with consolidation antifungal therapy. Three months after ART initiation the headaches and nausea returned along with fevers and emesis. A lumbar puncture revealed an opening pressure of 38 cm H_2O and CSF analysis revealed WBC 58 cells/µL. Laboratory data revealed a CD4+ count of 179/µL. CSF cryptococcal antigen was present and culture was negative. MRI of the brain was normal. CXR showed worsened nodular disease that appeared subtle on prior admission. Blood cultures were negative.

Question 1: What is the most likely diagnosis?

A. Cryptococcal meningitis recurrence
B. Antifungal therapy failure
C. "Unmasking" immune reconstitution inflammatory syndrome
D. Progressive multifocal leukoencephalopathy
E. "Paradoxical" immune reconstitution inflammatory syndrome (IRIS)

Question 2: Which of the following is NOT a risk factor for developing IRIS in the HIV population?

A. Degree of CD4 improvement after ART initiation
B. Initiation of ART with low CD4+ count
C. Previously treated mycobacteria tuberculosis or cryptococcus infection
D. Protease inhibitor-based ART regimen
E. The degree of decline in HIV viremia

Question 3: What is the predominant cell response and/or inflammatory cell infiltrate in this form of immune reconstitution disease?

A. CD8+
B. Granulomatous inflammation with increased number of T cells producing IFN-gamma
C. CD4+
D. Th17
E. B-cell response

CASE 5

A 45-year-old man with HIV presents for evaluation of progressive dyspnea with exertion and cough for 1 year. He denies fever, chills, night sweats, or weight loss. He is an active 12 pack-year smoker and reports no prior pulmonary infections. Spirometry reveals post-bronchodilator FEV_1/FVC ratio of 0.72 and FEV_1 78% predicted. DLco is 48% predicted. He has been noncompliant with his antiretroviral therapy. Chest CT shows diffuse emphysematous changes.

Question 1: What is the most important next step in management?

A. Smoking cessation
B. Change ART therapy
C. Start ICS
D. Start LABA/ICS
E. Start long acting muscarinic antagonist (LAMA)

Question 2: COPD in patients with HIV has been linked to airway colonization with which of the following microorganism?

A. *Streptococcus pneumoniae*
B. *Pneumocystis jirovecii*
C. *Influenza A/B*
D. *Escherichia coli*
E. *Pseudomonas aeruginosa*

Question 3: What was the most common pulmonary function abnormality in the HIV population prior to the availability of ART?

A. Decreased FEV_1
B. Decreased FEV_1/FVC ratio
C. Decreased DLco
D. Decreased FVC
E. Decreased TLC

CASE 6

A 48-year-old man with a 10-year history of HIV well controlled with antiretroviral therapy (CD4+ >500, undetectable HIV viral load) is seen in ambulatory clinic. He is an active 20 pack-year smoker and has never had pulmonary complications from HIV infection. He presents with worsening dyspnea with exertion for 15 months, but denies cough, fevers, chills, or weight loss. CXR is normal. Spirometry reveals post bronchodilator FEV_1/FVC ratio of 0.65, FEV_1 68% predicted, and DLco 65% predicted. Alpha-1 antitrypsin levels are normal.

Question 1: Which of the following have been associated with an annual decline of FEV$_1$ in the HIV population?

A. CD4+ <100 cells/μL and HIV viral load >75,000 copies/mL

B. CD4+ >100 cells/μL and HIV viral load <75,000 copies/mL

C. CD4+ <100 cells/μL and HIV viral load <75,000 copies/mL

D. CD4+ >100 cells/μL and HIV viral load >75,000 copies/mL

E. None of the above

Question 2: **Proposed mechanisms for HIV-related COPD and/or emphysema in the ART era include all of the following EXCEPT:**

A. Upregulation of matrix metalloproteinases

B. Direct effects of ART

C. Modified immune inflammatory response to colonizing pathogen

D. Decreased apoptosis

E. Direct cytotoxic effects of HIV

CASE 7

A 48-year-old man with HIV presents for evaluation regarding a chronic nonproductive cough. At the time of presentation he denied fevers, chills, or weight loss. He is a 15 pack-year smoker with a remote history of intravenous drug use in his early 20s. CXR reveals a nodular opacity in the left upper lobe and CT shows a spiculated 2.5 cm mass. His CD4+ count is 350/μL and he is compliant with his antiretroviral therapy. A percutaneous biopsy is consistent with malignancy.

Question 1: **What is the most likely histopathology on biopsy?**

A. Squamous cell carcinoma

B. Small-cell lung cancer

C. Adenocarcinoma

D. Hodgkin's Lymphoma

E. Neuroendocrine tumor

Question 2: **What is the median age at lung cancer diagnosis in the HIV patient population?**

A. Age 40

B. Age 50

C. Age 60

D. Age 70

E. Age 30

Question 3: **What is the most likely stage at the time of diagnosis for nonsmall cell lung cancer (NSCLC) in the HIV population?**

A. Stage I

B. Stage I/II

C. Stage II

D. Stage III

E. Stage III/IV

Question 4: **Which of the following have NOT been linked to the development of lung cancer in the HIV/AIDS population?**

A. Pulmonary infections

B. Cigarette smoking

C. Intravenous drug use

D. Diagnosis of AIDS defining malignancy

E. Age

CASE 8

A 32-year-old bisexual man who was recently diagnosed with HIV (prior CD4 cell count 113 cells/mm^3 and viral load of 5,000 copies/mL) and chronic obstructive pulmonary disease presents with a 2-week history of shortness of breath and cough. He was recently seen by his primary physician and completed a short course of antibiotics and prednisone. He also reported lesions on his legs that he had noticed for the past few months.

* *

On physical examination, he is tachycardic and tachypneic and pulmonary examination reveals decreased breath sounds at the bilateral bases with associated dullness to percussion. There are multiple moderately sized, raised, nontender, and violaceous lesions on the patient's trunk and upper extremities. Repeat laboratory values reveal normal white blood cell count, CD4 cell count 105 cells/mm^3 and viral load of 15,000 copies/mL.

* *

Chest radiograph is shown here:

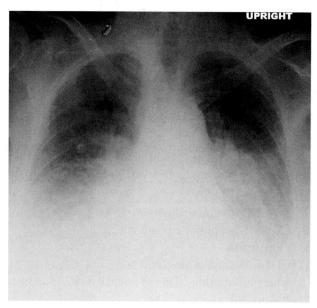

Plain chest radiograph.
Used with permission of Eric Kleerup, MD, Division of Pulmonary and Critical Care Medicine, David Geffen School of Medicine, UCLA.

Question 1: **What is the most likely cause for this patient's abnormal chest radiograph?**

A. Lymphoma
B. Human herpes virus-8
C. *Pneumocystis jirovecii pneumonia*
D. *Mycobacterium tuberculosis*
E. Congestive heart failure

Question 2: **What is the next best step?**

A. Bronchoscopy with bronchoalveolar lavage
B. CT chest
C. Sputum culture
D. Transthoracic echocardiogram
E. Skin biopsy

Question 3: **A large volume thoracentesis was performed. Pleural fluid was serosanguinous and free flowing. Analysis of the fluid revealed low nucleated cell counts with a monocyte predominant exudative effusion and an elevated LDH. Cytologic examination of the pleural fluid was unremarkable. What is the next best step?**

A. Restart prednisone at higher dose
B. Start clarithromycin and ethambutol
C. Initiate antiretroviral therapy
D. Start trimethoprim-sulfamethoxazole
E. Obtain echocardiogram

CASE 9

A 34-year-old man is admitted to the hospital with 3 weeks of worsening dyspnea on exertion, nonproductive cough, and fevers. The patient reports being sexually active with multiple male partners. On physical examination, he is febrile with a temperature of 38.6°C (101.5°F) with tachycardia and tachypnea. There are scattered white plaques in the oropharynx. Cardiopulmonary examination reveals tachycardia and diffuses crackles bilaterally. Chest radiograph reveals bilateral diffuse pulmonary infiltrates. Rapid HIV test is positive.

* *

Bronchoalveolar lavage is performed with microscopy of fluid shown:

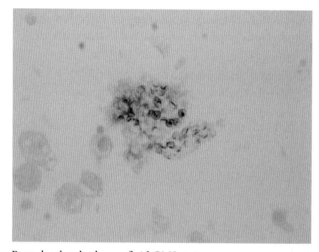

Bronchoalveolar lavage fluid GMS stain
Used with permission of Sharon Hirschowitz, MD, Division of Anatomic Pathology & Clinical Pathology, and Eric Kleerup, MD, Division of Pulmonary and Critical Care Medicine, David Geffen School of Medicine, UCLA.

Question 1: **What is the most likely diagnosis?**

A. Pulmonary candidiasis
B. *Pneumocystis jirovecii* pneumonia
C. *Mycobacterium tuberculosis*
D. *Mycobacterium avium* complex infection
E. CMV pneumonia

Question 2: **What is the next best step?**

A. Obtain high resolution CT of the chest
B. Obtain pulmonary function tests
C. Transthoracic echocardiogram
D. Measure venous blood gas
E. Measure arterial blood gas

Question 3: **What is the most appropriate treatment regimen?**

A. Clarithromycin and ethambutol
B. Fluconazole
C. Ganciclovir
D. Trimethoprim-sulfamethoxazole
E. Isoniazid, rifampin, pyrazinamide, and ethambutol

CASE 10

A 24-year-old student nurse is recently diagnosed with HIV after a healthcare-related exposure. She otherwise feels well and is without complaints. She denies cough, night sweats, fevers, chills, or weight loss. She is found to have a CD4+ T-lymphocyte count of 173 cells/mm^3.

Question 1: **For what opportunistic infection should prophylactic antibiotics be started in this patient?**

A. Toxoplasmosis
B. Pneumocystis jirovecii pneumonia (PCP)
C. Mycobacterium avium complex infection
D. Mycobacterium tuberculosis infection
E. None of the above

Question 2: **What is the preferred prophylactic regimen for this patient?**

A. Trimethoprim-sulfamethoxazole daily
B. Dapsone twice daily
C. Atovaquone daily
D. Azithromycin
E. None of the above

Question 3: **Which of the following are indications for initiating *pneumocystis jirovecii* pneumonia prophylaxis?**

A. Any AIDS-defining illness
B. CD4+ T-lymphocyte count <200
C. Oral thrush
D. CD4+ T-lymphocyte count >200 but <250 cells/μL where monitoring CD4 cell count every 3 months is not possible
E. All of the above

Answers

Question 1: C. Initiate RIPE therapy

HIV infection is the most important biologic risk factor for the development of *Mycobacterium tuberculosis*. In this clinical scenario, an HIV-positive patient with a CD4+ <50 presents with radiographic and clinical evidence compatible with disseminated tuberculosis. A diagnosis is not yet confirmed, but the patient clinically deteriorates despite treatment for community-acquired pneumonia for 3 days. According to the WHO algorithm for smear-negative TB suspects, early empirical TB therapy is recommended after 3 to 5 days of broad antibiotics.[1] This algorithm, which includes the avoidance of fluoroquinolones, has been shown to reduce mortality in seriously ill patients with HIV-related TB.[2]

* *

Although this patient is immunocompromised, there is no indication to broaden antimicrobials to cover hospital-acquired organisms based on clinical history. Pneumocystis pneumonia is less likely given the localized infiltrates/nodules, and serologies for the most likely fungal pathogens are negative making fungal pathogens much less likely.

Question 2: E. Lymph node biopsy and AFB blood cultures

Despite limited sensitivity, sputum culture for *Mycobacterium tuberculosis* remains the anchor for confirming pulmonary TB. The sensitivity of mycobacterial culture is not influenced by HIV coinfection, but confirmation may take several weeks. The sensitivity of sputum smear microscopy for acid-fast bacilli (AFB) for the detection of pulmonary TB is variable and depends on laboratory technique and resources. In this clinical scenario, the suspicion for pulmonary TB is high despite AFB smears being negative. Pulmonary and/or disseminated TB infection has not been effectively ruled out so the next most accessible site of infection should be pursued. In this patient with lymphadenopathy both needle aspiration of lymph tissue and mycobacterial blood cultures would be appropriate.

* *

The most common form of extrapulmonary *Mycobacterium tuberculosis* infection is TB lymphadenitis. Other extrapulmonary forms include disseminated TB (the second most common in HIV-TB), pleural TB, and TB meningitis. HIV-infected patients are more likely to develop extrapulmonary and disseminated disease than HIV-uninfected individuals. The risk of HIV-associated TB increases with lower CD4 counts as extrapulmonary disease can occur in up to 70% of patients with CD4 cell counts $<100/\mu L$.[3,6] For the diagnosis of HIV-associated TB lymphadenitis, wide needle aspiration for staining and histology can be pursued with sensitivity near 75%, but higher yields are reported with excisional samples.[4,5] In those with a CD4 count $<100/\mu L$ nearly half the blood cultures are positive for *Mycobacterium tuberculosis* thus confirming disseminated disease.[6]

* *

The diagnostic yield for sputum AFB collection has not been shown to increase beyond three samples, especially without radiographic evidence of cavitary disease. Although a CT scan of the chest would better characterize lung pathology, this would neither confirm nor refute pulmonary TB. Bronchoscopy with BAL in this scenario poses a great exposure risk to the bronchoscopist to infectious droplets with the immediate diagnostic yield estimated at only ~25%.[7] Lymph node biopsy and blood cultures are more accessible than transcutaneous pulmonary biopsy.

Question 3: A. RIPE therapy for 2 months followed by isoniazid and rifampin for 4 months

In addition, all patients receiving isoniazid should receive pyridoxine 50 mg daily to prevent peripheral neuropathy. The recommended treatment for HIV-associated TB is the same as non–HIV-associated disease. In this case, there is evidence for disseminated and extrapulmonary infection so the treatment would include 2 months of rifampin, isoniazid, pyrazinamide, and ethambutol (RIPE), followed by at least 4 months of rifampin and isoniazid. This treatment regimen is the same for pulmonary, pleural, pericardial, abdominal, or urogenital involvement. In addition, treatment of TB pericarditis includes 11 weeks of systemic corticosteroids and may require surgery if there is evidence of pericardial constriction.

* *

The American Thoracic Society (ATS), Centers for Disease Control and Prevention (CDC), the National Institutes of Health (NIH), and Infectious Diseases Society of America (IDSA) all recommend that HIV-related TB therapy be extended to 9 months for those with persistent sputum-positive cultures after 2 months of treatment, and 9 to 12 months when there is CNS or bone/joint involvement (see Table 21-1).[8,9] In TB meningitis, the treatment includes 2 months of rifampin, isoniazid, pyrazinamide, and streptomycin (or fluoroquinolone) followed by 7 to 10 months of rifampin and isoniazid. Treatment of TB meningitis also includes dexamethasone tapered over 6 to 12 weeks. TB involving the bone or joints is treated with 2 months of RIPE followed by 7 months of rifampin and isoniazid. Daily therapy in both the intensive (first 2 months) and continuation phase (>4 months) is considered optimal to prevent treatment relapse, failure, and drug resistance. An accepted alternative is daily therapy in the intensive phase and intermittent (three times weekly) under directly observed treatment (DOT) in the continuation phase.

Question 4: A. Within 2 weeks of starting RIPE therapy
The initiation of antiretroviral therapy (ART) concurrently with TB therapy improves overall survival for nonresistant, multidrug-resistant (MDR-TB), and extensively drug-resistant tuberculosis strains (XDR-TB).[10,11] The timing of ART with TB treatment is dependent on the level of immunosuppression and severity of illness. Based on US Department of Health and Human Services, for CD4 counts <50/μL the recommended time to start is within 2 weeks from TB therapy initiation. In three randomized controlled trials, early ART led to survival benefit despite increased incidence of immune reconstitution inflammatory syndrome (IRIS).[12-14] In those with CD4 counts >50/μL and severe clinical disease (low BMI, anemia, low albumin, low Karnofsky score, or organ dysfunction) the recommended time for starting ART is within 2 to 4 weeks of TB therapy initiation. If the CD4 count is >50/μL but without severe clinical disease ART should be started within 8 to 12 weeks of starting TB treatment.[15] TB meningitis is the only exception to initiating ART therapy within the first 2 weeks, regardless of CD4 count, given the increased risk of CNS IRIS and associated death.[16]

CASE 2

Question 1: C. TMP-SMX (PCP prophylaxis)
The WHO recommends that all HIV-positive TB patients in the developing world receive TMP-SMX at the time of TB diagnosis and throughout the duration of TB treatment. Prior studies have demonstrated

TABLE 21-1   TREATMENT FOR TUBERCULOSIS BASED ON LOCATION OF DISEASE

Site of Disease	Therapy	Other Recommendations
Pulmonary Pleural Lymphadenitis Abdominal Urogenital Disseminated Pericardium	RIPE × 2 months, then Rifampin/isoniazid × 4 months	Pericardial disease requires 11 weeks of prednisone taper and potential surgery if constrictive pericarditis
CNS (meningitis)	Rifampin, isoniazid, pyrazinamide, streptomycin (or fluoroquinolone) × 2 months, then Rifampin/isoniazid × 7–10 months	Dexamethasone tapered over 6–12 weeks Antiretroviral therapy should be delayed for at least 2 weeks and up to 8 weeks regardless of CD4 count
Bone or joint	RIPE × 2 months, then Rifampin/isoniazid × 7 months	Surgical decompression of spinal disease if evidence of cord compression

decreased mortality at prophylactic doses in this patient population.[21] The mechanism by which TMP-SMX accomplishes this is not clear, but TMP-SMX is known to prevent *Pneumocystis jirovecii*, malaria, and other infections. Other guidelines recommend TMP-SMX prophylaxis for HIV patients with CD4 cell counts <200/μL.

Question 2: B. CD4 cell count

In more advanced stages of HIV infection TB is associated with poor granuloma formation and failure to contain mycobacteria. This results in more aggressive disease characterized by more systemic symptoms and frequent dissemination to extrapulmonary sites when compared to HIV-negative individuals.[17] A weakened immune response, as seen in those with lower CD4 counts, often significantly alters findings on chest radiography. In particular, CD4 counts <200/μL are associated with atypical radiographic findings including lower lobe involvement, reticulonodular infiltrates, pleural effusions, and mediastinal lymphadenopathy.[6,18] When CD4 counts are >350/μL the presentation is more likely to resemble that of HIV-negative patients with upper lobe fibronodular and cavitary lesions. In HIV-positive patients with confirmed pulmonary TB, the chest radiograph may be normal in as many as 32% of patients in high-incidence areas.[19] In addition to a miliary pattern, disseminated TB may present with normal chest radiography in more than half of HIV-associated TB.[20]

Question 3: E. XDR-TB, mortality up to 90%

Multidrug-resistant TB (MDR-TB) is TB that is resistant to isoniazid and rifampin. Extensively drug-resistant TB (XDR TB) is MDR TB resistant also to fluoroquinolones and at least one of the following injectable drugs: capreomycin, kanamycin, or amikacin. Mortality rates can be as high as 90% for patients infected with XDR TB. As per WHO guidelines, drug susceptibility testing (DST) is recommended for all HIV-associated TB at the time of diagnosis. In resource poor regions this may not be feasible, so targeting patients that are higher risk for multidrug resistance including prior treatment failure, treatment relapse, and lower CD4 counts (<200/μL) is recommended.

Question 4: D. Induction of cytochrome P450 enzyme

Antiretroviral therapy typically includes two nucleoside reverse transcriptase inhibitors (NRTIs) combined with either a nonnucleoside reverse transcriptase inhibitor (NNRTI), a boosted protease inhibitor, or an integrase inhibitor. Rifampin has the most significant drug-drug interaction and induces cytochrome P450 3A4 (CYP3A4). This metabolizes protease inhibitors and NNRTIs. The exception is efavirenz (the most commonly used NNRTI), as no dose adjustments are required with rifampin. Protease inhibitors should not be used with rifampin because of extreme reductions in their levels despite ritonavir-boosting.[22] If protease inhibitors are required (i.e., NNRTI resistance), rifampin should be replaced with rifabutin, as rifabutin's pharmacokinetics are not significantly altered by protease inhibitors.[23,24] Integrase inhibitor levels are also decreased by rifampin by the induction of the enzyme responsible for the glucuronidation step of metabolism.[25]

CASE 3

Question 1: C. HIV-associated TB immune reconstitution inflammatory syndrome (IRIS)

Immune reconstitution inflammatory syndrome is relatively common in patients with TB initiated on ART. Similar to other forms of IRIS, HIV-associated TB with IRIS (TB-IRIS) reflects an exaggerated inflammatory response to opportunistic pathogen antigens. Signs may include new or worsening pulmonary infiltrates, enlarged lymph nodes, serositis, or abscess. The more severe type of IRIS is rare and up to one-third of HIV-associated TB[26–28] will develop a mild to moderate form.[29,30] TB-IRIS may present in two forms. In the "paradoxical" form, the patient presents with worsening of known TB, usually during the treatment period. In the "unmasking" version, the previously asymptomatic patient presents with new symptoms after ART initiation. The "unmasking" of TB is rare in the United States and more common in high-burden areas as in the case presented.[31,32] HIV-associated TB with IRIS typically presents within the first 3 months of ART initiation and is associated with low CD4 count (<100/μL), greater decline in HIV viral load, and early initiation of ART during TB treatment.[33] The "paradoxical" form of IRIS in HIV-associated TB is a diagnosis of exclusion. If "paradoxical" TB-IRIS is suspected, other potential causes must be excluded including drug toxicity, new infection, malignancy, and TB treatment failure. The timing of ART alone should not be used in the diagnosis of "paradoxical" IRIS.[34,35]

Question 2: C. Only if IRIS is life threatening

In most cases, ART can be safely continued without further intervention.[29] The severity of disease determines the need for intervention and typically involves nonsteroidal anti-inflammatory drugs and/or corticosteroids. A study conducted in South Africa revealed improved symptoms, reduction of invasive procedures and hospitalizations in TB-IRIS when a 4-week course of prednisone was compared to placebo.[36] IRIS may be life threatening if the inflammatory process leads to respiratory failure, CNS disease, or airway obstruction.[34,37-39] Further management of TB-IRIS may require drainage of abscesses/fluid collections or neurosurgical intervention for elevated intracranial pressures.

CASE 4

Question 1: E. "Paradoxical" immune reconstitution inflammatory syndrome (IRIS)

Diagnostic criteria for IRIS include: (1) the presence of low pretreatment CD4 count, (often less than 100/μL), (2) a positive virologic response to ART, (3) the absence of drug-resistance, adverse drug reactions, noncompliance, or bacterial superinfection, (4) temporal relationship with ART initiation and disease onset, and (5) signs and symptoms of an inflammatory condition.

* *

Cryptococcal-IRIS most commonly localizes to the CNS or lung and typically presents in "paradoxical" form. The onset of symptoms is variable, but often occurs within 2 months of ART initiation, but may be delayed beyond 6 months.[40-42] The "unmasking" of cryptococcal disease is rare and occurs in ~1% of asymptomatic patients starting ART for the first time.[77] IRIS-related cryptococcal meningitis often presents with a low CSF WBC count on lumbar puncture (<25/μL) at the time of initial diagnosis. On follow-up lumbar puncture, during development of IRIS, CSF WBC count often reveals a greater number of inflammatory cells. In one retrospective study, the median CSF WBC during IRIS was 56/μL compared to 12/μL for true cryptococcal meningitis.[43] In the same study, IRIS-related cryptococcal meningitis was also associated with greater median opening pressures on lumbar puncture (39 cm H_2O vs. 31 cm H_2O), lower median cryptococcal antigen (1:128 vs. 1:2,048), and greater median CD4 count (72/μL vs. 34/μL) than HIV-related cryptococcal meningitis without IRIS.

* *

Pulmonary complications related to IRIS include both infectious and noninfectious etiologies. Infectious causes include *Mycobacterium tuberculosis, Pneumocystis jirovecii, Cryptococcus neoformans,* and nontuberculous mycobacteria (NTM). Noninfectious etiologies include Kaposi's sarcoma and sarcoidosis. Pulmonary manifestations of cryptococcal-IRIS include nodular or cavitary lung disease, mediastinal adenopathy, hypoxia, ARDS, and respiratory failure. Pulmonary cryptococcal-IRIS may present isolated to the lung or more commonly as part of a disseminated disease process with CNS, lymph node, and skin involvement. When isolated to one organ, CNS disease is still the most common and fatal. Pulmonary cryptococcal-IRIS may mimic opportunistic infections or other forms of IRIS so further diagnostic workup (i.e., biopsy, culture, histology) is required to confirm a diagnosis.

* *

Pneumocystis jirovecii, the organism responsible for pneumocystis (PCP) pneumonia, is the second most common cause of pulmonary IRIS. PCP pneumonia IRIS (PCP-IRIS) can present in an "unmasking" or "paradoxical" form. Symptoms include the classic features of dry cough, dyspnea, and hypoxia. Initiation of antimicrobial therapy for pneumocystis pneumonia is often complicated by a paradoxical inflammatory response requiring corticosteroids for moderate to severe disease. PCP-IRIS may present with a similar inflammatory response, but typically, symptoms begin 1 to 3 weeks after ART initiation. As a way to ameliorate potential confusion, some experts propose waiting for clinical improvement after 4 to 7 days of antimicrobial therapy prior to ART.[76] The early initiation of ART is supported by a randomized study of 282 patients with HIV-related opportunistic infections that consisted of mostly PCP pneumonia (63% of study population) and excluded TB. Subjects were randomized to receive ART within the first 2 weeks of PCP therapy or waiting at least 4 weeks. The early treatment group showed a significant reduction in mortality and progression to AIDS when compared to the delayed method. The study excluded the severely ill and case reports of respiratory failure from PCP-IRIS following early ART initiation have been reported.[73,74]

* *

Worldwide, nontuberculous mycobacteria (NTM) is a rare cause of IRIS, and most cases are isolated to Europe or the United States. In the largest NTM-IRIS case series, 15 of 51 cases had pulmonary or thoracic disease represented by pulmonary infiltrates, cavitation, lung mass, endobronchial disease, and lymphadenopathy. In this case series, no deaths were related to pulmonary NTM-IRIS.

Most pulmonary NTM-IRIS is represented by *M. avium intracellulare* (MAC), but cases of *M. parascrofulaceum*, *M kansasii*, and *M. xenopi* have been described.[78–81]

* *

Noninfectious forms of pulmonary IRIS include Kaposi's sarcoma and sarcoidosis. Pulmonary Kaposi's sarcoma-IRIS is not uncommon and can be fatal.[83] Radiographic findings include worsening or recurrent reticular/reticulonodular opacities, consolidation, ground glass opacities, lymphadenopathy, and pleural effusions.[82,83] In general, the following risk factors were identified for developing Kaposi's sarcoma IRIS: detectable HHV-8 DNA, high plasma HIV viral load, hematocrit <30%, and a diagnosis of Kaposi's sarcoma that predates ART initiation.[84,85] The more common form of Kaposi's sarcoma IRIS is cutaneous disease including lymphedema or mucosal involvement. Most cases present 2 to 3 months after ART initiation.[84,86]

* *

Sarcoidosis is a CD4 T-cell–mediated chronic granulomatous process most commonly involving the lungs. Multiple reports of sarcoidosis developing during ART have been reported especially when the CD4 count increases to over 200/μL and/or after 12 months of therapy.[86] The clinical and radiological findings of HIV-infected patients are similar to the non-HIV population.

Question 2: D. Protease inhibitor-based ART regimen

There has been conflicting data regarding the use of a protease inhibitor-based ART regimen and risk for IRIS. In the most recent study, there was no difference in incidence of IRIS based on treatment with protease inhibitor versus NNRTI-based therapy.[44] In the same study, which did not include TB-IRIS, higher HIV RNA levels pretreatment, higher CD4 cell counts and lower RNA levels during treatment were associated with IRIS. Multiple retrospective studies have associated IRIS with low CD4 counts at the time of ART initiation.[45–47]

Question 3: B. Granulomatous inflammation with increased number of T cells producing IFN-gamma

Granulomatous inflammation can be caused by fungi (*Histoplasma* and *Cryptococci*), protozoa (*Leishmania* species), nontuberculous mycobacteria, or mycobacteria. In those with TB or cryptococcal IRIS, inflammation is associated with a Th1 immune response and increased number of circulating T cells that produce IFN-gamma.[48–50] In contrast, IRIS associated with viral infections (JC virus, HIV, CMV) is associated with an inflammatory response dominated by CD8+ T cells. The Th17 response has been implicated in tissue suppuration and is specific to mycobacteria infection.[51]

CASE 5

Question 1: A. Smoking cessation

Recommendations regarding treatment for HIV-related emphysema follow the same guidelines as for the HIV-negative population. In the case presented, the focus should be on smoking cessation as the first step. In the era prior to ART an emphysema-subtype characterized HIV-related COPD. The incidence of emphysema, based on HRCT imaging, was 15% in the HIV-positive group compared to 2% in the HIV-negative subjects, regardless of smoking status.[52] In the same study, the incidence in HIV-positive smokers was greater than 37% compared to 0% in HIV-negative smokers, suggesting a synergistic effect of smoking and HIV infection. Consistent with other studies prior to the ART era, there was minimal airflow obstruction found on spirometry.

Question 2: B. *Pneumocystis jirovecii*

In addition to pneumocystis pneumonia infection. A primate model demonstrated increased emphysematous changes on quantitative CT and increased airflow limitation by spirometry when compared to matched controls.[53] In a prospective human study, there was greater airflow obstruction in patients colonized with *Pneumocystis jirovecii* when compared to matched controls. The other responses have not been linked to HIV-related COPD.[54]

Question 3: C. Decreased DLco

In the largest prospective study prior to the availability of ART, pulmonary function testing was performed in HIV-positive subjects and matched controls.[55] Low DLco was the most common abnormality and was associated with emphysematous changes on computed tomography (CT). Although emphysema was the most commonly seen phenotype in the pre-ART era there were no significant findings of obstruction by spirometry. In addition, diffusing capacity was significantly lower in HIV-positive patients when CD4 count was <200/μL. Multiple studies in asymptomatic HIV-positive patients have demonstrated reduced diffusing capacity in 9% to 70% of cases.[56,57] The high prevalence of low DLco has also been observed after the availability of ART. In one study evaluating etiology of low DLco, 25% of never-smokers on ART showed a moderately low diffusion capacity (<60% predicted).[58] In these never-smokers there was no evidence of obstruction (FEV_1/FVC <0.7) or emphysema on CT imaging. In contrast, low DLco in ever-smokers was associated with low FEV_1/FVC ratio and emphysema on CT scanning. These findings suggest that multiple factors influence low DLco in HIV-positive patients on effective ART.

* *

There have been multiple studies assessing spirometry in HIV-positive outpatients with no history of pulmonary disease during the ART era. The prevalence of irreversible airflow obstruction was 21% in one observational study measuring pre- and post-bronchodilator spirometry.[59] In this same study a low DLco was the most common abnormality. In a separate cross-sectional study the prevalence of obstruction was 16.3% in a group of smokers and nonsmokers. The same study demonstrated the prevalence for never smokers was 13.6%.[72] In a prospective cohort study followed for 4.5 years, the prevalence of obstruction increased from 10% to 19%.[60] Almost all patients with a reduced FEV_1/FVC were smokers.

CASE 6

Question 1: A. CD4+ <100 cells/µL and HIV viral load >75,000 copies/mL

In the AIDS Linked to IntraVenous Experience (ALIVE) study, comprised intravenous drug users and mostly smokers (85%), it was shown in 303 HIV-positive patients that a high HIV viral load (>200,000 copies/mL) was associated with obstructive lung disease.[74] In a follow-up longitudinal study from the ALIVE cohort, serial PFTS and laboratory testing were performed over 3 years. High viral loads (>75,000 copies/mL) were associated with greater annual decline in FEV_1 and FVC when compared to HIV-negative subjects and HIV-positive individuals with viral loads £75,000 copies/mL. Low CD4 counts (<100 cells/uL) were also associated with greater annual decline in FEV_1 and FVC compared to HIV-negative and HIV-positive individuals with CD4 counts >200 cells/uL.[75]

Question 2: D. Decreased apoptosis

Apoptosis is one of the proposed mechanisms in the development of COPD. In non–HIV-infected patients, it has been hypothesized that lung endothelial and epithelial cell apoptosis are key steps in COPD development.[64,65]

Multiple studies have linked HIV proteins and HIV directly to increased apoptosis and thus may play a role in COPD.[66-68]

* *

Although the exact mechanism is unclear, ART is an independent risk factor for increased airway obstruction. A "modified" IRIS response after the initiation of ART has been proposed as a potential contributor to COPD.[69] Immune restoration during antiretroviral treatment may lead to a chronic inflammatory response without the obvious clinical symptoms seen in typical IRIS. It is postulated that colonizing organisms serve as antigens to further propagate inflammation leading to COPD development.[70]

* *

The upregulation of metalloproteinases (MMP) have also been linked to the development of HIV-related emphysema. One autopsy study showed evidence of HIV-1 RNA infection of alveolar macrophages in areas of emphysema.[71] The adjacent noninfected areas were found to have increased expression of MMP-9, an important mediator of matrix degradation in emphysema. In addition to increasing metalloproteinases, HIV showed direct cytotoxic effects on lung tissue as a potential cause of emphysema. In a separate study, HIV-infected patients colonized by pneumocystis were associated with airway obstruction and increased sputum levels of MMP-12.[54]

* *

Multiple risk factors and mechanisms have been attributed to HIV-related COPD. The prevalence of cigarette smoking is high in many HIV-infected populations. Approximately 75% of HIV-infected people have smoked at least 100 cigarettes in their lifetime, and about half are active smokers.[61,62] Intravenous drug use (IDU) is also common amongst HIV-positive patients but a direct causal relationship between IDU and emphysema remains unclear. One case control study of HIV-positive patients revealed the prevalence of emphysema was not significantly greater in those with a history of IDU.[63]

CASE 7

Question 1: C. Adenocarcinoma

Similar to the general population, adenocarcinoma is the most common histologic subtype, followed by squamous cell and small cell lung cancers.[92] A Veteran Affairs study reported adenocarcinoma accounting for 50% to 75%

of all HIV-related lung cancers in their patient population.[92]

* *

Since the initiation of antiretroviral therapy there has been a shift in malignancies diagnosed in the HIV/AIDS population. Antiretroviral therapy has significantly reduced the incidence of AIDS defining malignancies such as Kaposi's sarcoma and non-Hodgkin's lymphoma. Subsequently, the life expectancy of individuals with HIV and AIDS has increased, resulting in a greater number of non-AIDS defining illnesses. Many of these illnesses include non-AIDS defining cancers (NADC) which now account for 50% of all cancers in the HIV population. Lung cancer is the most prevalent and the risk is several fold greater than the general population, adjusted for age and smoking, suggesting other contributory mechanisms.[87–91]

Question 2: B. Age 50

The average age at the time of lung cancer diagnosis in the HIV population has ranged from 38 to 57 years in multiple case-control and longitudinal cohort studies.[93] In one study comparing the age at diagnosis of cancer between the HIV and the general population, the median age for lung cancer diagnosis was 50 in the HIV group compared to 70 in the general population. A statistical significance remained even after adjusting for several risk factors in both groups.

Question 3: E. Stage III/IV

In a review article that combined data from 19 case-control studies and longitudinal cohorts, the prevalence of advanced disease (stage III/IV) at the time of cancer diagnosis ranged from 33% to 100%.[93] Most of these patients were diagnosed with nonsmall cell lung cancer (NSCLC) and adenocarcinoma served as the dominant subtype in 15 of 19 studies. A separate study reported 87% of patients with HIV and NSCLC were staged III/IV at the time of diagnosis (compared to 68% in the general population). When adjusting for cancer stage however, there was no mortality difference between the HIV and the general population.[94]

Question 4: D. Diagnosis of AIDS defining malignancy

In the antiretroviral era, HIV infection has been found to be a risk factor for the development of lung cancer.[99] In addition to HIV infection, smoking, intravenous drug use (IDU), pulmonary infections, and age have also been linked to lung cancer in this population.

During the ART era there has been an inverse relationship between the development of AIDS defining cancers (ADC) and NADC. In comparing the time periods 1991–1995 to 2001–2005 the risk of ADC has decreased threefold while NADC has increased threefold.[96] ADC (i.e., Kaposi's sarcoma, non-Hodgkin's lymphoma) has not been recognized as a risk factor for the development of lung cancer in the HIV population.

* *

HIV infection has been recognized as an independent risk factor for lung cancer in multiple studies during the ART era.[93] The reason for the increased risk remains unclear. One explanation is the aging HIV population and the improved survival with ART. This has led to the development of more common diseases such as heart disease and cancer.[88,95] Adjusting for age, the risk of lung cancer remains several fold higher than the general population suggesting other factors are involved.

* *

Pulmonary inflammation secondary to smoking and infection has been implicated in lung cancer development in the HIV population. Smoking is considered an independent risk factor for the development of lung cancer in those infected with HIV.[97] In the United States, smoking is two to three times more likely among those with HIV, but does not fully account for the increased risk of lung cancer. In one study, the incidence of lung cancer was 2.5 times greater than the general population after adjusting for smoking.[98] In another prospective study examining HIV and intravenous drug users, the risk of lung cancer was doubled after controlling for smoking.[101] In addition to smoking, epidemiological data has suggested a link between lung infections (i.e., bacterial pneumonia, TB) and the development of lung cancer.[87] In the large HIV/AIDS Cancer Match study, a history of recurrent pneumonia was associated with a higher risk of lung cancer. When adjusted for smoking, the risk was no longer statistically significant suggesting the possibility of a synergistic effect of smoking and recurrent pneumonias.

* *

Intravenous drug use (IDU) has also been associated with an increased risk of lung cancer in multiple HIV studies. One study showed a sixfold increase in lung cancer for those with HIV and IDU compared to HIV and non-IDU.[100] The same study showed non-HIV patients with IDU had a greater risk of lung cancer than non-HIV patients without IDU. Other studies refute the association between illicit drug use and lung cancer.[100] One possible explanation for the discrepancy is the high concordance of smoking and IDU potentially masking the negative effects of IDU.

**

Among those with HIV, the risk of lung cancer increases almost exponentially with age. The risk of lung cancer at age 60 was 28 times the risk at age 30.[96]

CASE 8

Question 1: B. Human herpes virus-8

The lower extremity cutaneous findings are concerning for extensive Kaposi's sarcoma lesions. Given this patient's history of HIV, symptoms and the cutaneous lesions, the radiographic findings are most concerning for pulmonary involvement in AIDS-related Kaposi's sarcoma (KS). KS is an AIDS-related complication caused by human herpes virus-8.

**

Patients with pulmonary KS almost always have prior cutaneous disease. Pulmonary KS can involve the lung parenchyma, airways, pleura, or mediastinal lymph nodes. The two most common radiographic presentations of KS are findings of nodular densities of varying sizes throughout both lungs with hilar fullness or findings of linear densities following septal lines. Pleural effusions are seen in up to two-thirds of patients with parenchymal KS.[101]

**

Rapid progression of pulmonary KS can be precipitated by systemic glucocorticoids. Furthermore, a fall in CD4 count below 150 cells/mL, an increase in viral load above 10,000 copies/mL, and development of pleural effusions are often seen in progressive pulmonary KS. Therefore, given the patient's history of Kaposi's sarcoma, drop in CD4 count, increase in viral load, and recent glucocorticoid use, the clinical signs and symptoms are most consistent with pulmonary Kaposi's sarcoma.

**

Prior to the advent of highly active antiretroviral therapy (HAART), pulmonary KS was reported in approximately 10% of patients with AIDS and 25% of patients with cutaneous KS. Several large studies indicate that the incidence of KS in the United States and Europe is diminishing, particularly with the introduction of HAART combination therapy. There remains a greater incidence of KS in men who have sex with men, than in heterosexual men and women.[102-106]

Question 2: A. Bronchoscopy with bronchoalveolar lavage

Given this patient's history of HIV and lower extremity lesions, the clinical symptoms and radiographic findings are most concerning for Kaposi's sarcoma (KS). However, other infectious etiologies such as pneumocystis pneumonia must be ruled out prior to the diagnosis of pulmonary KS.[102] Furthermore, bronchoscopy is the best diagnostic test to examine the airways for endobronchial KS lesions and to obtain bronchoalveolar lavage samples for microbiologic stains and cultures, immunoassays for infectious agents, and cytologic examination for viral inclusions or tumors other than KS. Endobronchial and transbronchial biopsies have diagnostic yields of only 26% to 60% and should be performed with caution given the vascular nature of the tumor.[101] Histologic identification can be difficult due to the paucity of malignant features and biopsy findings may be misinterpreted as reactive fibrous tissue.[101]

Question 3: C. Initiate antiretroviral therapy

The clinical scenario and pleural fluid characteristics are consistent with intrathoracic KS. Cytologic examination is often unremarkable in patients with pulmonary KS. Therefore, the next best step is to initiate antiretroviral therapy. Antiretroviral therapy (ART) remains the mainstay in the treatment of pulmonary KS. Introduction of ART has been associated with regression of AIDS-associated KS. Discontinuation of glucocorticoids has also been associated with regression of KS and therefore restarting prednisone is contraindicated. There is no evidence of mycobacterium avium complex and therefore initiation of clarithromycin and ethambutol are unlikely to benefit this patient.[103-106]

**

In a randomized controlled study, patients given antiretroviral therapy and bleomycin, doxorubicin, and vincristine showed a higher overall KS response over 12 months. However, there was no difference found in overall survival. Therefore, initiation of chemotherapy is typically reserved for patients who do not show response to antiretroviral therapy or have symptomatic pulmonary KS.[107]

CASE 9

Question 1: B. *Pneumocystis jirovecii* pneumonia

This clinical scenario is most consistent with pneumocystis jirovecii pneumonia (PCP). PCP is characterized by a subacute onset of progressive dyspnea, fever, nonproductive cough, and chest discomfort that progresses within days to weeks. Symptoms are worsened with exertion. In mild cases, exertion will elicit examination changes of tachypnea, tachycardia, diffuse rales, and oxygen desaturation. Often, oral thrush will be seen as a co-infection. The most characteristic laboratory abnormality consists of hypoxemia with a notable alveolar-arterial O_2 difference (>35 mm Hg).

* *

Chest radiograph may feature diffuse, bilateral interstitial infiltrates. However, normal chest radiographs can be seen in early disease.[108] Factors associated with a higher risk of PCP include low CD4 counts, oral thrush, recurrent bacterial pneumonia, unintentional weight loss, and high viral loads.[109]

* *

The incidence of PCP has declined after the introduction of PCP prophylactic antibiotic use and antiretroviral therapy. The incidence among patients with AIDS in Western Europe and the United States is <1 case per 100 person-years.[110]

Question 2: E. Arterial blood gas

This clinical scenario and the bronchoalveolar lavage fluid findings are pathognomonic for PCP.[111] An arterial blood gas should be obtained to characterize the severity of illness. Patients with PCP and moderate-to-severe disease, defined by a room air paO_2 <70 mm Hg or Alveolar-arterial O_2 gradient ≥35 mm Hg, should receive adjunctive corticosteroids within 72 hours after starting specific PCP therapy.[112] Corticosteroids given in conjunction with appropriate antimicrobial therapy for pneumocystis decreases the incidence of respiratory failure and mortality.[113]

* *

A high-resolution computed tomography of the chest, pulmonary function testing, transthoracic echocardiogram, and venous blood gas are unlikely to be helpful in this patient.

Question 3: D. Trimethoprim-sulfamethoxazole

Trimethoprim-sulfamethoxazole (TMP-SMX) is the treatment of choice for PCP (grade AI). Patients with PCP and moderate-to-severe disease, defined by a room air paO_2 <70 mm Hg or Alveolar-arterial O_2 gradient ≥35 mmHg, should also receive adjunctive corticosteroids within 72 hours after starting specific PCP therapy. The recommended duration of therapy for PCP is 21 days.[112]

* *

Clarithromycin and ethambutol, fluconazole, ganciclovir, and RIPE therapy are ineffective for PCP.

CASE 10

Question 1: B. *Pneumocystis jirovecii* pneumonia (PCP)

Indications for prophylaxis to prevent a first episode of PCP include: a CD4 count <200 cells/µL; oropharyngeal candidiasis; CD4 <14%; history of AIDS-defining illness, or CD4 count >200 but <250 cells/µL if monitoring CD4 cell count every 3 months is not possible. This patient has a CD4 count <200 and, therefore, should be started on prophylaxis for PCP.[112]

* *

Indications for prophylaxis to prevent toxoplasma gondii encephalitis include toxoplasma IgG-positive patients with CD4 count <100 cells/µL. Seronegative patients receiving PCP prophylaxis not active against toxoplasmosis should have toxoplasma serology retested if CD4 count declines to <100. Prophylaxis should be initiated if seroconversion occurs.[112]

* *

The only indication for prophylaxis to prevent disseminated mycobacterium avium complex (MAC) disease is a CD4 count <50 cells/µL after ruling out active disseminated MAC disease based on clinical assessment.[112]

* *

According to the Infectious Diseases Society of America guidelines, there are no indications for mycobacterium tuberculosis (TB) prophylaxis. As per the guidelines, patients may be treated for latent TB infection (LTBI) or presumed LTBI in the setting of a positive screening test for LTBI with no evidence of active TB and no prior treatment for active TB or LTBI. Patients in close contact with a person with infectious TB without evidence of active TB may be treated for LTBI regardless of screening test results.[112]

Question 2: **A. Trimethoprim-sulfamethoxazole daily**

Dapsone and atovaquone are second-line agents used for PCP prophylaxis.[112] Azithromycin may be used for the treatment of MAC, but is not active against PCP.

Question 3: **E. All of the above**

Indications for prophylaxis to prevent first episode of PCP include: a CD4 count <200 cells/μL; oropharyngeal candidiasis; CD4 <14%; history of AIDS-defining illness, or CD4 count >200 but <250 cells/μL if monitoring CD4 cell count every 3 months is not possible. This patient has a CD4 count <200 and, therefore, should be started on prophylaxis for PCP.

REFERENCES

1. World Health Organization. *Stop TB Department. Treatment of Tuberculosis: Guidelines.* 4th ed. Geneva, Switzerland: World Health Organization; 2010.
2. Holtz TH, Kabera G, Mthiyane T, et al. Use of a WHO-recommended algorithm to reduce mortality in seriously ill patients with HIV infection and smear-negative pulmonary tuberculosis in South Africa: an observational cohort study. *Lancet Infect Dis.* 2011;11(7):533–540.
3. Chaisson RE, Schecter GF, Theuer CP, et al. Tuberculosis in patients with the acquired immunodeficiency syndrome clinical features, response to therapy, and survival. *Am Rev Respir Dis.* 1987;136(3):570–574.
4. Bem C, Patil PS, Elliott AM, et al. The value of wide-needle aspiration in the diagnosis of tuberculous lymphadenitis in Africa. *AIDS.* 1993;7(9):1221–1225.
5. Bekedam HJ, Boeree M, Kamenya A, et al. Tuberculous lymphadenitis, a diagnostic problem in areas of high prevalence of HIV and tuberculosis. *Trans R Soc Trop Med Hyg.* 1997;91(3):294–297.
6. Jones BE, Young SM, Antoniskis D, et al. Relationship of the manifestations of tuberculosis to CD4 cell counts in patients with human immunodeficiency virus infection. *Am Rev Respir Dis.* 1993;148(5):1292–1297.
7. Salzman SH, Schindel ML, Aranda CP, et al. The role of bronchoscopy in the diagnosis of pulmonary tuberculosis in patients at risk for HIV infection. *Chest.* 1992;102(1):143–146.
8. American Thoracic Society, Centers for Disease Control and Prevention and the Infectious Diseases Society. Treatment of tuberculosis. *Am J Respir Crit Care Med.* 2003;167(4):603–662.
9. Panel on Opportunistic Infections in HIV-Infected Adults and Adolescents. Guidelines for the prevention and treatment of opportunistic infections in HIV-infected adults and adolescents: recommendations from the Centers for Disease Control and Prevention, the National Institutes of Health, and the HIV Medical Association of the Infectious Diseases Society of America. 2013.
10. Abdool Karim SS, Naidoo K, Grobler A, et al. Timing of initiation of antiretroviral drugs during tuberculosis therapy. *N Engl J Med.* 2010;362(8):697–706.
11. Gandhi NR, Andrews JR, Brust JC, et al. Risk factors for mortality among MDR- and XDR-TB patients in a high HIV prevalence setting. *Int J Tuberc Lung Dis.* 2012;16(1):90–97.
12. Abdool Karim SS, Naidoo K, Grobler A, et al. Integration of antiretroviral therapy with tuberculosis treatment. *N Engl J Med.* 2011;365(16):1492–1501.
13. Blanc FX, Sok T, Laureillard D et al; CAMELIA (ANRS 1295–CIPRA KH001) Study Team. Earlier versus later start of antiretroviral therapy in HIV-infected adults with tuberculosis. *N Engl J Med.* 2011;365(16):1471–1481.
14. Havlir DV, KendallMA, Ive P, et al; AIDS Clinical Trials Group Study A5221. Timing of antiretroviral therapy for HIV-1 infection and tuberculosis. *N Engl J Med.* 2011;365(16):1482–1491.
15. United States Department of Health and Human Services. Guidelines for the use of antiretroviral agents in HIV-1-infected adults and adolescents. http://www.aidsinfo.nih.gov/contentfiles/lvguidelines/adultandadolescentgl.pdf. Accessed Nov 15, 2014.
16. Torok ME, Yen NT, Chau TT, et al. Timing of initiation of antiretroviral therapy in human immunodeficiency virus (HIV)–associated tuberculous meningitis. *Clin Infect Dis.* 2011;52(11):1374–1383.
17. Shafer RW, Kim DS, Weiss JP, et al. Extrapulmonary tuberculosis in patients with human immunodeficiency virus infection. *Medicine (Baltimore).* 1991;70(6):384–397.
18. Keiper MD, BeumontM, Elshami A, et al. CD4 T lymphocyte count and the radiographic presentation of pulmonary tuberculosis: a study of the relationship between these factors in patients with human immunodeficiency virus infection. *CHEST.* 1995;107(1):74–80.
19. Cain KP, McCarthy KD, Heilig CM, et al. An algorithm for tuberculosis screening and diagnosis in people with HIV. *N Engl J Med.* 2010;362(8):707–716.
20. Von Reyn CF, Kimambo S, Mtei L, et al. Disseminated tuberculosis in human immunodeficiency virus infection: ineffective immunity, polyclonal disease and high mortality. *Int J Tuberc Lung Dis.* 2011;15(8):1087–1092.
21. Wiktor SZ, Sassan-Morokro M, Grant AD, et al. Efficacy of trimethoprim-sulphamethoxazole prophylaxis to decrease morbidity and mortality in HIV-1-infected patients with tuberculosis in Abidjan Côte d'Ivoire: a randomised controlled trial. *Lancet.* 1999;353:1469–1475.
22. Barry M, Gibbons S, Back D, et al. Protease inhibitors in patients with HIV disease. Clinically important pharmacokinetic considerations. *Clin Pharmacokinet.* 1997;32(3):194–209.
23. Boulanger C, Hollender E, Farrell K, et al. Pharmacokinetic evaluation of rifabutin in combination with lopinavir-ritonavir in patients with HIV infection and active tuberculosis. *Clin Infect Dis.* 2009;49(9):1305–1311.
24. Sekar V, Lavreys L, Van de Casteele T, et al. Pharmacokinetics of darunavir/ritonavir and rifabutin coadministered in HIV-negative healthy volunteers. *Antimicrob Agents Chemother.* 2010;54(10):4440–4445.
25. Kassahun K, McIntosh I, Cui D, et al. Metabolism and disposition in humans of raltegravir (MK-0518), an anti-AIDS

drug targeting the human immunodeficiency virus 1 integrase enzyme. *Drug Metab Dispos.* 2007;35(9):1657–1663.

26. Narita M, Ashkin D, Hollender ES, et al. Paradoxical worsening of tuberculosis following antiretroviral therapy in patients with AIDS. *Am J Respir Crit Care Med.* 1998;158(1): 157–161.

27. Breen RA, Smith CJ, Bettinson H, et al. Paradoxical reactions during tuberculosis treatment in patients with and without HIV co-infection. *Thorax.* 2004;59(8):704–707.

28. Wendel KA, Alwood KS, Gachuhi R, et al. Paradoxical worsening of tuberculosis in HIV-infected persons. *Chest.* 2001;120(1):193–197.

29. Managing drug interactions in the treatment of HIV-related tuberculosis Atlanta, GA, Centers for Disease Control and Prevention, 2007. Available at www.cdc.gov/tb/publications/guidelines/TB_HIV_Drugs/PDF/tbhiv.pdf. Accessed Nov 15, 2014.

30. Guidelines for the programmatic management of drug-resistant tuberculosis: emergency update 2008. Geneva, World Health Organization; 2008 (WHO/HTM/TB/ 2008.402)

31. Novak RM, Richardson JT, Buchacz K, et al; HIV Outpatient Study (HOPS) Investigators. Immune reconstitution inflammatory syndrome: incidence and implications for mortality. *AIDS.* 2012;26(6):721–730.

32. Lawn SD, Wilkinson RJ, Lipman MC, et al. Immune reconstitution and "unmasking" of tuberculosis during antiretroviral therapy. *Am J Respir Crit Care Med.* 2008;177(7):680–685.

33. Dibyendu D, Sarkar RN, Phaujdar S, et al. Incidence and risk factors of immune reconstitution inflammatory syndrome in HIV-TB coinfected patients. *Braz J Infect Dis.* 2011;15(6):553–559.

34. Lawn SD, Bekker LG, Miller RF. Immune reconstitution disease associated with mycobacterial infections in HIV-infected individuals receiving antiretrovirals. *Lancet Infect Dis.* 2005;5(6):361–373.

35. Meintjes G, Lawn SD, Scano F, et al; International Network for the Study of HIV-associated IRIS. Tuberculosis-associated immune reconstitution inflammatory syndrome: case definitions for use in resource-limited settings. *Lancet Infect Dis.* 2008;8(8):516–523.

36. Meintjes G, Wilkinson RJ, Morroni C, et al. Randomized placebo-controlled trial of prednisone for paradoxical tuberculosis-associated immune reconstitution inflammatory syndrome. *AIDS.* 2010; 24(15):2381–2390.

37. Muller M, Wandel S, Colebunders R, et al. ; IeDEA Southern and Central Africa. Immune reconstitution inflammatory syndrome in patients starting antiretroviral therapy for HIV infection: a systematic review and meta-analysis. *Lancet Infect Dis.* 2010;10(4):251–261.

38. Burman W, Weis S, Vernon A, et al. Frequency, severity and duration of immune reconstitution events in HIV-related tuberculosis. *Int J Tuberc Lung Dis.* 2007;11(12):1282–1289.

39. Pepper DJ, Marais S, Maartens G, et al. Neurologic manifestations of paradoxical tuberculosis-associated immune reconstitution inflammatory syndrome: a case series. *Clin Infect Dis.* 2009;48(11):e96–e107.

40. Skiest DJ, Hester LJ, Hardy RD. Cryptococcal immune reconstitution inflammatory syndrome: report of four cases in three patients and review of the literature. *J Infect.* 2005;51:e289–e297.

41. Lortholary O, Fontanet A, Mémain N, et al. Incidence and risk factors of immune reconstitution inflammatory syndrome complicating HIV-associated cryptococcosis in France. *AIDS.* 2005;19:1043–1049.

42. Sungkanuparph S, Jongwutiwes U, Kiertiburanakul S. Timing of cryptococcal immune reconstitution inflammatory syndrome after antiretroviral therapy in patients with AIDS and cryptococcal meningitis. *J Acquir Immune Defic Syndr.* 2007;45:595–596.

43. Shelburne SA 3rd, Darcourt J, White AC Jr, et al. The role of immune reconstitution inflammatory syndrome in AIDS-related Cryptococcus neoformans disease in the era of highly active antiretroviral therapy. *Clin Infect Dis.* 2005;40:1049–1052.

44. Grant PM, Komarow L, Andersen J, et al. Risk factor analyses for immune reconstitution inflammatory syndrome in a randomized study of early vs. deferred ART during an opportunistic infection. *PLoS One.* 2010;5:e11416.

45. Ratnam I, Chiu C, Kandala NB, et al. Incidence and risk factors for immune reconstitution inflammatory syndrome in an ethnically diverse HIV type 1-infected cohort. *Clin Infect Dis.* 2006; 42:418–427.

46. Manabe YC, Campbell JD, Sydnor E, et al. Immune reconstitution inflammatory syndrome: risk factors and treatment implications. *J Acquir Immune Defic Syndr.* 2007;46:456–462.

47. Murdoch DM, Venter WD, Feldman C, et al. Incidence and risk factors for the immune reconstitution inflammatory syndrome in HIV patients in South Africa: a prospective study. *AIDS.* 2008;22:601–610.

48. Bourgarit A, Carcelain G, Martinez V, et al. Explosion of tuberculin specific Th1-responses induces immune restoration syndrome in tuberculosis and HIV co infected patients. *AIDS.* 2006;20:F1–F7.

49. Elliott JH, Khol V, Sarun S, et al. Investigation of the pathogenesis and diagnosis of tuberculosis-associated immune reconstitution inflammatory syndrome and antiretroviral therapy–associated tuberculosis using skin testing and a whole blood interferon-g release assay [abstract WEPE0201]. In: Program and abstracts of the XVII International AIDS Conference (Mexico City). 2008.

50. Tan DB, Yong YK, Tan HY, et al. Immunological profiles of immune restoration disease presenting as mycobacterial lymphadenitis and cryptococcal meningitis. *HIV Med.* 2008;9:307–316.

51. French, MA. HIV/AIDS: immune reconstitution inflammatory syndrome: a reappraisal. *Clin Infect Dis.* 2009; 48(1):101–107.

52. Diaz PT, King MA, Pacht ER, et al. Increased susceptibility to pulmonary emphysema among HIV-seropositive smokers. *Ann Intern Med.* 2000;132:369–372.

53. Shipley TW, Kling HM, Morris A, et al. Persistent pneumocystis colonization leads to the development of chronic obstructive pulmonary disease in a nonhuman primate model of AIDS. *J Infect Dis.* 2010;202(2):302–312.

54. Morris A, Alexander T, Radhi S. Airway obstruction is increased in pneumocystis-colonized human immunodeficiency virus-infected outpatients. *J Clin Microbiol.* 2009;47(11):3773–3776.

55. Rosen MJ, Lou Y, Kvale PA. Pulmonary function tests in HIV-infected patients without AIDS. Pulmonary Complications of HIV Infection Study Group. *Am J Respir Crit Care Med.* 1995;152(2):738–745.

56. Shaw RJ, Roussak C, Forster SM, et al. Lung function abnormalities in patients infected with the human immunodeficiency virus with and without overt pneumonitis. *Thorax.* 1988;43:436.

57. Crothers K, McGinnis K, Kleerup E, et al. HIV infection is associated with reduced pulmonary diffusing capacity. *J Acquir Immune Defic Syndr.* 2013;64:271–278.

58. Gingo MR, He J, Wittman C, et al. Contributors to diffusion impairment in HIV-infected persons. *Eur Respir J.* 2014;43:195–203.

59. Gingo MR, George MP, Kessinger CJ. Pulmonary function abnormalities in HIV-infected patients during the current antiretroviral therapy era. *Am J Respir Crit Care Med.* 2010;182(6):790–796.

60. Kristoffersen US, Lebech AM, Mortensen J. Changes in lung function of HIV-infected patients: a 4.5-year follow-up study. *Clin Physiol Funct Imaging.* 2012; 32(4):288–295.

61. Niaura R, Shadel WG, Morrow K, et al. Human immunodeficiency virus infection, AIDS, and smoking cessation: The time is now. *Clin Infect Dis.* 2000;31:808–812.

62. Gritz ER, Vidrine DJ, Lazev AB, et al. Smoking behavior in a low-income multiethnic HIV/AIDS population. *Nicotine Tob Res.* 2004;6:71–77.

63. Diaz PT, King MA, Pacht ER, et al. The pathophysiology of pulmonary diffusion impairment in human immunodeficiency virus infection. *Am J Respir Crit Care Med.* 1999;160:272–277.

64. Demedts IK, Demoor T, Bracke KR, et al. Role of apoptosis in the pathogenesis of COPD and pulmonary emphysema. *Respir Res.* 2006;7:53.

65. Kasahara Y, Tuder RM, Cool CD, et al. Endothelial cell death and decreased expression of vascular endothelial growth factor and vascular endothelial growth factor receptor 2 in emphysema. *Am J Respir Crit Care Med.* 2001;163:737–744.

66. Tuder RM, McGrath S, Neptune E. The pathobiological mechanisms of emphysema models: what do they have in common? *Pulm Pharmacol Ther.* 2003;16:67–78.

67. Micoli KJ, Mamaeva O, Piller SC, et al. Point mutations in the c-terminus of HIV-1 gp160 reduce apoptosis and calmodulin binding without affecting viral replication. *Virology.* 2006;344:468–479.

68. Micoli KJ, Pan G, Wu Y, et al. Requirement of calmodulin binding by HIV-1 gp160 for enhanced FAS-mediated apoptosis. *J Biol Chem.* 2000;275:1233–1240.

69. George MP, Kannass M, Huang L. Respiratory symptoms and airway obstruction in HIV-infected subjects in the HAART era. *PLoS One.* 2009;4(7):e6328.

70. Morris A, George MP, Crothers K. HIV and chronic obstructive pulmonary disease: is it worse and why? *Proc Am Thorac Soc.* 2011;8(3):320–325.

71. Yearsley MM, Diaz PT, Knoell D, et al. Correlation of HIV-1 detection and histology in AIDS-associated emphysema. *Diagn Mol Pathol.* 2005;14:48–52.

72. Hirani A, Cavallazzi R, Vasu T, et al. Prevalence of obstructive lung disease in HIV population: cross sectional study. *Respir Med.* 2011;105:1655–1661.

73. Jagannathan P, Davis E, JacobsonM, et al. Life-threatening immune reconstitution inflammatory syndrome after Pneumocystis pneumonia: a cautionary case series. *AIDS.* 2009;23:1794–1796.

74. Drummond MB, Kirk GD, Astemborski J, et al. Association between obstructive lung disease and markers of HIV infection in a high-risk cohort. *Thorax.* 2012;67(4):309–314.

75. Drummond MB, Merlo CA, Astemborski J, et al. The effect of HIV infection on longitudinal lung function decline among IDUs: a prospective cohort. *AIDS.* 2013; 27(8):1303–1311.

76. Miller RF, Huang L, Walzer PD. et al. Pneumocystis pneumonia associated with human immunodeficiency virus. *Clin Chest Med.* 2013;34(2):229–241.

77. Haddow LJ, Colebunders R, Meintjes G, et al. Cryptococcal immune reconstitution inflammatory syndrome in HIV-1-infected individuals: proposed clinical case definitions. *Lancet Infect Dis.* 2010;10:791–802.

78. Phillips P, Bonner S, Gataric N, et al. Nontuberculous mycobacterial immune reconstitution syndrome in HIV-infected patients: spectrum of disease and long-term follow-up. *Clin Infect Dis.* 2005;41:1483–1497.

79. Teruya H, Tateyama M, Hibiya K, et al. Pulmonary Mycobacterium parascrofulaceum infection as an immune reconstitution inflammatory syndrome in an AIDS patient. *Intern Med.* 2010;49:1817–1821.

80. Lawn SD. Acute respiratory failures due to Mycobacterium kansasii infection: immune reconstitution disease in a patient with AIDS. *J Infect.* 2005;51:339–340.

81. Leone S, Giglio S, Maio P, et al. Mycobacterium xenopi pulmonary infection resulting in self-limited immune reconstitution inflammatory syndrome in an HIV-1 infected patient. *New Microbiol.* 2009;32:415–417.

82. Martin J, Laker M, Clutter D, et al. Kaposi's sarcoma-associated immune reconstitution inflammatory syndrome (KSIRIS) in Africa: initial findings from a prospective evaluation. 16th Conference on Retroviruses and Opportunistic Infections; Montreal, Canada; 2009.

83. Godoy MC, Rouse H, Brown JA, et al. Imaging features of pulmonary Kaposi sarcoma-associated immune reconstitution syndrome. *AJR Am J Roentgenol.* 2007;189:956–965.

84. Letang E, Almeida JM, Miro JM, et al. Predictors of immune reconstitution inflammatory syndrome-associated with Kaposi sarcoma in Mozambique: a prospective study. *J Acquir Immune Defic Syndr.* 2010;53:589–597.

85. Bower M, Nelson M, Young AM, et al. Immune reconstitution inflammatory syndrome associated with Kaposi's sarcoma. *J Clin Oncol.* 2005;23:5224–5228.

86. Morris DG, Jasmer RM, Huang L, et al. Sarcoidosis following HIV infection: evidence for CD4. Lymphocyte dependence. *Chest.* 2003;124:929–935.

87. Alshafie MT, Donaldson B, Oluwole SF. Human immunodeficiency virus and lung cancer. *Br J Surg.* 1997;84(8): 1068–1071.

88. Engels EA, Pfeiffer RM, Goedert JJ, et al; for the HIV/AIDS Cancer Match Study. Trends in cancer risk among people with AIDS in the United States 1980–2002. *AIDS.* 2006;20(12):1645–1654.

89. Long JL, Engels EA, Moore RD, et al. Incidence and outcomes of malignancy in the HAART era in an urban cohort of HIV-infected individuals. *AIDS.* 2008;22(4):489–496.

90. Frisch M, Biggar RJ, Engels EA, et al; AIDS-Cancer Match Registry Study Group. Association of cancer with AIDS-related immunosuppression in adults. *JAMA.* 2001;285(13):1736–1745.

91. Shiels MS, Cole SR, Kirk GD, et al. A meta-analysis of the incidence of non-AIDS cancers in HIV-infected individuals. *J Acquir Immune Defic Syndr.* 2009;52(5):611–622.

92. Sigel K, Wisnivesky J, Gordon K, et al. HIV as an independent risk factor for incident lung cancer. *AIDS.* 2012;26(8):1017–1025.

93. Winstone TA, Man SF, Hull M, et al. Epidemic of lung cancer in patients with HIV infection. *Chest.* 2013;143(2):305–314.

94. Brock MV, Hooker CM, Engels EA, et al. Delayed diagnosis and elevated mortality in an urban population with HIV and lung cancer: implications for patient care. *J Acquir Immune Defic Syndr.* 2006;43(1):47–55.

95. Shiels MS, Pfeiffer RM, Gail MH, et al. Cancer burden in the HIV-infected population in the United States. *J Natl Cancer Inst.* 2011;103(9):753–762.

96. Guiguet M, Boué F, Cadranel J, et al; Clinical Epidemiology Group of the FHDHANRS CO4 cohort. Effect of immunodeficiency, HIV viral load, and antiretroviral therapy on the risk of individual malignancies: a prospective cohort study. *Lancet Oncol.* 2009;10(12):1152–1159.

97. Engels EA, Brock MV, Chen J, et al. Elevated incidence of lung cancer among HIV-infected individuals. *J Clin Oncol.* 2006;24(9):1383–1388.

98. Engels EA. Inflammation in the development of lung cancer: epidemiological evidence. *Expert Rev Anticancer Ther.* 2008;8(4):605–615.

99. Serraino D, Boschini A, Carrieri P, et al. Cancer risk among men with, or at risk of, HIV infection in southern Europe. *AIDS.* 2000;14(5):553–559.

100. Kirk GD, Merlo C, O'Driscoll P, et al. HIV infection is associated with an increased risk for lung cancer, independent of smoking. *Clin Infect Dis.* 2007;45(1):103–110.

101. Aboulafia DM. The epdiemiolgic, pathologic, and clinical features of AIDS-associated pulmonary Kaposi's sarcoma. *Chest.* 2000;117(4):1128–1445.

102. Morris A, Crothers K, Beck JM, Huang L. American Thoracic Society Committee on HIV Pulmonary Disease: an official ATS Workshop Report–emerging issues and current controversies in HIV-associated pulmonary diseases. *Proc Am Thorac Soc.* 2011;8(1):17–26.

103. Moore R, Keruly JC, Gallant J, et al. Decline in morbidity and opportunistic disease with combination antiretroviral therapy. Abstract 22374. Presented at: 12th World AIDS Conference; June 26–July 3, Geneva, Switzerland: 1998.

104. Jones J, Hanson DL, Dworkin JW, et al. Effect of antiretroviral and other antiviral therapies on the incidence of Kaposi's sarcoma and trends in Kaposi's sarcoma. Abstract 13241. Presented at: 12th World AIDS Conference; June 26–July 3, Geneva, Switzerland: 1998.

105. Stebbing J, Sanitt A, Nelson M, et al. A prognostic index for AIDS-associated Kaposi's sarcoma in the era of highly active antiretroviral therapy. *Lancet* 2006;367:1495–1502.

106. Gill J, Bourboulia D, Wilkinson J, et al. Prospective study of the effects of antiretroviral therapy on Kaposi sarcoma–associated herpesvirus infection in patients with and without Kaposi sarcoma. *J Acquir Immune Defic Syndr.* 2002;31:384–390.

107. Mosam A, Shaik F, Uldrick TS, et al. A randomized controlled trial of highly active antiretroviral therapy versus highly active antiretroviral therapy and chemotherapy in therapy-naïve patients with HIV associated Kaposi sarcoma in South Africa. *J Acquir Immune Defic Syndr.* 2012;60(20):150–157.

108. Selwyn PA, Pumerantz AS, Durante A, et al. Clinical predictors of Pneumocystis carinii pneumonia, bacterial pneumonia and tuberculosis in HIV-infected patients. *AIDS.* 1998;12(8):885–893.

109. Kaplan JE, Hanson DL, Navin TR, et al. Risk factors for primary Pneumocystis carinii pneumonia in human immunodeficiency virus-infected adolescents and adults in the United States: reassessment of indications for chemoprophylaxis. *J Infect Dis.* 1998;178(4):1126–1132.

110. Buchacz K, Baker RK, Palella FJ Jr, et al. AIDS-defining opportunistic illnesses in US patients, 1994–2007: a cohort study. *AIDS.* 2010;24(10):1549–1559.

111. Baughman RP, Dohn MN, Frame PT. The continuing utility of bronchoalveolar lavage to diagnose opportunistic infection in AIDS patients. *Am J Med.* 1994;97(6):515–522.

112. Masur H, Brooks JT, Benson CA, et al. Prevention and treatment of opportunistic infections in HIV-infected adults and adolescents: Updated Guidelines from the Centers for Disease Control and Prevention, National Institutes of Health, and HIV Medicine Association of the Infectious Diseases Society of America. *Clin Infect Dis.* 2014;58(9):1308–1311.

113. Briel M, Bucher HC, Boscacci R, et al. Adjunctive corticosteroids for Pneumocystis jiroveci pneumonia in patients with HIV infection. *Cochrane Database Syst Rev.* 2006 ;(3):CD006150.

22

Critical Care

Ronaldo Collo Go MD, Michael Silverberg MD, Rafael Yunen MD,
Amar Anantdeep Singh Sarao MD, Charanya Sivaramamkrishnan MD,
Vikram Dhawan MD, and Roopa Kohli-Seth MD

CASE 1

A 30-year-old man with Crohn's disease comes in to the emergency department feeling weak and tired. He reports a history of diarrhea for the last 10 days. His chemistry blood work done in the emergency department shows a sodium level of 145 milliequivalents per liter (mEq/L), potassium of 3.5 mEq/L, chloride of 105 mEq/L, bicarbonate of 14 mEq/L with minimally elevated BUN and creatinine levels.

Question 1: **What is his expected pCO_2 in mm Hg on an arterial blood gas if no additional metabolic or primary respiratory acid–base disorders are present?**

A. 22
B. 18
C. 37
D. 29
E. None of the above

Question 2: **An arterial blood gas shows a pH of 7.32, pCO_2 of 60 mm Hg with a bicarbonate level of 30 mEq/L. Which of the following statements best explains the current acid–base disorder?**

A. Acute respiratory acidosis with metabolic compensation
B. Chronic respiratory acidosis with complete metabolic compensation
C. Chronic respiratory acidosis with incomplete metabolic compensation
D. Acute respiratory alkalosis with metabolic acidosis
E. Acute respiratory acidosis with metabolic acidosis

CASE 2

A 55-year-old man who is currently admitted for diabetic ketoacidosis has been recently transitioned from insulin drip to lantus and SQ insulin. He complains of substernal chest pain. He is started on aspirin, clopidogrel, bivalirudin, and statin. Electrocardiogram is nonspecific and serial cardiac enzymes are negative.

Question 1: **What further diagnostic and/or therapeutic steps would you take to best manage this gentleman's current condition?**

A. Arrange for diagnostic angiography
B. Arrange for exercise stress test
C. Order for a transthoracic echocardiogram to assess cardiac function
D. Order a CT angiogram of the chest to rule out aortic dissection and pulmonary embolism
E. Send the patient for myocardial perfusion study

Question 2: **About 2 hours after you last saw the patient, he reports another episode of chest discomfort, which is much worse than his previous episode. His chest discomfort fails to respond to three doses of sublingual nitroglycerin. Over the next half an hour he develops shortness of breath, and his examination reveals diffuse rales bilaterally. His neck veins are distended. His heart rate is unchanged, blood pressure drops to 85/45, RR is 25. Cardiac auscultation is unremarkable. ECG remains unchanged. His cardiac biomarkers have remained unremarkable thus far. Your next course of action is:**

A. Administer streptokinase or recombinant TPA at therapeutic dose
B. Arrange for an emergent angiography

C. Restart the ACE inhibitor which was held overnight

D. Start nitroglycerin infusion for refractory angina

E. Start low-dose metoprolol and administer furosemide for pulmonary vascular congestion

Question 3: What is the most likely pathophysiological mechanism for the disease process described above?

A. An occlusive thrombus atop an unstable atherosclerotic plaque with no collateral circulation

B. Coronary artery dissection

C. A nonocclusive thrombus on top of an unstable atherosclerotic plaque

D. Anomalous origin of coronary artery

E. Fat emboli

CASE 3

A 60-year-old woman with Crohn's disease, chronic diarrhea, hypertension, and hyperlipidemia is admitted to the ICU with severe generalized weakness with inability to walk or stand. Her potassium is 1.4 at the time of admission. ECG shows normal sinus rhythm (NSR) with T-wave flattening. Her potassium is corrected over the ensuing 2 days with a normal basic metabolic panel at present. Her strength returns to baseline. This morning around 8 am she reports diffuse chest discomfort accompanied by shortness of breath and nausea. Blood pressure is 70/40, HR 120, and RR 22. Lungs are clear with distended neck veins. ECG is shown below.

Question 1: What is the next best step?

A. Aspirin 325 mg, clopidogrel 300 mg, nitroglycerine 5 mg sublingual (repeat twice more if needed)

B. Fluid bolus, aspirin 325 mg, emergent angiography with plan for primary PCI

C. Medical stabilization first with fluids, inotropic support and then PCI once stable

D. Emergent fibrinolytic therapy using rTPA with rescue PCI if fibrinolytic therapy fails

E. None of the above

Question 2: A few hours later, the patient is in distress. Her blood pressure is 60/30 and her heart rate is 130. She is barely arousable, with dilated neck veins, clear lungs, and diminished heart sounds on auscultation. Extremities are cold with barely palpable femoral pulses.

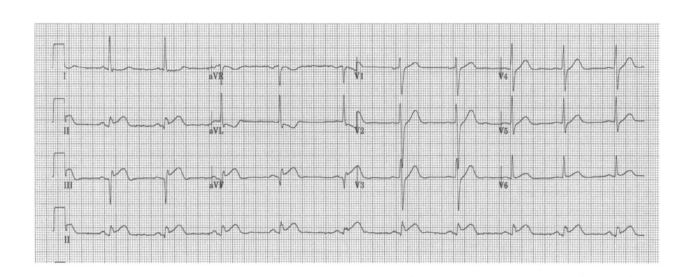

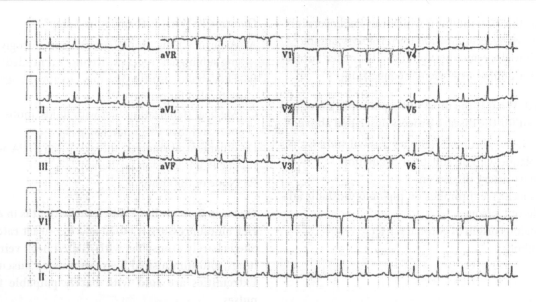

A bedside echocardiogram (see above) was ordered and it showed:

A. Severe regurgitant jet across the mitral valve
B. Evidence of turbulent blood flow from left ventricle to the right through the interventricular septum
C. Severe regurgitant flow across the aortic valve
D. Hypoechoic fluid in the pericardial sac with evidence of RV diastolic collapse
E. None of the above

CASE 4

A 58-year-old man with a history of hypertension and diabetes collapses after an argument. EMS is called and he is found in ventricular fibrillation. Return of spontaneous circulation is achieved after two rounds of chest compressions, epinephrine, and defibrillation. Patient is intubated in the field and is now seen in the emergency department. His blood pressure is 100/45, HR 110, RR 16 on mechanical ventilation, and extremities show no edema. His heart examination reveals no audible murmur or any other adventitious heart sounds. Lung examination reveals basilar crackles bilaterally. Pupils are equal, mid-dilated, and reactive to light. No obvious movement can be elicited as a response to painful stimulus. ECG shows normal sinus rhythm with no definite ST elevation or depression. Nonspecific ST-T wave changes, however, are noted. The QTc and other intervals are within normal limits. ABG shows metabolic acidosis with a pH of 7.25 and a lactate of 10. His routine chemistry blood work done last week at his doctor's office is unremarkable with an A1C of 6.5. Point-of-care glu-

cose is 110. His medications are glargine 20 units qHS and enalapril 2.5 mg daily. STAT echocardiography is done which shows globally decreased contractility with focal hypokinesis of the anterior wall of the left ventricle. You have decided to proceed with therapeutic hypothermia for this patient. His chemistry panel is unremarkable except for a serum bicarbonate level of 14 mEq/L. His cardiac biomarkers are minimally above the upper limit of normal.

Question 1: Which of the following should be part of the management for this patient?

A. Emergent head CT to rule out intracranial bleed as the cause of his condition
B. Discussion with an interventional cardiologist to discuss the value of an emergent coronary angiography
C. STAT chest CT angiogram to rule out pulmonary embolism
D. Administer amiodarone bolus followed by a continuous infusion
E. Start D_5W 1 L containing 150 mEq of sodium bicarbonate at 100 cc/h

Question 2: **Which of the following statements best summarizes the current evidence of the role of temperature control or management in preserving overall and/or neurological outcome after cardiac arrest?**

A. Therapeutic hypothermia has been conclusively shown to improve neurological outcomes after cardiac arrest

B. Therapeutic hypothermia has been shown to worsen the neurological outcomes after cardiac arrest

C. There is sufficient evidence to show that hyperthermia or fever worsens neurological outcomes whereas the role of hypothermia continues to be debated in literature based on current evidence

D. Therapeutic hypothermia is detrimental to overall outcomes with increased all-cause mortality after cardiac arrest due to increased incidence of infection and coagulopathy

E. None of the above

CASE 5

A 70-year-old man with COPD and systolic congestive heart failure with an EF 20% comes in complaining of shortness of breath. He is noted to be hypotensive, BNP 1,000, Hemoglobin 15 mg/dL, chest radiograph shows bilateral opacities, ECG shows a known LBBB, and creatinine is 2 mg/dL.

Question 1: **Which of the following would suggest that he would benefit from crystalloid bolus?**

A. SVV 10

B. SVI 12

C. Ultrasound visualization of the IVC with 2 cm diameter with no respiratory variation

D. PPV 10

E. SVI 9

Question 2: **A pulmonary artery catheter is placed. The cardiac output 4, PCWP 12, mixed venous oxygen saturation is 50%. What would be the next best step?**

A. Dobutamine

B. Crystalloid bolus

C. Transfusion of red blood cells

D. Norepinephrine

E. Repeat blood gas from triple-lumen catheter

CASE 6

A 58-year-old woman is admitted with fever from the emergency department. Her vital signs are a blood pressure of 70/60, heart rate of 128, respiratory rate of 28, temperature of 39°C, and oxygen saturation of 95% on room air.

Question 1: **According to the Surviving Sepsis Campaign guidelines, what are the resuscitation parameters one should target in this patient?**

A. MAP >60, CVP 6–10, $ScVO_2$ >70, urine output >0.5 cc/kg/h

B. MAP >60, CVP 6–10, SVO_2 >70, urine output >0.5 cc/kg/h

C. MAP >60, CVP 8–12, SVO_2 >70, urine output >1 cc/kg/h

D. MAP >65, CVP 10–14, $ScVO_2$ >75, urine output >0.5 cc/kg/h

E. MAP >65, CVP 8–12, SVO_2 >65, urine output >0.5 cc/kg/h

Question 2: **She receives 3 L of crystalloid and is placed on a mechanical ventilator for work of breathing. Her laboratory results are the following: WBC 28,000, hemoglobin 13 mg/dL, and platelets are 550,000. Chemistry shows a sodium level of 149 mEq/L, potassium level of 3.9 mEq/L, bicarbonate of 18 mEq/L, blood urea nitrogen level of 35 mg/dL, and creatinine of 1.5 mg/dL. She has a lactic acid level of 4 mmol/L. Blood pressure is 80/40, heart rate 110, respiratory rate of 30, and oxygen saturation is 100% on FiO_2 30%. Her CVP is 9 mm Hg. Central venous oxygen saturation from the right IJ you placed earlier shows 60%.**

According to SSC guidelines, what additional measure can you take in order to reach your resuscitation targets?

A. Start dobutamine at 30 μg/min only as the patient is adequately fluid resuscitated

B. Start norepinephrine at 10 μg/min only as the patient is adequately fluid resuscitated

C. Administer stress dose steroids for refractory shock

D. Transfuse 1 unit of packed RBCs to increase the oxygen-carrying capacity

E. Administer additional fluid boluses until a CVP of 12 to 15 mm Hg is reached

CASE 7

An 80-year-old man with history of coronary artery disease and severe systolic heart failure, who was recently discharged from the hospital for decompensated heart failure, complains of fatigue and shortness of breath. His blood pressure is 70/35, HR is 115, and he is breathing at 22 breaths per minute. His lung examination reveals minimal crackles at the bases. Examination of the extremities reveals no edema but they are cold to touch with faint pulses. An echocardiogram done reveals an EF of 20%, poor diastolic function, LV hypertrophy, no pericardial effusion, and minimal mitral regurgitation. ECG shows sinus tachycardia, LBBB, LVH, old q waves in lead 1 and AVL. His lactate is 3 mmol/L, sodium is 140 mEq/L, and potassium is 4 mEq/L, BUN 40 mg/dL, Cr 1.9 mg/dL from a level of 1.5 (2 days ago). His medications upon discharge include metoprolol 25 mg PO BID, enalapril 2.5 mg daily, spironolactone 25 mg daily and furosemide 40 mg daily. A pulmonary artery catheter is inserted and shows a cardiac index of 2.1 L/min/m². Pulmonary capillary wedge pressure is 18 mm Hg. His cardiac biomarkers are not elevated. Chest x-ray shows mostly clear lungs with basilar atelectasis. He has not taken this medication in the last 24 hours.

Question 1: **What is the next step in the management of this patient?**

A. Administer a fluid challenge to improve the patient's blood pressure and organ perfusion
B. Arrange with the cardiology consultant to place an intra-aortic balloon pump counter-pulsation device or an impella device
C. Start the patient on dobutamine infusion
D. Start milrinone infusion
E. Arrange for cardiac resynchronization therapy

Question 2: **In a patient with cardiogenic shock after an acute MI, which of the following statements best summarizes the pathophysiology of cardiogenic shock?**

A. It is only the necrotic myocardial tissue that contributes to the poor myocardial function. Areas of myocardium with intact flow restored with PCI do not contribute to cardiogenic shock.
B. After an acute myocardial infarction, in addition to necrotic myocardial tissue, areas of myocardium which have had normal perfusion restored can also contribute to poor myocardial function.

C. Areas of myocardium, which have had normal perfusion, restored after intervention and if they are contributing to cardiogenic shock can be recruited using pharmacological means.
D. Areas of nonnecrotic myocardium, which have very poor blood flow, can also contribute to cardiogenic shock. These areas can however be recruited if appropriate interventions are undertaken to restore blood blow to these segments.
E. B,C, and D.

CASE 8

A 23-year-old man was involved in a horse-riding accident. He was found to have a heart rate 55, BP 80/40, and RR 20. His lungs and heart were unremarkable, and his pulses were 1+ on the radial and dorsalis pedis arteries. His neurological examination revealed no discernible sensation in his extremities or the rest of the body. His arms and legs lacked any motor strength. His mentation was intact. His laboratory results were unremarkable.

Question 1: **According to the current evidence, which of the following represents the blood pressure target for this patient?**

A. MAP >55
B. MAP >65
C. MAP >75
D. MAP >85
E. MAP >100

CASE 9

Question 1: **Which of the following figures represents the arterial wave form in the dorsalis pedis?**

A.

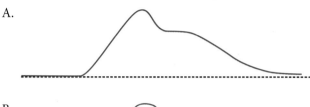

B.

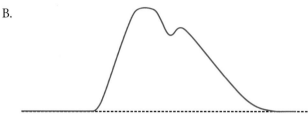

C.

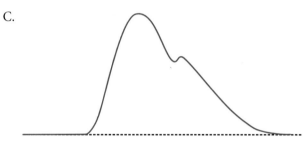

D.

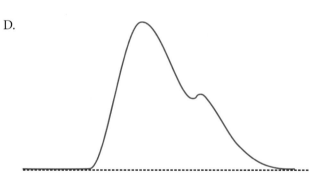

E.

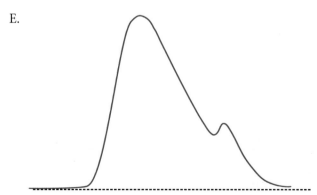

Reproduced with permission from McGhee BH, Bridges EJ. Monitoring arterial blood pressure: what you may not know. *Crit Care Nurse.* 2002;22(2):60–64.

Question 2: **Which of the following scenarios result in this type of wave form?**

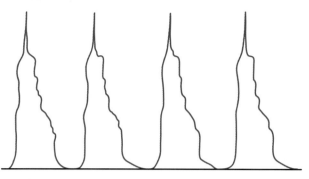

A. Hypertension
B. Low cardiac output
C. Hypovolemia
D. Nitroglycerin
E. All of the above

Question 3: **Stroke volume variation (SVV) is utilized to determine fluid responsive hypotension in a 50-year-old woman who is intubated for severe sepsis from a urinary tract infection. Her current vital signs are 60/40 with heart rate 80-140 in atrial fibrillation, and respiratory rate at 16. Her ventilator is set at a rate of 16, tidal volume at 8 mL/kg, FiO₂ 50 and PEEP 5. Which of the following parameters limit the utilization of SVV in this patient?**

A. Atrial fibrillation
B. Tidal volume 8 mL/kg
C. Positive pressure ventilation
D. PEEP 5
E. Synchrony with ventilation

CASE 10

The following waveforms are obtained from the pulmonary artery catheter inserted in a patient while in your ICU.

Question1: **Which of the following waveforms most likely represents a pressure tracing taken from the pulmonary artery? Please note that the lower line on all the graphics represents a pressure of zero and the scale is the same in all the graphics.**

A.

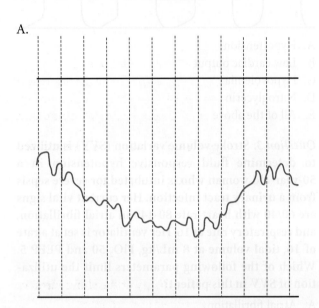

C.

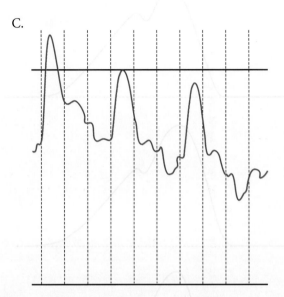

B.

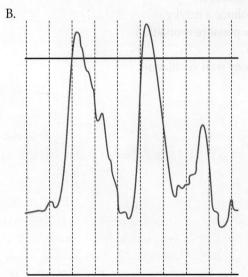

D.

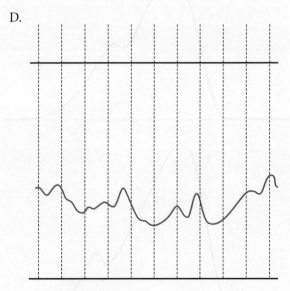

E. None of the above

Adapted with permission from Hall JB, Schmidt GA, Wood LDH. Principles of critical care. 3rd ed. New York, NY: McGraw-Hill Companies; 2005.

Question 2: The following is from the pulmonary artery catheter. At the top of the figure is the ECG tracing, and the bottom is the pulmonary artery occlusion tracing.

What is the most likely diagnosis?

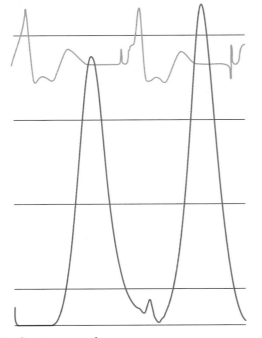

A. Cardiac tamponade
B. Interventricular septum rupture
C. Mitral stenosis
D. Mitral regurgitation
E. Pericarditis

CASE 11

A 25-year-old man whose ideal body weight is 70 kg is involved in a motor vehicle accident and suffers a closed-head injury. Upon admission he is found to be 70 kg and appears to have good nutritional status. Over the course of a week in the neurological intensive care unit he in unable to tolerate any enteral nutrition.

Question 1: **You plan to initiate total parenteral nutrition. Which of the following choices represent daily target goals for the macronutrients?**

A. Dextrose 160 g, lipid 88 g, and protein 195 g
B. Dextrose 360 g, lipid 58 g, and protein 105 g
C. Dextrose 460 g, lipid 28 g, and protein 45 g
D. Dextrose 260 g, lipid 38 g, and proteins 100 g
E. Dextrose 220 g, lipid 48 g, and proteins 110 g

CASE 12

A 66-year-old man comes in with a 5-hour history of right-sided weakness and slurred speech. He has a history of hypertension, diabetes mellitus, and osteoarthritis. He is currently on hydrochlorothiazide, metformin, and aspirin. On physical examination he is drowsy but arousable to voice. Blood pressure is 230/120 mm Hg, pulse rate is 86/min and irregular, and respiration rate is 16/min. No papilledema is detected. Neurologic examination findings include slurred speech, a lack of movement in the right arm, trace antigravity movement in the right leg, and profound sensory loss to all modalities on the right side. Results of the laboratory studies reveal INR 1.3, platelet count of 230,000/μL and serum creatinine of 1.5 mg/dL. Urine toxicology is negative. A CT scan of the head shows a left thalamic intracerebral hemorrhage with intra ventricular extension and mild enlargement of the ventricles.

Question 1: **Which of the following is the most appropriate next step in management?**

A. External ventricular drain placement
B. Platelet infusion
C. Labetalol infusion
D. Fresh-frozen plasma
E. Repeat CT scan

Question 2: **Most likely etiology of the above bleed is:**

A. Aspirin
B. Coagulopathy
C. Uncontrolled hypertension
D. Arteriovenous malformation
E. None of the above

CASE 13

A 30-year-old woman, with history of hypertension on hydrochlorothiazide, is evaluated in the emergency department for acute onset of a severe headache.

* *

On physical examination, blood pressure is 170/100 mm Hg, pulse rate is 86/min, and respiration rate is 12/min. General medical examination findings are normal. Neurologic examination shows that she is somnolent but arousable, with symmetric and briskly reactive pupils and a left arm drift. Results of routine laboratory studies are normal.

* *

A CT scan of the head shows a subarachnoid hemorrhage, with a thick clot in the right sylvian fissure, but no hydrocephalus or cerebral edema. Angiography shows a 10-mm right-middle cerebral artery aneurysm.

**

The patient undergoes urgent aneurysmal clipping with no complications. She is transferred to the intensive care unit and has no further symptoms until 7 days after initial evaluation, when she is less responsive and has new left arm paralysis on neurologic examination.

Question 1: **What is the most likely etiology of the patient's change in neurological status?**

A. Aneurysmal rupture
B. Cerebral vasospasm
C. Hydrocephalus
D. Postoperative meningitis
E. None of the above

Question 2: **Which is the next best diagnostic study?**
A. MRI brain
B. Electroencephalography
C. Lumbar puncture
D. CT angiography
E. None of the above

Question 3: **Which of the following has been shown to improve overall outcome?**
A. Tranexamic acid
B. Clazosentan
C. Nimodipine
D. Transluminal balloon angioplasty
E. None of the above

CASE 14

A 62-year-old man is admitted to the intensive care unit following repair of ruptured abdominal aortic aneurysm. Intraoperatively he has received 4 PRBC, 2 FFP, and 3 L of crystalloids. He is on invasive mechanical ventilation with a FiO_2 100% and PEEP of 10 cmH_2O and pressures. Urine output is gradually diminishing with an indwelling bladder catheter in place. He has been started on vancomycin and imipenem postoperatively. Temperature is 37.2°C (98.9°F), blood pressure is 91/52 mm Hg, pulse rate is 108/min, and respiration rate on ventilation is 14/min. BMI is 35. On physical examination his abdomen is distended, tense with hypoactive bowel sounds and edematous abdominal wall. There are decreased breath sounds in the bases of his lungs; tachycardia is noted on cardiac examination with pitting peripheral edema. His

laboratory results are significant for WBC of 28,000/μL, BUN 45 mg/dL, serum creatinine 2.68 mg/dL (baseline 0.91). Ultrasound of the kidneys reveals normal-sized kidneys with no hydronephrosis.

Question 1: **Which of the following is the most likely cause of the patient's kidney failure?**

A. Vancomycin-induced nephrotoxicity
B. Abdominal compartment syndrome
C. Obstructive uropathy
D. Prerenal azotemia
E. None of the above

Question 2: **All the following are risk factors of the above etiology, EXCEPT:**

A. High BMI
B. Massive blood transfusion
C. Mechanical ventilation
D. Positive fluid balance
E. Pressors

CASE 15

A 35-year-old woman who is 32-weeks pregnant comes to the ED with complaints of dyspnea, fatigue, and non-productive cough worsening over the last 5 days. She appears confused with a fluctuating neurological status. Her vital signs in the ED reveal a temperature of 37.9°C, BP 80/54 mm Hg, HR 122/min, RR 22/min, SpO_2 86% on RA. On examination there is a visible jugular venous distension, S3 and S4 gallop, B/L rales heard diffusely in the lung fields and palpable hepatomegaly. Her extremities are cool and clammy. She is intubated for worsening hypoxia and poor mental status.

Question 1: **Which of the following is the best next step with regard to her hypotension?**

A. Intravenous fluid resuscitation
B. Norepinephrine
C. Nitroprusside
D. Dobutamine
E. Milrinone

Question 2: **The above patient is admitted to the ICU and hemodynamically stabilized. A transthoracic echocardiogram reveals an ejection fraction of 28%. Which of the following is the drug of choice?**

A. Low–molecular-weight heparin
B. Enalapril
C. Warfarin

D. Immunosuppressive therapy

E. None of the above

CASE 16

After a 911 call from neighbors who heard a gunshot, a 46-year-old man is found bleeding by EMS on the stairs of the apartment building. He has penetrating wounds to the back and abdomen. He is cold, clammy, and only withdraws to pain. He is immediately intubated at the scene, started on lactated Ringers via an intraosseous line and brought to the ED. In the emergency room, the patient is found with BP 60/38 mm Hg, HR 132, T 96°F, intubated, and an unchanged mental status. His abdomen is distended and dull to percussion, and there is minimal active bleeding from the abdominal and back wounds. EMS tells you that there is considerable blood loss at the scene and that he has received only about a 500 mL of crystalloid because the intraosseous line is not working well. Two 18-gauge peripheral lines are established and initial laboratory results are sent. The blood bank is notified for a massive transfusion protocol. Meanwhile, the laboratory panel reveals a hematocrit of 17, Plt 256, INR 1.6, and PTT 47.

Question 1: Which of the following interventions is likely to result in an adverse outcome in this patient?

A. Immediate transfer to the operating room for a damage control laparotomy, transfusion of tranexamic acid within 1 hour, packed cells, plasma, and platelets in a ratio of 1:1:1 with a goal of bringing the MAP to greater than 65 after surgery

B. Immediate transfusion of Ringer's lactate boluses to bring the MAP to 65 followed by transfer to the operating room for damage control laparotomy, and transfusion of tranexamic acid within 1 hour, with transfusion of packed cells, plasma, and platelets in a ratio of 1:1:1

C. Immediate thromboelastography (TEG), transfusion of tranexamic acid followed by transfer to the operating room for damage control laparotomy and transfusion of packed cells, plasma and platelets in a ratio of 1.4:1:1 with a goal of bringing the MAP to 60 to 65 after intraoperative hemostasis is achieved

D. Immediate transfer to the operating room for a damage control laparotomy, intraoperative thromboelastography (TEG), transfusion of tranexamic acid within 3 hours, Ringers lactate boluses, packed cells, and platelets in a ratio of 1:1:1 with a goal of achieving a urine output of about 0.5 mL/kg/h after surgery

E. None of the above

Question 2: Which of the following is not an indication for permissive hypotension?

A. Intracranial bleeding

B. Penetrating abdominal trauma

C. Penetrating thoracic trauma

D. Dissecting aortic aneurysm

E. None of the above

CASE 17

A 26-year-old man is brought to the hospital after a jogger finds him in the woods and needing medical attention. Patient is lethargic and not very coherent and therefore not able to provide good history. His vital signs include respiratory rate 24, heart rate 50, blood pressure 100/50, and temperature 33°C. On his examination, he appears to be stiff and cold to touch. His laboratory results are unremarkable except for a positive urine toxicology screen for marijuana.

Question 1: What is the next appropriate step to take in his management?

A. Warm blankets

B. CT scan of the head

C. Intravenous fluids

D. Narcan

E. None of the above

Question 2: What of the following can be seen in such patients?

A. Atrial fibrillation

B. Prolonged PR interval

C. J waves

D. Sinus bradycardia

E. All of the above

CASE 18

Question 1: **What type of renal replacement therapy is depicted below?**

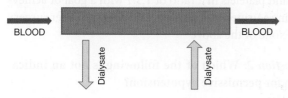

A. SCUF
B. CVVH
C. CVVHD
D. CVVHF
E. None

CASE 19

A 25-year-old woman with history of antiphospholipid syndrome is complaining of shortness of breath. Chest CTA is ordered to rule out a pulmonary embolism. She has no allergies to contrast creatinine 0.30.

Question 1: **Which of the following is an appropriate prophylaxis for contrast-induced nephropathy?**

A. Normal saline
B. Normal saline and PO NAC
C. Normal saline and IV NAC
D. Normal saline and lasix
E. Sodium bicarbonate

Question 2: **CTA is negative for malignancy but it is positive for mediastinal adenopathy which is positive for cancer. She is scheduled to receive chemotherapy. Which of the following is an appropriate prophylaxis to prevent tumor lysis syndrome–induced AKI?**

A. Normal saline
B. Normal saline and rubicase
C. Normal saline, lasix, rubicase, and allopurinol
D. Normal saline, lasix, allopurinol, and sodium bicarbonate
E. Normal saline, lasix, rubicase, and sodium bicarbonate

CASE 20

A 39-year-old morbidly obese woman, G3P4, 35 weeks age of gestation (AOG) is complaining of vaginal bleeding and shortness of breath. Vaginal ultrasound shows the placenta partially covering the cervical OS.

Question 1: **Which of the following does NOT change with pregnancy?**

A. Tidal volume
B. Hemoglobin
C. Residual volume
D. Vital capacity
E. Functional residual capacity

Question 2: **Patient has an operative vaginal delivery. She subsequently complains of worsening shortness of breath and increased vaginal bleeding. Her blood pressure and heart rate drops. Fluid resuscitation is started. She is noted to have seizures. Laboratory results show hemoglobin 9, platelets 88,000, and fibrinogen 200 mg/dL. A pulmonary artery catheter is inserted and studies from the catheter show squamous cells, trophoblastic cells, mucin, and lanugo.**

A. Preeclampsia
B. Amniotic fluid embolism syndrome
C. Pulmonary embolism
D. Congestive heart failure
E. Myocardial infarction

CASE 21

A 25-year-old man returned 5 days ago from a trip that involved air travel. Since then, he has been complaining of progressive shortness of breath, chills, and fever. Upon arrival to the emergency room, he is noted to have an oxygen saturation of 85% on room air and respiratory rate of 35. He is placed on NRB and his oxygen saturation improves to 90%. Chest radiograph shows diffuse bilateral infiltrates. Arterial blood gas on nonrebreather shows pH 7.30/60/55/25/90%. Because of the progression of his symptoms he is subsequently intubated.

Question 1: **He is 5 ft 6 in and weighs 150 lb. What would be his initial ventilator settings?**

A. TV 510/RR 14/PEEP 5/FiO$_2$ 100
B. TV 255/RR 14/PEEP 10/FiO$_2$ 100
C. TV 600/RR 14/PEEP 5/FiO$_2$ 100
D. TV 400/RR 14/PEEP 10/FiO$_2$ 100
E. TV 340/RR 14/PEEP 5/FiO$_2$ 100

Question 2: **Which mode of mechanical ventilation is represented in the picture below?**

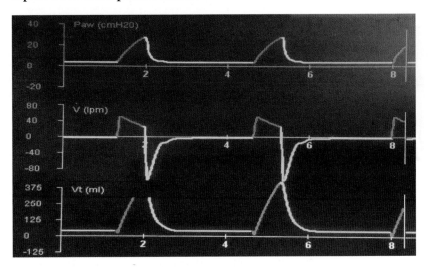

A. PRVC pressure–regulated volume control
B. Pressure control
C. Pressure support
D. Volume control
E. APRV

Question 3: **Which of the following therapies have been shown to have improved outcomes in ARDS?**

A. Cisatracurium early in the course for 48 hours
B. Glucocorticoids after 14 days of the disease
C. GMCSF
D. Prostacyclin
E. Antioxidant therapy

CASE 22

A 35-year-old man is admittted for management of respiratory failure requiring mechanical ventilation. Patient is now on pressure support trial. In an effort to increase patient ventilator synchrony, it is decided to try a novel therapy similar to pressure support called proportional assist ventilation (PAV). Unlike pressure support, this novel therapy is characterized by:

A. Amount of PEEP is limited
B. Ends breath by time-cycling mechanism
C. Adjust inspiratory pressure in response to patient effort
D. Mortality benefit
E. Beneficial in critical illness polyneuropathy

CASE 23

A 42-year-old man is on mechanical ventilation for community-acquired pneumonia. The ventilator graph is shown below:

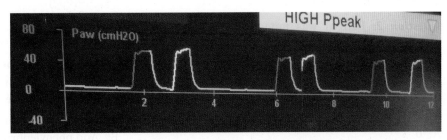

Question 1: **What would be the next step?**

A. Increase respiratory rate
B. Increase tidal volume
C. Decrease sedation
D. Switch to pressure support
E. Do nothing

Question 2: The next day, his ventilator graph is shown below:

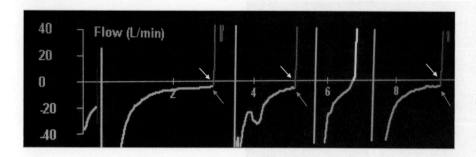

Question 2: **What should be the next step?**

A. Decrease respiratory rate
B. Decrease inspiratory time
C. Improve flow
D. Improve rise time
E. All of the above

CASE 24

A 40-year-old man with history of alcohol abuse was noted to be unresponsive at home. Rapid sequence intubation was completed in the emergency department.

Question 1: **Which of the following NMBA depolarizes the plasmatic membrane of the muscle?**

A. Succinylcholine
B. Rocuronium
C. Cisatracurium
D. Pancuronium
E. All of the above

Question 2: **Patient was noted to have aspirated. Despite higher levels of oxygen supplementation and PEEP, he continued to be dyssynchronous with the ventilator. He was started on NMBA infusion. Two twitches on the peripheral nerve stimulator suggest what percentage of the receptors are blocked?**

A. 0
B. <75%
C. 75% to 80%
D. 90%
E. 100%

CASE 25

Question 1: **What is the hemodynamic profile of septic shock?**

A. PAOP increase, CO decrease, SVR increase, SvO_2 decrease
B. PAOP decrease, CO decrease, SVR increase, SvO_2 decrease
C. PAOP decrease or normal, CO decrease, normal or increase, SVR decrease, SvO_2 increase
D. PAOP increase, CO decrease, SVR increase, SvO_2 decrease
E. PAOP decrease or normal, CO decrease, SVR increase, SvO_2 decrease

Question 2: **A patient was started on norepinephrine for persistent hypotension. Which receptors are involved with norepinephrine?**

A. A_1B_1
B. B_1B_2
C. $A_1B_1B_2D_1$
D. $A_1B_1B_2$
E. A_1

Question 3: **After the norepinephrine was started, the current vital signs are BP 80/60 HR 120 RR 22. Lactate is still 4. What is the next step?**

A. Switch to dopamine
B. Add phenylephrine
C. Switch to vasopressin
D. Give a bolus of hexastarch
E. Start a corticosteroid infusion

CASE 26

A 50-year-old man with 50 pack-year smoking history was complaining of hemoptysis. He was admitted to the ICU and was noted to have a pulmonary embolism with infarction, right upper lobe mass and diffuse mediastinal adenopathy on CTA. He had recently lost his daughter in a car accident.

Question 1: **His family members did not want to disclose the possibility of cancer to the patient. What would be the next best step?**

A. Inquire why the family wishes to withhold information
B. Inform the patient
C. Do nothing
D. Negotiate with the family members
E. Proceed with an EBUS

Question 2: **The patient has a cardiac arrest from a massive pulmonary embolism. The family has decided to proceed for comfort measures only and he was started on a morphine drip. This act is what type of principle?**

A. Autonomy
B. Beneficence
C. Nonmaleficence
D. Justice
E. Double effect

CASE 27

A 59-year-man with a history of colon cancer presented to the emergency department with syncope. He complained of dizziness and shortness of breath. His initial vital signs were temperature 99.3, HR 122, BP 88/50, saturation 80% on RA and 88% on NRB. He appeared uncomfortable and tachypneic. His lungs were clear and his cardiac examination only revealed tachycardia. He was intubated and given fluid boluses. His repeat BP was 80/42 and a central line was placed. Norepinephrine was started. His chest x-ray showed the endotracheal tube and right triple-lumen catheter were in place and no acute parenchymal disease.

Question 1: **The next day the patient was still hemodynamically unstable and was not responsive despite holding sedation. There was concern of an intracranial event. Which of the following seen on ultrasound would make you less concerned for elevated intracranial pressure?**

A. An optic nerve diameter of 4.2 mm
B. A difference in the optic nerve diameter between both eyes of 0.3 mm
C. An optic nerve sheath diameter of 6.1 mm
D. An optic nerve sheath diameter of 4.9 mm
E. An optic nerve diameter of 5.3 mm

CASE 28

A 72-year-man complains of shortness of breath on exertion. He says he was told by his doctor to come to the hospital because he had a white out of his lung. On examination there are decreased BS on the right. You perform a bedside ultrasound to determine cause of the "white out." Based on the ultrasound below what do you expect to see on the chest x-ray?

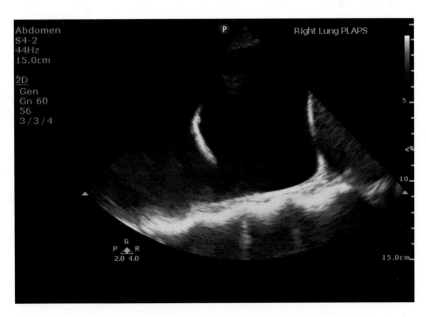

A. Multiple opacities in both lungs
B. Opacification of the entire right lung with shift of mediastinum away from the right
C. Opacification of the entire right lung with shift of mediastinum toward the right
D. Pneumothorax on the right
E. None of the above

CASE 29

A 72-year-old woman on chemotherapy and radiation for breast cancer complains of chest pain and shortness of breath. She reports that over the past 2 days she has been having increased shortness of breath and chest pain. She denies fevers. On physical examination she appears uncomfortable and appears to have difficulty breathing. Vital signs reveal a temperature of 37°C, a heart rate of 110, a respiratory rate of 24, and a blood pressure of 102/54. Her lungs are clear to auscultation bilaterally. Cardiac examination reveals muffled heart sounds and jugular venous distention.

Question 1: **Based on the suspected diagnosis what do you expect to see on the cardiac ultrasound?**

A. Hypoechoic area behind the heart that crosses the aorta on PSLA view with collapse of the RV during diastole
B. Hypoechoic area behind the heart that stops at the aorta on PSLA view with collapse of the RV during diastole
C. Hypoechoic area behind the heart that crosses the aorta on PSLA view with collapse of the RV during systole
D. Hypoechoic area behind the heart that stops at the aorta view with collapse of the RV during systole
E. None of the above

CASE 30

A 58-year-old man with DM and HTN presents to the emergency department with fevers up to 103.4. He is found to have a heart rate of 150 and a blood pressure of 60/50. He is resuscitated with fluids and vasopressors and intubated due to hemodynamic instability. The next day he has 4/4 bottles that are growing *Staphylococcus aureus*. On talking to his friends you find out that he has been abusing IV drugs. His blood pressure is 98/55 on norepinephrine. A bedside ultrasound is performed.

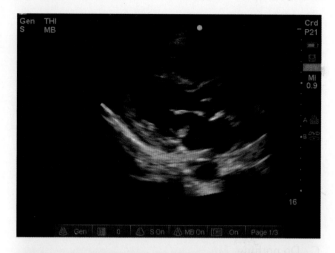

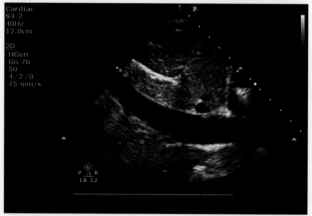

Question 1: **What is your next step in management?**

A. Give more fluids
B. Increase the dose of vasopressors
C. Add dobutamine
D. Cardiac surgery consult
E. Give hydrocortisone

Question 2: **This patient has received 6 L of IVF. His vasopressor requirements have improved and his lactate decreases from 8 to 2.2. However, the nurses are concerned that his urine output has decreased. Renal and bladder ultrasound is performed. What is your conclusion?**

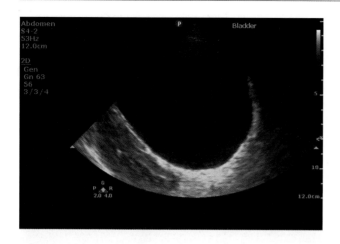

A. The patient needs more IVF
B. The patient is in renal failure due to ATN
C. The patient is in renal failure due to poor cardiac output
D. The patient has an obstructing renal stone
E. The patient's foley is misplaced

CASE 31

A 65-year-old man with diabetes mellitus, hypertension, and end-stage renal disease presents to the hospital 2 days ago with pneumonia. You are consulted because the patient continues to have fevers up to 102.8 and a WBC of 24 with 90% neutrophils on vancomycin, cefepime, and levofloxacin. A chest x-ray shows bilateral effusions with the left-sided effusion much larger than the right-sided effusion. You perform a bedside lung ultrasound and see the following image. What is the preferred therapy?

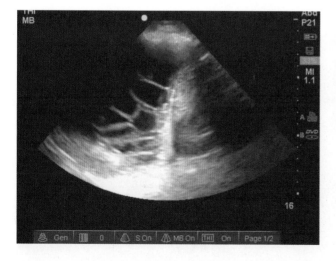

A. Place a chest tube
B. Broad-spectrum antibiotics
C. Take off more fluid on dialysis
D. Perform a thoracentesis
E. Increase furosemide

CASE 32

A 34-year-old man with alcoholism, diabetes mellitus, and intravenous drug use has been in the intensive care unit for acute respiratory failure requiring invasive mechanical ventilation and sepsis secondary to gram-positive bacteremia. He has already been given 1 L of crystalloid but is still hypotensive.

Question 1: **Which of the following is the best indicator that this patient doesn't need fluids?**

A. The IVC collapses 40% with inspiration
B. The IVC measures 1.8 cm
C. The IVC distends 20% with inspiration
D. The IVC measures 2.8 cm
E. None of the above

Question 2: **The patient's peripheral IV access has been insufficient and triple-lumen catheter has been suggested. Ultrasound of the internal jugular vein is shown below. Which of the following is correct?**

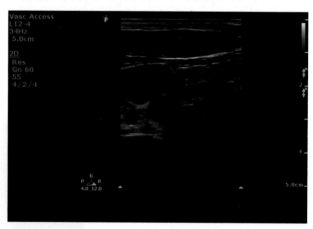

A. The screen is set at the correct depth.
B. The IJ is well centered on the screen
C. This view confirms that there is no clot in the vessel
D. The artery is in the ideal place for IJ placement
E. The IJ is about 1.2 cm below the skin surface

CASE 33

An 18-year-old man is an unrestrained passenger involved in a front end motor vehicle collision. On arrival the patient is awake, but confused. He appears intoxicated and is not complaining of any injuries. On examination he is protecting his airway, has no respiratory distress, and has a strong pulse. Vital signs are temperature 36.5°C, HR 118, BP 110/76, respiratory rate 18, and pulse ox 100%. He has a 3-cm laceration to the left forehead. He has bilateral breath sounds and his lungs are clear. His abdomen is soft. He has a right lower extremity fracture. You decide to perform a FAST examination.

Question 1: Which of the following statements about the FAST examination are correct?

A. If you have a positive FAST examination you are required to perform a diagnostic peritoneal lavage (DPL)

B. Fluid seen on a FAST examination is 100% specific for intra-abdominal trauma

C. One view of the bladder is sufficient in a male patient

D. The FAST examination includes at a minimum a perihepatic view, a perisplenic view, pelvic view, and a subxiphoid cardiac view

E. Views of the lung to exclude pneumothorax should not be included on the FAST examination because a chest x-ray is a better way to diagnose pneumothorax

Question 2: Right before you begin your FAST examination, the nurse says that the patient's HR is now 142 and his blood pressure is 68/40. You continue giving the patient fluids. Your FAST examination shows the following image. What is the best approach to management?

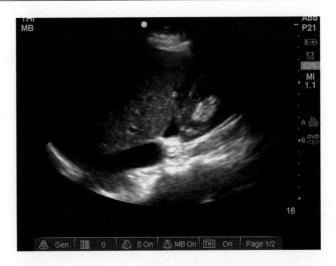

A. CT scan to confirm your findings

B. Place a chest tube on the left

C. Pericardiocentesis

D. Surgical exploration

E. Conservative management with fluid and blood products

CASE 34

A 36-year-old man presents to the emergency department with shortness of breath. You perform a lung ultrasound (see below) and on every area of the lung you see horizontal lines between the rib shadows that are artifactual reflections of the pleural surface. Based on this information you conclude that the most appropriate treatment for this patient would be?

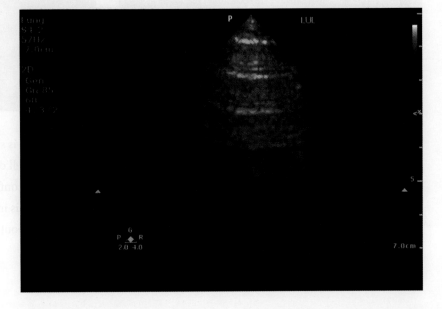

A. Antibiotics
B. Diuresis
C. Thoracentesis
D. Albuterol and steroids
E. Chest tube placement

CASE 35

A 50-year-old man with history of diabetes and hypertension is involved in a motor vehicle accident. He sustains a subdural hematoma and high cervical lesion. He is unresponsive and is intubated.

Question 1: Which of the following statements is true?

A. The patient's capacity will not change over time
B. Patients with psychiatric illnesses do not have capacity
C. Competency is a legal definition made in part with patient's capacity
D. Physician judgment bypasses surrogate's consent
E. None of the above

Question 2: There has not been any change regarding the patient's condition after 72 hours. His blood pressure is 120/80 and temperature is 98°C. He is currently on no sedation and requires norepinephrine to maintain MAP >65. He appears to have fixed and dilated pupils. He has absence of the following reflexes: corneal, pupillary, and gag. He appears to have fasciculations in the muscles supplied by the facial nerves and adduction of the shoulders.

His laboratory tests including drug screen are unremarkable. The physician has discussed with the family regarding brain death protocol. What is the next step to determine brain death?

A. Apnea test
B. Brain death cannot be determined because of the movements of the muscles supplied by the facial nerve and adduction of the shoulders
C. Brain death cannot be determined yet because he is on norepinephrine.
D. Cerebral angiography
E. Brain death cannot be determined because the observation period is insufficient

Answers

CASE 1

Question 1: D. 29

Whenever primary metabolic acidosis occurs, the body responds with respiratory compensation via elimination of carbon dioxide. This can be calculated via Winter's formula, which is $pCO_2 = 1.5 \times HCO_3 + 8 \ (+2)$.[1] Another formula is a change in pCO_2 in mm Hg $= 1.2 \times$ change in bicarbonate in mEq/L.[1] Thus expected pCO_2 for bicarbonate of 14 mEq/L would be 27 to 31 mm Hg.

Question 2: C. Chronic respiratory acidosis with incomplete metabolic compensation

The metabolic compensatory changes for respiratory acidosis are summarized below:[1]

* *

Primary acute respiratory acidosis: compensatory change in bicarbonate = + 1 mEq/L for every 10 mm Hg rise in pCO_2.

* *

Primary chronic respiratory acidosis: compensatory change in bicarbonate = +(4–5) mEq/L for every 10 mm Hg rise in pCO_2.

* *

In the question, the pH is acidotic with an elevated pCO_2. The primary process is respiratory acidosis with metabolic compensation. If this was acute respiratory acidosis with metabolic compensation the expected bicarbonate would be ~26. If this was chronic respiratory acidosis, with complete metabolic compensation, the expected bicarbonate would be close to 34. A chronic respiratory acidosis with incomplete metabolic compensation would definitely fit this ABG. The expected bicarbonate is in the range of 26 to 34. An acute respiratory acidosis with an expected metabolic compensation would bring the bicarbonate level to close to 26.

CASE 2

Question 1: C. Order for a transthoracic echocardiogram to assess cardiac function

The diagnosis shown in this case is unstable angina (UA)/non-ST elevation myocardial infarction (NSTEMI). Cardiac biomarkers remain negative in UA and are positive in NSTEMI.[2]

* *

A typical 12- to 24-hour observation period is indicated to rule out myocardial necrosis using serial cardiac biomarkers.[2] After a period of clinical stability a noninvasive stress test is often done to evaluate the extent of coronary artery disease and to look for high-risk features. Prior to the noninvasive stress testing, an evaluation of the cardiac function is carried out using a transthoracic echocardiogram. If there is compromised cardiac function such as new LVEF <40%, one proceeds straight to coronary angiography without first going through noninvasive stress testing.[2]

* *

It is not advisable, thus, to stress the myocardium during an episode of ongoing UA or myocardial infarction. Because of no hypoxia or tachycardia, pulmonary embolism is unlikely. The use of fibrinolytic therapy is contraindicated in the setting of UA/NSTEMI.

Question 2: B. Arrange for an emergent angiography

The presence of hemodynamic instability, heart failure, unstable rhythm, or ongoing chest discomfort even after maximal medical therapy in the setting of UA/NSTEMI mandates early invasive approach namely angiography with an intention to perform primary PCI of the culprit lesion.[2] Use of nitroglycerin infusion in setting of low blood pressure is not advisable. Similarly, use of beta blockers or ACE inhibitors would be contraindicated in the setting of low blood pressure. Fibrinolytic therapy remains contraindicated in the setting of UA/NSTEMI. The patient meets criteria to be taken for angiography and possibly PCI.

Question 3: C. A nonocclusive thrombus on top of an unstable atherosclerotic plaque

The pathogenesis of UA/NSTEMI involves a mismatch between demand and supply of oxygen to the myocardium. Most commonly this involves a nonocclusive thrombus that develops atop a disrupted atherosclerotic plaque. An occlusive thrombus can also lead to UA/NSTEMI provided there are collateral vessels supplying some blood to the affected myocardium. Prinzmetal's angina is a coronary artery dissection or focal spasm of an epicardial coronary artery. Another mechanism of oxygen supply and demand mismatch to the myocardium commonly seen in the critical care setting is the onset of conditions which increase myocardial oxygen demand in a patient with underlying atherosclerotic coronary artery disease. These patients often have baseline chronic stable angina. Conditions that precipitate such a mismatch between oxygen supply and demand in this set of patients include hypotension, fever, tachycardia, thyrotoxicosis, acute blood loss, or hypoxemia.

**

The most likely mechanism of UA/NSTEMI is the formation of a nonocclusive thrombus on top of an unstable atherosclerotic coronary artery plaque. An occlusive coronary artery plaque usually results in STEMI. Although anomalous coronary artery and spontaneous coronary artery dissection are both known causes of acute coronary syndrome they are both very rare causes.

CASE 3

Question 1: B. Fluid bolus, aspirin 325 mg, emergent angiography with plan for primary PCI

This patient has an ST elevation myocardial infarction (STEMI) complicated by cardiogenic shock. The next step in the management of this patient is urgent coronary angiography with the intention to perform primary PCI of the infarct vessel.[2] Prescribing ASA and clopidogrel may be prudent in a case of STEMI but nitroglycerin in this patient is not advisable. Medical stabilization versus emergent PCI in a STEMI complicated by shock was evaluated in the SHOCK trial which showed higher all-cause mortality at 6 months in the group assigned to medical stabilization first versus those assigned to emergency PCI.[3]

Question 2: D. Hypoechoic fluid in the pericardial sac with evidence of RV diastolic collapse

The ECG of the patient shows evidence of electrical alternans suggestive of cardiac tamponade. The patient has ventricular free wall rupture, which is a known complication of a myocardial infarction and has a very high mortality. On echocardiogram, one may see significant pericardial fluid with evidence of cardiac tamponade on echocardiography, namely collapse of the right-sided cardiac chambers during diastole.

CASE 4

Question 1: B. Discussion with an interventional cardiologist to discuss the value of an emergent coronary angiography

The most common etiology for an out-of-hospital cardiac arrest in adults older than 38 years is underlying coronary artery disease. His bedside echocardiogram reveals globally decreased myocardial function, a finding that is not uncommon after cardiac arrest. The focal wall motion abnormality in the anterior wall of the left ventricle, however, coupled with an initial rhythm of ventricular fibrillation in addition to an antecedent history of chest pain strongly point toward an acute coronary syndrome as the triggering event for this patient's cardiac arrest. Lack of ST elevation on ECG does not rule out the presence of an acute coronary syndrome after cardiac arrest. In the 2010 guidelines on the acute coronary syndrome, the American Heart Association recommends that primary PCI after ROSC in cases cardiac arrest of presumed cardiac etiology of ischemic nature, even in the absence of clearly defined STEMI, may be reasonable. These recommendations are guided by the fact that for out-of-hospital cardiac arrests about one-half of the patient population was found to have acute coronary occlusion upon early angiography.

**

Although an intracranial bleed is possible, the patient's examination is nonfocal with symmetrical pupils. His immediate history was suggestive of chest pain and not of any focal deficits or headache. An intracranial pathology is unlikely given the clinical scenario. His echocardiogram showed no RV dilation to suggest a massive PE but is remarkable however for focal wall motion abnormality suggestive of ACS. The patient did have an episode of V. Fib, which is likely of ischemic origin. He is in sinus rhythm and it is acceptable to observe for now without the use of amiodarone. His bicarbonate is low likely from lactic acidosis from decreased perfusion during arrest and is likely to correct with time. He is not acidotic to the point of needing a bicarbonate infusion at this time.

Question 2: **C. There is sufficient evidence to show that hyperthermia or fever worsens neurological outcomes whereas the role of hypothermia continues to be debated in literature based on current evidence**

Therapeutic hypothermia to 32–34°C for 12–24 hours post cardiac arrest, usually for ventricular fibrillation, has been shown to improve functional status and mortality rates.[4,5] It is hypothesized that hypothermia reduces cerebral metabolism, excitatory amino acids, oxygen free radicals, lipid peroxidation and inflammatory mechanisms that may lead to ischemia and apoptosis. Inclusion criteria includes: initiation within 6 hours of arrest, SBP >90 with or without pressures, and in a coma. Exclusion criteria includes: DNR, Surgery within 2 weeks, sepsis, and bleeding disorders. However, recent studies have suggested could not corroborate the beneficial effects of therapeutic hypothermia.[6–10]

CASE 5

Question 1: **B. SVI 12**

Hemodynamic measurements are crucial in the critically ill patients. Pulmonary artery catheters directly measure cardiac pressure and estimate cardiac output, systemic vascular resistance and pulmonary vascular resistance but no study has demonstrated improved outcome. It also raises concerns whether patients with these catheters have poorer outcomes. The following are noninvasive approaches to determine if the patient is fluid responsive.[11,12]

Methods		Fluid Responsiveness If:
Pulse contour analysis	Bioimpedance	Pulse pressure variation (PPV) or stroke volume variation (SVV) ≥12–13%
NICOM	Bioreactance	Stroke volume index (SVI) ≥10% after 500 mL bolus or passive leg raise
Ultrasound	Surrogate for CVP/RAP	IVC is collapse or IVC diameter is <2 cm or 50% respiratory variation

Question 2: **A. Dobutamine**

The cardiac output (Q or CO) is the volume of blood pumped from a cardiac ventricle in 1 minute. In males, the average resting CO is 5.6 L/min and in females, the average resting CO is 4.9 L/min. There are multiple approaches to measuring cardiac output such as pulmonary artery thermodilution, echocardiography, pulse

pressure methods, impedance cardiography, and magnetic resonance imaging.

* *

Oxygen delivery is the rate at which oxygen is sent to the tissues.[1,13] It is calculated as DO_2 (mL/min) = CO × CaO_2. CaO_2 is the arterial oxygen content which is CaO_2 (mL O_2/dL) = (1.34 × hemoglobin concentration × SaO_2) + (0.0031 × PaO_2). Mixed venous oxygen or CvO_2 (mL O_2/dL) is derived from the right atrium and calculated as (1.34 × hemoglobin concentration × CvO_2) + (0.0031 × PaO_2). Ideal CvO_2 is >70% if obtained from triple-lumen catheter or >65% from pulmonary artery catheter. Oxygen extraction is the relationship of DO_2 and VO_2. It is the portion of oxygen that is removed from the blood and derived from this ratio (CaO_2–CvO_2)/CaO_2. Normal ratios are 0.25 to 0.30.

* *

In the critically ill condition, tissue anoxia might be secondary to poor extraction or poor oxygen delivery. In patient appears to have decreased cardiac output. Dobutamine with its inotropic effects might improve the cardiac output.

CASE 6

Question 1: **E. MAP >65, CVP 8–12, SVO$_2$ >65, urine output >0.5 cc/kg/h**

The initial resuscitation goals, according to the 2012 SSC guidelines, are MAP >65, CVP 8 to 12 mm Hg, SVO$_2$ >65 or ScVO$_2$ >70, urine output >0.5 cc/kg/h.[7]

Question 2: **E. Administer additional fluid boluses until a CVP of 12 to 15 mm Hg is reached**

Although using CVP to guide fluid resuscitation in someone has been an area of debate and this is recognized by the guidelines writing committee, it is, however, an easily measurable parameter. The recommendation from the 2012 SSC guidelines are to fluid resuscitate a nonintubated patient in septic shock until a CVP of 8 to 12 mm Hg is achieved.[7] The goal for CVP in a patient on mechanical ventilation in septic shock, however, is 12 to 15 mm Hg.[14] Other conditions which may elevate the CVP include pulmonary hypertension and abdominal compartment syndrome. The optimum threshold for blood transfusion in septic shock has not been determined. However, a hemoglobin concentration of 13 g/dL does not indicate a need for transfusion. Starting vasoactive medications anytime during shock can be reasonable especially when it takes time to fluid resuscitate a patient but this patient can certainly be more fluid resuscitated.

CASE 7

Question 1: A. Administer a fluid challenge to improve the patient's blood pressure and organ perfusion

A bedside diagnosis of cardiogenic shock can often be made in the presence of hypotension, documented poor LV function with clinical evidence of poor perfusion of end organs such as mental status, oliguria, cold extremities in the absence of pulmonary embolism, septic shock, ongoing bleeding, and hypovolemia. Cardiogenic shock has a cardiac index <2.2 L/min/m^2 with high filling pressures such as pulmonary artery occlusion pressure of >15 mm Hg.[15]

* *

Patients with history of ischemic coronary heart disease and especially those with left ventricular diastolic dysfunction may need higher filling pressure, >15 mm Hg, to have optimal cardiac output. In a patient with hypotension and low pressure it is prudent to give a fluid challenge and gauge the patient's hemodynamic response unless florid pulmonary edema is present. If however the patient does not respond to the fluid challenge, inotropic agents and/or mechanical circulatory support with IABP or LVADs may be employed while the heart recovers from the acute episode. Cardiac resynchronization therapy is typically indicated in a patient with heart failure with EF $<35\%$ with NYHA class 2, 3, 4 and QRS >150 ms.[15]

Question 2: E. B, C, and D

Knowing the pathophysiology of cardiogenic shock after an acute myocardial infarction is vitally important as interventions based on this understanding can lead to improved outcomes. After an acute myocardial infarction, areas of myocardial infarction with restored blood flow, which are viable but demonstrate no function, are termed "stunned."[8] These areas of myocardium are, however, amenable to be recruited using inotropic agents. Areas of myocardium with no demonstrable function even though having very poor blood flow can be recruited provided appropriate intervention are undertaken to restore flow. The areas of myocardium are termed "hibernating."

CASE 8

Question 1: D. MAP >85

This patient most likely has neurogenic or spinal shock. Based on the examination this patient likely has ASIA grade "A" injury of spinal cord, likely at the cervical spine level. An ASIA grade "A" injury for cervical spine portends a poor prognosis (see Table 22-1).[16] The mechanism of hypotension in neurogenic shock is mediated from a decreased sympathetic tone with decreased peripheral vascular resistance. Hypotension with relative bradycardia is usually seen.

* *

Early aggressive therapy includes maintaining perfusion to the injured cord, preventing and treating pulmonary complications. Pulmonary complications are more common in patients with more severe injury and those with injury at higher cervical cord level especially above C4. The current recommendation from the Congress of Neurological Surgeons is to maintain a MAP of 85 to 90 for the first 7 days following spinal cord injury.[16]

Table 22-1   SCALE (AIS) AMERICAN SPINAL INJURY ASSOCIATION (ASIA) IMPAIRMENT

ASIA Grade	Clinical Presentation
A	*Complete cord injury*: no motor or sensory function below S4–5
B	*Incomplete sensory*: Motor function is not preserved but sensory is preserved below the neurologic level and includes the sacral segments (light touch or pin prick at S4–5 or deep anal pressure)
C	*Incomplete motor*: Motor function is preserved below the neurologic level and has a muscle grade 0 to 2
D	*Incomplete motor*: Same as Grade C but motor strength more than or equal to 3
E	*Normal cord function*: Both motor and sensory preserved to pre-injury level

CASE 9

Question 1: **E.**

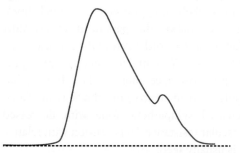

The arterial catheter carries the pressure waves from left ventricular contractions, through column-filled tubes, and into the transducer which converts the mechanical pressure into an electronic signal. The arterial wave form (see figure below) consists of A: systolic upstroke or anacrotic limb; B: anacrotic shoulder with the peak reflecting the systolic pressure and its rounded contour reflecting displacement of volume; C: dicrotic notch reflecting closure of aortic valve and retrograde flow; and D: the downward limb of the wave.[17] The placement of the dicrotic notch is lower in hypovolemic patients and in more distal branches of arterial tree.[17]

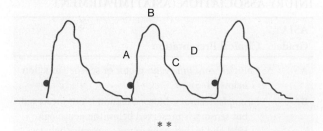

**

The wave form is a combination of pulse pressure and impedance from blood flow and bifurcation of arteries. The reflected waves are higher in the more peripheral vessels, leading to taller systolic upstrokes. The answer choices represent A: aorta, B: brachial artery; C: radial artery; D: femoral artery; and E: dorsalis pedis. However, the contribution of reflected waves might not be evident in patients with hypotension or hypovolemia.

Question 2: **A. Hypertension**
Damping is necessary; otherwise the arterial line waveform would lose its contour. When it is over damped, the waveform becomes rounder, losing its dicrotic notch. This can also occur in aortic stenosis, low cardiac output, and shock. When it is under damped, this will result in falsely high systolic pressures and falsely low diastolic pressures. This can be found in hypertension, vasoconstriction, or aortic regurgitation.

Question 3: **A. Atrial fibrillation**
The utility of using stroke volume variation (SVV) in determining fluid responsive hypotension has strict requirements to determine its predictability. This includes synchrony with mechanical ventilation, 8 to 10 mL/kg tidal volume, and sinus rhythm. Any deterrents from these parameters would render it unpredictable.

CASE 10

Question 1: **C.**

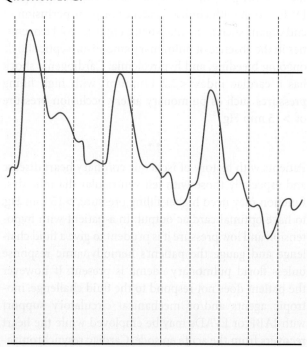

Choices A and D both represent atrial type waveforms with choice A likely the right atrial waveform. Choice D is the pulmonary capillary wedge waveform with baseline changes due to respirations. Although the right atrial and the pulmonary capillary wedge tracings can be hard to distinguish from one another they are certainly very different than the right ventricular or the pulmonary artery tracings. Choices B and C both have a systolic peak and a diastolic trough which can either reflect the right ventricle or pulmonary artery. To distinguish between the two, there is a diastolic step-up seen as the catheter moves from the right ventricle to the pulmonary artery.

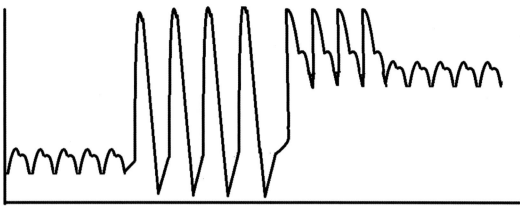

Right Atrial Pressure = 0–7 mm Hg

Right Ventricular Pressure
Systolic (RVSP) = 15–25 mm Hg
Diastolic (RVDP) = 3–12 mm Hg

Pulmonary Artery Pressure
Systolic (PASP) = 15–25 mm Hg
Diastolic (DASP) = 8–15 mm Hg

Pulmonary Artery Occlusion Pressure
6–12 mm Hg

PULMONARY ARTERY CATHETER READINGS

RA/CVP	0–7 mm Hg	Elevated in right ventricular infarction, pulmonary hypertension, pulmonary stenosis, tricuspid stenosis, left to right shunts, volume overload, restrictive cardiac disease, cardiac tamponade Loss of a wave form in atrial fibrillation or saw tooth in atrial flutter
RV	15–25 mm Hg/ 3–12 mm Hg	Cannon a waves with atrioventricular dissociation
PA	15–25 mm Hg/ 8–15 mm Hg	Elevated RV systolic pressure in pulmonary hypertension, pulmonic stenosis, pulmonary embolism
PCWP (estimate of left ventricular end-diastolic pressure and not left ventricular end-diastolic volume)	6–15 mm Hg	Elevated RV diastolic pressure in RV infarction, restrictive cardiac disease, pulmonary hypertension
Cardiac Index, L/min/m^2	3.4 (2.8–4.2)	Elevated in volume overload, left heart failure, mitral valve disease, pulmonary embolism, hypoxemia, left to right shunts, pulmonary arterial hypertension
Stroke volume Index, mL/m^2/beat	47 (30–65)	Elevation in a wave seen in increased left ventricular filling resistance such as mitral stenosis, systolic dysfunction, diastolic dysfunction, volume overload, and infarction
Arteriovenous oxygen difference, mL per liter of blood	38 (30–48)	Elevation in v wave seen in mitral regurgitation or acute septal defect

**

Cardiac output (CO) is determined via thermodilution or the Fick equation. The Fick equation is CO = oxygen consumption/(10 × arteriovenous oxygen difference). Arteriovenous oxygen difference calculation is 1.34 × hemoglobin concentration × (arterial oxygen saturation – mixed venous oxygen saturation). Systemic vascular resistance is calculated as (mean arterial pressure – right atrial pressure)/CO × 80 and pulmonary vascular resistance is calculated as (mean pulmonary artery pressure – left atrial pressure)/CO × 80.

**

Pulmonary arterial catheters can also detect left to right intracardiac shunt by "step-up."[13] This is >10% increase in oxygen saturation with blood in RA, RV, or PA is compared to mixed venous oxygen saturation. Mixed venous saturation at rest can be calculated as (3 × [O$_2$ saturation from SVC + O$_2$ saturation from IVC])/4.[1,13]

Question 2: D. Mitral regurgitation

The tall peak waves, which present after the T wave on the ECG, represent the V waves of mitral regurgitation and correlate to left ventricular systole. The smaller wave present between the two tall wave is the A wave from the left atrial contraction.

CASE 11

Question 1: B. Dextrose 360 g, lipid 58 g, and protein 105 g

Estimated daily total non-protein calorie needs for this man who is 70 kg is 70 kg × 25 kcal/kg = 1,750 kcal. Protein requirements vary according to the level of physiological stress a person is experiencing such that a minimal or no stress mandates ~0.8 g/kg where as a critically ill person, most would agree, needs ~1.5 g/kg of protein daily. With this in mind, the daily protein requirement for this patient is about 70 kg × 1.5 g/kg = 105 g. Thirty percent to fifty percent of the total caloric intake is provided by fat or lipid emulsions in the parenteral nutrition. Assuming 30% of total caloric intake is provided by the lipid emulsion, this amounts to 1,750 kcal × 0.3 = 525 kcal. Since a gram of lipid emulsion contains 9 kcal, it would take ~58 g of lipids to provide the 525 kcal. The remaining calories are to be provided by carbohydrates, usually in the form of dextrose. Thus 1,750 – 525 = 1,225 kcal are to be provided by dextrose. Each gram of dextrose provides 3.4 kcal. One needs about 360 g of dextrose to provide the 1,225 kcal. This makes choice B the correct answer.

CASE 12

Question 1: C. Labetalol infusion

Uncontrolled hypertension is a major risk factor for hematoma expansion, which is principal predictor of poor prognosis in intracerebral hemorrhage. In ICH, the antihypertensive treatment of acute cerebral hemorrhage (ATACH) trial and intensive blood pressure reduction in acute cerebral hemorrhage trial (INTERACT) have demonstrated that systolic BP reduction to 140 is well tolerated and associated with attenuation of hematoma expansion.[18,19] The impact of BP reduction on outcomes is being evaluated in the ongoing phase III ATACH II and INTERACT 2 trials. No evidence exists to recommend definitive BP management strategies in acute SAH, although hypertension should likely be avoided before an aneurysm is secured, and hypotension should be avoided altogether.[11] Placement of an external ventricular drain is inappropriate in this interactive patient. If the patient were to develop impaired consciousness, then cerebrospinal fluid shunting may be necessary to reduce elevated intracranial pressure. Platelet transfusions have not shown to have an improvement in outcome or decrease in hematoma expansion in

patients with intracerebral hemorrhage taking aspirin. Fresh-frozen place is not indicated in this patient with relatively normal INR.

Question 2: C. Uncontrolled hypertension

Hypertensive vasculopathy is the most common etiology of spontaneous ICH.[20] Cerebral amyloid angiopathy is the most common cause of nontraumatic lobar ICH in the elderly, while vascular malformations are the most common cause of ICH in children. Additional causes of nontraumatic ICH include:

- Hemorrhagic infarction (including venous sinus thrombosis)
- Septic embolism, mycotic aneurysm
- Brain tumor
- Bleeding disorders, anticoagulants, and thrombolytic therapy
- Central nervous system (CNS) infection (e.g., herpes simplex encephalitis)
- Vasculitis

**

Drugs (cocaine, amphetamines, phenylpropanolamine in appetite suppressants, and cold remedies) may be an independent risk factor for intracranial hemorrhage.[21-23]

CASE 13

Question 1: B. Cerebral vasospasm

The complications after subarachnoid hemorrhage are classified as early or late.[24-28] In the first 48 hours after hemorrhage, aneurysm re-rupture and hydrocephalus are the principal causes of neurologic deterioration. At 72 hours, the risk of cerebral arterial vasospasm emerges. This complication typically presents with a decline on neurologic examination and may lead to cerebral infarction, which may worsen already existing brain injury. The risk is greater in women, younger age group, and GCS less than 8.

**

Subarachnoid hemorrhage (SAH)-induced vasospasm is a complex entity caused by vasculopathy, impaired autoregulation and hypovolemia, causing a regional reduction of cerebral brain perfusion, which can then induce ischemia.[25] Cerebral vasospasm can present either asymptomatically, detected only radiologically or symptomatically (delayed ischemic neurologic deficit).

* *

Large-vessel vasospasm, autoregulatory dysfunction, inflammation, genetic predispositions, microcirculatory failure, and spreading cortical depolarization are aspects of delayed neurologic deterioration that have been described in the literature.

* *

Experimental evidence suggests that oxyhemoglobin release secondary to blood clot elimination may initiate the cascade involving vasoactive substances such as endothelium-derived nitrite oxide and endothelin-1, which leads to cerebral vasospasm.[25] Further research is needed to clarify the pathophysiology of vasospasm after BAVM rupture and to explain the different impacts of subarachnoid and intraventricular clots on the genesis of vasospasm.

Question 2: D. CT angiography
CT angiography can directly visualize arterial narrowing. Digital subtraction angiography (DSA) is usually the gold standard for the diagnosis of cerebral vasospasm. However transcranial Doppler is commonly the first-screening method for the detection of cerebral vasospasm. Because of the common association between clinical deterioration from DCI and angiographic vasospasm, arterial narrowing on angiography and increased blood flow velocities on TCD ultrasound examination are often used as surrogate diagnostic tool.

* *

Previous studies have shown that electroencephalogram (EEG) can detect blood flow changes associated with DCI sooner than other modalities potentially leading to earlier diagnosis. However, continual monitoring with raw EEG requires significant expertise and effort, and may be difficult due to the intermittent need for MRI studies in these patients.

* *

Lumbar puncture and MRI brain have not shown to be of benefit in diagnosing cerebral vasospasm in aneurysmal subarachnoid hemorrhage.

Question 3: C. Nimodipine
Nimodipine, a calcium channel blocker, is still the only medicine shown to improve neurologic outcomes in a multicenter, double blind, placebo-controlled trial.[24-28] Tranexamic acid decreased early rebleeding of unsecured aneurysms but no improvement in functional outcome or mortality. Clazosentan, an endothelin receptor antagonist, demonstrated a dose-dependent reduction in moderate or severe angiographic vasospasm but in phase III trial failed to demonstrate improvement in functional outcome despite a 65% reduction in angiographic vasospasm.[29] In addition to drug therapy, a study of prophylactic transluminal balloon angioplasty to prevent delayed ischemia demonstrated no difference in functional outcome despite a significantly lower incidence of vasospasm.

CASE 14

Question 1: B. Abdominal compartment syndrome
As per the World Society of Abdominal Compartment Syndrome, it is defined as intra-abdominal pressure greater than 20 mm Hg with new organ dysfunction.[30] A clause within the definition includes that it may occur with or without an abdominal perfusion pressure (APP = mean arterial pressure − intra-abdominal pressure) <60 mm Hg. Normal intra-abdominal pressure is 0 to 5 mm Hg secondary to compliance of abdominal wall. Intra-abdominal hypertension is defined as intra-abdominal pressure exceeding 12 mm Hg. Categories within the definition include primary IAH/ACS in which there is a direct abdominal-pelvic injury and secondary IAH/ACS where there is not.

* *

There are multiple pathophysiological mechanisms that can explain the symptomatology of ACS.[30-36] There is compression of the inferior vena cava causing decreased preload and cardiac output. Afterload is further increased because of a parallel increase in aortic impedance and reduced stroke volume. Decreased extrathoracic compliance leads to variable increase in shunt fraction, dead space, and transalveolar pressures. Hypoperfusion leads to splanchnic-hepatic dysfunction/failure, increased transmitted intracerebral pressure, and particularly cessation of renal filtration gradient.

* *

Vancomycin can cause nephrotoxicity, however the patient has received only one dose of the drug. Although obstruction may have similar pathophysiology to ACS, the presence of an indwelling bladder catheter and lack of hydronephrosis on ultrasound suggest an alternate etiology of the AKI. Pre-renal azotemia is unlikely given the fact that the patient is minimally responsive to fluids and appears clinically fluid overloaded.

Question 2: **E. Pressors**
Considering medical patients without causal abdominal pathology, patient characteristics predisposing toward IAH are high body mass index, invasive mechanical ventilation, positive fluid balance (>5 L), massive blood product transfusion, and high sequential organ failure assessment (SOFA)/acute physiology and chronic health evaluation II (APACHE II) scores. Epidemiologic studies in surgical intensive care unit (ICU) populations have estimated that IAH/ACS incidence is 4% to 81%. Intra-abdominal hypertension/ACS has demonstrated to be independently associated with worse patient-related outcomes (ICU and hospital mortality, higher SOFA scores including delta SOFA, increased ICU length of stay, mechanical ventilator days plus mechanical ventilator weaning failures).[30–36]

CASE 15

Question 1: **D. Dobutamine**
Women with acute heart failure benefit from intravenous administration of positive inotropic agents such as dobutamine and milrinone, none of which are contraindicated in pregnancy.[37] Positive inotropic agents improve cardiac performance, facilitate diuresis, preserve end-organ function, and promote clinical stability. Dobutamine requires beta receptors for its inotropic effects, whereas milrinone does not, an important distinction in planning care for a patient who is being treated with beta-blocking drugs. Milrinone has vasodilating properties for both the systemic and the pulmonary circulation; a mechanism that may be of marked benefit over other inotropic agents. In women with systolic blood pressure less than 90 mm Hg, dobutamine may be preferred over milrinone.[37] Vasodilatory drugs such as nitroglycerin and nitroprusside also may be of benefit. Nitroprusside should be used with caution in pregnant women because the toxic effects of thiocyanate to the fetus. Clinicians should not focus therapy on a specific blood pressure value that might or might not indicate hypotension; rather, they should focus on signs and symptoms associated with poor cardiac output and hypoperfusion, such as cold clammy skin, cool upper and lower extremities, decreased urine output, and altered mental status. Inotropic agents are of greatest value in women who have relative hypotension and intolerance or no response to vasodilators and diuretics. Regardless, if invasive monitoring of hemodynamic status is used, once the clinical status of the woman has stabilized, every effort should be made to devise an oral regimen that can maintain symptomatic improvement and reduce the subsequent risk of any deterioration in her condition

Question 2: **A. Low–molecular-weight heparin**
Left ventricular thrombus is common in women with peripartum cardiomyopathy (PPCM) whose ejection fraction is less than 35%.[37,38] Warfarin should be given to postpartum women whose ejection fraction is 35% or less, and heparin or a low–molecular-weight heparin should be given to women who are pregnant and have a similar ejection fraction of 20 to 35. Anticoagulation therapy should be continued until left ventricular function is normal according to echocardiographic findings.[29] Angiotensin-converting enzyme inhibitors and angiotensin receptor blockers should be avoided during pregnancy because of severe adverse neonatal effects.[37] Warfarin can cause spontaneous fetal cerebral hemorrhage in the second and third trimesters and therefore is generally contraindicated during pregnancy. Immunosuppressive therapy does not yet have a fully proven role, but it could be considered in patients with proven myocarditis. Given the various etiologic mechanisms of peripartum cardiomyopathy, it is unlikely that immunosuppression will help all patients. Furthermore, without a large randomized trial, treatment successes may merely reflect the natural course of the disease.

CASE 16

Question 1: **B. Immediate transfusion of Ringer's lactate boluses to bring the MAP to 65 followed by transfer to the operating room for damage control laparotomy, and transfusion of tranexamic acid within 1 hour, with transfusion of packed cells, plasma, and platelets in a ratio of 1:1:1**
Trauma is one of the world's leading causes of death and disability. Forty percent of deaths in trauma are related with massive hemorrhage. Massive hemorrhage is defined as loss of the entire blood volume of the body in 24 hours or half the blood volume in 3 hours. Damage control resuscitation has emerged has the hallmark of management in patients with hemorrhagic shock. The components of damage control resuscitation include permissive hypotension, early damage control surgery, involving initial hemostasis and prevention of contamination and delay of definitive surgery after resuscitation. The third strategy, which has shown benefit, has been transfusion of packed cells, plasma and platelets in a low

ratio to one another. Transfusion of only packed cells, or a high ratio of plasma cells to packed cells has resulted in worsening coagulopathy and complications. Recently, the CRASH-2 and MATTER-2 trials have shown that tranexamic acid has an important place in the management of massive hemorrhage if administered within 3 hours of the trauma.[39,40] Thromboelastography (TEG) has been shown to be better at assessing coagulopathy in trauma than conventional tests and may be used to guide therapy with tranexamic acid, but there are no established guidelines regarding this. Some of the complications of massive hemorrhage and resuscitation include adult respiratory distress syndrome, sepsis syndrome, acute renal failure, coagulopathy, wound infection, and pneumonia. Permissive hypotension is one of the interventions, which showed a survival benefit in hemorrhagic shock. A landmark study published by Bickell et al. in 1994 showed a clear advantage for delayed resuscitation in both survival, length of stay and incidence of complications.[41] For adequate tissue oxygenation to be maintained, traditional approaches included early and aggressive fluid administration to restore blood volume. This approach however was suggested to increase the hydrostatic pressure on the wound, resulting in dislodgement of blood clots, and diluting the coagulation factors as well as causing hypothermia. The concept of low-volume fluid resuscitation, or permissive hypotension avoids the adverse effects of early aggressive resuscitation while maintaining a level of tissue perfusion that, although lower than normal, is adequate for short periods. In the prehospital period, there is a clear benefit to restricting administration of IV fluids as demonstrated from analysis of the German Trauma registry. Evidence for the restricted initial administration of intrahospital fluid is clearer now, and a recently published prospective randomized trial demonstrated a benefit for the initial intrahospital hypotensive resuscitation strategy.

Question 2: A. Intracranial bleeding

Permissive hypotension, MAP 50-60, has been shown to improve outcomes in penetrating abdominal trauma.[42] In case of blunt injuries of the thorax and abdomen, its utility is less clear, considering there have been studies, which showed no improvement in outcomes. In abdominal aortic aneurysm rupture, permissive hypotension is contraindicated in traumatic brain injury and spinal injuries, because an adequate perfusion pressure is crucial to ensure tissue oxygenation of the injured central nervous system. Multiple studies have shown the utility of controlled fluid resuscitation in abdominal aortic

aneurysm rupture. A systolic BP of at least 110 must be achieved in order to maintain adequate cerebral perfusion. In addition, the concept of permissive hypotension should be carefully considered in the elderly patients, and may be contraindicated if the patient suffers from chronic arterial hypertension.

CASE 17

Question 1: A. Warm blankets

Hypothermia occurs on exposure to cold environment for prolonged periods of time. It is divided into three categories: mild, moderate, and severe which are 32° to 35°C, 28° to 32°C, or below 28°C, respectively. Hypothermia affects almost all organs in the body, see table below:[39-48]

Organ system	Effect
Central nervous system (CNS)	<u>Mild</u>: loss of fine to gross motor function
	<u>Moderate</u>: decrease in mental status and pupillary dilation
	<u>Severe</u>: comatose with flat EEG at 19–20°C
Cardiovascular system (CVS)	<u>Mild</u>: tachycardia and later bradycardia
	<u>Moderate</u>: atrial fibrillation
	<u>Severe</u>: ventricular fibrillation with asystole with further lowering of temperature
Respiratory system	First increase in minute ventilation later decrease in MV. Also increase mucus production and depressed ciliary function leads to pulmonary edema
Renal	Cold diuresis due to increased cardiac output and decreased tubular function

This patient has mild hypothermia and is hemodynamically stable. Mild hypothermia can be treated with passive rewarming by using blankets and preventing further loss of heat. Wet clothing should be removed. Rewarming should occur at a rate of 0.5° to 2.0°C. If not successful then active rewarming methods should be employed. This patient may have intracranial pathology for his mental status change but in view of his temperature and no focal deficits, CT scan initially is not a good option. Although BP seems to be low normal and these patients usually are dehydrated due to cold diuresis, intravenous fluids should be given. The main focus is to treat hypothermia. Patient with drug toxicity can exhibit change in mental status, this patient has negative toxin screen for benzodiazepines and hence Narcan is not needed.

Question 2: E. All of the above
Patients with hypothermia can have all types of arrhythmias. J wave is not pathognomonic of hypothermia but usually seen in 25% to 30% of cases.[49-58] Patients with hypothermia have prolongation of PR, QRS, and QT interval due to slowed impulse conduction of potassium channels.[48-57] As hypothermia progresses patients present with different rhythms.

CASE 18

Question 1: C. CVVHD
There are two approaches for the nomenclature of renal failure: RIFLE which includes changes within 7 days and Acute Kidney Injury Network (AKIN) which includes changes within 48 hours. Predisposing factors in the critical setting to acute renal failure include age, sepsis, contrast, medications, cardiac surgery, diabetes, preexisting renal failure, and shock. There is no known prophylaxis to prevent AKI although it is generally believed that maintaining MAP >65 and adequate fluid resuscitation seems to be key. Fluid resuscitation with hypooncotic fluids such as crystalloids, 4% albumin, or gelatin have been shown safe and effective and no risk for renal dysfunction. However, over-resuscitation with any fluid can predispose to acute renal failure in the form of abdominal compartment syndrome.

ACUTE RENAL FAILURE CLASSIFICATION

RIFLE	Creatinine (Cr) and GFR	Urine Output (UO)
Risk	Increase Cr baseline ≥1.5 or decrease GFR ≥25%	<0.5 mL/kg/h for ≥6 h
Injury	Increase Cr from baseline ≥2.0 or decrease GFR ≥50%	<0.5 mL/kg/h for ≥12 h
Failure	Increase Cr from baseline ≥3.0 or decrease GFR ≥75% or serum Cr ≥4 (354 μmol/L) with acute rise ≥0.5 mg/dL (44 μmol/L)	<0.3 mL/kg/h for ≥24 h or anuria ≥12 h
Loss	Loss of function for >4 weeks (requiring dialysis)	
Endstage	Loss of function for >3 months (requiring dialysis)	
AKIN		
Stage 1	Increase Cr baseline ≥0.3 mg/dL (26.2 μmol/L) or increase ≥150–199% from baseline	<0.5 mL/kg/h for ≥6 h
Stage 2	Increase Cr 200–299% from baseline	<0.5 mL/kg/h for ≥12 h
Stage 3	Increase Cr ≥300% from baseline Serum Cr ≥4 (≥354 μmol/L) with acute rise ≥0.5 mg/dL (44 μmol/L)or initial of RRT	<0.3 mL/kg/h for ≥24 h or anuria ≥12 h

Reproduced with permission from Bagshaw SM, George C, Bellomo R, et al. A comparison of the RIFLE and AKIN criteria for acute kidney injury in critically ill patients. *Nephrol Dial Transplant.* 2008;23(5):1569–1574.

* *

The two processes in RRT are diffusion and convection. Diffusion is where solutes move from higher concentration to a lower concentration. In this process, blood with the high concentration of solutes moves on the opposite direction of dialysate across a semipermeable membrane or filter. The other process, convection (ultrafiltration), involves a solute carried across the semipermeable membrane in response to a transmembrane pressure gradient called solvent drag. This process can remove middle molecules causing uremia and cytokines propagating sepsis.

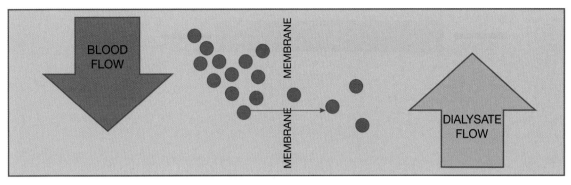

DIFFUSION

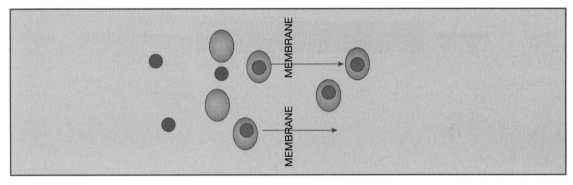

CONVECTION

* *

Indications for RRT in the critical care setting might not necessarily be the same as indications for RRT in patients with chronic renal failure. These include: fluid overload, refractory hypertension, hyperkalemia (K >6.5), dysnatremia (Na <115 or >160), uremia (BUN >70), metabolic acidosis, oliguria <200 mL/12 h, and pericarditis.[59-61]

* *

The optimal time for initiation of RRT in the critical care setting is unknown and unnecessary RRT may worsen renal function and prolong recovery. Optimal dose has not also been determined although RRT dose of >3.6 Kt/Vd in intermittent HD and 20 mL/kg/h in continuous RRT are considered adequate.[59-61]

* *

The advantages of intermittent hemodialysis include rapid clearance, no need for anticoagulation, lower costs, less removal of amino acids, and cofactors. The disadvantages include hemodynamic instability, disequilibrium syndrome, and brain edema. The advantages of continuous RRT include less hemodynamic instability and less need for fluid restrictions. Disadvantages include slow removal of toxins, need for frequent monitoring, continuous exposure to artificial membranes, masks fever continuously, need for anticoagulation, and increase removal of amino acids and cofactors.

* *

There are several approaches to CRRT. Slow continuous ultrafiltration (SCUF) is used to remove fluid with no clearance of toxins since there is no replacement fluid. Continuous venovenous hemofiltration (CVVH) dilutes plasma with fluid and uses convection to remove toxins and ultrafiltrate. Continuous venovenous hemodialysis (CVVHD) uses dialysate to remove toxins. Continuous venovenous hemofiltration (CVVHDF) uses both convection and diffusion.

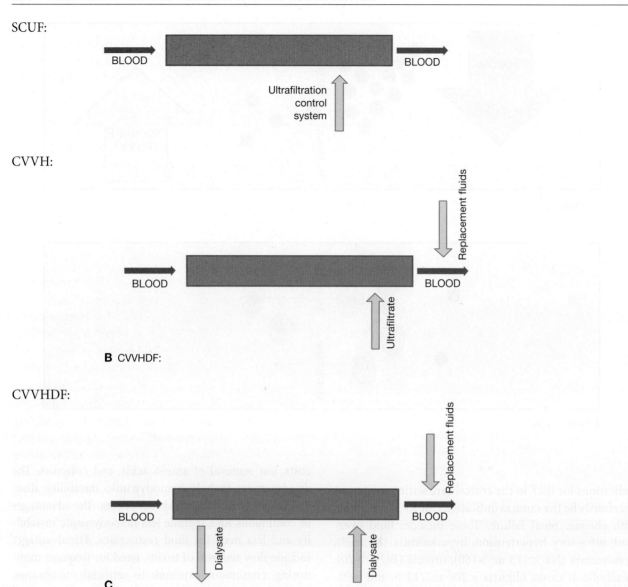

Modified with permission from Ronco C, Bellomo R, Kellum J. *Critical Care Nephrology*. 2nd ed. Philadelphia, PA: Saunders/Elsevier; 2009.

TYPES OF RENAL REPLACEMENT THERAPY

RRT	Blood Flow (Qb)	Ultrafiltration Rate (QF)	Clearance (K)	Dialysate Flow (Qd)	Plasma filtrate Flow (Pf)
SCUF	100 mL/min	2–8 mL/min			
CVVH	100–200 mL/min	10–30 mL/min	15–45 L/24 h		
CVVHD	100–200 mL/min	2–4 mL/min	15–45 L/24 h	10–30 mL/min	
CVVHDF	100–200 mL/min	10–30 mL/min	20–50 L/24 h	10–30 mL/min	
CPE-PE	100–200 mL/min				20–30 mL/min
CVVHD-SLEDD	100–200 mL/min	2–8 mL/min	40–60 L/24 h	50–200 mL/min	
CHP	100–200 mL/min				

CASE 19

Question 1: A. Normal saline

Contrast-induced nephropathy (CIN) is defined as increase in creatinine 0.5 mg/dL or 25% above baseline within 48 hours of contrast administration. Administration of IV NAC have been found to prevent CIN in high-risk patients although sufficient data is still lacking to have a strong recommendation.[59] NAC also has potential complications like hypotension, angioedema, bronchospasm, seizure, and hyponatremia. The same has been said regarding sodium bicarbonate.

Question 2: B. Normal saline and rubicase

Tumor lysis syndrome (TLS) is a syndrome that describes the metabolic derangements, hypocalcemia, hyperkalemia, hyperuricemia, and AKI. It usually occurs after chemotherapy for cancer but can occur spontaneously. In preventing AKI, high urine output with saline and diuretics are advocated. Rubicase is found superior to allopurinol in preventing complications from TLS and urine alkalinization is not recommended.[59] Sodium bicarbonate promotes calcium phosphatase deposition in the kidneys and other tissues.

CASE 20

Question 1: D. Vital capacity

Pregnancy associated pulmonary changes include: (1) airway mucosal hyperemia and increased respiratory secretions secondary to increased estrogen production, particularly in the third trimester; (2) elevation of the diaphragm up to 4 cm and widening of lower rib cage; (3) pulmonary function changes such as decreased RV, FRC and TLC, increased IC, TV, DLco, and minute ventilation; (4) cardiac changes with increased cardiac output and decreased systemic vascular resistance; and (5) increased blood and plasma volume.[62,63] Vital capacity does not change.[62,63] Dyspnea is common secondary to progesterone induced brainstem stimulation and hyperventilation, anemia, unmasking of heart disease; and mechanical obstruction from uterus.[62,63]

Question 2: B. Amniotic fluid embolism syndrome

Amniotic fluid emboli syndrome consists of amniotic fluid entering maternal circulation either through endocervical veins, placental insertion, or site of trauma during labor or shortly after labor.[64,65] This prompts cardiogenic shock, hypoxemic respiratory failure, and inflammatory response leading to DIC. Risk factors include multiparity, precipitous labor, placenta previa, placenta abruption, eclampsia, lacerations, instrumental delivery, and fetal distress. Amniotic fluid debris, which consists of squamous cells, trophoblastic cells, mucin, and lanugo, is not uncommon in patients with amniotic fluid emboli although its presence along with the clinical picture can help in the diagnosis. Treatment is largely supportive.

* *

Preeclampsia is new onset hypertension on a woman at least 20 weeks age of gestation (either two occasions where BP >140/90 at least 4 hours apart or BP >160/110) with proteinuria >0.3 g/24 h or protein/creatinine ratio >0.3.[66-68] If proteinuria is absent, new onset hypertension presence of either thrombocytopenia (<100,000), creatinine >1.1 or doubled from baseline, elevated liver function tests to twice baseline, pulmonary edema, or cerebral symptoms is still diagnostic. Developmental abnormalities in placental vasculature lead to placental hypoperfusion and hypoxia.[66-68] This prompts antiangiogenic factors causing maternal endothelial dysfunction. Hemolysis, elevated liver enzymes, and low platelet count (HELLP) might be considered the severe form of preeclampsia. Treatment for preeclampsia without severe features would consist of serial blood work and assessment of fetal well-being. Antihypertensives are generally not needed if BP <160/110.[66-68] Definitive treatment for severe preeclampsia is delivery and to start magnesium sulfate for seizure prophylaxis. Calcium gluconate is administered in the event of magnesium toxicity, which is manifested by loss of deep tendon reflexes, respiratory failure, and cardiac arrest. If there is preeclampsia, and less than 34 weeks age of gestation, antenatal glucocorticoids are recommended.[66-68] Gestational hypertension is new onset hypertension after 20 weeks age of gestation and resolves by 12-week postpartum.[66-68] Signs and symptoms of preeclampsia are absent. Preexisting hypertension is found if the patient has hypertension prior to 20 weeks age of gestation or lasts longer than 12-week postpartum. Preeclampsia can be superimposed on preexisting hypertension if there is new proteinuria after 20 weeks age of gestation or there if there is worsening hypertension or end-organ damage.[66-68]

**

Peripartum cardiomyopathy is the development of left ventricular dysfunction, EF <45%, toward the end of pregnancy or a few months postpartum with the exclusion of other causes. The pathophysiology is multifactorial, leading some to hypothesize myocarditis, angiogenic imbalance, altered procalcitonin processing, and an inflammatory response. Diagnosis is based on clinical and laboratory findings which might include abnormal BNP, ECG, and echocardiogram. Treatment would include diuretics, vasodilators, and avoidance of ACEI/ARB.

CASE 21

Question 1: A. TV 510/RR 14/PEEP 5/FiO₂ 100

ARDS is defined as progressive hypoxemia, cyanosis, and dyspnea within 1 week of inciting event.[69] Objective parameters for definition includes bilateral opacities on chest radiograph or chest computed tomography, exclusion of cardiac or volume overload with a normal BNP or echocardiogram, and hypoxemia with elevated A–a gradient. According to the Berlin definition, there are three levels of severity: Mild = PaO_2/FiO_2 200 ≤300 mm Hg on PEEP or CPAP ≥5 cm H_2O; moderate = PaO_2/FiO_2 100 to 200 mm Hg on PEEP ≥5 cm H_2O or severe = PaO_2/FiO_2 ≤100 mm Hg on PEEP ≥5 cm H_2O. Risk factors include: aspiration, trauma, pneumonia, transfusions, drugs, genetics such as mutations to surfactant protein B and mutations to angiotensin-converting enzyme (ACE), obesity, cigarettes, thoracic surgery, pancreatitis, near drowning, and blood type A.[69]

**

According to ARDSNET protocol, the initial ventilator setting is focused on low lung volume strategy with initial tidal volumes = 8 mL/kg PBW and reduced by 1 mL/kg ≤2 hours to maintain 6 mL/kg PBW. PBW or predicted body weight is defined for males as 50 + 2.3 [height in inches − 60] and for females as 45.5 + 2.3 [height in inches − 60].[69]

**

The goals are to maintain PaO_2 55 to 88 mm Hg or SpO_2 88% to 95%, plateau pressures ≤30 cm H_2O and pH 7.30 to 7.45.[69] To achieve these goals, the following is advised: (1) lower oxygen – high PEEP or high oxygen and low PEEP strategy; (2) for plateau pressures >30 cm H_2O, tidal volume is decreased by 1 mL/kg to a minimum of

4 mL/kg or if plateau pressure <30 but dyssynchrony, tidal volume can be increased up to 8 mL/kg as long as plateau pressure <30; and (3) if pH 7.15 to 7.30, increase respiratory rate until pH 7.30 or if pH remains <7.15, may increase tidal volume and add sodium bicarbonate.[69]

Question 2: D. Volume control

Volume control is based on a measured volume set by the clinician.[70-74] Main advantage is guaranteed minute ventilation. There is a considerable difference between mandatory and spontaneous breaths. In mandatory, the patient is a passive object receiving gas determine by the ventilator at a set rate and volume (or pressure in PC). The example below depicts a mandatory breath type, VC.

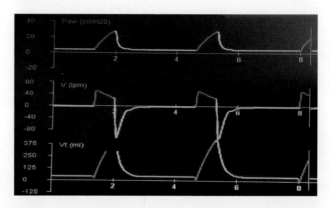

Pressure control ventilation is based on a positive pressure set by the clinician with a variable tidal volume.[70-74] A pressure-limited breath is delivered at a set rate with a tidal volume determined by the preset pressure limit. Inspiratory time is also set by clinician. As shown in the graph, pressure limited and the flow waveform is always decelerating as flow slows as it reaches the pressure limit. Disadvantage: minute ventilation is not guaranteed.

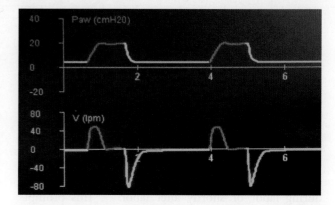

* *

PRVC combines a pressure limit with a volume assurance over the course of several breaths. It does it by mechanically manipulating Ti and flow. It is a duel control mode of ventilation. It utilizes pressure-limited, volume targeted, time cycled breaths that can be ventilator or patient triggered. The Pip can vary on a breath-to-breath basis to achieve a tidal volume set by the clinician. The ventilator automatically adjusts the inspiratory pressure to maintain a target volume. The advantage is guaranteed minute ventilation.

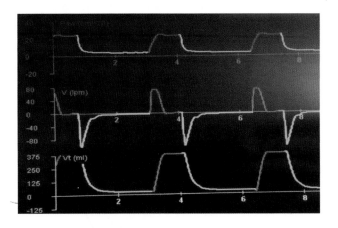

* *

APRV is time-cycled alternate between two levels of positive airway pressure, with the main time on the high level and a brief expiratory release to facilitate ventilation.[29,75,76] Utilized as a type of inverse ratio ventilation, exhalation time shortened in order to maintain alveoli open.

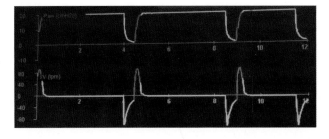

* *

SIMV, like A/C guarantees a set number of positive breaths. Unlike A/C, if patient's respiratory rate exceeds this guaranteed breaths, the ventilator provides assisted breaths up to the set rate and then allowed unassisted or flow cycled. If patient's respiratory rate is below the guarantee, ventilator will again make up the difference

with mandatory controlled breaths. Picture below shows volume SIMV.

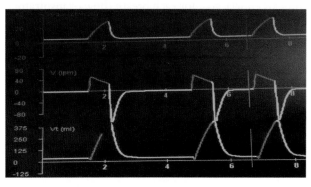

* *

High flow oscillation (HFO) can use respiratory rates four times the normal value (>150 breaths per minute) with very small volumes. Studies have shown that in comparison to more conventional mechanical ventilation in ARDS, there is improvement in oxygenation but no mortality benefit.[77,78]

* *

Pressure support is a method of assisting spontaneous breathing patients. The patient controls all parts of the breath except the pressure limit. Breath can be provided as a stand-alone mode without any guarantee breaths. Many modern stand-alone PS systems also have so-called apnea ventilation-backup algorithms (usually volume control mode setting) for safety when patient respiratory efforts are suddenly reduced or absent.

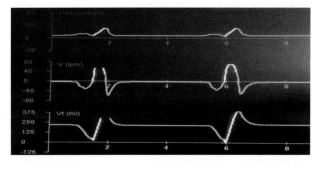

* *

As mentioned, the ventilator displays of pressure and flow yield significant information about both ventilator settings and respiratory system mechanical properties. Breaths can be either controlled entirely by the ventilator or interactive with patient efforts.

* *

The breath in each mode is characterized by the trigger (time or effort), goal for each breath (flow or inspiratory pressure) and what cycle off the breath (volume, flow, or time).[70–74] A timer triggers all controlled breaths. Assisted breaths are triggered by the effort. Volume breaths are volume cycle and pressure breaths are time cycle.

Ventilator Mode	Breath Initiation	Breath Target	Breath Cycle
VC	Time	Volume	Volume/time
PC	Time	Pressure	Time
PRVC	Time	Volume	Volume
PS	Pressure/flow	Pressure	Flow
VS	Pressure/flow	Volume	Flow
CPAP	Pressure/flow	Pressure	Flow
SIMV	Time/pressure/flow	Volume	Volume/time

Question 3: A. Cisatracurium early in the course for 48 hours

There are several novel therapies that are thought to improve outcome in ARDS.[69] Glucocorticoids at a dose of 1 mg/kg per day and given early and no later than 14 days, have been shown to reduce length of ICU stay, ventilator days, and mortality. Although still debatable, antioxidants delivered through tube feeds eicosapentaenoic acid and gamma linolenic acid resulted in fewer ventilator and ICU days. Granulocyte-monocyte colony stimulating factor improve macrophage host defenses although routine use warrants further investigation. Inhaled vasodilators such as nitric oxide and prostacyclin have been shown to improve oxygenation but not improve outcomes. Early use of neuromuscular blockers, particularly cisatracurium, for 48 hours, have been shown to improve adjusted 90-day survival, ventilator free days, and reduce barotrauma probably secondary to improved chest compliance, elimination of patient dyssynchrony, reduce oxygen consumption, and reduce inflammatory cell release.

CASE 22

Question 1: C. Adjust inspiratory pressure in response to patient effort

Novel therapies have emerged in an effort to increase patient ventilator synchrony and promote an interac-

tive ventilator support. Examples are proportional assist ventilation (PAV) and neutrally adjusted ventilator assist (NAVA).[79] Both adjust flow dependent on patient effort. Unlike pressure support, they also adjusts inspiratory pressure in response to patient efforts. PAV monitors continuous patient flow demand and adjust pressure/flow according to a clinician set proportion of required work of breath. NAVA in particular measures diaphragmatic electromyographic signals and adjust pressure and flow in proportion to the intensity of the signal. Breath is cycled when sensed effort has ceased, not a timed cycling process. PEEP is not limited and can be added as with all other modes. Disadvantage is that unlike pressure support a very weak patient will result in a little support from the ventilator. In contrast with PS where even with minor efforts it will always deliver the set inspiratory pressure for the duration of the effort. To date no RCTs have been created to show superiority over other conventional modes of ventilation.

CASE 23

Question 1: B. Increase tidal volume

The patient has double trigger which is the delivery of two consecutive cycles separated by a short expiratory time. This is secondary to the ventilation's inspiratory time being shorter than the patient's inspiratory time. Approaches to improve this would include increasing inspiratory time or tidal volumes, switching to a mode with variable flow delivery such as pressure control ventilation, or increasing sedation.[73,80]

Question 2: E. All of the above

Auto-PEEP can be secondary to shortened expiratory time, which might be a consequence of the underlying disease, inadequate flow or inadequate rise time. Approaches to improve this would be to decrease respiratory rate, decrease inspiratory time, improve flow or improve rise time.[73–81]

CASE 24

Question 1: A. Succinylcholine

Rapid sequence intubation is for patients who have not fasted or have a high risk of aspiration. It involves pretreatment, rapid induction to unconsciousness, and neuromuscular blockade. Bag valve mask (BVM) ventilation is not necessary. Pretreatment is to decrease the physiologic response to intubation. Agents used include: lidocaine, opioids, atropine, or defasciculating dose (10% of the actual dose) of a nondepolarizing NMBA. Rapid induction includes: etomidate (0.3 mg/kg IV) which is not associated with significant hypotension and safest for neuro-patients; ketamine (1–2 mg/kg IV) which is advised for asthma and anaphylaxis; propofol (2 mg/kg IV) which is safe for neuro-patients; or versed (0.3 mg/kg IV) which has the slowest onset.

* *

Depolarizing agents such as succinylcholine, bind to the postsynaptic acetylcholine receptors. This leads to continuous stimulation, fasciculations, and then paralysis. They can cause hypertension, hyperkalemia, arrhythmias, and increased intracranial pressure. In addition, it is advised not to use this agent in rhabdomyolysis, severe burns, crush injuries, infections with exotoxin, and denervating diseases. Nondepolarizing NMBA generally has a slower onset than succinylcholine and they block the binding of acetylcholine to its receptors. Examples include atracurium, cisatracurium, mivacurium, pancuronium, and vecuronium.

Question 2: C. 75% to 80%

The concern for prolonged use of neuromuscular blockers is ICU neuropathy. Other complications include corneal abrasions, decubitus ulcers, apnea, bronchospasm, hypotension or hypertension, rash, and increased incidence of deep venous thrombosis. One approach

to monitor its use is train of four or peripheral nerve stimulator (PNS). PNS is typically performed either in the ulnar nerve where the adductor pollicis muscle (thumb) is observed for twitching; facial nerve where the orbicularis oculi muscle (above eye brow) is observed; or posterior tibial nerve where the flexor halluces brevis muscle (great toe) is observed.[80,82]

* *

A low amplitude, usually 10 to 20 mA with increases of 10 mA is continued until four twitches are noted. Four twitches suggest 0% receptors are blocked, three twitches suggest that <75% receptors are blocked, two twitches suggest 75% to 80% receptors are blocked, one twitch suggests that 90% of receptors are blocked, and no twitch suggests that 100% of receptors are blocked.[80,82] If no twitch is seen, the circuit and attachments are first checked before decreasing or holding the dose of NMBA. Monitoring continues every 15 to 30 minutes until twitches are noted. Once the NMBA infusion is no longer needed and discontinued, four twitches are normally seen after 2 hours.

CASE 25

Question 1: C. PAOP decrease or normal, CO decrease, normal or increase, SVR decrease, SvO$_2$ increase

The table below lists the different types of shock and their hemodynamic profile.[83,84]

TYPES OF SHOCK

	Pulmonary Artery Occlusion Pressure	Cardiac Output	Systemic Vascular Resistance	Mixed Venous Oxygen Saturation
Cardiogenic shock	Increase	Decrease	Increase	Decrease
Hypovolemic shock	Decrease	Decrease	Increase	Decrease
Distributive shock (sepsis or neurogenic)	Decrease or normal	Decrease, normal or increase	Decrease	Increase
Obstructive shock—tamponade	Increase	Decrease	Increase	Decrease
Obstructive shock—pulmonary embolism	Decrease or normal	Decrease	Increase	Decrease

***Question 2:* A. A₁B₁**

Alpha receptors are located in vascular walls and causes vasoconstriction. They are also located in the cardiac muscle where they prolong duration of contraction. Beta 1 receptors are located in the cardiac muscle where they have inotropic and chronotropic effects. Beta 2 receptors cause vasodilation. Dopamine receptors cause vasodilation in the renal, mesenteric, coronary, and neurovascular circulation. Vasopressin receptor 1 causes vasoconstriction; vasopressin 2 has antidiuretic effects. The table below lists the different pressors and their receptors.[83,84]

	Receptor
Dopamine	
0.5–2 μg/kg/min	$B_1B_2D_1$
2–10 μg/kg/min	$A_1B_1B_2D_1$
10–20 μg/kg/min	$A_1B_1B_2D_1$
Norepinephrine	A_1B_1
Phenylephrine	A_1
Dobutamine	B_1B_2
Epinephrine	$A_1B_1B_2$
Vasopressin	$V_1V_2V_3$

***Question 3:* E. Start a corticosteroid infusion**

According to the current guidelines from Levy et al., severe sepsis is defined as sepsis-induced hypotension, elevated lactate, urine output <0.5 mL/kg/h for at least 2 hours despite adequate resuscitation, acute lung injury (at least <PaO_2/FiO_2 <250) in the absence of pneumonia, creatinine >2.0 mg/dL, bilirubin >2 mg/dL, platelet <100,000 μL, and coagulopathy (INR >1.5).[14]

* *

Initial resuscitation includes the following goals within the first 6 hours for sepsis-induced hypoperfusion or elevated lactate >4 mmol/L: (1) CVP 8 to 12 mm Hg, MAP >65 mm Hg, UO >0.5 mL/kg/h, and central venous or mixed venous oxygen saturation 65% to 70%; and (2) normalization of lactate.[14] Crystalloids are preferred with a goal of 30 mL/kg and albumin can be substituted for crystalloids. Cultures should be obtained if no significant delay (>45 minutes) and empiric antibiotics are

administered within the first hour. Empiric antibiotics should be continued for no more than 3 to 5 days and attempts to de-escalate as soon as possible.

* *

Norepinephrine (Grade 1B) is the initial vasopressor of choice.[14] Dopamine (Grade 2 C) is an alternative to norepinephrine if no tachycardia or if there is bradycardia.[14] If inadequate, epinephrine (Grade 2B) or vasopressin can be added to norepinephrine.[14] Phenylephrine (Grade 1 C) is used as a salvage vasopressor.[14] Dobutamine is started if there is known cardiac dysfunction or signs of ongoing hypoperfusion (Grade 1 C).[14] Corticosteroids are considered if the patient has refractory hypotension despite pressors and fluid resuscitation as a continuous infusion to avoid hyperglycemia with a dose of 200 mg per day (Grade 2 C).[14] ACTH stimulation test should be used to guide the selection of which patients need corticosteroids (Grade 2B).[14]

CASE 26

***Question 1:* A. Inquire why the family wishes to withhold information**

The family requests to withhold information to a competent patient in an effort to protect him, but negates his sense of autonomy. It is important to maintain a relationship with both patient and family and determine the patient's desire for such information.

* *

Approaches to this dilemma include inquiring the family why they want to withhold that information and their perspective on what the patient would want, determining how much medical information the patient wishes, stating personal views, and negotiating a clinical approach.[85]

***Question 2:* E. Double effect**

There are four major principles in medical ethics. Autonomy is the individuals' right to make an informed decision regarding medical choices.[85] Beneficence mandates that clinicians act in the best interest of the patient.[85] Nonmaleficence mandates that no harm should come to the patient.[85] Justice implies that all patients should be treated equally.[85] Double effect is defined as an action leading to two consequences, usually both beneficence and nonmaleficence, such as this patient.[85]

CASE 27

Question 1: **D. An optic nerve sheath diameter of 4.9 mm**

The optic nerve sheath diameter can be used to estimate elevated intracranial pressure. The cutoff for elevated pressure varies between 5 and 5.8 mm depending on the studies.[86,87] The optic nerve diameter does not correlate with increased intracranial pressure. You may see a difference in optic nerve sheath diameter with a mass impinging on the nerve but the difference would likely be larger. The gold standard for monitoring intracranial pressure is invasive intracranial devices. The optic nerve is surrounded by cerebrospinal fluid and elevated intracranial pressure will be transmitted to the optic nerve sheath. An optic nerve sheath diameter >5 mm suggests an elevated intracranial pressure. The measurement is done 3 mm posterior to the globe.

CASE 28

Question 1: **B. Opacification of the entire right lung with shift of mediastinum away from the right**

The ultrasound below shows a large simple pleural effusion. Ultrasound has a sensitivity of 97% and a specificity of 97% to detect pleural effusions. On ultrasound, a simple pleural effusion is a hypoechoic. A more complex effusion may appear to have particulate matter or even have septations and appear to be a very complex

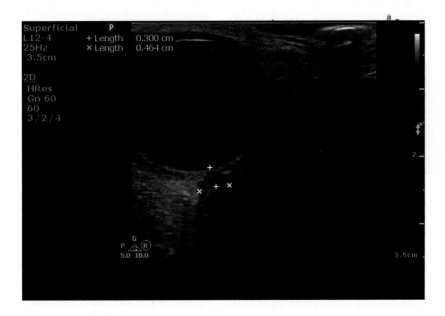

space. Atelectasis on ultrasound will appear as consolidated lung.

* *

Ultrasound has a sensitivity of 92% to 100% in detecting pneumothorax.[88–91] A supine chest x-ray has a sensitivity of 36% to 75% to diagnose pneumothorax.[88–91] The specificity of ultrasound is 78% up to 100% when a lung point is identified.[88–91] A pneumothorax will show an absence of sliding lung and possibly a lung point. Pneumothorax should be accessed on the anterior chest. The examiner should first look for lung sliding which is evidence that the lung is not against the chest wall. M-mode will not show a seashore sign when lung sliding is not present. The presence of lung sliding or B line on ultrasound will rule out pneumothorax.

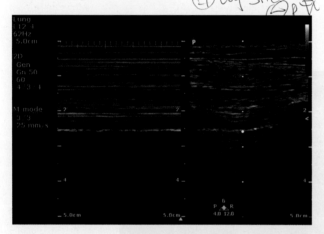

CASE 29

Question 1: **B. Hypoechoic area behind the heart stops at the aorta on PSLA view with collapse of the RV during diastole**
Fluid in the pericardium will stop at the aorta. Fluid that crosses the aorta is more likely due to a pleural effusion. With severe cardiac tamponade, the RV may collapse during diastole. Clinical symptoms can lack specificity to diagnose pericardial tamponade. Hypotension is uncommon in patients with subacute (medical) tamponade who accumulate pericardial effusion over days to weeks. Ultrasound is important for the diagnosis of pericardial effusions and for assessing for hemodynamic compromise. Right atrial or right ventricular collapse indicates that pericardial pressure is greater than intracardiac pressures. Right ventricular collapse is more

specific but less sensitive. Right atrial collapse that lasts more than one-third of the cardiac cycle is more specific.

* *

On 2D ultrasound look for the following to diagnose pericardial tamponade:

1. Collapse of the right atrium during diastole (best seen on apical four chamber view or subcostal view)

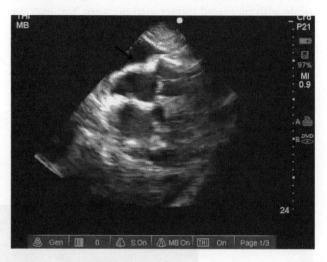

2. Collapse of the right ventricular during beginning and middle of diastole (best seen of subcostal or parasternal short axis)
3. A septal shift toward the left ventricle in inspiration and toward the right ventricle in expiration(best seen on apical four chamber view)
4. Enlarged noncollapsible IVC
5. Left atrial or even left ventricle collapse can occur in localized effusion. Care must be taken in pulmonary hypertension patients because pericardial effusions are a poor prognostic indicator. Due to increased right-sided pressures there may be no collapse of the RV or RA. Collapse of the left-sided chambers can be important in these patients

CASE 30

Question 1: **D. Cardiac surgery consult**
The image shows a vegetation on the mitral valve and warrants a cardiac surgery consultation. If the patient had a small IVC it would suggest need for more fluid. There is no indication that he needs more vasopressors. Dobutamine may be used with evidence of poor perfusions due to decreased cardiac function. There is no

evidence of decreased contractility in this case. Hydrocortisone may be used for patients unresponsive to fluids and pressors and there is no indication that this patient has any evidence of adrenal insufficiency.

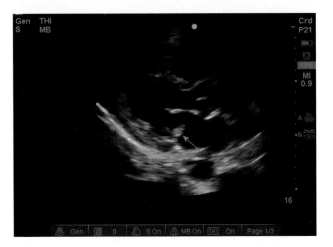

Question 2: E. The patient's foley is misplaced

The image shows a large distended bladder. The kidney appears normal. The foley is misplaced or the patient has no foley. The patient appears to be adequately resuscitated and is otherwise improving. The following image shows a foley balloon within the bladder. It is important to look for balloon placement in the bladder if you are concerned about foley misplacement.

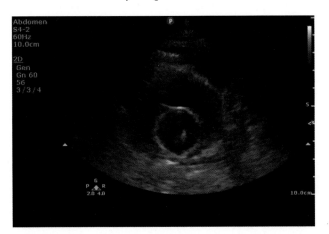

CASE 31

Question 1: A. Place a chest tube

A patient who has fevers and a loculated effusion has an empyema until proved otherwise. Performing a thoracentesis first and placing a chest tube based on the results may be an option in some cases. However, loculations suggest a complicated effusion and this thoracentesis

alone is insufficient therapy. Antibiotics alone also would not be sufficient.

CASE 32

Question 1: D. The IVC measures 2.8 cm

Measurements of the IVC should be taken at the level of the hepatic vein. If a patient is passive on a ventilator then you can use the distensibility as a marker of fluid responsiveness. It has been shown that if the IVC distended >18% it suggests that the patient is fluid responsive.[92-95] The diameter to suggest fluid non-responsiveness is not clear. An IVC diameter >2 likely means sufficient volume status and an IVC diameter <1 cm likely suggests decreased intravascular volume. A patient with IVC diameter between 1 and 2 cm is not clearly in either group. It is not clear how well the collapse of the IVC correlates to fluid responsiveness. IVC collapse has never been shown to predict fluid responsiveness in spontaneously breathing patients. Studies that showed a correlation to fluid responsiveness have used a cutoff of >50% collapse in order to be significant.[92-95] A visual estimate of IVC collapse may be as good as more detailed measurement and a patient with a "virtual IVC" likely needs fluids. It can be helpful to use M-mode to measure the IVC and look for respiratory variation.

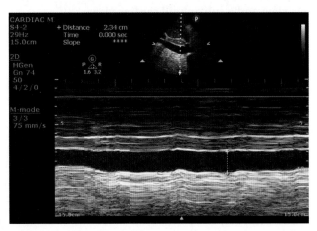

Question 2: E. The IJ is about 1.2 cm below the skin surface

It is important to understand the internal jugular anatomy to improve your chances of successful catheter placement in the internal jugular vein. Using the marks on the right side of the screen we can see that the vessel is just below the first big tick mark which indicates 1 cm. The screen should be set to the lowest depth possible in order to see surrounding important structures especially the carotid artery. This image is slightly too deep and will not have optimal resolution. The IJ is not centered on the screen which allows you to see all structures on either side. In order to confirm that there is no clot, multiple areas of the vessel need to be checked, and the vessel should be compressed. The artery ideally should be to the side of the vein in order to avoid going through the vein into the artery.

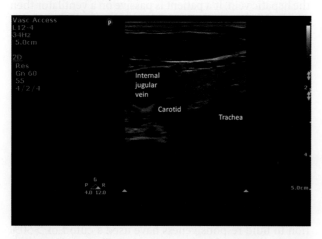

CASE 33

Question 1: **D. The FAST examination includes at a minimum a perihepatic view, a perisplenic view, pelvic view, and a subxiphoid cardiac view**

The FAST examination is used to rule out intra-abdominal bleeding as well as cardiac injury leading to pericardial effusion or tamponade.[96] The perihepatic view examines the Morrison's pouch, the recess between the liver and right kidney. The perisplenic view examines the space between the spleen and left kidney. The pelvic view looks for any fluid around the bladder or uterus. The subxiphoid cardiac view is used to rule out pericardial effusion/tamponade. Other views can be done including examining the anterior chest for lung sliding to rule out pneumothorax which is more sensitive than chest x-ray for pneumothorax. This is sometimes referred to as eFAST (extended FAST). Other cardiac views can be done as well if the subxiphoid view is difficult. A positive FAST examination means that there is fluid in the abdomen and therefore a DPL is not needed but may be performed in certain situations. The FAST examination is not specific for intra-abdominal bleeding from trauma as ascites and peritoneal dialysis would show similar images.

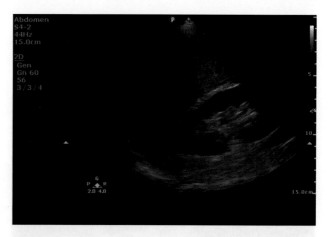

Question 2: **D. Surgical exploration**

This patient has a dropping blood pressure and his ultrasound shows fluid in the Morrison's pouch. It must be assumed that this is blood. The most appropriate treatment would be surgical exploration. The patient is becoming unstable with worsening vital signs. It would not be appropriate to delay treatment with a CT scan. If the patient was more stable a CT would be appropriate to better define the injuries. The patient has evidence of bleeding and worsening vital signs so conservative treatment would not be appropriate. The ultrasound image shows fluid between the liver and kidney. There is no evidence of fluid in the pleural or pericardial space.

CASE 34

Question 1: **D. Albuterol and steroids**

A lines with sliding lung represent normal lung parenchyma. A patient with asthma will have a normal lung ultrasound. Therefore choice D albuterol and steroids is the best answer. The other diagnosis to consider with a normal lung ultrasound would be a pulmonary embolism or nonpulmonary causes of shortness of breath. Ultrasound findings of pneumonia will be either consolidated lung or focal B lines. Therefore choice A antibiotics is incorrect. Pulmonary edema would show diffuse B lines on ultrasound therefore choice B diuresis is incorrect. A pleural effusion which shows a hypoechoic area and would not have normal A lines in the area of effusion therefore choice C thoracentesis is incorrect. A chest tube would be the treatment for a pneumothorax and the finding would be the absence of sliding lung or a lung point.

CASE 35

Question 1: C. Competency is a legal definition made in part with patient's capacity

Capacity is the ability to make informed decisions, which may change over time.[85] Patients with psychiatric diseases do not necessarily lack capacity.[85] Competency is a legal definition that is made in part with the patient's capacity.[85] Patient's surrogate's decisions should be honored.

Question 2: D. Cerebral angiography

Brain death can be diagnosed clinically provided that several prerequisites are fulfilled including: (1) presence of a catastrophic event; (2) exclusion of complicating medical conditions; (3) no drug intoxication or poisoning; and (4) vital signs include temperature >36°C and SBP >100 mm Hg.[97–99] The neurologic examination must have absence of reflexes (corneal, pupillary, jaw jerk, gag or sucking, or cough with tracheal suctioning). Even though the patient should be comatose, patients might have movements originating from peripheral nerves or spinal cord. These include rhythmic movements from muscles supplied by facial nerve, finger flexors movements, adduction of shoulders, elbow flexion, supination or pronation of the wrists, trunk flexion, neck and abdominal muscle contraction, flexion of knee, hip, and ankle with foot stimulation, upper limb pronation extension reflex, and widespread fasciculations.[77–99]

* *

The apnea test is contraindicated in high cervical lesions, neuromuscular blocker use, or chronic CO_2 retainers.[97–99] In adults, it is typically performed after >6 hours of observation, >24 hours for hypoxic encephalopathy, and >72 hours for patients who were placed on the hypothermic protocol after cardiac arrest. The apnea test is performed after preoxygenation for 10 minutes to eliminate nitrogen stores. The patient is disconnected from the ventilator and placed on 6 L nasal cannula or 12 L/min T piece. After 10 minutes, a blood gas is drawn and considered positive if $PaCO_2$ >60 mm Hg or 20 mm Hg greater than baseline. Apnea test is aborted if the patient becomes hypotensive, hypoxic (O_2 sat <85% for >30 seconds), or develop arrhythmias.

* *

Ancillary tests, such as cerebral angiography, transcranial Doppler, magnetic resonance angiography, computed tomographic angiography, electroencephalograph, or evoke potentials, are utilized if the apnea test is not valid, patient is on sedation, multiorgan failure, or neurologic examination is inconclusive.[97–99]

REFERENCES

1. Marino PL, eds. Chapter 28: Acid-base interpretations. *The ICU Book*. 3rd ed. Lippincott Williams & Wilkins; 2007.

2. O'Connor RE, Brady W, Brooks SC, et al. Part 10: acute coronary syndromes: 2010 American Heart Association Guidelines for Cardiopulmonary Resuscitation and Emergency Cardiovascular Care. *Circulation*. 2010;122(18 Suppl 3):S787–S817.

3. Hochman JS, Sleeper LA, Webb JG, et al. for the SHOCK Investigators. Early revascularization in acute myocardial infarction complicated by cardiogenic shock. *N Engl J Med*. 1999;341:625–634.

4. Seupaul RA, Wilbur LG. Evidence-based emergency medicine. Does therapeutic hypothermia benefit survivors of cardiac arrest? *Ann Emerg Med*. 2011;58(3):282–283.

5. Hyperthemia after cardiac arrest study group. Mild Therapeutic Hypothermia to improve the neurologic outcome after cardiac arrest. *N Engl J Med*. 2002.346(8):549–556.

6. Nolan JP, Morley P, Hoek V, et al. Therapeutic hypothermia after cardiac arrest. *Circulation*. 2003;108:118–121.

7. Kim F, Nichol G, Maynard C, et al. Effect of prehospital inducion of mild hypothermia on survival and neurological status among adults with cardiac arrest: A randomized clinical trial. *JAMA*. 2014;311(1):45–52.

8. Diao M, Huang F, Guan K, et al. Prehospital therapeutic hypothermia after cardiac arrest: A systemic review and meta-analysis of randomized controlled trials. *Resuscitation*. 2013;84(8):1021–1028.

9. Bernard SA, Smith K, Cameron P et al. Induction of therapeutic hypothermia by paramedics after resuscitation from out-of-hospital ventricular fibrillation cardiac arrest: A randomized controlled trial. *Circulation*. 2010;122(7):737–742.

10. Bernard SA, Smith K, Cameron P, et al. Induction of prehosptial therapeutic hypothermia after resusciation from nonventricular fibrillation cardiac arrest. *Crit Care Med*. 2012;40(3):747–753.

11. Marik PE. Noninvasive cardiac output monitors: A state-of-the-art review. *J Cardiothorac Vasc Anesth*. 2013;27(1):121–134.

12. Marik PE, Levitov A, Young A, et al. The use of bioreactance and carotid doppler to determine volume responsiveness and blood flow redistribution following passive leg raising in hemodynamically unstable patients. *Chest*. 2013;143(2):364–370.

13. Silvestry FE. *Pulmonary Artery Catheterization: Interpretation of Tracings*. http://www.uptodate.com/contents/pulmonary-artery-catheterization-interpretation-of-tracings?source=search_result&search=pulmonary+artery+catheter&selectedTitle=1%7E150. Accessed on January 2015.

14. Dellinger RP, Levy MM, Rhodes A, et al. Surviving sepsis campaign: international guidelines for management of severe sepsis and septic shock: 2012. *Crit Care Med*. 201341(2):580–637.

15. Hollenberg M., Parrillo J. Cardiogenic shock. *Critical Care Medicine : Principles of Diagnosis and Management in the Adult.* 4th ed. Elsevier/Saunders; 2014:325–337.

16. Ryken T, Hurlbert RJ, Hadley MN, et al. The acute cardiopulmonary management of patients with cervical spinal cord injuries. *Neurosurgery.* 2013;72(3):84–92.

17. McGhee BH, Bridges ME. Monitoring arterial blood pressure: What you may not know. *Crit Care Nurse.* 2002;22(2): 60–79.

18. Anderson CS, Huang Y, Wang JG, et al. Intensive blood pressure reduction in acute cerebral haemorrhage trial (INTERACT): a randomised pilot trial. *Lancet Neurol.* 2008;7(5):391–399.

19. Qureshi AI, Palesc YY. Antihypertensive Treatment of Acute Cerebral Hemorrhage (ATACH) II: design, methods, and rationale. *Neurocrit Care.* 2011;15(3):559–576.

20. Grise EM, Adeoye O. Blood pressure control for acute ischemic and hemorrhagic stroke. *Curr Opin Crit Care.* 2012r;18(2):132–138.

21. Beslow LA, Licht DJ, Smith SE, et al. Predictors of outcome in childhood intracerebral hemorrhage: a prospective consecutive cohort study. *Stroke.* 2010;41(2):313–318.

22. Martin-Schild S, Albright KC, Hallevi H, et al. Intracerebral hemorrhage in cocaine users. *Stroke.* 2010;41(4): 680–684.

23. Kernan WN, Viscoli CM, Brass LM, et al. Phenylpropanolamine and the risk of hemorrhagic stroke. *N Engl J Med.* 2000;343(25):1826–1832.

24. Chhor V, Le Manach Y, Clarençon F, et al. Admission risk factors for cerebral vasospasm in ruptured brain arteriovenous malformations: An observational study. *Crit Care.* 2011;15(4):R190.

25. Suhardja A. Mechanisms of disease: roles of nitric oxide and endothelin-1 in delayed cerebral vasospasm produced by aneurysmal subarachnoid hemorrhage. *Nat Clin Pract Cardiovasc Med.* 2004;1:110–116.

26. Brallier JW, Deiner SG. Use of the bilateral BIS monitor as an indicator of cerebral vasospasm in ICU patients. *Middle East J Anesthesiol.* 2013;22(2):161–164.

27. Goodman DJ, Kumar MA. Evidence-based neurocritical care. *Neurohospitalist.* 2014;4(2):102–108.

28. Allen GS, Ahn HS, Preziosi TJ, et al. Cerebral arterial spasm—a controlled trial of nimodipine in patients with subarachnoid hemorrhage. *N Engl J Med.* 1983;308(11): 619–624.

29. Myers TR, MacIntyre NR. Respiratory controversies in critical care setting: does APRV offer important new advantages in mechanical ventilatory support? *Resp Care.* 2007;52(4):452–458.

30. Kirkpatrick AW, Roberts DJ, De Waele J, et al. Intra-abdominal hypertension and the abdominal compartment syndrome: updated consensus definitions and clinical practice guidelines from the World Society of the Abdominal Compartment Syndrome. *Intensive Care Med.* 2013; 39(7): 1190–1206.

31. Ortiz-Diaz E, Lan CK. Intra-abdominal hypertension in medical critically ill patients: a narrative review. *Shock.* 2014;41(3):175–180.

32. De Waele JJ, Hoste EA, Malbrain ML. Decompressive laparotomy for abdominal compartment syndrome-a critical analysis. *Crit Care.* 2006;10(2):R51.

33. Caldwell CB, Ricotta JJ. Changes in visceral blood flow with elevated intraabdominal pressure. *J Surg Res.* 1987;43 (1):14–20.

34. Lee SL, Anderson JT, Kraut EJ, et al. A simplified approach to the diagnosis of elevated intra-abdominal pressure. *J Trauma.* 2002;52(6):1169–1172.

35. Ridings PC, Bloomfield GL, Blocher CR, et al. Cardiopulmonary effects of raised intra-abdominal pressure before and after intravascular volume expansion. *J Trauma.* 1995; 39(6):1071–1075.

36. Deeren DH, Dits H, Malbrain ML. Correlation between intra-abdominal and intracranial pressure in nontraumatic brain injury. *Intensive Care Med.* 2005;31(11):1577–1581.

37. Johnson-Coyle L, Jensen L, Sobey A. Peripartum Cardiomyopathy: Review and Practice Guidelines. *Am J Crit Care.* 2012;21(2):89–98.

38. James AH. Venous thromboembolism: Mechanisms, treatment, and public awareness. *Arterioscler Thromb Vasc Biol.* 2009;29:326–331.

39. Shakur H, Roberts I, Bautista R, et al. Effects of tranexamic acid on death, vascular occlusive events, and blood transfusion in trauma patients with significant haemorrhage (CRASH-2): a randomised, placebo-controlled trial. *Lancet.* 2010;376:23–32.

40. Morrison JJ, Dubose JJ, Rasmussen TE, et al. Military Application of Tranexamic Acid in Trauma Emergency Resuscitation (MATTERs) Study. *Arch Surg.* 2012;147(2): 113–119.

41. Bickell WH, Wall MJ Jr, Pepe PE, et al. Immediate versus delayed fluid resuscitation for hypotensive patients with penetrating torso injuries. *N Engl J Med.* 1994;17:1105–1109.

42. Morrison CA, et al. Hypotensive resuscitation strategy reduces transfusion requirements and severe postoperative coagulopathy in trauma patients with hemorrhagic shock: Preliminary results of a randomized controlled trial. *Trauma.* 2011;70(3):652–653.

43. Rossaint R, Bouillon B, Cerny V, et al. Management of bleeding following major trauma: an updated European guideline. *Crit Care.* 2010;14:R52.

44. Dutton RP, Mackenzie CF, Scalea TM. Hypotensive resuscitation during active hemorrhage: impact on in-hospital mortality. *J Trauma.* 2002;17:1141–1146.

45. Maegele M, Lefering R, Yucel N, et al. Early coagulopathy in multiple injury: an analysis from the German Trauma Registry on 8724 patients. *Injury.* 2007;17:298–304.

46. Berry C, Ley EJ, Bukur M, et al. Redefining hypotension in traumatic brain injury. *Injury.* 2012;17:1833–1837.

47. Sampalis JS, Tamim H, Denis R, et al. Ineffectiveness of on-site intravenous lines: is prehospital time the culprit? *J Trauma.* 1997;17:608–615.

48. Hamilton H, Constantinou J, Ivancev K. The role of permissive hypotension in the management of ruptured abdominal aortic aneurysms. *J Cardiovasc Surg (Torino).* 2014;55(2):151–159.

49. Ulrich AS, Rathlev NK. Hypothermia and localized cold injuries. *Emerg Med Clin North Am.* 2004;22:281–298.

50. Jolly BT, Ghezzi KT. Accidental hypothermia. *Emerg Med Clin North Am.* 1992;10:311–327.

51. McCulough L, Arora S. Diagnosis and treatment of hypothermia. *Am Fam Physician.* 2004;70(12):2325–2332.

52. Danzl DF, Pozos RS. Accidental hypothermia. *N Engl J Med.* 1994;331:1756–1760.

53. Soar J, Perkins GD, Abbas G, et al. European Resuscitation Council Guidelines for Resuscitation 2010 Section 8. Cardiac arrest in special circumstances: Electrolyte abnormalities, poisoning, drowning, accidental hypothermia, hyperthermia, asthma, anaphylaxis, cardiac surgery, trauma, pregnancy, electrocution. *Resuscitation.* 2010;81(10): 1408–1410.

54. Keller R, Schnider TW, Nerdhart P. Deep accidental hypothermia and cardiac arrest—Rewarming with forced air. *Acta Anesthesiol Scand.* 1997;41:1359–1364.

55. Steele MT, Nelson MJ, Sessler DI, et al. Forced air speeds rewarming in accidental hypothermia. *Ann Emerg Med.* 1996;27:479–484.

56. Lloyd EL. Accidental hypothermia. *Resuscitation.* 1996;32: 111–124.

57. Slouis CM, Bachvarov HL. Heated inhalation treatment of hypothermia. *Am J Emerg Med.* 1984;2:533–536.

58. Kjaerguard B, Back P. Warming of patients with accidental hypothermia using warm water lavage. *Resuscitation.* 2006; 68:203–207.

59. Brochard L, Abroug F, Brenner M, et al. An Official ATS/ERS/SICM/SCCM SRLF Statement: Prevention and Management of Acute Renal Failure in the ICU Patient: an international consensus conference in intensive care medicine. *Am J Respir Crit Care Med.* 2010;181(10):1128–1155.

60. Deepa C, Muralidhar K. Renal replacement therapy in ICU. *J Anaesthesiol Clin Pharmacol.* 2012;28(3):386–396.

61. O'Reilly P, Tolwani A. Renal replacement therapy III: IHD, CRRT, SLED. *Crit Care Clin.* 2005;(21):367–378.

62. Wise RA, Polito AJ, Kirshnan V. Respiratory physiologic changes in pregnancy. *Immunol Allergy Clin North AM.* 2006;26(1):1–12.

63. Hegewald MJ, Crapo RO. Respiratory physiology in pregnancy. *Clin Chest Med.* 2011;32(1):1–13.

64. Ito F, Akasaka J, Koike N, et al. Incidence, diagnosis, and pathophysiology of amniotic fluid embolism. *J Obstet Gynaecol.* 2014;34(7):580–584.

65. Fletcher SJ, Parr MJ. Amniotic fluid embolism: A case report and review. *Resuscitation.* 2000;43(2):141–146.

66. Higgins JR, deSwiet M. Blood pressure measurement and classification in pregnancy. *Lancet.* 2001;357(9250): 131–135.

67. Edlow JA, Caplan LR, O'Brien K, et al. Diagnosis of acute neurologic emergencies in postpartum women. 2013;12(2): 175–185.

68. Steegers EA, Von Dadelszen P, Duvekott JJ, et al. Preeclampsia. *Lancet.* 2010;376(9741):631–644.

69. http://www.ardsnet.org/ardsnet_publications_public. Accessed on January 2015.

70. Lellouche F, Brochard L. Advanced closed loops during mechanical ventilation. *Best Pract Research Clin Anaesth.* 2009;23:81–93.

71. Branson RD, Davis K. Dual control modes: combining volume and pressure breaths. *Resp Care Clin North Am.* 2001; 7:397–401.

72. Maung AA, Kaplan LJ. Airway pressure release ventilation in acute respiratory distress syndrome. *Crit Care Clin.* 2011;27(3):501–509.

73. Hess DR. Applied respiratory physiology: Use of ventilator waveforms and mechanics in the management of critically Ill patients. *Respir Care.* 2005;50(1):26–27.

74. Chatburn RL. *Fundamentals of Mechanical Ventilation.* Cleveland Heights, OH: Mandu Press;2003.

75. Stawicki SP, Goyal M, Sarani B, et al. HFOV and APRV: a practical guide. *J Intensive Care Med.* 2009;24(4):215–229.

76. Kallet RH. Patient-ventilator interaction during acute lung injury, and the role of spontaneous breathing: part 2. airway pressure release ventilation. *Resp Care.* 2011;56(2): 190–203.

77. Derdak S, Mehta S, Stewart TE, et al; Multicenter Oscillatory Ventilation For Acute Respiratory Distress Syndrome Trial (MOAT) Study Investigators. High-frequency oscillatory ventilation for ARDS in adults: a randomized, controlled trial. *Am J Respir Crit Care Med.* 2002;166:801–808.

78. Ferguson ND, Cook DJ, Guyatt GH, et al. High-frequency oscillation in early acute respiratory distress syndrome. *N Engl J Med.* 2013;368(9):795–805.

79. Kacmarek RM. Proportional assist ventilation and neutrally adjusted ventilator assist. *Respir Care.* 2011;56(2):140–148.

80. Corso L. Train of four results and observed muscle movements in children during continuous neuromuscular blockade. *Crit Care Nurse.* 2008;28(3):30–38.

81. Nilsestuen JO, Hargett KD. Using ventilator graphics to identify patient-ventilator asynchrony. *Respir Care.* 2005;50(2):202–234.

82. Tietze KJ. Use of Neuromuscular Blocking Medications in Critically Ill Patients. http://www.uptodate.com/contents/use-of-neuromuscular-blocking-medications-in-critically-ill-patients?source=search_result&search=train+of+four&selectedTitle=1%7E35#H15. Accessed on January 2015.

83. Finfer SR, Vincent JL. Circulatory shock. *N Engl J Med.* 2013;369:1726–1734.

84. Stratman RC, Wiesner AN, Smith KM, et al. Hemodynamic management after spinal cord injury. *Orthopedics.* 2008;31(3):252–255.

85. Truog R, Campbell M, Curtis JR, et al. Recommendations for end-of-life care in the intensive care unit: a consensus statement by the American College of Critical Care Medicine. *Crit Care Med.* 2008;36(4):953–963.

86. Soldatos T, Karakitsos D, Chatzimichail K, et al. Optic Nerve Sonography in the Diagnostic Evaluation of Adult Brain Injury. *Critical Care.* 2008;12(3):R67.

87. Lichtenstein D. Ultrasound in the management of thoracic disease. *Crit Care Med.* 2007;35(Suppl 5):S250–S261.

88. Lichtenstein D. Lung ultrasound in the critically ill. *Curr Opin Crit Care.* 2014 20(3):315–322.

89. Lichtenstein DA, Mezière G, Lascols N, et al. Ultrasound diagnosis of occult pneumothorax. *Crit Care Med.* 2005; 33(6):1231–1238.

90. Blavais M, Lyon M, Duggard S. A prospective comparison of supine chest radiography and bedside ultrasound for the diagnosis of traumatic pneumothorax. *Acad Emerg Med.* 2005;12:844–849.

91. Soldati D, Testa A, Sher S, et al. Occult traumatic pneumothorax: diagnostic accuracy of lung ultrasonography in the emergency department. *Chest.* 2008;133:204–211.

92. Barbier C, Loubières Y, Schmit C, et al. Respiratory changes in inferior vena cava diameter are helpful in predicting fluid responsiveness in ventilated septic patients. *Intensive Care Med.* 2004;30:1740–1746.

93. Feissel M, Michard F, Faller JP, et al. The respiratory variation in inferior vena cava diameter as a guide to fluid therapy. *Intensive Care Med.* 2004;30:1834–1837.

94. Nagdev AD, Merchant RC, Tirado-Gonzalez A, et al. Emergency department bedside ultrasonographic measurement of the caval index for noninvasive determination of low central venous pressure. *Ann Emerg Med.* 2010;55(3): 290–295.

95. Dipti A, Soucy Z, Surana A, et al. Role of inferior vena cava diameter in assessment of volume status: a meta-analysis. *Am J Emerg Med.* 2012 ;30(8):1414–1419.

96. American Institute of Ultrasound in Medicine. AIUM Practice Guideline for the Performance of the Focused Assessment With Sonography for Trauma (FAST) Examination. *J Ultrasound Med.* 2014;33:2047–2056. DOI:10.7863/ultra.33.11.2047.

97. Dhanani S, Hornby L, Ward R, et al. Variability in the determination of death after cardiac arrest: a review of guidelines and statements. *J Intensive Care med.* 2012;27 (4):238–252.

98. Smilevitch P, Lonjaret L, Fourcade O, et al. Apnea test for brain death determination in a patient on extracorporeal membrane oxygenation. *Neurocrit Care.* 2013;19(2):215–217.

99. Wijdicks EF, Rabinstein AA, Manno EM, et al. Pronouncing brain death: Contemporary practice and safety of the apnea test. *Neurology.* 2008;71(16):1240–1244.

23

Biostatistics

Michael Elias MD and Roopa Kohli-Seth MD

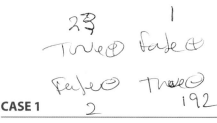

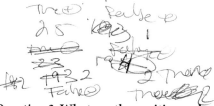

CASE 1

To determine the diagnostic accuracy of lung ultrasound in the diagnosis of pneumothorax in trauma patients in the emergency department, a research team conducted the following experiment:

All the patients admitted to the emergency department with a suspicion of pneumothorax (PTX) had a chest radiograph followed by a spiral chest CT scan and a lung ultrasound. Twenty-five traumatic pneumothoraces were detected by spiral CT scan in 218 hemithoraces; 13 of 25 PTXs were revealed by chest radiograph, while 23 of 25 PTXs were identified by lung US with one false-positive result.[1]

Question 1: What are the sensitivity and specificity of lung US in the diagnosis of traumatic pneumothorax?

A. Sensitivity: 92%, specificity: 100%
B. Sensitivity: 52%, specificity: 87%
C. Sensitivity: 48%, specificity: 97%
D. Sensitivity: 89%, specificity: 93%
E. Sensitivity: 92%, specificity: 99.4%

Question 2: What are the sensitivity and specificity of chest x-ray in the diagnosis of traumatic PTX?

A. Sensitivity: 92%, specificity: 99.4%
B. Sensitivity: 52%, specificity: 100%
C. Sensitivity: 99.4%, specificity: 92%
D. Sensitivity: 100%, specificity: 99.4%
E. Sensitivity: 76.5%, specificity: 87%

Question 3: What are the positive and negative predictive values of lung US in the diagnosis of traumatic PTX?

A. PPV: 95.83%, NPV: 98.96%
B. PPV: 98.99%, NPV: 94.15%
C. PPV: 99.4%, NPV: 92%
D. PPV: 94.15%, NPV: 95.83%
E. PPV: 93.76%, NPV: 90%

Question 4: What are the positive and negative predictive values of chest x-rays in the diagnosis of traumatic PTX?

A. PPV: 94.5%, NPV: 95.83%
B. PPV: 98.99%, NPV: 94.45%
C. PPV: 100%, NPV: 94.15%
D. PPV: 94.15%, NPV: 95.83%
E. PPV: 93%, NPV: 85%

Question 5: What is the prevalence of PTX?

A. 11%
B. 11.46%
C. 11.97%
D. 12.95%
E. 13.10%

Question 6: Increasing the number of patients in the study will result in which of the following?

A. Improve the accuracy
B. Improve the precision
C. Improve both the accuracy and precision
D. Worsen both the accuracy and precision
E. Will have no effect with either accuracy or precision

Question 7: **What is the accuracy of lung US in the diagnosis of traumatic PTX?**

A. 88.07%

B. 88.53%

C. 88.99%

D. 98.62%

E. 99.55%

CASE 2

To evaluate the diagnostic accuracy of D-dimer test in suspected pulmonary embolism patients, 30 patients with clinical and radiological signs suspicious for PE were included in a study.[2] Each subject was submitted to a clinical probability by Revised Geneva Score, a plain chest x-ray, a CT pulmonary angiography (CTPA), and a D-dimer assay.

* *

The results of D-dimer test for cases with low, intermediate, and high clinical probability of PE are reported in the following table:

	Low Probability		Intermediate Probability		High Probability	
	PE	No PE	PE	No PE	PE	No PE
+ D-dimer	0	0	10	5	10	0
− D-dimer	0	3	0	0	2	0

Question 1: **What is the NPV for both low and intermediate clinical probabilities?**

A. 37.5%

B. 66.6%

C. 81.4%

D. 89.3%

E. 100%

Question 2: **Based on the table above, the D-dimer is a valid diagnostic tool to exclude the diagnosis of low-intermediate probability of PE based on which of the following?**

A. The sensitivity

B. The specificity

C. The PPV

D. The NPV

E. None of the above

CASE 3

A study is conducted on a population of 1,500 people. At the start of the study, 127 cases of disease X are detected. Over the next 18 months, 32 new cases are diagnosed.

Question 1: **What is the prevalence rate per 1,000 people of the disease X being studied at the start of the study**

A. 16.27 per 1,000 people

B. 21.34 per 1,000 people

C. 41.33 per 1,000 people year

D. 74.66 per 1,000 people year

E. 84.66 per 1,000 people

Question 2: **What is the incidence rate per 1,000 people/year?**

A. 15.5 per 1,000 people/year

B. 21.3 per 1,000 people/year

C. 32.7 per 1,000 people/year

D. 42.6 per 1,000 people/year

E. 48.8 per 1,000 people/year

CASE 4

Question 1: **Match the following terms to their appropriate definition:**

1. Birth rate	A. Infants deaths per 1,000 live births; [Infants deaths/live births × 1,000]
2. Fertility rate	B. Maternal death per 100,000 live births; [Maternal deaths/live births × 100,000]
3. Mortality rate	C. Death from a specific cause compared to all causes of deaths; [Death from a specific cause/total of all deaths × 100] in%
4. Infant mortality rate	D. Births per 1,000 women of childbearing age; [Live births/childbearing age women × 1,000]
5. Maternal mortality rate	E. Deaths from a specific cause per number of persons with the disease; [Deaths/cases × 100] in%
6. Cause specific mortality rate	F. Birth per 1,000 population; [Live births/population × 1,000]
7. Case fatality rate	G. Deaths from a specific cause per population
8. Proportionate mortality rate	H. Deaths per 1,000 population; [Deaths/population × 1,000]

CASE 5

The following table represents the number of deaths per age group for two diseases X and Y:

Age Groups	Disease X		Disease Y	
	Cases	Death	Cases	Deaths
0–20	3	2	4	3
20–40	40	4	35	3
40–60	60	6	38	4
60–80	187	15	67	11
>80	110	23	105	19

Question 1: **What is the case fatality rate for disease X?**

A. 8.5%
B. 12.5%
C. 17.8%
D. 23.1%
E. 26.4%

Question 2: **What is the proportionate mortality rate for disease Y?**

A. 44.44%
B. 53.4%
C. 62.87%
D. 64.36%
E. 69.89%

CASE 6

Question 1: **A randomized trial was conducted to determine if a macrolide antibiotic, such as azithromycin, would decrease the frequency of exacerbations in COPD patients at risk of exacerbations.[3] The use of azithromycin in the prevention of COPD exacerbation consists of which of the following?**

A. Primary prevention
B. Secondary prevention
C. Tertiary prevention

CASE 7

To determine whether lung screening with low-dose CT scan could reduce lung cancer mortality, the National Lung Screening Trail (NLST) was conducted from 2002 to 2004 on 53,454 persons with high-risk factors for lung cancer.[4] 26,722 participants were randomly assigned to three annual screening with a low-dose CT, while 26,732 were assigned to three annual chest radiography. Data was collected through December 31, 2009.

Question 1: **According to the abstract above, the use of low-dose CT scan in the prevention of lung cancer consists of which of the following?**

A. Primary prevention
B. Secondary prevention
C. Tertiary prevention

CASE 8

An analysis of over 112 studies on second-hand smoking among teenagers who never smoked showed a significant association between exposure to environmental tobacco smoke and lung-cancer risk.

Question 1: **According to the statement above, prevention of environmental tobacco smoke exposure consists of which of the following?**

A. Primary prevention
B. Secondary prevention
C. Tertiary prevention

CASE 9

The ENDORSE study was a multinational survey designed to assess both the prevalence of venous thromboembolism (VTE) risk in the acute hospital care setting as well as the proportion of at-risk patients who received effective prophylaxis.[5] 68,183 patients were enrolled; 30,827 (45%) were surgical patients, and 37,356 (55%) were medical patients. 11,613 (58.5%) of the surgical patients at risk received recommended VTE prophylaxis by the American College of Chest Physicians, compared with 6,119 (39.5%) at-risk medical patients.

Question 1: **According to this abstract, the ENDORSE study is:**

A. A case report
B. A case series report
C. A cross-sectional observational study
D. A case-control observational study
E. A cohort observational study

CASE 10

Many COPD exacerbations are believed to be due to upper and/or lower respiratory tract viral infections. Some investigators conducted an experiment to evaluate the incidence of these infections in patients with COPD.

Respiratory syncytial virus, influenza A and B, parainfluenza 3 and picornaviruses were detected by polymerase chain reaction (PCR) in upper and lower respiratory tract specimens. Patients hospitalized with acute exacerbation of COPD and patients with stable COPD admitted for other medical reasons were studied.[6]

Question 1: This experiment is which of the following?

A. A case report
B. A case series report
C. A cross-sectional observational study
D. A case-control observational study
E. A cohort observational study

Question 2: What is the odd of dying from a pulmonary embolus if the mortality associated is 10%?

A. 1/7
B. 1/8
C. 1/9
D. 1/10
E. 1/11

CASE 11

Question 1: A study that starts with the risk factors or exposures and follows the population over time to assess the incidence of the disease to demonstrate an association is which one of the following?

A. A case report
B. A case series report
C. A cross-sectional observational study
D. A case-control observational study
E. A cohort observational study

CASE 12

To determine the incidence of bacterial pneumonia in a population of intravenous drug users (IVDUs), and to examine the association with HIV, a team of investigators prospectively studied 433 IVDUs without AIDS. These patients were enrolled in a longitudinal study of HIV infection in an out-patient methadone maintenance program. At enrollment, 144 (33.3%) subjects were HIV-seropositive and 289 (66.7%) were seronegative. Over a 12-month period, 14 out of 144 (9.7%) seropositive subjects were hospitalized for community-acquired bacterial pneumonia, compared with 6 out of 289 (2.1%) seronegative subjects.[7]

Question 1: According to the abstract, this observational study is which one of the following?

A. A case report
B. A case series report
C. A cross-sectional observational study
D. A case-control observational study
E. A cohort observational study

Question 2: According to abstract above, what is the relative risk?

A. 5.4
B. 9.7
C. 12.3
D. 13.8
E. 15.9

CASE 13

To identify the risk factors associated with bronchiolitis, a case-control study was conducted on 53 infants with bronchiolitis. These 53 subjects were matched with two controls with no bronchiolitis.

The results are shown in the following table.[8]

Predictors		Number of Subjects	Bronchiolitis Developed (%)
Breast fed	No	103	38 (36.9)
	Yes	56	15 (26.8)
Crowding index (number of persons/ number of rooms)	>0.6	76	33 (43.4)
	≤0.6	83	20 (24.1)
Family history of allergy	Yes	83	28 (33.7)
	No	76	25 (32.9)
Family history of asthma	Yes	34	16 (47.1)
	No	125	37 (29.6)
Older siblings	Any	99	43 (43.4)
	None	60	10 (16.7)
Smoking in household:			
Any	Yes	108	44 (40.7)
	No	51	9 (17.6)
Mother	Yes	68	30 (44.1)
	No	91	23 (25.3)
Father	Yes	82	32 (39)
	No	77	21 (27.3)
Socioeconomic index	Low	86	34 (39.5
	High	73	19 (26)

Question 1: According to the table above, what is the odds ratio of being exposed to smoke among children with bronchiolitis compared to healthy children?

A. 3.20
B. 2.33
C. 2.11
D. 1.50
E. 0.96

Question 2: What interpretation can be best made of the odds ratio calculated in Question 1?

A. The odd of developing bronchiolitis is 2.33 times more important in the infants exposed to smoke.
B. The odd of being exposed to smoke is 1.5 times more important in infants with bronchiolitis.
C. The odd of being exposed to smoke is 2.11 times more important in infants with bronchiolitis than in infants without bronchiolitis.
D. The odd of being exposed to smoke is 3.2 times more important in infants with bronchiolitis than the odd of being exposed to smoke in infants without bronchiolitis.
E. The odd of developing bronchiolitis is 4.7 times more important in infants exposed to smoke.

CASE 14

Question 1: What are the relative risk (RR), the absolute risk reduction (ARR), and the relative risk reduction (RRR) if the control treatment mortality rate is 15% and the experimental treatment mortality rate is 25% in a randomized controlled trial?

A. RR = 0.6, ARR = +10%, RRR = +66%
B. RR = 0.6, ARR = +10%, RRR = −66%
C. RR = 0.6, ARR = −10%, RRR = +66%
D. RR = 1.6, ARR = −10%, RRR = +66%
E. RR = 1.6, ARR = −10%, RRR = −66%

CASE 15

Question 1: Calculate the Number Needed to Treat (NNT) if, in a randomized controlled trial, the control treatment mortality rate is 34% and the experimental treatment mortality rate is 31%.

A. 10
B. 33
C. 115
D. 208
E. 212

CASE 16

Question 1: Calculate the Number Needed to Harm (NNH) if, in a randomized controlled trial, the control treatment mortality rate is 15% and the experimental treatment mortality rate is 25%.

A. 10
B. 50
C. 100
D. 200
E. 300

CASE 17

A randomized controlled trial comparing the effect of a new combination of vasopressin-epinephrine and corticosteroid supplementation during and after CPR on return of spontaneous circulation (ROSC) and survival to hospital discharge was performed The first outcome, measured as the return of spontaneous circulation (ROSC) lasting more than 20 minutes, is shown on the following table.[9]

Question 1: According to the following table, calculate the relative risk, the absolute risk reduction, and the relative risk reduction:

	EPI	VASO + EPI + STEROID
ROSC ≥20 min	91	109
ROSC <20 min	47	21
Total	138	130

A. RR = 1.23, ARR = 25%, RRR = −15%
B. RR = 1.27, ARR = −18%, RRR = −27%
C. RR = 2.29, ARR = 12%, RRR = 34%
D. RR = 3.09, ARR = −29%, RRR = 22%
E. RR = 3.12, ARR = 26%, RRR = −12%

Question 2: The second outcome, measured as the survival at discharge with good neurologic outcome, is shown in the table below.[9] Calculate the relative risk, the absolute risk reduction, and the relative risk reduction for the second outcome:

	Epinephrine Group	Vasopressin + Epinephrine + Steroid Group
Survived neurologic outcome at discharge with good	7	18
Survived at discharge with poor neurologic outcome	131	112

A. RR = 1.76, ARR = 8.8%, RRR = +0.76
B. RR = 0.36, ARR = 13%, RRR = 1
C. RR = 0.28, ARR = 22%, RRR = 76%
D. RR = 2.76, ARR = −8.8%, RRR = 1.76
E. RR = 3.25, ARR = 17%, RRR = 1

CASE 18

Question 1: The survival rate for an experimental treatment was studied in two randomized controlled trials. Which trial is more precise?

A. RCT A: Survival rate = 15% with a 95% CI [0% to 30%]
B. RCT B: Survival rate = 15% with a 95% CI [15% to 17%]
C. RCT C: Survival rate = 15% with a 95% CI [5% to 25%]
D. RCT D: Survival rate = 15% with a 95% CI [10% to 21%]
E. RCT E: Survival rate = 15% with a 95% CI [16% to 20%]

CASE 19

Question 1: The absolute risk reduction for several studies are mentioned below. Which study is statistically significant at the 5% level?

A. Study A: ARR = 0.018 with 95% CI [−0.044 to 0.079]
B. Study B: ARR = 0.023 with 95% CI [−0.028 to 0.073]
C. Study C: ARR = 0.076 with 95% CI [0.049 to 0.103]
D. Study D: ARR = 0.024 with 95% CI [0 to 0.045]
E. Study E: ARR = 0.043 with 95% CI [−0.001 to 0.086]

CASE 20

The relative risks for two randomized controlled trials are reported. In the OSCILLATE trial,[10] the relative risk of death with high-frequency oscillatory ventilation (HFOV) group as compared to conventional low tidal volume ventilation is RR = 1.33, 95% CI [1.09 to 1.64], p = 0.005. In the ACURASYS trial,[11] the risk ratio for death at 90 days in the cisatracurium group as compared with the placebo group in patients with severe ARDS is RR = 0.68, 95% CI [0.48 to 0.98], p = 0.04.

Question 1: According to the information above, which item is true in ARDS patients?

A. High-frequency oscillatory ventilation decreases the risk of death while cisatracurium increases the risk of death.
B. High-frequency oscillatory ventilation increases the risk of death while cisatracurium increases the risk of death.
C. High-frequency oscillatory ventilation decreases the risk of death while cisatracurium decreases the risk of death.
D. High-frequency oscillatory ventilation increases the risk of death while cisatracurium decreases the risk of death.
E. High-frequency oscillatory ventilation increases the risk of death while no conclusion can be made for cisatracurium.

CASE 21

According to the ARDSnet 2000 trial, lower tidal volume mechanical ventilation improved mortality compared to traditional tidal volumes in patients suffering from acute lung injury (ALI)/ acute respiratory distress syndrome (ARDS).[12] The mortality was 31% in the lower tidal volume group (experiment) versus 39.8% in the traditional tidal volume group (control) with 95% CI for the difference between groups [2.4% to 15.3%], p = 0.007.

Question 1: **Calculate the number needed to treat NNT with the 95% confidence interval.**

A. NNT = 5, 95% CI [1 to 15]
B. NNT = 7, 95% CI [3 to 26]
C. NNT = 9, 95% CI [5 to 33]
D. NNT = 11, 95% CI [6 to 41]
E. NNT = 13, 95% CI [8 to 62]

CASE 22

Question 1: **The following diagram was published in a meta-analysis of randomized controlled trials; which trial has more weight, power and precision?**

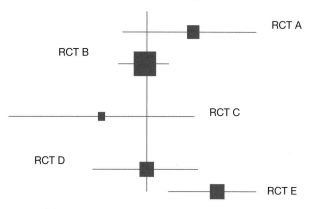

A. RCT A
B. RCT B
C. RCT C
D. RCT D
E. RCT E

Answers

CASE 1

Question 1: E. Sensitivity: 92%, specificity: 99.4%

In the clinical practice, a diagnostic test is used to establish whether or not a patient is likely to have a disorder. A new diagnostic test is compared to a reference test, called a gold standard, often impractical to use because they can be invasive, expensive, or time consuming. The diagnostic value of a test varies and its performance is based on four measures: the sensitivity (sen), the specificity (sp), the positive predictive value (PPV), and the negative predictive value (NPV).

* *

The four possible outcomes (true-positive, false-positive, true-negative, and false-negative) can be represented in a 2 × 2 table.

	Gold Standard		Total
New test being evaluated	Disease +	Disease −	
+ Diagnostic test	(True +) a	(False +) b	a + b
− Diagnostic test	(False −) c	(True −) d	c + d
	a + c	b + d	N

The sensitivity represents the proportion of patients with the disease who tested positive by the new test being evaluated. Mathematically, sensitivity is = a/a + c. If a test has a high sensitivity (>90%), the test has high true-positive values and few false-negative values thus it can be used to rule out a disease when negative.

* *

The specificity is the proportion of people without the disease who are correctly tested negative. Mathematically, specificity = d/b + d. If a test has a high specificity (>90%), the test has high true-negative and few false-positive and can be used to rule in the disease.

Ideally tests should have both sensitivity and specificity close to 100%.

* *

In our study, the number of PTX diagnosed by the new diagnostic test (here lung US) is compared to the gold standard (CT scan).

	Gold Standard		Total
New test being evaluated	PTX (+ CT)	No PTX (− CT)	
+ Lung US	23	1	24
− Lung US	2	192	194
	25	193	218

The sensitivity is 23/25 × 100 = 92% and the specificity is 192/193 × 100 = 99.48%

Question 2: B. Sensitivity: 52%, specificity: 100%

Using the same table, we calculate the sensitivity and specificity of chest x-ray in the diagnosis of PTX in ED patients.

	Gold Standard		Total
New test being evaluated	PTX (+ CT)	No PTX (− CT)	
+ chest x-ray	13	0	13
− chest x-ray	12	193	205
	25	193	218

The sensitivity is 13/25 × 100 = 52% and the specificity is 193/193 × 100 = 100%

Question 3: A. PPV: 95.83%, NPV: 98.96%

The sensitivity and specificity are characteristics of the test and are not affected by the prevalence of the disease. On the other hand, the PPV and NPV vary with the prevalence of the disease. The PPV gives the probability that the patient is truly positive when tested positive. The NPV gives the probability that the patient is truly negative when tested negative.

	Gold Standard		Total
New test being evaluated	Disease +	Disease –	
+ Diagnostic test	(True +) a	(False +) b	a + b
– Diagnostic test	(False –) c	(True –) d	c + d
	a + c	b + d	N

In mathematical term, the PPV is the proportion of patients with the disease among all the patients who test positive: PPV = a/a + b.

* *

The NPV is the proportion of patients who do not have the disease among all the patients who tested negative: NPV = d/c + d.

	Gold Standard		Total
New test being evaluated	PTX (+ CT)	No PTX (– CT)	
+ Lung US	23	1	24
– Lung US	2	192	194
	25	193	218

The PPV is 23/24 × 100 = 95.83% and the NPV is 192/194 × 100 = 98.96%

Question 4: C. PPV: 100%, NPV: 94.15%

Using the 2×2 table, we calculate the PPV and NPV of chest x-ray in the diagnosis of PTX in ED patients.

	Gold standard		Total
New test being evaluated	PTX (+ CT)	No PTX (– CT)	
+ chest x-ray	13	0	13
– chest x-ray	12	193	205
	25	193	218

The PPV is 13/13 × 100 = 100% and the NPV is 193/205 × 100 = 94.14%.

Question 5: B. 11.46%

The prevalence is the proportion of patients diagnosed with the disease by the gold standard at a given time. This should not be confused with the incidence which is a measure of the risk of developing a disease over a specific period of time.

* *

Using the 2×2 table, the prevalence is defined mathematically by a + c/N.

	Gold Standard		Total
New test being evaluated	Disease +	Disease –	
+ Diagnostic test	(True +) a	(False +) b	a + b
– Diagnostic test	(False –) c	(True –) d	c + d
	a + c	b + d	N

When applying this table to our experiment we can easily establish the prevalence:

	Gold Standard		Total
New test being evaluated	PTX (+ CT)	No PTX (– CT)	
+ Lung US	23	1	24
– Lung US	2	192	194
	25	193	218

The prevalence is 25/218 × 100 = 11.46%.

Question 6: B. Improve the precision

Accuracy and precision are two different concepts. A diagnostic test can be accurate but not precise, or precise but not accurate, both accurate and precise or neither. For example, if a diagnostic test contains a systematic error, increasing the number of subjects being studied will increases the precision but not the accuracy since the systematic error will repeat. Eliminating the systematic error improves accuracy but does not change precision.

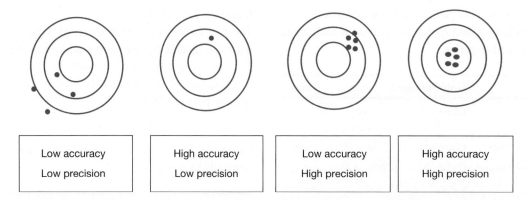

| Low accuracy | High accuracy | Low accuracy | High accuracy |
| Low precision | Low precision | High precision | High precision |

Question 7: D. 98.62%

The accuracy of a test is the proportion of all screened people who are correctly classified by the new screening test. However, in the real clinical setting, the accuracy is not practically used and does not provide the clinician with useful information. Using a 2 × 2 table, it is defined mathematically by the (true-positive + true-negative)/N

	Gold Standard		Total
	PTX (+ CT)	No PTX (− CT)	
New test being evaluated			
+ Lung US	23	1	24
− Lung US	2	192	194
	25	193	218

The accuracy is = (23 + 192)/218 × 100 = 98.62%.

CASE 2

Question 1: E. 100%

When combining the low and intermediate clinical probabilities in a 2 × 2 table, the NPV can be easily calculated:

	Low and Intermediate Probability		High Probability	
	PE	No PE	PE	No PE
+ D-dimer	10	5	10	0
− D-dimer	0	3	2	0
	10	8	12	0

For low and intermediate probabilities of PE, the NPV is 3/(3 + 0) × 100 = 100%. For comparison, the NPV is 0% for high clinical probability of PE.

Question 2: D. The NPV

Because of an excellent NPV (100%), the D-dimer is a valuable tool to exclude the diagnosis of PE only in the setting of low or intermediate clinical probabilities of PE. In the setting of high clinical probability of PE, the NPV is low and does not allow to rule out safely the diagnosis of PE.

CASE 3

Question 1: E. 84.66 per 1,000 people

The prevalence rate is defined by the proportion of all individuals with the disease at a specific time. It is mainly related to chronic conditions. In our case, the prevalence is 127/1,500 = 0.0846 which is 84.66 per 1,000 people.

Question 2: A. 15.5 per 1,000 people/year

The incidence rate is defined by the proportion of new individuals who develop the new disease during a period of time. It is mainly focused on acute condition. Over an 18-month period it is 32/(1,500 − 127) = 0.0233. Over 12 months, the incidence rate is 12 × 0.0233/18 = 0.0155; which is 15.5 per 1,000 people per year.

CASE 4

Question 1: 1-F, 2-D, 3-H, 4-A, 5-B, 6-G, 7-E, 8-C

CASE 5

Question 1: B. 12.5%

The case fatality rate for the disease X is defined by the proportion of cases that lead to death.

* *

It is $(2 + 4 + 6 + 15 + 23)/(3 + 40 + 60 + 187 + 110)$ $= 50/400 = 0.125 = 12.5\%$.

Question 2: A. 44.44%

The proportionate mortality rate for disease Y is defined by the proportion of deaths from disease Y compared to all causes. It is defined by the total deaths from disease Y/total deaths from disease X and Y $= (3 + 3 + 4 + 11 + 19)/[(3 + 40 + 60 + 187 + 110) + (3 + 3 + 4 + 11 + 19)] = 40/[40 + 50] = 44.44\%$.

CASE 6

Question 1: C. Tertiary prevention

There are three types of preventive healthcare strategies: primary, secondary, and tertiary. Primary prevention consists in promoting the health of a population by preventing the onset of at risk behaviors and exposure to risk factors and environmental hazards. Primary prevention such as vaccine immunization or antismoking campaign decreases the incidence of the disease.

* *

Secondary prevention consists of screening for risk factors and early detection of asymptomatic or mild disease, allowing early effective interventions and potentially curative treatments. Secondary prevention decreases disease prevalence. Once the patient has the risk factors, secondary prevention consists in detecting the patients with asymptomatic disease in order to prevent the onset of symptoms. The treatment of asymptomatic hypertension and cancer screening are examples of secondary prevention strategies.

* *

Once the patient has the disease or an advanced stage of the disease, the goal of tertiary prevention is to prevent disability, mortality and further decline in quality of life by preventing recurrence of symptomatic illness, slowing the progression of the disease, and reducing the long-term impairments. An example of tertiary prevention would be the placement of a defibrillator in severe heart failure patients or palliative surgeries to stop the progression of cancer.

CASE 7

Question 1: B. Secondary prevention

Please refer to the answer of Question 1 of Case 6.

CASE 8

Question 1: A. Primary prevention

Please refer to the answer of Question 1 of Case 6.

CASE 9

Question 1: C. A cross-sectional observational study

A cross-sectional study is a prevalence study. It aims at assessing the data of a sample population at a particular time point (i.e., the number of western Africans affected by the EBOLA virus at a given time). Such a study demonstrates an association between the risk factors or exposure and the disease. It does not necessarily demonstrate any cause-effect relation.

CASE 10

Question 1: D. A case-control observational study

A study that starts with the disease and looks back retrospectively in time to assess the risk factors is a case control. A case-control observational study is usually retrospective. It compares two groups of individuals, those with the disease (the case) versus those without (the control) and tries to identify the risk factors that caused the disease.

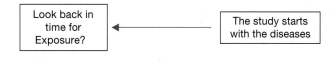

* *

The main advantage is that there is no need for a lengthy follow-up in time since it is retrospective. The disadvantage is that the quality of the data collected retrospectively might not be optimal since it depends on how the data was registered prior to the study. It is particularly useful to study rare diseases or to define the risk factors of an outbreak. A case-control study establishes an association between the exposure and the disease. This relationship might not necessarily be statistically significant.

	Disease + (Case)	Disease − (Control)
+ Risk factors, + exposure	A	B
− Risk factors, − exposure	C	D

A 2 × 2 table allows calculation of the odds ratio (OR) which is defined by:

$$OR = \frac{\text{The odd to have the risk factor in the case group}}{\text{The odd to have the risk factor in the control group}}$$

The odd is defined by a ratio of two probabilities:

$$Odd = \frac{\text{The probability the event happens}}{\text{The probability the event does not happen}} = \frac{P}{1-P}$$

We can calculate the odds for both groups:

$$\text{Odd of having the risk factor in the case group} = \frac{\dfrac{A}{A+C}}{\dfrac{C}{A+C}} = \frac{A}{C}$$

$$\text{Odd of having the risk factor in the control group} = \frac{\dfrac{B}{B+D}}{\dfrac{D}{B+D}} = \frac{B}{D}$$

Thus the odds ratio is defined by:

$$OR = \frac{\dfrac{A}{C}}{\dfrac{B}{D}} = \frac{A \times D}{B \times C}$$

If OR = 1, there is no association, the exposure does not affect the risk of getting the disease. If the OR is >1, the exposure increases the risks of getting the disease (higher odds of outcome), while it decreases the risk if OR is <1 (lower odds of outcome).

Question 2: C. 1/9

The odd of dying of a PE is the ratio of two probabilities. It is the probability of dying divided by the probability of not dying, this is equal to $P/(1 - P) = 10\%/(1 - 10\%) = 0.1/0.9 = 1/9$.

CASE 11

Question 1: E. A cohort observational study

A cohort observational study is a prospective study which follows healthy subjects with potential risk factors for the appearance of the disease. It can establish an

association between the exposure and the disease. The disadvantage is the length and expensive since it might take years for a disease to develop.

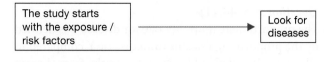

* *

The cause effect relationship between the exposure or risk factor and the disease is assessed using the relative risk (RR) or attributable risk (AR) (also called absolute risk reduction).

	Disease +	Disease −	Incidence:
+ Risk factors, exposure	A	B	I_1 (exposed)
− Risk factors, exposure	C	D	I_0 (not exposed

* *

The relative risk is a ratio of incidences $RR = I_1/I_0$. The attributable risk is a difference of incidences $AR = I_1 - I_0$. If RR = 1 or AR = 0, there is no association or cause-effect relationship between the exposure and the disease. If the RR >1 or AR >0, the exposure increases the risk of the disease. If the RR <1 or AR <0, the exposure decreases the risk of developing the disease. It is important to know that not all cohort studies are prospective. Some can be retrospective when the investigator monitor the incidence of disease over time and identify risk factors.

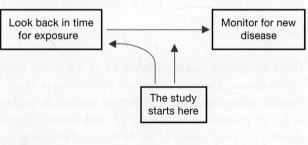

CASE 12

Question 1: E. A cohort observational study

A cohort study starts with healthy subjects exposed to a risk factor. The subjects are followed over time to establish the incidence of the disease. (For more detailed explanations of the other answers choices, please refer to Question 1 of Cases 9 to 12).

Question 2: A. 5.4

From the abstract, we can easily draw a 2 × 2 table that will help us to establish the incidences and thus calculate the relative risk. The total number of patient observed is 433. One hundred and forty-four are seropositive while 289 are seronegative. Fourteen of the 144 seropositive patients developed a pneumonia compared to 6 of the 289 seronegative patients.

	PNA	No PNA	Incidence:
+ HIV (w/o AIDS)	14	130	I_1 (exposed) = 14/130 = 0.107
– HIV	6	283	I_0 (not exposed = 6/283 = 0.020

The relative risk is RR = I_1/I_0 = 0.107/0.02 = 5.4. Thus, according to that study, being HIV+ (without AIDS) multiplies the risk of developing pneumonia by 5.4.

CASE 13

Question 1: A. 3.20

This is a case-control study. Using a 2 × 2 table we can easily apply the rules of the odds ratio explained earlier in the answer of Case 10 Question 1. From the table, we can see that among the total number of subjects exposed to smoke (108), 44 developed a bronchiolitis, thus our case has 44 subjects and our control group has 108 – 44 = 64 subjects. Among the 51 subjects not exposed to smoke, 9 were diagnosed with bronchiolitis therefore our case population has 9 subjects and our control has 51 – 9 = 42 subjects who did not have a bronchiolitis.

	+ Bronchiolitis (Case)	– Bronchiolitis (Control)
smoke exposition (exposure)	44	64
no smoke exposition (no exposure)	9	42

The odd ratio is [44 × 42]/[9 × 64] = 3.20.

Question 2: D. The odd of being exposed to smoke is 3.2 times more important in infants with bronchiolitis than the odd of being exposed to smoke in infants without bronchiolitis.

The odds ratio calculated in Question 1 is 3.20. This is interpreted as the following:

$$\text{The OR} = \frac{\text{The odd of being exposed to smoke among bronchiolitis infants (case)}}{\text{The odd of being exposed to smoke among healthy infants (control)}} = 3.20$$

The odds of being exposed in the bronchiolitis group (case) are 3.20 times the odd of being exposed in the healthy infants group (control).

CASE 14

Question 1: E. RR = 1.6, ARR = – 10%, RRR = – 66%

The relative risk (RR), the absolute risk reduction (ARR) and the relative risk reduction (RRR) measure the importance of the effect of a treatment. The relative risk provides how many times more likely an event will occur in the experimental group compared to the control group. It is defined by the ratio of two risks: the risk of outcome in the experimental group (experimental event rate)/the risk of outcome in the control group (control event rate). If the RR = 1, there is no difference between groups and therefore the experimental treatment has no effect. If the RR is <1, the treatment decreases the risk of outcome. If the RR is >1, the treatment increases the risk of outcome. In our case, the RR = EER/CER = 25%/15% = 1.6; the experimental treatment increases the mortality.

* *

The absolute risk reduction (ARR) also called the absolute risk difference is the difference between the risks of outcome in the control group (CER) minus the risk of outcome in the experimental group (EER). ARR = CER – EER. If the ARR = 0, there is no difference between both treatments. If the ARR <0, CER < EER, the experimental treatment increases the risk of outcome. If the ARR >0, CER > EER, the experimental treatment decreases the risk of outcome. In our case, the ARR = 15% – 25% = −10%, the experimental treatment increases the risk of mortality by an absolute value of 10%.

* *

The relative risk reduction is a reduction in the rate of the outcomes between both groups. It is defined as RRR = 1 – RR = 1 – EER/CER = [CER – EER]/CER = ARR/CER. In our case, the RRR = 1 – 1.66 = −10%/15% = −0.66 = −66%. Therefore the experimental treatment increases the risk of death by 66% relative to the control treatment. The RRR is the most reported value in

RCT however it is less relevant than the ARR because it tends to amplify the benefit of an RCT. For example, if the EER = 1% and the CER is 2%, the ARR = CER – EER = 2% – 1% = 1% but the RRR = ARR/CER = 1%/2% = 0.5 = 50%. The RRR will give the "impression" that the experimental treatment has an important effect since it has decreased the mortality by 50% relative to the control group while in absolute it is only 1% and is irrelevant.

CASE 15

Question 1: B. 33
The number needed to treat (NNT) represents the number of patients needed to treat with the experimental treatment to prevent one bad outcome. It is defined by NNT = 1/ARR. NNT = 1/[EER – CER] = 1/[34% – 31%] = 1/3% ≈ 33. Therefore, 33 patients need to be treated with the new experimental treatment in order to prevent the death of 1 patient.

* *

The NNT is useful to the clinician; it helps to consider how much of a benefit a clinician would expect for his patients.

CASE 16

Question 1: A. 10
Similarly to the number needed to treat, the number needed to harm (NNH) represents the number of patients needed to be exposed to a risk factor or a detrimental effect of a treatment to harm one patient with a bad outcome.

* *

The NNH = 1/ARR = 1/[EER – CER] = 1/[15% – 25%] = 1/– 10% = 10; therefore 10 patients need to be exposed to the experimental treatment to provoke the death of one patient.

CASE 17

Question 1: B. RR = 1.27, ARR = – 18%, RRR = – 27%
Unlike the other observational studies mentioned previously, a randomized controlled trial represents the highest level of evidence. It is an experimental study in

which the subjects are randomized into groups to ensure unbiased allocation to different treatments. The first step consists in reorganizing the information provided into a 2 × 2 table into the following fashion:

Treatments Groups	Outcome Measured		Calculated Event Rates
	Positive Effect	Negative Effect	
New experimental treatment	a	B	Experimental event rate EER = a/(a + b)
Old control treatment	c	D	Control Event Rate CER = c/(c + d)

* *

Applying the data to our tables gives us the following event rates:

Treatments Groups	Outcome Measured		Calculated Event Rates
	ROSC ≥20 min (+ outcome)	ROSC <20 min	
(Experiment) epinephrine + vasopressin + steroids	109	21	EER = 109/(109 + 21) = 84%
(Control) epinephrine	91	47	CER = 91/(91 + 47) = 66%

The relative risk is RR = EER/CER = 84%/66% = 1.27.

* *

The absolute risk reduction (or absolute risk difference) ARR = EER – CER = 66% – 84% = –18%. The experiment treatment reduces the risk (a return of spontaneous circulation lasting less than 20 minutes) by an absolute value of 18%.

* *

The relative risk reduction RRR = 1 – RR = 1 – 1.27 = – 0.27 = – 27%. The new experimental treatment reduces the risk (of ROSC lasting less than 20 minutes) by 27% relative to the control treatment.

Question 2: D. RR = 2.76, ARR = – 8.8%, RRR = 1.76
Reorganizing the data into a 2 × 2 table will allow calculating the event rates:

	Outcome		
	Survived at Discharge with Good Neurologic Outcome	**Survived at Discharge with Poor Neurologic Outcome**	**Calculated Event Rates**
(Experiment): vasopressin + epinephrine + steroids	18	112	EER = 18/(18 + 112) × 100 = 13.8%
(Standard) epinephrine	7	131	CER = 7/(7 + 131) × 100 = 5%

The relative risk is RR = EER/CER = 13.8%/5% = 2.76. The experimental treatment increases the rate of event (here the rate of survival with good neurological outcome at discharge).

* *

The Absolute risk reduction (or absolute risk difference) ARR = EER − CER = 13.8% − 5% = 8.8%; the experimental treatment decreases the rate of survival with poor neurological outcome by an absolute value of 8.8%. The relative risk reduction RRR = 1 − RR = 1 − 2.76 = ARR/CER = − 8.8%/5% = − 1.76. The experimental treatment multiply the "risk" of survival at discharge with a good neurological outcome by 1.76; which is equivalent to an increase by 76% (since 1 + 0.76 = 1 + 76%) relative to the control treatment.

CASE 18

Question 1: **B. RCT B: Survival rate = 15% with a 95% CI [15% to 17%]**
The "importance" of the effect of a treatment is evaluated using the relative risk, the absolute risk and the relative risk reduction. However, these values are useless if not provided with their 95% confidence interval which measures the "precision" of the measured effect. Since only a random sample is used in clinical studies, the true effect of a treatment on the general population is not known and can only be estimated. If our confidence interval is narrow, our central estimate is precise. On the other hand, if our sample population is small, our confidence interval is wide and our central estimate is not precise and could take any value within that interval. Thus, in RCT A, the survival rate measured could be any value from 0% to 30%. In RCT B, the survival rate is any value between 15% and 17%. We are confident that if we were to repeat our experiment 100 times, 95 times the estimated survival rate would be between (and including) 15% and 17%.

* *

For proportions, the 95% CI is defined by: [p − 1.96 × SE(p); p + 1.96 × SE (p)] where p is the proportion in% or decimal, the standard error is SE (p) = √[p(1 − p)/n] with n being the sample size.

* *

For means, the 95% CI is defined by: [mean − 1.96 × SE (mean); mean + 1.96 × SE (mean)]. The standard error is SE (mean) = SD/ √n where SD is the standard deviation and n the sample size.

* *

If the sample size n increases, both the standard error SE and the confidence interval decrease.

CASE 19

Question 1: **C. Study C: ARR = 0.076 with 95% CI [0.049 to 0.103]**
In studies A, B, D, and E, the 95% CI includes the 0, therefore the ARR (the difference between the events rates EER-CER) can be 0. Study C shows an ARR with a 95% CI that does not include the 0. We are 95% confident that the measured ARR is >0, therefore the treatment C has an effect and that effect is statistically significant. The same reasoning applies to the relative risk and odds ratio. If the 95% CI for the relative risk RR includes 1, the RR can be 1 and there would be no difference between the treatments.

CASE 20

Question 1: **D. High-frequency oscillatory ventilation increases the risk of death while cisatracurium decreases the risk of death.**

In the OSCILLATE trial, the 95% CI for the relative risk RR does not include 1, therefore the RR is >1, the experimental treatment HFOV increases the mortality. In the ACURASYS trial, the 95% CI for the relative risk does not include 1, therefore the RR is <1. We can conclude that the cisatracurium decreases the risk of mortality.

CASE 21

Question 1: **D. NNT = 11, 95% CI [6 to 41]**

The number needed to treat is defined by NNT = 1/ARR = 1/[CER – EER] = 1/[39.8% – 31%] = 11.36. The number needed to treat with low tidal volume ventilation to avoid one death in patients with ARDS is 11.

**

The difference in mortality risks between groups represents the absolute risk difference (ARR). The 95% CI for the ARR = [2.4% to 15.3%]. The 95% CI for the NNT = [1/15.3% to 1/2.4%] = [6.5 to 41]. The NNT is 11 but in reality it could take any values from 6 to 41 patients.

CASE 22

Question 1: **B. RCT B**

The larger the number of patients included, the smaller the confidence interval and thus the more precise the study. The RCT B has a higher number of patients, thus a small CI of 95%; this study is more precise and carries more weight when compared to other RCT listed in the meta-analysis.

REFERENCES

1. Soldati G, Testa A, Sher S, et al. Occult traumatic pneumothorax diagnostic accuracy of lung ultrasonography in the emergency department. *Chest.* 2008;133(1):204–211.

2. Youssf ARI, Ismail MF, ElGhamry R, et al. Diagnostic accuracy of D-dimer assay in suspected pulmonary embolism patients. *Egypt J Chest Dis Tuberc.* 2014;63(2):411–417.

3. Albert RK, Connett J, Bailey WC, et al. Azithromycin for prevention of exacerbations of COPD. *N Engl J Med.* 2011;365(8):689–698.

4. Aberle DR, Tapson VF, Bergmann JF, et al. Reduced lung-cancer mortality with low-dose computed tomographic screening. *N Engl J Med.* 2011;365(5):395–409.

5. Cohen AT, Tapson VF, Bergmann JF, et al. Venous thromboembolism risk and prophylaxis in the acute hospital care setting (ENDORSE study): a multinational cross-sectional study. *Lancet.* 2008;371(9610):387–394.

6. Rohde G, Wiethege A, Borg I, et al. Respiratory viruses in exacerbations of chronic obstructive pulmonary disease requiring hospitalisation: a case-control study. *Thorax.* 2003;58(1):37–42.

7. Selwyn PA, Hartel D, Wasserman W, et al. Impact of the AIDS epidemic on morbidity and mortality among intravenous drug users in a New York City methadone maintenance program. *Am J Public Health.* 1989;79(10):1358–1362.

8. McConnochie KM, Roghmann KJ. Parental smoking, presence of older siblings, and family history of asthma increase risk of bronchiolitis. *Am J Dis Child.* 1986;140(8):806–812.

9. Mentzelopoulos SD, Zakynthinos SG, Tzoufi M, et al. Vasopressin, epinephrine, and corticosteroids for in-hospital cardiac arrest. *Arch Inter Med.* 2009;169(1):15–24.

10. Malhotra A, Drazen JM. High-frequency oscillatory ventilation on shaky ground. *N Engl J Med.* 2013;368(9):863–865.

11. Papazian L, Forel JM, Gacouin A, et al. Neuromuscular blockers in early acute respiratory distress syndrome. *N Engl J Med.* 2010;363(12):1107–1116.

12. Ventilation with lower tidal volumes as compared with traditional tidal volumes for acute lung injury and the acute respiratory distress syndrome. *N Engl J Med.* 2000;342(18):1301–1308.

24

Hyperbaric Medicine

Nagendra Madisi MD, Ronaldo Collo Go MD, and Roopa Kohli-Seth MD

CASE 1

A 24-year-old man went on a ski trip to the Swiss Alps. He had a mild, nonproductive cough without fever, a couple days prior which he attributed to a viral illness. He usually runs 6 miles a week and is a nonsmoker. On day 1, he camped at 1,800 m. On day 2, he reached 2,800 m and decided to ski at this level for the rest of his vacation but later that afternoon he developed severe shortness of breath. His colleagues observed the use of accessory muscles of respiration, tachycardia with a regular rhythm, and rales were heard on lung examination bilaterally. He was rushed to the ER; CXR showed bilateral opacification and EKG was normal.

Question 1: A simple respiratory unit is depicted below, with the circular unit as your alveoli and the arrow as your blood flow. The areas in red highlight the mechanism of hypoxia. Which of the following illustrations depict the etiology of his symptoms?

A.

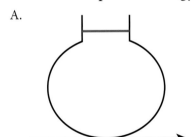

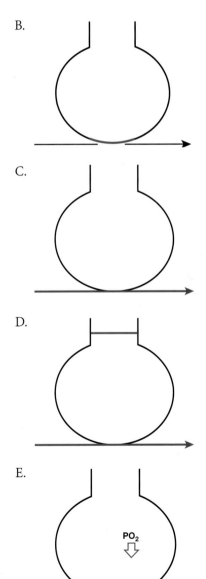

Question 2: **What is your diagnosis?**

A. High-altitude pulmonary edema (HAPE)
B. High-altitude cerebral edema (HACE)
C. Acute mountain sickness
D. Chronic mountain sickness
E. Periodic breathing of high altitude

Question 3: **What is the best initial management for this condition?**

A. Rapid descent to a lower altitude
B. Intravenous diuretics
C. Corticosteroids
D. Oral acetazolamide
E. Oxygen

Question 4: **What is the best pharmacological agent to prevent his disease?**

A. Dexamethasone
B. Oral acetazolamide
C. Oral furosemide
D. Nifedipine
E. Tadalafil

CASE 2

A 55-year-old woman from Baltimore visits her cousin in Aspen, Colorado for Christmas and plans to spend the New Year's Eve skiing. Twelve hours after arrival she is brought to the emergency department complaining of acute onset of headache, confusion, nausea, and vomiting. On physical examination, she is noted to have an ataxic gait.

Question 1: **What is the best diagnostic test?**

A. CT head
B. CT chest
C. MRI of the brain
D. Lumbar puncture
E. V/Q scan

Question 2: **Which of the following measures is life saving in patients with high-altitude cerebral edema (HACE) when the descent is delayed?**

A. Dexamethasone
B. Hyperbaric oxygen
C. Diuretics
D. A and B
E. A, B, and C

CASE 3

A 56-year-old man comes to your clinic for follow-up after a recent hospitalization for acute STEMI a week ago. His other medical history includes hypertension and hyperlipidemia. His blood pressure is 132/86 mm Hg; pulse is 88/min, respiratory rate of 16/min and temperature of 37.7°C (100°F). On physical examination he has no jugular venous distension or pedal edema, normal S1, S2 with clear breath sounds on auscultation. Echocardiography done during a recent hospitalization showed mild MR with an LVEF of 56% and no valvular abnormalities. He is planning on flying to Europe with his wife next week.

Question 1: **What is your advice to the patient on air travel following a recent cardiac event?**

A. Air travel after 3 days
B. Air travel after 10 days
C. Air travel after 3 months
D. No reservations regarding flight
E. Patient cannot fly ever

Question 2: **Which of the following patients need oxygen for air travel?**

A. A 66-year-old chronic smoker with a hypoxic air challenge test result of PaO_2 >6.6 kPa (>50 mm Hg) or SpO_2 >85%
B. An obese patient with a home oxygen requirement flow rate of 5 L/min
C. Pneumothorax
D. A 34-year-old cystic fibrosis patient with resting room air SpO_2 <92% at sea level
E. None of the above

CASE 4

A 43-year-old diver arrives at the emergency department with complaints of severe abdominal pain, right-leg paresthesia and weakness. The night prior he had been diving in Hawaii and flew back home this morning. His past medical history is positive for GERD only and the only medication he uses is pantoprazole on and off. He is alert and oriented, and physical examination is remarkable for diffuse abdominal tenderness and right leg weakness.

Question 1: **Which of the following laws explain his disease?**

A. $P_1V_1 = P_2V_2$
B. $V_1/V_2 = T_1/T_2$
C. $P_{total} = P_1 + P_2 + P_N$
D. $P = k_H c$
E. $V_1/N_1 = V_2/N_2$

Question 2: **What is the most appropriate management for the above condition?**

A. 100% oxygen and hyperbaric therapy
B. Intravenous antibiotics
C. Emergency laparotomy
D. CT abdomen
E. MRI of the brain

CASE 5

Question 1: **A 37-year-old overenthusiastic man is very excited to go scuba diving for the first time. During the training, the instructor reminds him that the most common complication from scuba diving is:**

A. Ear barotrauma
B. Air emboli
C. Nitrogen narcosis
D. Decompression syndrome
E. Hypothermia

Question 2: **During the dive, the man appears sluggish to follow the instructions of the dive and subsequently becomes unresponsive. The instructor slowly brings him up to the surface where he slowly regains consciousness. What did he have?**

A. Nitrogen narcosis
B. Air emboli
C. Decompression syndrome
D. Hypothermia
E. Malingering

Question 3: **Which of the following is the occupational hazard for professional divers and personnel exposed to hyperbaric stressors?**

A. Aseptic bone necrosis
B. Coronary artery disease
C. Parkinsonism
D. Strokes
E. None of the above

CASE 6

A 65-year-old man was rescued from his burning house and rushed to the emergency room. Upon arrival he was awake but confused. He was not oriented to place, name, or situation. He was a former smoker and had history of CAD and hypertension. His vital signs were BP 138/98, HR 102, oxygen saturation 95% on room air, and RR 24. His physical examination showed carbonaceous material around his nostrils. The pharynx was observed and noted to have some edema. Lungs appear to be clear in auscultation. Oxygen was started. Labs including arterial blood gas, chest radiograph, and CT head were unremarkable. The carboxyhemoglobin (COHgb) was 18%.

Question 1: **What should be the next step?**

A. Intubate
B. Corticosteroids
C. Observation
D. Laryngoscopy
E. None of the above

Question 2: **The disease entity above will move the oxygen dissociation curve to which direction?**

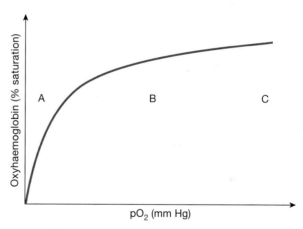

A. A
B. B
C. C
D. A or C
E. None

Question 3: Which of the following conditions is NOT an indication for hyperbaric oxygen therapy in carbon monoxide poisoning?

A. Pregnant woman with carboxyhemoglobin (COHgb) of >20

B. A 33-year-old man with COHgb of >25

C. A 54 year-old man with EKG changes consistent with ischemia

D. Exposure of >24 hours of carbon monoxide

E. A 45 year-old man with history of smoking and COHgb of >15

Question 4: What is the absolute contraindication for using hyperbaric oxygen therapy (HBO therapy)?

A. COPD patients with blebs on chest x-ray

B. Seizure disorder

C. Pneumothorax

D. Pregnancy

E. Claustrophobia

Question 5: Concomitant cyanide poisoning is also suspected. Which of the following treatments of cyanide poisoning should be avoided?

A. Sodium thiosulfate

B. Hydroxycobalamin

C. Sodium nitrite

D. Methylene blue

E. Dicobalt acetate

Answers

CASE 1

Question 1: E.

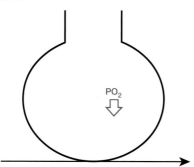

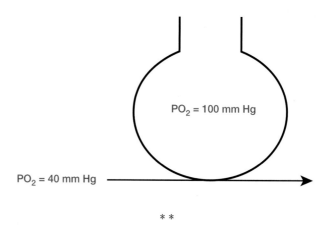

* *

The normal respiratory unit is depicted at right. Oxygen transportation from the atmosphere to the red blood cells is dependent on the delivery of oxygen into the alveoli, the integrity of the alveoli membrane, adequate time for the red blood cells (RBC) to pass through the alveoli to collect the oxygen, the affinity of oxygen to the ferrous component of hemoglobin in the red blood cells, and the inspired partial pressure of oxygen. The partial pressure of oxygen is defined by the calculation: $PiO_2 \times FiO_2$ ($Pb - 47$ mm Hg). Pb is the barometric pressure. Pb decreases with increasing altitude and decreasing temperature. There is a direct correlation with Pb and oxygen availability.

* *

Normally, the PO_2 of inspired oxygen is 100% at sea level. The PO_2 of a RBC coming in the respiratory unit is 40 mm Hg. As the RBC travels through the capillaries in the respiratory unit, the large pressure gradient causes diffusion of oxygen from the alveoli into the RBC. A RBC spends 0.75 seconds in the respiratory unit. In normal resting conditions, the alveolar PO_2 is almost the same as capillary PO_2 by 0.33 seconds.

In patients with hypobaric hypoxemia such as found in high-altitude illness, there is a decrease in the oxygen pressure gradient; therefore there is less oxygen being diffused into the capillaries.[1-4] In exertion, this is worse since the red blood cells have less time to spend in the respiratory unit. Hypoxia inducible factor 1a (HIF-1a) is responsible for compensatory changes in high altitude, which includes: (1) hyperventilation, which causes decrease in PCO_2 and decrease in serum bicarbonate as a renal compensatory mechanism with subsequent diuresis; (2) increase in heart rate, cardiac output, and blood pressure; and (3) increased 2,3-DPG and red blood cell production.[1-4]

* *

The body's compensatory mechanism is called acclimatization. It starts within minutes and takes weeks to complete. The following illustrations depict the other types of hypoxia.

451

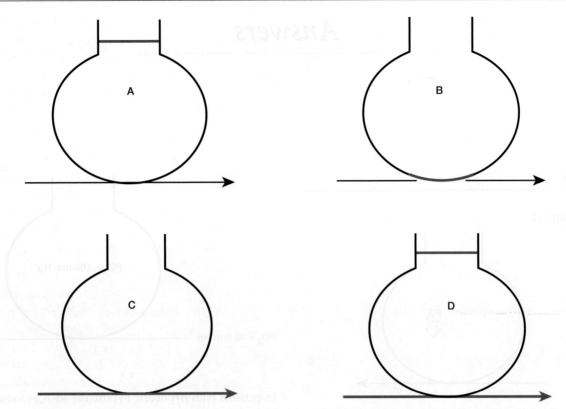

A: Atelectasis or pneumonia with decreased delivery of oxygen in the respiratory unit. **B:** Interstitial lung disease with decreased diffusion of oxygen via abnormalities with the alveolar membrane. **C:** Pulmonary hypertension with decreased transit time for red blood cells in the respiratory unit. **D:** ARDS. Multifactorial.

Question 2: A. High-altitude pulmonary edema (HAPE)
Symptoms related to this high-altitude illness resulting from hypobaric hypoxia begin within 6 to 12 hours in altitudes starting at 1,500 m but more common at >2,500 m.[3–5] Risk factors include prior history of HAI, vigorous exercise prior to ascent, substance abuse such as alcohol and other sedatives, neuromuscular or circulatory disease. Symptoms include headaches, dizziness, nausea, vomiting, malaise, paresthesias, and insomnia.[3–5] Progression of symptoms can lead to HAPE within 48 hours with bilateral infiltrates and secondary to mean pulmonary arterial pressure >40. High-altitude cerebral edema (HACE) can manifest with HAPE or manifest independently. Chronic mountain sickness or Monge's disease is the result of living at altitudes of >3,500 m for years and is characterized by polycythemia and hypoxia.[3–8] Periodic breathing of high altitude is a form of cheynnes stokes and is a neurologic response to hypoxia and respiratory alkalosis.

Question 3: A. Rapid descent to a lower altitude
Prevention of HAI includes: adequate rest prior to ascent, avoidance of alcohol and drugs, and acetazolamide 24 hours prior to ascent. For altitudes >2,500 to 3,000 m, it is recommended that patients can climb high but would have to descend >300 m to sleep. This is repeated multiple times until the patient is acclimated.

**

Mild symptoms can be treated with a day of rest and NSAIDS for headache, but progression to HAPE warrants descent and supplemental oxygen.

**

Initial treatment of HAPE includes oxygen supplementation, warmth and rest, and descent to <3,000 m. When descent is not possible or as an adjunct treatment, nifedipine, which acts to reduce pulmonary artery pressures and vascular resistance are given. Tadalafil and sildenafil have been given as treatment but their effectiveness is not fully studied. There is no role for diuretics in the treatment of high-altitude pulmonary edema. Dexamethasone is indicated severe high-altitude cerebral edema, and nifedipine or PDE 5 inhibitors are indicated for high-altitude pulmonary edema; treatment with these agents should be followed by descent as soon as possible.

Question 4: B. Oral acetazolamide
The use of acetazolamide can reduce the development of acute mountain sickness by as much as 75% and help in treatment. The optimal dose is unknown but it is generally recommended that 125 mg PO BID 24 hours before the ascent and continued for 48 hours. Higher doses may be used for ascents greater than 4,300 but generally not recommended due to higher risk of side effects such as paresthesias, polyuria, nausea, and sleepiness.

* *

Dexamethasone, 2 mg every 6 hours or 4 mg every 12 hours, can be used as an adjunct or alternative to acetazolamide, but generally less preferred because it doesn't allow acclimatization. Higher doses are recommended for >4,000 m.

* *

Other agents that can be used to reduce high-altitude pulmonary edema (HAPE) are nifedipine in a slow-release formulation at a dose of 30 mg twice per day, tadalafil (a phosphodiesterase-5 inhibitor) at a dose of 10 mg twice per day, and dexamethasone at a dose of 8 mg twice per day. They lower pulmonary-artery pressure and reduce the incidence of HAPE. Inhaled salmeterol, a long-acting β_2-agonist, at a high dose of 5 puffs (125 µg) twice per day, appears to be less effective.

CASE 2

Question 1: C. MRI of the brain
This patient's symptoms are consistent with high-altitude cerebral edema (HACE). This occurs in individuals with acute mountain sickness (AMS) and/or high-altitude pulmonary edema (HAPE) at elevations over 3,000 to 3,500 m.[9-10] The onset is usually delayed for 6 to 12 hours following arrival at high altitude, but can occur as rapidly as 1 to 2 hours or as late as 24 hours.[9-10] Symptoms include irritability, confusion, ataxia, stupor, and finally coma. Clinical examination may reveal papilledema, ataxia, retinal hemorrhages, and, occasionally, focal neurological deficits. WBC count may be elevated and the lumbar puncture may be bland except for an increased opening pressure. A chest radiograph may reveal pulmonary edema with hypoxemia on ABG. Computerized tomography (CT) of the brain may show cerebral edema and attenuation of signal more in the white matter than gray matter. MRI is more revealing and shows characteristic intense T2 signal in the white matter, especially in splenium of the corpus callosum. Since MRI may remain abnormal for days to weeks, it can be useful to establish the diagnosis of HACE even after recovery. Hemosiderin deposits may be present on MRI years after HACE.

Question 2: D. A and B
High-altitude cerebral edema (HACE) is a life-threatening condition and needs immediate medical management. Treatment is immediate descent >1,000 m, oxygen, and dexamethasone. Dexamethasone at an initial dose of 8 to 10 mg orally, intramuscularly (IM), or intravenously (IV), followed by 4 mg every 6 hours until complete descent is achieved. Symptoms can recur once the drug is stopped if descent has not been accomplished. Sufficient oxygen should be given to maintain the SpO_2 above 90%, flow of 2 to 4 L/min by facemask or nasal cannula is generally adequate. If descent is not possible, hyperbaric therapy chamber is utilized. It is a lightweight, manually inflated hyperbaric chamber that is common in remote mountain clinics and on expeditions. They are capable of simulating a descent of 2,500 m or more. Hyperbaric treatment should be combined with dexamethasone and supplemental oxygen to augment the effectiveness.

CASE 3

Question 1: A. Air travel after 3 days
According to the British Thoracic Society, patients who have had an acute STEMI with no signs of heart failure, age <60 years, and restored TIMI on angiography are considered low risk.[11] These patients can travel 3 days after onset of the acute event. Patients who had uncomplicated coronary artery bypass grafting are allowed to travel after 14 days of surgery only after pneumothorax is excluded on an x-ray because a pneumothorax is an absolute contraindication for air travel.[11-13] During ascent to high altitude there is air trapping which leads to expansion of gas during reduction in pressure that causes the pneumothorax to convert to tension

pneumothorax causing cardiopulmonary complications. Patients who undergo elective PTCA can fly 2 days after the procedure. Patients with NSTEMI should undergo angiography and revascularization before considering air travel. Unstable angina patients are advised not to fly until the issues are addressed. NYHA class IV patients are advised to refrain from air travel, but if it is absolutely necessary that these patients travel will need 2 L of in-flight oxygen and a wheelchair.[11–15]

Question 2: **D. A 34-year-old cystic fibrosis patient with resting room air SpO$_2$ <92%**

Contraindications to commercial air travel: (1) infectious tuberculosis; (2) pneumothorax with persistent air leak; (3) major hemoptysis; and (4) usual oxygen requirement at sea level at a flow rate exceeding 4 L/min. Patients with oxygen saturation <92% on room air at sea level require oxygen supplementation. Further testing such as hypoxia air challenge test is warranted if the oxygen saturation is between 92 to 95% with one of the following risk factors: (1) chest pain or dyspnea or prior air travel; (2) inability to walk 50 m without dyspnea; (3) hypercapnia; (4) FEV1 <50; (5) low DLCO; (6) restrictive lung disease, coronary artery disease, cerebrovascular disease, or pulmonary hypertension; and (7) recent hospitalization for respiratory disease. Hypoxic air challenge test might also be warranted if the patient has chronic respiratory disease despite oxygen saturation >95%. The hypoxia air challenge test, also called as hypoxia altitude simulation test (HAST), the high-altitude simulation test and hypoxia inhalation test, is used to assess the in-flight oxygen requirements during air travel.[14] During this procedure the patient is asked to breathe a mixture of gases via mask (15.1% oxygen mixed with nitrogen at sea level will correspond to an altitude of 8,000 ft). Arterial blood gases are obtained before and after the procedure. If the oxygen saturation remains at 88 or above or PaO$_2$ is greater than 55 mm Hg (7.4 kPa, approximately an SpO$_2$ of 88), supplemental oxygen is NOT required for air travel. If the PaO$_2$ decreases to <50 mm Hg (6.6 kPa, approximately an SpO$_2$ of 85), supplemental oxygen is advised for future air travel. If the PaO$_2$ is 50 to 55 mm Hg (6.6–7.4 kPa) the test is considered borderline. Additional testing is required that includes arterial blood gas sample or pulse oxygen saturation with mild exertion (e.g., walking) or 6-minute walk. Pneumothorax is an absolute contraindication for air travel. During ascent to high altitude, air trapping leads to expansion of gas. The reduction in pressure causes the pneumothorax to convert to tension pneumothorax.

CASE 4

Question 1: **D. P = k$_H$C**

The patient has decompression sickness (DCS). When a diver is exposed to pressures greater than 1 atm, the tissue uptake of inert gases, like nitrogen, is elevated and the pressure gradient develops as they ascend to the surface. Nitrogen leaves the tissue, dissolving into the blood and passing to the lungs, where it is exhaled. With rapid ascent a sheer pressure gradient develops leading to the formation of intravascular nitrogen gas bubbles that pass through vital organs causing symptoms.[16–17] This is explained by Henry's law which states that at a constant temperature, the amount of a given gas that dissolves in a given type and volume of liquid is directly proportional to the partial pressure of that gas in equilibrium with that liquid. The equation is P = k$_H$C where P = pressure, C is concentration and k$_H$ is a constant.

* *

There are two types of decompression sickness: type I with rash, localized pain usually in elbow or shoulder, lymphadenopathy or edema and type II with neurologic manifestations such as paresthesias, weakness, and progression to paraplegia, shortness of breath and chest pain as venous air embolism travels to the pulmonary and cardiac circulation system. Symptoms can occur within 1 hour in 75% of cases, but 90% occur within 12 hours.[18–21]

* *

The other answer choices are as follows: Boyle's law (P$_1$V$_1$ = P$_2$V$_2$) which states that the product of pressure and volume of a gas is constant as long as temperature is constant. This can be found in barotrauma and air embolism. Dalton's law (P$_{total}$ = P$_1$ + P$_2$ + P$_N$) states that the total pressure is the sum of partial pressures of individual gases. Charles' law (V$_1$/V$_2$ = T$_1$/T$_2$) states that at a constant pressure, gas expands in proportion to temperature increase. Avogadro's law (V$_1$/N$_1$ = V$_2$/N$_2$) states that equal volumes of different gases contain the same number of molecules at constant temperature and pressure.

* *

Risk factors include fast ascent, right to left shunt, male, and air travel. The current recommendations from Divers Alert Network (DAN) and underwater and hyperbaric medicine guidelines regarding air travel after diving include: (1) at least 12 hours after a single dive and (2) at least 24 hours after repetitive, multiple diving.[18–23] Diving after prolonged flying also increases risk for DCS.

DAN recommends a period of at least 12 hours (ideally 24 hours) after the flight, with appropriate rest, nutrition, and hydration, before diving.

* *

Prevention includes an ascent rate of 10 m per minute, breathing mixtures with less inert gas after the dive, and pre-breathing oxygen before the dive to remove excess nitrogen.

Question 2: A. 100% oxygen and hyperbaric therapy

The treatment of decompression sickness includes hydration; administration of 100% oxygen once there is a clinical suspicion of decompression sickness/illness. An oxygen administration decrease the nitrogen concentration and volume of bubbles and occasionally symptoms may resolve but frequently recur therefore oxygen is not a replacement for hyperbaric oxygen (HBO). Delay in transferring the patients to center that provides HBO can result in poor outcomes. Trendelenburg position is no longer advocated since it can lead to cerebral edema. The supine position is desired in a conscious patient because the rate of nitrogen washout is greater compared to sitting. Other measures include frequent examination, hydration and normothermia. The mainstay of treatment of is therapeutic recompression while the patient is breathing oxygen. The patient should be recompressed as soon as possible; however, patients should be considered for recompression even after several days delay. Treatments should be repeated if possible until symptoms have either resolved or stabilized. Appropriate hydration is essential; the use of HBO is generally safe, relatively nontoxic. Pharmacologic agents (e.g., anticoagulants, antiplatelet agents, corticosteroids) may be useful adjuncts to recompression therapy. Intravenous isotonic fluids without glucose are recommended because dehydration is common and hydration may increase the washout of gases.

* *

Hyperbaric oxygen therapy (HBO) decreases the volume and the size of air bubbles and in the blood. Most HBO treatments are performed at 2 to 3 atmospheres absolute (ATA). In air embolism and decompression sickness, where pressure is directly proportional to therapeutic effect, treatments frequently start at 6 ATA. At 5 atm, a bubble is reduced to 20% of its original volume and 60% of its original diameter. This additional pressure, when associated with inspiration of high levels of oxygen, substantially increases the level of oxygen dissolved into blood plasma. The hyperoxia is the second beneficial effect of hyperbaric oxygen therapy, which increases oxygenation. In addition, plasma nitrogen concentration decreases, increasing the gradient of nitrogen from bubble to plasma, thus accelerating the absorption of bubbles.

* *

Hyperbaric therapy should be undertaken for at least 4 hours, since bubble elimination may be poor in areas of reduced blood flow.

CASE 5

Question 1: A. Ear barotrauma

Barotrauma is a consequence of pressures in air filled body cavities failing to equilibrate following environmental changes. Barotrauma can manifest as pulmonary edema, pulmonary hemorrhage, pneumomediastinum, and pneumothorax.[24,25] Air can embolize to venous circulation. This can lead to ischemic consequences such as myocardial infarction and cerebrovascular accident. Middle-ear barotrauma is the most common complication from diving. The symptoms are pressure, pain, hearing loss, nausea, and vomiting.

Question 2: A. Nitrogen narcosis

Nitrogen narcosis mimics alcohol intoxication/sedative abuse causing loss of motor function and decision-making ability. It is caused by the raised partial pressure of nitrogen in nervous system tissue and occurs at depths >100 ft. At depths >300 ft the diver can become unconscious. Treatment would be a gradual ascent. Risk factors include hypercapnia, alcoholism, fatigue, and hypothermia.

Question 3: A. Aseptic bone necrosis

Aseptic bone necrosis is also called dysbaric osteonecrosis (DON) and seen in personnel working in high-pressure environments like professional divers, instructors, tunnel workers/dive masters and less commonly in recreational SCUBA divers. The most common bones that are affected are the femur, humerus, and tibia. It is a consequence of nitrogen bubbles that enter bone marrow and obstruction of circulation. This triggers the coagulation cascade and causes increased thrombosis leading to decreased blood flow and osteonecrosis. Other theories include fat embolism, increase in the plasma levels of plasminogen activator inhibitor-1 (PAI-1) that may also result in thrombus formation and thus contribute to the development of ischemia.[26]

**

Patients may present asymptomatically, and typical radiographic findings include decalcification of bone, cystic lesions, osteosclerotic patterns, nontraumatic fractures and a subchondral crescent sign. Treatment options are less promising and often require joint replacement. Rehabilitation, physical therapy and bisphosphonate therapies are effective to an extent as well.

**

The best treatment is prevention by using the safest decompression possible to avoid adverse after effects.

CASE 6

Question 1: A. Intubate

Securing the airway with a large endotracheal tube is mandatory if there is evidence of stridor, wheeze, facial burns, and edema or blisters in oropharynx because of the risk of developing severe edema. Observation is warranted with the absence of these signs. If there is erythema in the oropharynx, laryngoscopy is option to further investigate the pharynx. Corticosteroids show no benefit and can predispose patients to infections, particularly *Staphylococcus aureus* and *Pseudomonas aeruginosa*.

Question 2: A. A

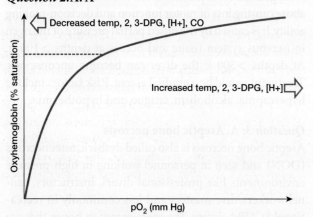

Reproduced with permission from West JB. Respiratory physiology: The essentials. 8th edition. Baltimore, MD: Lippincott Williams & Wilkins; 2012.

**

Oxyhemoglobin dissociation curve illustrates oxygen's tendency to bind to hemoglobin.

**

Bohr effect is a phenomenon which states the hemoglobin's binding affinity for oxygen is lessen with increased production of carbon dioxide and subsequently acidosis. This releases more oxygen into tissues. It begins with increased metabolic rate of tissues increasing production of carbon dioxide. Carbon dioxide then interacts with H_2O to bicarbonate through the equation:

$$CO_2 + H_2O = H_2CO_3 = H^+ + HCO_3^-$$

This process is accelerated by carbonic anhydrase. The abundance of oxygen and subsequent binding to hemoglobin causes release of protons or [H+] which binds to bicarbonate and carbon dioxide is released via exhalation. 2,3-Diphosphoglycerate (2,3-DPG) is formed in RBC as a response to hypoxia and anemia. It allows more unloading of oxygen into tissues. At the same time, deoxygenated hemoglobin has increased affinity for carbon dioxide which is defined as the Haldane effect.

**

The diagnosis of carbon monoxide (CO) poisoning is clinical. It is suspected if: (1) recent history of carbon monoxide poisoning/exposure; (2) symptoms consistent with CO poisoning that include headache, nausea/vomiting, confusion, dizziness, fatigue, chest pain, arrhythmia, loss of conscious; and (3) elevated carboxyhemoglobin levels. Carboxyhemoglobin threshold for CO monoxide poisoning includes: 3% above baseline in nonsmokers and 15% above baseline in smokers.[27-29] Venous or arterial samples can be used to assess the carboxyhemoglobin levels. Pulse oximetry is not a reliable measure of oxygenation in carbon monoxide poisoning because the pulse oximeter cannot differentiate between carboxyhemoglobin and oxyhemoglobin because of similar absorbance at wavelength 660 nm.[29] Therefore, the patient would have falsely elevated oxygen saturation.

Question 3: E. A 45-year-old man with history smoking and COHgb of >15

The treatment for CO poisoning is 100% oxygen in every patient and hyperbaric oxygen in few individuals who have symptoms of severe carbon monoxide poisoning. The patients that would benefit from HBO therapy include:[30]

- Carboxyhemoglobin level >25% or base excess lower than −2 mmol/L
- Asymptomatic patients with carboxyhemoglobin levels exceeding 40%
- Individuals with loss of consciousness due to CO poisoning
- Prolonged period of exposure to carbon monoxide poisoning
- Evidence of end organ damage

- Metabolic acidosis with pH <7.1
- Myocardial ischemia
- Pregnant patients with COHgb of >20%

**

The HBO therapy is delivered at 2.5 to 3.0 atm, which increases the dissolved oxygen content and increases the removal of carbon monoxide from the blood. It also avoids long-term morbidity from neurocognitive deficits associated with severe carbon monoxide poisoning. This therapy prevents lipid peroxidation in the brain, decreases inflammation, preserves adenosine triphosphate functionality and helps attention/concentration/memory deficits and is beneficial if given with 6 hours of exposure.

Question 4: C. Pneumothorax

The only absolute contraindication to hyperbaric oxygen (HBO) therapy is pneumothorax which can progress to tension pneumothorax. In these conditions the pneumothorax has to be decompressed before starting HBO therapy with a chest tube placement. There are multiple relative contraindications like COPD, asthma, sinus infections, recent ear or thoracic surgery, high-grade fever, and claustrophobia. In these conditions, the treating clinician should weigh the benefits of the treatment to avoid life-threatening neurological complications/adverse outcomes. Diseases like COPD and asthma may be at high risk of having pneumothorax. Pregnancy was once believed to represent a contraindication to HBO but no proven evidence to toxicity to fetus. Patients with seizure disorder are at increased risk of complications from central nervous system toxicity from high oxygen concentrations and also lower the seizure threshold. Patients on medications like doxorubicin (adriamycin), bleomycin, cisplatin are relative contraindications. Doxorubicin paired with oxidative stress might worsen cardio toxicity. Oxygen therapy and bleomycin can cause pulmonary toxicity, it is not clear if the effect of pulmonary toxicity is a synergistic effect of oxygen and the medication. HBO with cisplatin therapy impairs wound healing. Disulfiram (antabuse) blocks the production of superoxide dismutase, which protects against oxygen toxicity.

Question 5: C. Sodium nitrite

Cyanide poisoning can occur concurrently with carbon monoxide poisoning. It is associated with the following exposures: domestic fires, metal extraction in mining, plastics and rubber manufacturing, pesticides, amygdalin, sodium nitroprusside, and diets consisting of bitter almond, apricot, plum, peach, pear, apple, and cassava root.[31-33] Cyanide binds to the ferric ion of cytochrome oxidase A3, preventing the shuttling of electrons through the electron transport chain and the formation of ATP, and leading to lactic acidosis. Cyanide also neutralizes antioxidants leading to accumulation of oxygen-free radicals. It inhibits glutamic acid decarboxylase (GAD), which decreases GABA and can lead to seizures. Cyanide is rapidly absorbed through the respiratory tract, gastrointestinal tract, and skin. Patients can develop neurologic complications such as headaches, seizures, coma, delayed onset parkinsonism, tropical ataxic neuropathy particularly from cassava ingestion, shock, arrhythmias, pulmonary edema, abdominal pain, dermatitis, flushing and then cyanosis, renal failure, rhabdomyolysis, and hepatic failure.

**

Tests that can lead to a diagnosis of cyanide poisoning include elevated lactate levels, venous hyperoxia, and cyanide levels. A couple of caveats: (1) There is elevated central venous oxygen because of abundance of oxygen from lack of extraction of tissues but this is nonspecific and can be seen in carbon monoxide poisoning and hydrogen sulfide; and (2) Cyanide levels can take time to obtain.

**

Detoxification involves two processes to convert cyanide to water soluble molecules: (1) rhodanese, an enzyme found abundantly in liver and muscles, converts cyanide to thiocyanate via thiosulfate as a sulfur donor; and (2) hydroxocobalamin combines with cyanide to form cyanocobalamin. Antidotes include sodium thiosulfate at 50 mL of 25% solution and hydroxycobalamin at 70 mg/kg IV or dicobalt edetate 1.5% of 20 mL solution IV. Side effects include: (1) psychosis, arthralgias, vomiting, and myalgias for thiosulfate levels >10 mg/dL; (2) rash, headache, chest pain, and dysphagia for hydroxycobalamin; and (3) seizures, arrhythmias, hypotension with dicobalt edetate.

**

Another treatment is to induce methemoglobinemia. This allows an alternative binding site for cyanide and formation of cyanomethemoglobin which is less toxic. This can be performed with administration of amyl nitrite which induces 5% methemoglobinemia, and sodium nitrite which induces 15% to 20% methemoglobinemia, or dimethylaminophenol. This strategy is contraindicated in patients with concomitant carbon monoxide toxicity. The reason is that methemoglobin furthers shifts the oxygen-hemoglobin dissociation curve to the left, preventing more oxygen deliver to tissues. Antidote for methemoglobinemia, methylene blue, is avoided because it can release cyanide.

REFERENCES

1. West JB. High-altitude medicine. *Am J Respir Crit Care Med*. 2012;186(2):1229–1237.

2. Bärtsch P, Swenson E. Acute high-altitude illnesses. *N Engl J Med*. 2013;368:2294–2302.

3. Maggiorini M et al. High-altitude pulmonary edema is initially caused by an increase in capillary pressure. *Circulation*. 2001;103:2078–2083.

4. Basnyat B, Murdoch DR. High-altitude illness. *Lancet*. 2003;361(9373):1967–1974.

5. Hopkins SR, Garg J, Bolar DS, et al. Pulmonary blood flow heterogeneity during hypoxia and high-altitude pulmonary edema. *Am J Respir Crit Care Med*. 2005;171(1):83–87.

6. Frisancho R. Developmental functional adaptation to high altitude: Review. *Am J Hum Biol*. 2013;25:151–168.

7. Arias-Stella J, Krüger H, Recavarren S, et al. Pathology of chronic mountain sickness. *Thorax*. 1973;28;701–708.

8. Wang GD, Fan RX, Zhai W, et al. Genetic convergence in the adaptation of dogs and humans to the high altitude environment of the Tibetan plateau. *Genome Biol Evol*. 2014;6(8):2122–2128.

9. Wilson MH, Newman S, Imray CH. The cerebral effects of ascent to high altitudes. *Lancet Neurol*. 2009;8(2):175–191.

10. Hackett PH, Yarnell PR, Hill R, et al. High-altitude cerebral edema evaluated with magnetic resonance imaging: clinical correlation and pathophysiology. *JAMA*. 1998;280:1920–1925.

11. British Thoracic Society Standards of Care Committee. Managing passengers with respiratory disease planning air travel: British Thoracic Society recommendations. *Thorax*. 2002;57:289–304.

12. Graeme CP, Kennedy AM, Paterson E, et al. A chronic pneumothorax and fitness to fly. *Thorax*. 2007;62(2):187–189.

13. Hu X, Cowl CT, Baqir M, et al. Air travel and pneumothorax. *Chest*. 2014;145(4):688–694.

14. Dine CJ, Kreider ME. Hypoxia altitude simulation test. *Chest*. 2008;133(4):1002–1005.

15. Edvardsen A, Akerø A, Christensen CC, et al. Air travel and chronic obstructive pulmonary disease: a new algorithm for pre-flight evaluation. *Thorax*. 2012;67(11):964–969.

16. West JB, Schoene RB, Milledge JS. *High Altitude Medicine and Physiology*. Hodder Arnold, London; 2007.

17. Hackett PH, Roach RC. High-altitude medicine. In: Auerbach PS eds. *Wilderness Medicine*. 5th ed. Philadelphia, PA: Mosby; 2007.

18. Vann RD, Gerth WA, Denoble PJ, et al. Experimental trials to assess the risks of decompression sickness in flying after diving. *Undersea Hyperb Med*. 2004 Winter;31(4):431–444.

19. https://www.diversalertnetwork.org/research/projects/fad/index.asp Accessed on December 10, 2014.

20. Lindholm P, Lundgren CE. The physiology and pathophysiology of human breath-hold diving. *J Appl Physiol(1985)*. 2009;106(1):284–292.

21. Vann RD, Butler FK, Mitchell SJ, et al. Decompression illness. *Lancet*. 2011;377(9760):153–164.

22. Bove AA. Diving medicine. *Am J Respir Crit Care Med*. 2014;189(12):1479–1486.

23. Gempp E, Blatteau JE. Risk factors and treatment outcome in SCUBA divers with spinal cord decompression sickness. *J Crit Care*. 2010;25(2):236–242.

24. DeGorordo A, Vallejo-Manzur F, Chanin K, et al. Diving emergencies. *Resuscitation*. 2003;59(2):171–180.

25. McMullin AM. SCUBA diving: What you and your patients need to know. *Cleve Clin J Med*. 2006;73(8):711–716.

26. Miyanishi K, Kamo Y, Ihara H, et al. Risk factors for dysbaric osteonecrosis. *Rheumatology (Oxford)*. 2006;45(7):855–858.

27. Weaver LK, Valentine KJ, Hopkins RO. Carbon monoxide poisoning: risk factors for cognitive sequelae and the role of hyperbaric oxygen. *Am J Respir Crit Care Med*. 2007;176:491–497.

28. Simini B. Cherry-red discoloration in carbon monoxide poisoning. *Lancet*. 1988;352:1154.

29. Hampson NB. Pulse oximetry in severe carbon monoxide poisoning. *Chest*. 1998;114:1036–1041.

30. Lindell K. Weaver, hyperbaric oxygen for acute carbon monoxide poisoning *N Engl J Med*. 2002;347:1057–1067.

31. Hamel J. A review of acute cyanide poisoning with a treatment update. *Crit Care Nurse*. 2011;31(1)):72–81.

32. Borron SW, Baud FJ, Megarbane B, et al. Hydroxocobalamin for severe acute cyanide poisoning by ingestion or inhalation. *Am J Emerg Med*. 2007;25(5):551–558.

33. Hall AH, Dart R, Bogdan G. Sodium thiosulfate or hydroxocobalamin for the empiric treatment of cyanide poisoning? *Ann Emerg Med*. Jun. 207;49(6):806–813.

25

Cardiothoracic Surgery

Stephen Spindel MD and Dong-Seok Lee MD

CASE 1

Question 1: **The Chamberlain procedure is used for which lymph node stations?**

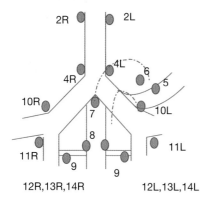

A. 5, 6
B. 12R, 13R, 14R
C. 7, 8, 9
D. 2R, 4R, 10R
E. 5, 10 L,11 L

CASE 2

A 60-year-old man with history of COPD is noted to have a left lower lobe mass with an enlarged lymph node at station 4R.

Question 1: **What is the TNM stage?**

A. Stage I
B. Stage II
C. Stage IIIA
D. Stage IIIB
E. Stage IV

He opts to undergo mediastinoscopy and develops fevers to 39.5°C, chest pain, subcutaneous emphysema, and has a WBC of 17,000. Computed tomography image is below.

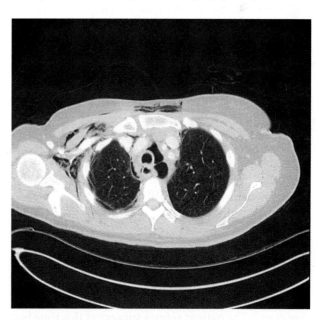

Question 2: **What is the best next step?**

A. CT angiography
B. Esophagram
C. Oral antibiotics
D. Continuous positive airway pressure (CPAP)
E. Serial chest radiographs for 24 hours

Question 3: Which answer is correct when comparing cervical mediastinoscopy to endobronchial ultrasound-guided needle aspiration (EBUS-NA) in patients with nonsmall cell lung cancer and mediastinal lymphadenopathy?

A. Cervical mediastinoscopy clearly shows superior specificity
B. EBUS-NA clearly shows superior specificity
C. The specificity for cervical mediastinoscopy and EBUS-NA is similar
D. Cervical mediastinoscopy shows clear superior sensitivity
E. EBUS-NA shows clear superior sensitivity

CASE 3

A 46-year-old man has been treated with antibiotics multiple times for recurrent lingular pneumonia over the past year. He is sent to a pulmonologist who orders a CT scan showing a spherical 2- × 1-cm solid endoluminal mass with complete obstruction of the lingular division of the left upper lobe bronchus, collapse of the lingula, and no mediastinal lymphadenopathy. A fusion PET/CT shows the endoluminal mass as being minimally hypermetabolic with no hypermetabolic mediastinal lymph nodes. Bronchoscopy with biopsy is performed, showing a smooth red-brown endobronchial mass isolated to the lingular bronchus with minimal involvement of the upper division of the left upper lobe bronchus. The biopsy results are consistent with typical carcinoid tumor.

Question 1: Which of the following is the most appropriate procedure for this patient?

A. Wedge resection
B. Lobectomy
C. Sleeve lobectomy
D. Pneumonectomy
E. Chemotherapy

Question 2: The patient refuses surgery at this time but returns 1 year later after more episodes of pneumonia. Bronchoscopy now shows the mass completely obstructs the left upper lobe bronchus and protrudes into the left mainstem bronchus with sparing of the lower lobe bronchus. Bronchoscopic image is below. No mediastinal lymphadenopathy is seen on CT scan.

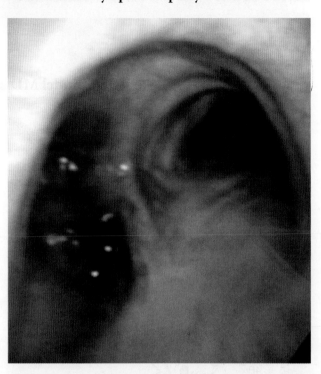

What is the most appropriate intervention?

A. Wedge resection
B. Lobectomy
C. Sleeve lobectomy
D. Pneumonectomy
E. The mass is unresectable

Question 3: On postoperative day 1, the patient's pain is poorly controlled. He is tachypneic with a poor cough and oxygen saturation of 84% on room air. His temperature is 38.2°C and WBC is 12,000. Physical examination reveals rales more prominent on the right hemithorax. Chest physiotherapy and bronchodilators have little effect. Chest tube output is appropriate and there is no air leak. Below are his images immediately postoperatively and on postoperative day 1.

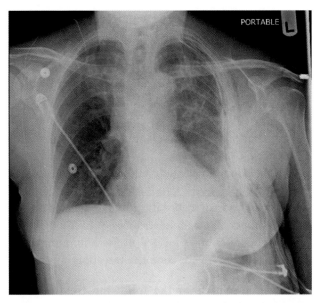

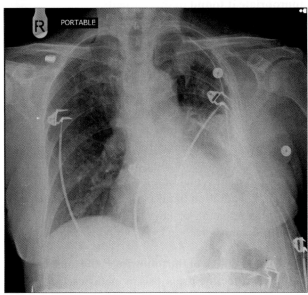

What is the best next step?

A. Serial troponins
B. CT angiography
C. Insertion of right-sided chest tube
D. Bedside awake bronchoscopy
E. Removal of left-sided chest tube

Question 4: **Which of the following is true regarding the US Preventive Services Task Force (USPSTF) recommendations for lung cancer screening?**

A. This patient should have been screened with yearly CT scans prior to his diagnosis
B. A 56-year-old male with 35 pack-years smoking history should undergo yearly CT scans

C. Semi-annual CT scans are recommended for a 63-year-old female with 45 pack-years smoking history
D. USPSTF recommends biannual CT scans for 60-year-old patients with smoking history greater than 40 pack-years
E. An 87-year-old female should undergo biannual CT scans if her smoking history is greater than 30 pack-years

CASE 4

A 77-year-old former heavy smoker with heart disease undergoes a low-dose CT scan showing a 1-cm peripheral, spiculated ground glass nodule in the right lower lobe which appears not to involve the visceral pleura and there is no mediastinal lymphadenopathy. A PET scan proves the lesion is hypermetabolic and the mediastinum has no FDG uptake. His cardiologist has cleared him for surgery and his pulmonary function test (PFT) results show 45% and 29% of predicted values for predicted postoperative forced expiratory volume in 1 second (PPO FEV_1) and predicted postoperative diffusing capacity for carbon monoxide (PPO DLco), respectively. His preoperative vital signs are heart rate of 72, blood pressure of 118/82, oxygen saturation of 94% on room air, and body mass index of 25.

Question 1: **What is the most appropriate initial procedure to diagnose this lung lesion?**

A. Open-wedge resection
B. Open lobectomy
C. CT-guided transthoracic needle biopsy
D. Endoscopic ultrasound guided needle aspiration
E. Elevated serum CA-125

Question 2: **With this patient's pulmonary function test results, what is the next step after the diagnosis is made?**

A. Shuttle-walk test
B. Formal cardiopulmonary exercise test
C. Proceed directly to surgery
D. Chemotherapy
E. Observation with biannual CT scans

Question 3: **If the lesion is positive for nonsmall cell lung cancer and his maximal oxygen consumption (VO_2 max) is 9 mL/kg/min, which of the following is the most appropriate option for this patient?**

A. VATS wedge resection
B. Open lobectomy

C. Sleeve lobectomy

D. Preoperative chemotherapy followed by either wedge resection or lobectomy

E. Chemotherapy without surgery

Question 4: **What risk factor is most associated with postoperative atrial fibrillation in lung resection patients?**

A. Diabetes mellitus

B. Female gender

C. Age

D. Smoking history

E. Obesity

CASE 5

A 45-year-old healthy woman nonsmoker has bloody stools and undergoes CT scan and colonoscopy showing colon adenocarcinoma. She receives appropriate treatment including resection and chemotherapy, but 6 months later a new 1-cm smooth spherical nodule is found in the periphery of the right middle lobe during screening CT scan. Full-body PET scan shows the nodule is hypermetabolic, no FDG uptake in the mediastinum with normal-sized nodes, and no signs of metastatic lesions elsewhere. The abdomen appears free from disease. Results from fine-needle aspiration prove the lesion to be adenocarcinoma of colonic origin. Her pulmonary function test shows FEV_1 110% of predicted and DLco 108% of predicted. Computed tomography image is below.

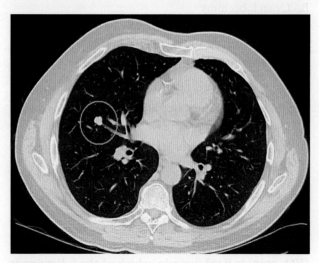

Question 1: **What is the best next step?**

A. Cervical mediastinoscopy

B. Wedge resection

C. Lobectomy

D. Palliative medical treatment only; no surgery

E. Observation with biannual CT scan

Question 2: **What finding would make a metastasectomy a contraindication in this patient?**

A. Right pleural fluid cytology positive for adenocarcinoma

B. An additional metastatic nodule located in the same lobe

C. An additional metastatic nodule located in the left upper lobe

D. Two additional metastatic nodules located in the right upper and right lower lobes

E. The single lesion is located in the hilum, requiring pneumonectomy for complete resection

Question 3: **Which of the following treatments is appropriate if found in this patient?**

A. Wedge resection of lung plus hepatic resection for single metastasis found on liver in addition to the peripheral lung lesion

B. Wedge resection of lung plus parietal pleurectomy for diffuse pleural tumor seeding found in addition to the peripheral lung lesion

C. Wedge resection of lung if abdominal carcinomatosis found in addition to the peripheral lung lesion

D. Wedge resection of lung plus pericardiectomy for discontinuous metastatic lesions on pericardium found in addition to the peripheral lung lesion

E. Wedge resection of lung plus prophylactic parietal pleurectomy

Question 4: **Which of the following is the most important factor affecting prognosis in metastasectomy?**

A. Age

B. Complete versus incomplete resection of lesion

C. Unilateral versus bilateral disease

D. Wedge resection versus lobectomy

E. Smoking history

CASE 6

A malnourished 59-year-old IV drug abuser with diabetes mellitus presents to the emergency department with a productive cough and dyspnea for 3 days. He is febrile to 38.7°C and his WBC is 14,000. A chest CT scan shows right lower lobe pneumonia with a moderate-sized right pleural effusion. There is no rim enhancement and no signs of loculations in the effusion. Thoracentesis is performed and pleural fluid studies sent, which show pH 7.10 and glucose 30 mg/dL.

Question 1: What is the best treatment at this time?

A. Outpatient treatment with oral antibiotics
B. Inpatient treatment with oral antibiotics
C. Inpatient treatment with IV antibiotics alone
D. Inpatient treatment with IV antibiotics and insertion of a chest tube
E. Posterolateral thoracotomy and decortication

Question 2: The patient refuses treatment and leaves the hospital against medical advice. He returns 3 weeks later with a temperature of 39.1°C and WBC of 17,000. Computed tomography shows a very large right loculated pleural effusion with bubbles of air, positive rim enhancement, and thickened parietal pleura. Intravenous antibiotics are initiated. Computed tomography images are below.

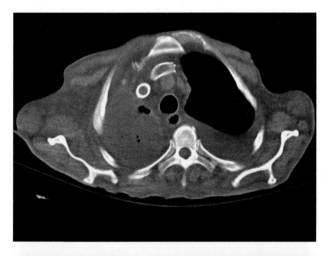

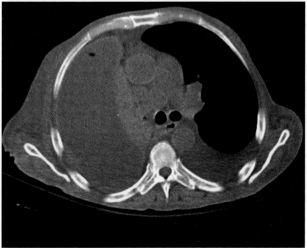

Which treatment will be most effective for this patient?

A. Bronchoscopy
B. Insertion of a chest tube alone
C. Insertion of a chest tube and bedside talc pleurodesis
D. Open-window thoracostomy via modified Eloesser flap
E. Posterolateral thoracotomy and decortication

Question 3: Surgery is performed, but the patient is unable to be extubated in the operating room. After 2 weeks postoperatively, he requires a tracheostomy and remains with persistent fevers up to 39.5°C, WBC of 19,000, and radiographs showing poor lung expansion. His albumin is 2.1 g/dL and total protein is 5.2 g/dL. What is the best treatment at this time?

A. Extrapleural pneumolysis via Lucite-ball plombage
B. VATS decortication
C. Open-window thoracostomy via modified Eloesser flap
D. Posterolateral thoracotomy and decortication
E. Prolonging current course of IV antibiotics

Question 4: What is the most common cause of empyema?

A. Iatrogenic
B. Thoracic trauma
C. Subphrenic abscess
D. Pneumonia
E. Diverticulitis

CASE 7

A 77-year-old male smoker with diabetes mellitus is 3 weeks postoperatively from a right pneumonectomy with preoperative chemoradiation for nonsmall cell lung cancer. His course was complicated by prolonged intubation requiring tracheostomy. He now develops an acute onset productive cough with copious serosanguinous fluid. He is afebrile, normotensive, and has a WBC of 9,000. Below are his chest radiographs before and after this new event.

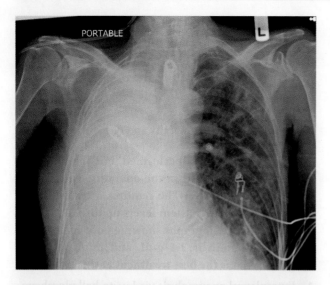

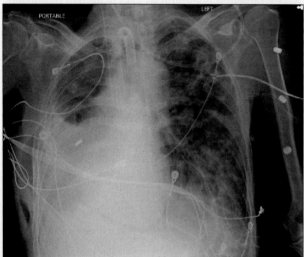

Question 1: **Which of the following is the best method for diagnosis?**

A. Esophagram
B. Exploratory thoracotomy
C. Bronchogram
D. Bronchoscopy
E. Repeat chest radiograph

Question 2: **What is the best initial treatment?**

A. Tube thoracostomy and intravenous antibiotics
B. Esophageal stent and intravenous antibiotics
C. Tracheal stent and intravenous antibiotics
D. Intravenous antibiotics alone
E. Daily therapeutic bronchoscopy to clear secretions

Question 3: **What is the recommended surgical treatment for this patient?**

A. Endobronchial valve placement
B. Endobronchial fibrin plug
C. Thoracotomy with debridement and additional chest tube placement (closed chest tube drainage)
D. Thoracotomy with debridement, muscle flap transposition, and open thoracic window
E. Thoracotomy with debridement and creation of esophageal spit fistula

Question 4: **Which of the following is true?**

A. Radiotherapy is not a risk factor for bronchopleural fistula
B. Candida species are the most common causative organisms for postpneumonectomy empyema
C. Right-sided postpneumonectomy bronchopleural fistulas are more common than left-sided ones
D. Postpneumonectomy esophagopleural fistulas have an incidence of 5%
E. Aggressive treatment including esophagectomy is indicated in most postpneumonectomy esophagopleural fistulas

Answers

CASE 1

Question 1: A. 5, 6

Mediastinal staging is a key aspect when investigating lung cancer, especially when the probability of mediastinal nodal metastases (i.e., clinical N2 disease) is high. De Langen et al.[1] showed that CT scan results with mediastinal lymph nodes measuring 1.0 to 1.5 cm correspond to a 29% probability of mediastinal nodal metastasis and nodes greater than 1.5 cm in size demonstrate a 66% probability of mediastinal nodal metastasis. Therefore, invasive staging is recommended to rule out N2 disease in these patients. Meanwhile, Meyers[2] showed that clinical stage I lung cancer patients with mediastinal and hilar nodes less than 1.0 cm in size have only a 6% chance of mediastinal metastasis and thus benefit little from routine invasive mediastinal staging techniques. In general, the indications for invasive mediastinal staging for non-small cell lung cancer include lymph nodes greater than 1 cm (short axis on CT scan), hypermetabolic uptake on PET scan, or possible need for induction therapy.[3]

* *

Many options exist for invasive mediastinal staging techniques, including endobronchial ultrasound-guided needle aspiration (EBUS-NA), cervical mediastinoscopy, anterior mediastinotomy, and open or VATS mediastinal lymph node sampling. The choice depends on the location of suspicious lymph nodes. The lymphatic drainage of left lower lobe tumors heads first to the subcarinal lymph nodes and then either contralateral or ipsilateral paratracheal nodes. On the other hand, left upper lobe tumors drain into the aorto-pulmonary window nodes first then usually to the left paratracheal lymph nodes. Right-sided lymphatic pathways mainly drain to ipsilateral nodal stations and less often contralaterally.[4] Cervical mediastinoscopy can access nodal stations 2, 3, 4, and 7; while left anterior mediastinotomy (Chamberlain procedure) can access the aorto-pulmonary window lymph nodes.[5] In this patient with suspicious nodal levels 4R and 7, a cervical mediastinoscopy would be best to assess for N2 and N3 diseases. The Chamberlain procedure and left mediastinal lymph node sampling cannot assess 4R. The lymphatic system of the lungs does not drain into the axillary lymph nodes.

CASE 2

Question 1: D. Stage IIIB

Using TNM classification from the American Joint Committee on Cancer (AJCC) staging manual,[6] a positive contralateral mediastinal lymph node (N3 disease) in a patient with no evidence of systemic metastasis is classified as Stage IIIB. Positive contralateral nodes greatly decreases survival rates and is overwhelmingly considered a contraindication to surgery. A 0% 3-year survival rate for patients with N3 disease who underwent chemoradiation with surgical resection was demonstrated by the Southwest Oncology Group.[7]

Question 2: B. Esophagram

Although complications from cervical mediastinoscopy are uncommon, the results can often be disastrous. Major complications include massive hemorrhage, esophageal perforation, and stroke due to innominate artery compression. Clinical presentation of an esophageal perforation is often nonspecific, including acute chest pain, abdominal pain, dyspnea, subcutaneous emphysema, and fever. Thus, suspicion should be high after any procedure involving or adjacent to the esophagus. An esophagram confirms the diagnosis of perforation[8] but more recently the use of CT scanning with oral contrast has increased as the diagnostic modality of choice.[9] Early use of intravenous antibiotics should be initiated and the patient should be kept nil by mouth.[8] These patients often require surgical repair.

Question 3: C. The specificity for cervical mediastinoscopy and EBUS-NA is similar

Endobronchial ultrasound needle aspiration is a transbronchial minimally invasive mediastinal staging technique which is seeing increased application and acceptance

465

in the preoperative evaluation of lung cancer. With the exception of stations 5, 6, 8, and 9, EBUS-NA can assess all other mediastinal nodes, as well as hilar nodes at levels 10, 11, and part of 12, making it a useful tool in detecting N1, N2, and N3 diseases.[10] While EBUS-NA can successfully access superior mediastinal lymph nodes, endoscopic ultrasound-guided needle aspiration (EUS-NA) can better access the posterior and inferior mediastinal nodes. EUS-NA deploys a transesophageal route sampling stations 5, 7, 8, and 9, and is often combined with EBUS-NA for near-complete evaluation of the mediastinum.[11] There is increasing evidence of EBUS and EUS being equally effective as mediastinoscopy for staging of nonsmall cell lung cancer, with prospective studies by Ernst[12] showing 87% sensitivity and 100% specificity of EBUS, and Larsen et al.[13] publishing 78% sensitivity and 100% specificity of EUS. Other studies have shown lower sensitivity in EBUS and EUS versus mediastinoscopy, but specificity remains 100%. Mediastinoscopy has an 81% sensitivity and 100% specificity, and remains the gold standard.[14] For evaluating mediastinal lymphadenopathy not associated with lung cancer, mediastinoscopy remains the gold standard but recent evidence shows endoscopic techniques having comparative effectiveness for diagnosing sarcoidosis, lymphoma, and infectious causes of lymphadenopathy.[15–16]

CASE 3

Question 1: B. Lobectomy

There are four subtypes of pulmonary neuroendocrine tumors: typical carcinoid, atypical carcinoid, large cell neuroendocrine carcinoma, and small cell lung carcinoma.[17] Although only about 1% of lung cancers are carcinoid tumors,[18] they are usually centrally located with 75% originating from lobar bronchi. Thus, patients with these tumors are usually symptomatic with cough, hemoptysis, and pneumonia,[19] but carcinoid syndrome (flushing, diarrhea, wheezing, valvular cardiac disease) is a rarity.[20] Due to location, diagnosis is often confirmed by bronchoscopic biopsy but can be difficult to distinguish typical from atypical carcinoid tumors.[21] CT scanning can aid in diagnosis since most typical carcinoids are spherical and centrally located, while most atypical carcinoids are peripheral and may have calcifications.[22] Due to the low prevalence of recurrence, typical carcinoid tumors do not require a wide margin of resection; therefore, lung-sparing operations, such as wedge resections and segmentectomies, are preferred.[23] Treatment of

atypical carcinoid tumors is more aggressive, such as lobectomy and pneumonectomy with mediastinal nodal dissections, due to higher rates of recurrence.[24] Consequently, prognosis is greater in typical carcinoids versus atypical carcinoids, with 10-year survival rates of 82% and 56%, respectively.[20]

* *

In this patient with a spherical endobronchial mass and biopsy consistent with a typical carcinoid tumor, a lung-sparing operation is optimal. A crucial step in sublobar and lobar resections is identifying the bronchus and noting its distance from the tumor. This patient's tumor protrudes from the base of the lingular bronchus (i.e., outside the anatomical boundary of resection), so a segmentectomy or wedge resection with negative surgical margins is highly unlikely. Yet, the tumor does not completely obstruct the upper division of the left upper lobe bronchus, allowing significant distance between the lesion and the left mainstem bronchus. A lobectomy would be most appropriate here since the likelihood of a negative margin is high and the lower lobe would be preserved. Sleeve lobectomies (anatomic lobectomy with bronchoplasty) are performed when the tumor protrudes from an upper lobe into the mainstem bronchus (i.e., a negative margin would be unlikely with an anatomic lobectomy). When bronchoplasty cannot be performed due to risk of positive margins on centrally located tumors, a pneumonectomy is undertaken.

Question 2: C. Sleeve lobectomy

The tumor now protrudes into the mainstem bronchus yet spares the lower lobe bronchus, therefore a sleeve lobectomy should provide a negative margin and avoid the morbidity of a pneumonectomy.

Question 3: D. Bedside awake bronchoscopy

Respiratory failure is the most common complication after thoracic surgery with an incidence of 15%[25] and is often due to atelectasis, retained secretions, pneumonia, and pulmonary edema. Early implementation of chest physiotherapy, ambulation, postural drainage, and incentive spirometry are crucial in preventing atelectasis and clearing mucous secretions to prevent pneumonia. When suspicion for pneumonia arises, early bronchoscopy can be used to remove thick secretions, open clogged airways, and procure cultures for antibiotic adjustments.[26] Based on this patient's chest x-ray findings of right middle lobe consolidation and his history, he likely has near-complete lobar collapse secondary to mucous plugging. The incidence of PE after thoracic surgery is around 2%[27] and more commonly occurs in larger anatomical resections such as lobectomy and pneumonectomy than sublobar resections.[28] Myocardial infarction is an uncommon postoperative complication with an incidence of 1%.[29] This patient has no pneumothorax and does not need a new chest tube.

Question 4: B. A 56-year-old male with 35 pack-years smoking history should undergo yearly CT scans

The USPSTF recommends lung cancer screenings with annual low-dose CT scanning for individuals aged 55 to 80 years with smoking history of 30 pack-years or more and are current smokers or have quit smoking within the past 15 years.[30,31] These recommendations are primarily based on the National Lung Screening Trial (NLST). This randomized controlled trial enrolled over 53,000 patients aged 55 to 74 years with 30 or more pack-years smoking history and either continued to smoke or quit within the past 15 years. The individuals were randomized to annual low-dose CT scan or annual chest radiograph for 3 years. The results showed a relative reduction in mortality from lung cancer of 20% with annual low-dose CT scanning compared to the radiography group.

CASE 4

Question 1: C. CT-guided transthoracic needle biopsy

After appropriate imaging is performed, invasive modalities are the next step for diagnosing lung cancer. Percutaneous transthoracic needle biopsy is a high yield diagnostic tool which can be performed via fluoroscopy or, more commonly, CT guidance. CT-guided techniques deploy either a core needle or a fine needle aspiration, both with similar accuracies,[32] can target small lesions under 2 cm, and can differentiate viable versus necrotic areas in larger ones. Its usefulness in diagnosing pulmonary nodules is proven with a sensitivity of 90% and 96% for nodules less than 2 cm and ones greater than 2 cm, respectively. Rates of complications vary but are mainly comprised pneumothoraces (about 15%, of which about 2% requires treatment) and hemoptysis (about 5%).[33] Due to the risks of pneumothorax and hemoptysis, relative contraindications include contralateral pneumonectomy, severe COPD, bleeding disorders, and severe pulmonary hypertension.[34] While a VATS wedge resection is an option, the morbidity of a thoracotomy

during an open wedge resection outweighs its benefits and is deployed after other modalities have failed. Endoscopic ultrasound-guided needle aspiration (EUS-NA) is a transesophageal approach, limiting its usefulness to diagnose peripheral lung nodules.

Question 2: B. Formal cardiopulmonary exercise test

The 2013 guidelines by the American College of Chest Physicians recommend all lung cancer patients being considered for surgery undergo lung function tests specifically focused on forced expiratory volume in 1 second (FEV_1) and diffusing capacity for carbon monoxide (DLco). The predicted postoperative (PPO) values should be calculated for both FEV_1 and DLco using either the anatomic method for lobectomy via a formula based on the number of lung segments to be resected or the perfusion method for pneumonectomy via a formula based on results from the quantitative radionuclide perfusion scan. If PPO FEV_1 and PPO DLco are >60% predicted, no further testing is needed and the patient is deemed low risk for complications and mortality. If either value is between 60% and 30% of predicted, a low technology exercise test (stair-climb or shuttle-walk test) is recommended. Patients with either PPO FEV_1 or PPO DLco <30% predicted or a failed low technology exercise test should undergo formal cardiopulmonary exercise test (CPET) with measurement of maximal oxygen consumption (VO_2 max). VO_2 max values <10 mL/kg/min or <35% of predicted correlate to a high risk for complications and mortality in patients undergoing major anatomic lung resections through a thoracotomy. The best options for these patients include minimally invasive surgery, sublobar resections, or nonoperative treatment.[35]

Question 3: A. VATS wedge resection

Peripheral T1 nonsmall cell lung cancer with negative mediastinal PET imaging can be classified as clinical stage I and do not require invasive mediastinal staging prior to lung resection, according to the European Society of Thoracic Surgeons guidelines.[14] The optimal therapy for clinical stage I nonsmall cell lung cancer is controversial in patients with borderline or poor pulmonary function. Although historically wedge resections have shown higher recurrence rates versus lobectomies, more recent studies have positive results with these sublobar resections for treatment of clinical stage I nonsmall cell lung cancer. The main three considerations for performing sublobar resections are surgical margins (distance from the tumor to the cut margin), tumor size, and lymph node assessment. Schuchert[36] showed sublobar resection patients with local recurrence had an average surgical margin of about 1.3 cm, while those without recurrence had about 1.9-cm margin. Therefore, a 2-cm margin is generally preferred. In addition, sublobar resection patients with tumors less than 2 cm in size have similar survival rates to lobectomy patients with the same size. The survival rates diverge in tumors larger than 2 cm for the two groups.[37] Studies have shown that tumors under 2 cm in size have about a 7% chance of lymph node metastases, so hilar and mediastinal lymph node sampling or dissection is suggested with intraoperative frozen-section pathology and a lobectomy is indicated if these results are positive.[38,39] The 2013 guidelines by the American College of Chest Physicians recommend lung cancer patients with a maximal oxygen consumption (VO_2 max) <10 mL/kg/min or <35% of predicted undergo minimally invasive surgery, sublobar resections, or nonoperative treatment for their disease.[35] The patient in this scenario has a VO_2 max of 9 mL/kg/min and a peripherally located clinical stage I nonsmall cell lung cancer. The best surgical option for this patient is a minimally invasive sublobar resection. There is no role for preoperative chemotherapy in clinical stage I nonsmall cell lung cancer.

Question 4: C. Age

Supraventricular arrhythmias, particularly atrial fibrillation, are the most common cardiac complications after thoracic surgery and have an incidence between 10% and 20% after lobectomy and up to 40% after pneumonectomy.[40,41] Atrial fibrillation is generally transient and often resolves with rate-control medications alone, usually beta blockers or calcium channel blockers.[42] Initiating oral metoprolol preoperatively and continuing it postoperatively has been shown to reduce incidence of atrial fibrillation to 7%.[43] Amar showed preoperative diltiazem reduced the incidence of postoperative arrhythmias from 15% to 25% in patients undergoing either lobectomy or pneumonectomy.[44] Prophylactic use of amiodarone has also decreased the incidence of arrhythmias in thoracic patients[45] but concerns arise over their association with postoperative respiratory complications. Age, specifically over 60 years, is the strongest independent risk factor in postoperative atrial fibrillation. Male gender, a history of atrial fibrillation, and preexisting cardiac conditions such as valvular disease and heart failure have also been shown to be predictors of atrial fibrillation.[46,47]

CASE 5

Question 1: B. Wedge resection

Although the role of surgery for metastatic cancers in general is usually very limited, there are clear advantages for surgical treatment of metastases to the lung. Since the location of metastases to lungs is usually peripheral and nonobstructive, 75% to 90% of patients are asymptomatic and found radiographically either during routine follow-up or incidentally. Dyspnea, cough, or hemoptysis can be the presenting symptoms and usually relate to large centrally located lesions, multiple lesions replacing lung parenchyma, or pleural effusions.[48] CT scan is the gold standard imaging modality and generally shows well-circumscribed spherical nodules characterizing metastatic lesions, while irregular spiculated lesions are more likely primary lung tumors.[49] Tissue diagnosis of the lesion is advantageous by distinguishing primary versus metastatic lesions and may affect therapeutic options. Fine-needle aspiration is usually the first attempted modality with thoracoscopic approaches reserved if diagnosis remains indeterminate.[50]

* *

The general criteria for performing a metastasectomy include control of the primary cancer, resectability of all metastatic lesions, no extrathoracic metastases, and the patient's overall ability to safely undergo pulmonary resection.[51] The primary objective of the operation is to completely resect the metastatic lesion with intentions to maximally preserve unaffected lung tissue since future metastasectomies may be required.[52] Therefore, wedge resections are indicated for the majority of lesions, while lobectomies and occasionally pneumonectomies are reserved for central and bulky lesions in which a sublobar resection cannot provide adequate surgical margins.[53,54] Metastases to the lung rarely spread to the mediastinal nodes and a formal lymph node dissection is generally not indicated unless radiographic evidence suspects mediastinal disease, in which case invasive mediastinal assessment should be performed prior to pulmonary resection.[48] The operation can be performed open via a unilateral thoracotomy, staged bilateral thoracotomy, or sometimes median sternotomy or thoracosternotomy (clamshell) for bilateral lesions, but also can be addressed through a unilateral or bilateral VATS approach. The VATS approach to metastasectomy has been shown to provide similar long-term survival as open approaches and has the benefits of reduced pain and shorter hospital length of stay.[55,56] Contraindications for pulmonary resection include malignant pleural or pericardial effusions and disseminated spread (discontinuous lesions) to the pleura or pericardium.[48]

* *

The three main factors affecting survival rates after surgery are resectability of the lesion, greater than 36-month disease-free interval, and absence of multiple metastatic lesions. Regardless of histology, a complete resection of the lesion is the most important factor for prognosis and inability to perform this may preclude surgery since 5-year survival drops to 13%. Patients with all three of these prognostic factors have a 5-year survival rate of 61%, but this rate drops to 24% in patients with disease-free interval less than 36 months and presence of multiple metastases. In general, patients with germ cell tumors have the best prognosis, followed by epithelial tumors and sarcomas being about equivalent, and the worst prognosis belonging to patients with melanoma.[53] Although multiple metastatic pulmonary lesions is a negative prognostic indicator, good results have still been shown with several metastasectomies performed in one setting[53,57] and there is no overall consensus as to the maximum number that would prohibit surgery.

* *

In this patient with a solitary small peripheral metastatic nodule and no extrathoracic disease, a wedge resection is the most appropriate treatment and preferred over lobectomy in order to preserve unaffected lung tissue. No preoperative invasive mediastinal assessment is needed due to lack of evidence for mediastinal disease seen on PET scan. In a patient meeting the above criteria, metastasectomy is superior to nonsurgical treatment alone.

Question 2: A. Right pleural fluid cytology positive for adenocarcinoma

As described above, malignant pleural effusion is a contraindication to metastasectomy.[48] While the presence of multiple metastases decreases survival, resection of these lesions provides a survival benefit. This healthy patient with good lung function can likely tolerate a pneumonectomy and evidence shows the procedure will be beneficial versus a nonsurgical approach.[53,54]

Question 3: A. Wedge resection of lung plus hepatic resection for single metastasis found on liver in addition to the peripheral lung lesion

An exception to the above criteria which prohibits metastasectomy in patients with extrathoracic lesions,

aggressive surgery for colorectal cancer metastases to both liver and lung shows better survival than chemotherapy alone. Complete resection of both the pulmonary and the hepatic lesions is the key prognostic factor.[58,59] Surgery is not indicated in patients with disseminated spread to the pleura, pericardium, or abdomen.[48,51]

Question 4: B. Complete versus incomplete resection of lesion

Age, unilateral versus bilateral metastatic lesions, and wedge resection versus lobectomy are factors that do not affect the prognosis.[48]

CASE 6

Question 1: D. Inpatient treatment with IV antibiotics and insertion of a chest tube

Parapneumonic effusions are common causes of pleural effusions and occur in about 40% to 57% of patients with community-acquired pneumonia. Of these effusions, 5% to 10% develop into empyemas.[60] Diagnosis and classification of parapneumonic effusions and empyemas are based on pleural fluid studies, pleural fluid Gram stain and culture, and CT scan findings. The American College of Chest Physicians classifies parapneumonic effusions into four categories with each category representing an increased risk of a poor outcome. Categories 1 and 2 are simple parapneumonic effusions, which mainly differ in size of the effusion. Category 3 is a complicated parapneumonic effusion and is characterized by at least one of the following: loculated or thickened parietal pleura, positive gram stain or culture, or pleural fluid pH <7.2 or glucose<60 mg/dL. Category 4 is empyema and defined by frank pus in the pleural space.[61] Empyemas are further classified by the American Thoracic Society into three stages. Stage I, the acute exudative stage, usually occurs within the first week and consists of a thin exudative fluid and no loculations. Stage II, the fibrinopurulent phase, occurs within 1 to 2 weeks and consists of frankly purulent fluid and loculations, but lung reexpansion without surgery is still likely. Stage III, the chronic organizing phase, occurs within 3 to 4 weeks and consists of very thick pus and fibrous peel encompassing the lungs making reexpansion without surgery unlikely. Stages I and II are also known as acute empyema, while stage III is known as chronic empyema.[62] Empyemas are often symptomatic and patients usually complain of dyspnea, cough, chest pain, and fever.[63]

* *

Treatment of parapneumonic effusions and empyemas varies depending on the developmental stage. For parapneumonic effusions, categories 1 and 2 are often solely treated with antibiotics and do not require tube thoracostomy. For categories 3 and 4, the American College of Chest Physicians recommends antibiotics, tube thoracostomy, likely intrapleural fibrinolytics, and/or surgery.[61]

* *

Acute versus chronic empyemas are managed with differing degrees of aggressiveness, yet the gold standard in both remains surgical removal of the infection with adequate drainage of the pleural space. Compared to stages II and III, the thinner pleural fluid and lack of loculations in stage I empyemas allow for greater intrapleural concentrations of antibiotics and more effective drainage with tube thoracostomy alone. The combination of chest tube and broad-spectrum intravenous antibiotics has a greater success in treatment of stage I empyemas versus stages II and II.[64,65] Tube thoracostomy can be attempted for treatment of stage II empyemas, but due to their increased failure rate and the higher success rate of surgery a more aggressive surgical approach is often advocated.[67] With a thinner pleural peel and greater rate of lung reexpansion compared to stage III empyemas, stage II empyemas are effectively treated with VATS decortication. The VATS technique for acute empyemas shows equivalent success versus formal thoracotomy and has the added benefit of less postoperative pain and dysfunction.[68] Use of intrapleural fibrinolytics has also shown some success in resolving stage II empyemas. Intrapleural urokinase with its greater safety profile than streptokinase can lyse loculations and allow for adequate pleural drainage via tube thoracostomy.[69,70] However, other evidence shows increased efficacy, shorter hospital stay, and decreased cost with an early VATS approach versus intrapleural fibrinolytics.[71] If no significant improvement with fibrinolytics is seen after 3 to 5 days, surgery is recommended.[68] When an empyema has evolved to the chronic organizing phase, tube thoracostomy is ineffective and surgery is the sole option. Formal thoracotomy and decortication is the preferred treatment for stage III empyemas since it provides full lung reexpansion and complete debridement of the infected pleural space.[72] For patients who fail initial surgical interventions or debilitated, high-risk patients, open-window thoracostomy and thoracoplasty are treatment options generally reserved for chronic empyema patients who fail initial surgical interventions or debilitated, high-risk patients.

Open-window thoracostomy is often performed via a modified Eloesser flap by rib resection and skin flap sewn to the base of the empyema cavity allowing effective long-term irrigation and drainage. The window can be left open permanently, closed with muscle flaps, or spontaneously closed from granulation tissue and reepithelialization. Open-window thoracostomy is an effective method in treating chronic complicated empyemas and limits mortality to about 5%.[73] Thoracoplasty is a collapse therapy accomplished by rib resection which decreases the size of the thorax and helps to obliterate the infected space. Due to its morbidity, this procedure is now uncommonly used but still effective, particularly in postpneumonectomy empyemas.[74]

* *

For the patient in this vignette, the pleural fluid studies and CT scan results suggest a category 3 parapneumonic effusion or early stage I empyema and tube thoracostomy is the recommended treatment.

Question 2: E. Posterolateral thoracotomy and decortication

A 3-week history of positive pleural fluid studies and symptoms plus CT scan findings all suggest a stage III chronic organizing empyema and surgery is the best option. As discussed above, tube thoracostomy alone would likely be ineffective. Talc pleurodesis is currently not recommended for the treatment of infected pleural effusions, but reports of its use have shown some success in select patients with stage II empyema.[75] Open-window thoracostomy is generally reserved for failed treatment or in debilitated, high-risk patients.

Question 3: C. Open-window thoracostomy via modified Eloesser flap

The patient is debilitated, failed initial surgical therapy, and has a continued infection. Open-window thoracostomy is indicated. Lucite-ball plombage is a collapse therapy originally deployed to treat tuberculosis by inserting methyl methacrylate Lucite balls extrapleurally and collapsing the parietal pleura, obliterating the infected space. The use of foreign bodies with its increased infection risk and introduction of antituberculosis antibiotics are two of the main reasons this technique is no longer in use.[76]

Question 4: D. Pneumonia

The main three causes of empyema include pneumonia (70%), iatrogenic (20%) which is mainly due to thoracic surgery, chest tube insertion, and thoracentesis, and traumatic (3%) often due to hemothoraces becoming secondarily infected. Subphrenic abscess, diverticulitis, and mediastinitis are less common etiologies of empyema.[60]

CASE 7

Question 1: **D. Bronchoscopy**

Pneumonectomy is one of the less common pulmonary resection surgeries and the majority of these are performed for treatment of nonsmall cell lung cancer. Complication rates are higher compared to lobar and sublobar resections and are mainly due to supraventricular tachyarrhythmias and respiratory complications. The mortality rate for pneumonectomy patients is about 6% with the main causes being respiratory failure, postpneumonectomy pulmonary edema, adult respiratory distress syndrome, and bronchopleural fistula. In particular, postpneumonectomy bronchopleural fistula with an overall incidence of 8% is a major factor contributing to this morbidity and mortality.[77] One reason for this is its high association with empyema. The majority of postpneumonectomy empyemas are caused by bronchopleural fistulas. Surgical technique, preoperative chemoradiation, diabetes, nutritional status, underlying lung disease, and right-sided pneumonectomy are all major risk factors.[78] Postpneumonectomy bronchopleural fistula and empyema can present days to weeks to years postoperatively. Symptoms include general signs of infection as well as expectorating serosanguinous fluid and aspiration pneumonitis in the contralateral lung. Bronchoscopy confirms the diagnosis of bronchopleural fistula and a CT scan can help assess for empyema. Initial treatment is insertion of a chest tube along with intravenous antibiotics. Placing the patient in the lateral decubitus position helps facilitate drainage from the chest tube and helps prevent aspiration into the contralateral lung. If there is a large-sized fistula and mechanical ventilation is required, a double lumen endotracheal tube should be used to protect the airways.[79] After initial treatment with tube thoracostomy, the general recommendation is thoracotomy with debridement, transposition of muscle flaps to cover the bronchial stump, and creation of an open thoracic window such as a modified Eloesser flap.[77-79] Using this method, about 84% of patients are treated successfully.[80]

* *

As noted above, bronchoscopy is the best method to diagnose postpneumonectomy bronchopleural fistula and CT scan can help assess for empyema. Esophagram is the best modality used to diagnose esophagopleural fistulas. Postpneumonectomy esophagopleural fistula is an uncommon complication of pneumonectomy with and incidence of about 0.5%. They typically present either immediately postoperatively due to intraoperative esophageal injury or months to years later from local recurrence of disease or infection. The majority are associated with empyema and this combination results in a very high mortality rate making treatment focus on conservative measures such as esophageal stenting and tube thoracostomy for empyema resolution.[81]

Question 2: **A. Tube thoracostomy and intravenous antibiotics**

As discussed above, for postpneumonectomy bronchopleural fistulas, it is universally recommended that all patients initially undergo tube thoracostomy for treatment of the operative side and to help prevent aspiration to the contralateral lung. Although there is increasing evidence of success with tracheal stenting for treatment of postpneumonectomy bronchopleural fistulas, the gold standard for initial treatment remains tube thoracostomy.[82]

Question 3: **D. Thoracotomy with debridement, muscle flap transposition, and open thoracic window**

As noted above, this intervention provides the greatest chance for successful treatment of postpneumonectomy bronchopleural fistulas and empyemas.[80] Successful bronchoscopic treatments for bronchopleural fistulas have been reported, including use of endobronchial valves and sealants such as fibrin glue and gel foam. However, results are variable and the level of evidence is low. These methods are generally reserved for very poor surgical candidates or temporizing treatments for unstable patients.[83,84]

Question 4: **C. Right-sided postpneumonectomy bronchopleural fistulas are more common than left-sided ones**

The overall incidence of postpneumonectomy bronchopleural fistula is about 8%, with 13% for right pneumonectomies and 5% for left pneumonectomies. Unlike the right side, the left mainstem bronchial stump retracts into the mediastinum resulting in the lower incidence of a fistula. For the right side, the pericardial fat pad, mediastinal pleura, intercostal muscle flap, or omental flap can be used to cover the bronchial stump and promote healing in order to reduce the occurrence of a postoperative bronchopleural fistula.[77] *Staphylococcus aureus* and *Pseudomonas aeruginosa* are the most common culprits of postpneumonectomy bronchopleural fistula and empyema.[79] Postpneumonectomy esophagopleural fistula has an incidence of about 0.5%.[81] Radiotherapy is a known risk factor for postpneumonectomy bronchopleural fistula and empyema.[78]

REFERENCES

1. de Langen AJ, Raijmakers P, Riphagen I, et al. The size of mediastinal lymph nodes and its relation with metastatic involvement: a meta-analysis. *Eur J Cardiothorac Surg.* 2009;36:440–445.

2. Meyers BF, Haddad F, Siegel BA, et al. Cost-effectiveness of routine mediastinoscopy in computed tomography–and positron emission tomography–screened patients with stage I lung cancer. *J Thorac Cardiovasc Surg.* 2006;131(4): 822–829.

3. Vallieres E, Waters PF. Incidence of mediastinal node involvement in clinical T1 bronchogenic carcinomas. *Can J Surg.* 1987;30(5):341–342.

4. Riquet M, Manac'h D, Dupont P, et al. Anatomic basis of lymphatic spread of lung carcinoma to the mediastinum: anatomo-clinical correlations. *Surg Radiol Anat.* 1994;16(3): 229–238.

5. Hammoud ZT, Anderson RC, Meyers BF, et al. The current role of mediastinoscopy in the evaluation of thoracic disease. *J Thorac Cardiovasc Surg.* 1999;118(5):894–899.

6. Frederick LG. *AJCC Cancer Staging Manual.* 6th ed. Vol. 1. New York, NY: Springer; 2002.

7. Albain KS, Rusch VW, Crowley JJ, et al. Concurrent cisplatin/etoposide plus chest radiotherapy followed by surgery for stages IIIA (N2) and IIIB non-small-cell lung cancer: mature results of Southwest Oncology Group phase II study 8805. *J Clin Oncol.* 1995;13(8) 1880–1892.

8. Goldstein LA, Thompson WR. Esophageal perforations: a 15 year experience. *Am J Surg.* 1982;143(4):495–503.

9. Hogan BA, Winter DC, Broe D, et al. Prospective trial comparing contrast swallow, computed tomography and endoscopy to identify anastomotic leak following oesophagogastric surgery. *Surg Endosc.* 2008;22(3):767–771.

10. Ernst A, Feller-Kopman D, Herth FJ. Endobronchial ultrasound in the diagnosis and staging of lung cancer and other thoracic tumors. *Semin Thorac Cardiovasc Surg.* 2007;19:201–205.

11. Wallace MB, Pascual JM, Raimondo M, et al. Minimally invasive endoscopic staging of suspected lung cancer. *JAMA.* 2008;299(5):540–546.

12. Herth FJ, Eberhardt R, Krasnik M, et al. Endobronchial ultrasound-guided transbronchial needle aspiration of lymph nodes in the radiologically and positron emission tomography-normal mediastinum in patients with lung cancer. *J Thorac Oncol.* 2008;3:577–582.

13. Larsen SS, Vilmann P, Krasnik M, et al. Endoscopic ultrasound guided biopsy versus mediastinoscopy for analysis of paratracheal and subcarinal lymph nodes in lung cancer staging. *Lung Cancer.* 2005;48(1):85–92.

14. De Leyn P, Lardinois D, Van Schil PE, et al. ESTS guidelines for preoperative lymph node staging for non-small cell lung cancer. *Eur J Cardiothorac Surg.* 2007;32(1):1–8.

15. Senturk A, Babaoglu E, Kilic H, et al. Endobronchial ultrasound-guided transbronchial needle aspiration in the diagnosis of lymphoma. *Asian Pac J Cancer Prev.* 2014; 15(10):4169–4173.

16. Choi YR, An JY, Kim MK, et al. The diagnostic efficacy and safety of endobronchial ultrasound-guided transbronchial needle aspiration as an initial diagnostic tool. *Korean J Intern Med.* 2013;28(6):660–667.

17. Beasley MB, Brambilla E, Travis WD. Travis. The 2004 World Health Organization classification of lung tumors. *Semin Roentgenol.* 2005;40(2):90–97.

18. Institute TUNC: Surveillance Epidemiology and End Results (SEER) data base, 1973–2004. http://seercancer-gov/2007, 2007.

19. Davila DG, Dunn WF, Tazelaar HD, et al. Bronchial carcinoid tumors. *Mayo Clin Proc.* 1993;68(8):795–803.

20. Fink G, Krelbaum T, Yellin A, et al. Pulmonary carcinoid: Presentation, diagnosis, and outcome in 142 cases in Israel and review of 640 cases from the literature. *Chest.* 2001;119(6):1647–1651.

21. Beasley MB, Thunnissen FB, Brambilla E, et al. Pulmonary atypical carcinoid: predictors of survival in 106 cases. *Hum Pathol.* 2000;31(10):1255–1265.

22. Marty-Ané CH, Costes V, Pujol JL, et al. Carcinoid tumors of the lung: do atypical features require aggressive management? *Ann Thorac Surg.* 1995;59(1):78–83.

23. Ferguson MK, Landreneau RJ, Hazelrigg SR, et al. Long-term outcome after resection for bronchial carcinoid tumors. *Eur J Cardiothorac Surg.* 2000;18(2):156–161.

24. Mezzetti M, Raveglia F, Panigalli T, et al. Assessment of outcomes in typical and atypical carcinoids according to latest WHO classification. *Ann Thorac Surg.* 2003;76(6): 1838–1842.

25. Agostini P, Cieslik H, Rathinam S, et al. Postoperative pulmonary complications following thoracic surgery: are there any modifiable risk factors?. *Thorax.* 65(9):815–818.

26. Ferdinand B, Shennib H. Postoperative pneumonia. *Chest Surg Clin North Am.* 1998;8(3):529–539.

27. Nagahiro I, Andou A, Aoe M, et al. Intermittent pneumatic compression is effective in preventing symptomatic pulmonary embolism after thoracic surgery. *Surg Today.* 2004; 34:6–10.

28. Ziomek, S, Read RC, Tobler HG, et al. Thromboembolism in patients undergoing thoracotomy. *Ann Thorac Surg.* 1993;56:223–226.

29. von Knorring J, Lepäntalo M, Lindgren L, et al. Cardiac arrhythmias and myocardial ischemia after thoracotomy for lung cancer. *Ann Thorac Surg.* 1992;53:642–647.

30. www.uspreventiveservicestaskforce.org

31. Aberle DR, Adams AM, Berg CD, et al.; National Lung Screening Trial Research Team. Reduced lung-cancer mortality with low-dose computed tomographic screening. *New Engl J Med.* 2011;365(5):395–409.

32. Greif J, Marmur S, Schwarz Y, et al. Percutaneous core cutting needle biopsy compared with fine needle aspiration in the diagnosis of peripheral lung malignant lesions. *Cancer.* 1998;84(3):144–147.

33. Laurent F, Latrabe V, Vergier B, et al. CT-guided transthoracic needle biopsy of pulmonary nodules smaller than 20 mm: results with an automated 20-gauge coaxial cutting needle. *Clin Radiol.* 2000;55(4):281–287.

34. Klein JS, Zarka MA. Transthoracic needle biopsy: an overview. *J Thorac Imaging*. 1997;12(4):232–249.

35. Brunelli A, Kim AW, Berger KI, et al. Physiologic evaluation of the patient with lung cancer being considered for resectional surgery: Diagnosis and management of lung cancer: American College of Chest Physicians evidence-based clinical practice guidelines. *Chest*. 2013;143(5 Suppl):e166S–e190S.

36. Schuchert MJ, Pettiford BL, Keeley S, et al. Anatomic segmentectomy in the treatment of stage I non-small cell lung cancer. *Ann Thorac Surg*. 2007;84(3):926–933.

37. Okada M, Nishio W, Sakamoto T, et al. Effect of tumor size on prognosis in patients with non–small cell lung cancer: the role of segmentectomy as a type of lesser resection. *J Thorac Cardiovasc Surg*. 2005;129(1)):87–93.

38. Okada M, Koike T, Higashiyama M, et al. Radical sublobar resection for small-sized non–small cell lung cancer: a multicenter study. *J Thorac Cardiovasc Surg*. 2006;132(4):769–775.

39. Miller DL, Rowland CM, Deschamps C, et al. Surgical treatment of non-small cell lung cancer 1 cm or less in diameter. *Ann Thorac Surg*. 2002;73(5):1545–1551.

40. Asamura H, Naruke T, Tsuchiya R, et al. What are the risk factors for arrhythmias after thoracic operations? *J Thorac Cardiovasc Surg*. 1993;106:1104–1110.

41. Amar D. Cardiac arrhythmias. *Chest Surg Clin North Am*. 1998;8:479–493.

42. Rena O, Papalia E, Oliaro A, et al. Supraventricular arrhythmias after resection surgery of the lung. *Eur J Cardiothorac Surg*. 2001;20:688–693.

43. Jakobsen CJ, Bille S, Ahlburg P, et al. Perioperative metoprolol reduces the frequency of atrial fibrillation after thoracotomy for lung resection. *J Cardiothorac Vasc Anesth*. 1997;11:746–751.

44. Amar D, Roistacher N, Rusch VW, et al. Effects of diltiazem prophylaxis on the incidence and clinical outcome of atrial arrhythmias after thoracic surgery. *J Thorac Cardiovasc Surg*. 2000;120(4):790–798.

45. Tisdale JE, Wroblewski HA, Wall DS, et al. A randomized trial evaluating amiodarone for prevention of atrial fibrillation after pulmonary resection. *Ann Thorac Surg*. 2009;88(3):886–895.

46. Amar D, Zhang H, Leung DH, et al. Older age is the strongest predictor of postoperative atrial fibrillation. *Anesthesiology*. 2002;96(2):352–356.

47. Vaporciyan AA, Correa AM, Rice DC, et al. Risk factors associated with atrial fibrillation after noncardiac thoracic surgery: analysis of 2588 patients. *J Thorac Cardiovasc Surg*. 2004;127(3):779–786.

48. Pass HI, Donington JS. Metastatic cancer of the lung. In: De Vita V, Hellman S, Rosenberg SA, eds. *Principles and Practice of Oncology*. Philadelphia, PA: JB Lippincott; 1997:2436–551.

49. Crow J, Slavin G, Kreel L. Pulmonary metastasis: a pathologic and radiologic study. *Cancer*. 1981;47(11):2595–2602.

50. Mack MJ, Hazelrigg SR, Landreneau RJ, et al. Thoracoscopy for the diagnosis of the indeterminate solitary pulmonary nodule. *Ann Thorac Surg*. 1993;56(4):825–832.

51. Rusch VW. Pulmonary metastasectomy current indications. *Chest*. 1995;107(6 Suppl):322S–331S.

52. Downey RJ. Surgical treatment of pulmonary metastases. *Surg Oncol Clin N Am*. 1999;8(2):341–354.

53. Pastorino U, Buyse M, Friedel G, et al; International Registry of Lung Metastases. Long-term results of lung metastasectomy: prognostic analyses based on 5206 cases. *J Thorac Cardiovasc Surg*. 1997;113(1):37–49.

54. Spaggiari L, Grunenwald DH, Girard P, et al. Pneumonectomy for lung metastases: indications, risks, and outcome. *Ann Thorac Surg*. 1998;66(6):1930–1933.

55. Lin JC, Wiechmann RJ, Szwerc MF, et al. Diagnostic and therapeutic video-assisted thoracic surgery resection of pulmonary metastases. *Surgery*. 1999;126(4):636–642.

56. Landreneau RJ, De Giacomo T, Mack MJ, et al. Therapeutic video-assisted thoracoscopic surgical resection of colorectal pulmonary metastases. *Eur J Cardiothorac Surg*. 2000; 18(6)):671–677.

57. Martini N, McCormack PM, Bains MS, et al. Surgery for solitary and multiple pulmonary metastases. *N Y State J Med*. 1978;78(11):1711–1714.

58. Barlow AD, Nakas A, Pattenden C, et al. Surgical treatment of combined hepatic and pulmonary colorectal cancer metastases. *Eur J Surg Oncol*. 2009;35(3):307–312.

59. Imdahl A, Fischer E, Tenckhof C, et al. [Resection of combined or sequential lung and liver metastases of colorectal cancer: indication for everyone?]. *Zentralbl Chir*. 2005; 130(6):539–543.

60.. Rahman NM, Davies RJ. Effusions from infections: Parapneumonic effusion and empyema. In: Light RW, Lee YCG, eds. *Textbook of Pleural Disease*. 2nd ed. London: Hodder & Stoughton; 2008:341–366.

61. Colice GL, Curtis A, Deslauriers J, et al. Medical and surgical treatment of parapneumonic effusions: an evidence-based guideline. *Chest*. 2000;118:1158–1171.[Erratum in: *Chest*. 2001;119:319.]

62. Cohen RG, DeMeester TR, Lafontaine E. The pleura. In: Sabiston DC, Spencer FC, eds. *Surgery of the Chest*. 6th ed. Philadelphia, PA: WB Saunders; 1995.

63. Varkey B, Rose HD, Kutty CP, et al. Empyema thoracis during a ten-year period. Analysis of 72 cases and comparison to a previous study (1952 to 1967). *Arch Intern Med*. 1981;141(13):1771–1776.

64. Bergeron MG. The changing bacterial spectrum and antibiotic choice in thoracic surgery: Surgical management of pleural diseases. In: Deslauriers J, Lacquet LK, eds. *International Trends in General Thoracic Surgery*. St. Louis, MO: Mosby-Year Book; 1990: Vol 6. P197–P207.

65. Moran JF. Surgical management of pleural space infections. *Semin Respir Infect*. 1988;3(4):383–394.

66. Crouch JD, Keagy BA, Delany DJ. Pigtail catheter drainage in thoracic surgery. *Am Rev Respir Dis*. 1987;136:174–175.

67. Pothula V, Krellenstein DJ. Early aggressive surgical management of parapneumonic empyemas. *Chest*. 1994;105(3):832–836.

68. Silen ML, Naunheim KS. Thoracoscopic approach to the management of empyema thoracis. Indications and results. *Chest Surg Clin N Am*. 1996;6(3):491–499.

69. Bouros D, Schiza S, Patsourakis G, et al. Intrapleural streptokinase versus urokinase in the treatment of complicated parapneumonic effusions: a prospective, double-blind study. *Am J Respir Crit Care Med.* 1997;155(1):291–295.

70. Lopez-Rivero L, Lopez-Pujol J, Quevedo S, et al. Urokinase in the management of loculated intrapleural effusion. Abstracts from the 2nd European Conference on General Thoracic Surgery. In: E.S.T.S. Gotti G, Elias S, Paldini P, eds. *Universita degli Studi di Siena.* Siena, Italy: Cattedra de Chirugia Toracia; 1994.

71. Wait MA, Sharma S, Hohn J, et al. A randomized trial of empyema therapy. *Chest.* 1997;111(6):1548–1551.

72. Martella AT, Santos GH. Decortication for chronic postpneumonic empyema. *J Am Coll Surg.* 1995;180(5):573–576.

73. Thourani VH, Lancaster RT, Mansour KA, et al. Twenty-six years of experience with the modified Eloesser flap. *Ann Thorac Surg.* 2003;76(2):401–406.

74. Nakaoka K, Nakahara K, Iioka S, et al. Postoperative preservation of pulmonary function in patients with chronic empyema thoracis: a one-stage operation. *Ann Thorac Surg.* 1989;47(6):848–852.

75. Weissberg D, Kaufman M. The use of talc for pleurodesis in the treatment of resistant empyema. *Ann Thorac Surg.* 1986;41(2):143–145.

76. Brantigan OC, Rigdon HL. Extrapleural pneumonolysis with Lucite ball plombage. *Chest.* 1950;18(4):277–290.

77. Darling GE, Abdurahman A, Yi QL, et al. Risk of a right pneumonectomy: role of bronchopleural fistula. *Ann Thorac Surg.* 2005;79(2):433–437.

78. Panagopoulos ND, Apostolakis E, Koletsis E, et al. Low incidence of bronchopleural fistula after pneumonectomy for lung cancer. *Interact Cardiovasc Thorac Surg.* 2009;9(4):571–575.

79. Abbas Ael-S, Deschamps C. Postpneumonectomy empyema. *Curr Opin Pulm Med.* 2002;8(4):327–333.

80. Pairolero PC, Arnold PG, Trastek VF, et al. Postpneumonectomy empyema. The role of intrathoracic muscle transposition. *J Thorac Cardiovasc Surg.* 1990;99(6):958–966.

81. Massard G, Ducrocq X, Hentz JG, et al. Esophagopleural fistula: an early and long-term complication after pneumonectomy. *Ann Thorac Surg.* 1994;58(5)::1437–1440.

82. Andreetti C, D'Andrilli A, Ibrahim M, et al. Effective treatment of post-pneumonectomy bronchopleural fistula by conical fully covered self-expandable stent. *Interact Cardiovasc Thorac Surg.* 2012;14(4):420–423.

83. Lois M, Noppen M. Bronchopleural fistulasan overview of the problem with special focus on endoscopic management. *Chest.* 2005;128(6):3955–3965.

84. Gasanov AM, Pinchuk TP, Danielian ShN, et al. The effectiveness of the valve bronchial occlusion in case of bronchopleural fistulas. *Khirurgiia (Mosk).* 2013;(2):22–24.

26

Pulmonary Pathology

Abul Ala Syed Rifat Mannan MD and Songyang Yuan MD

CASE 1

Question 1: **Identify the structure at the center of image:**

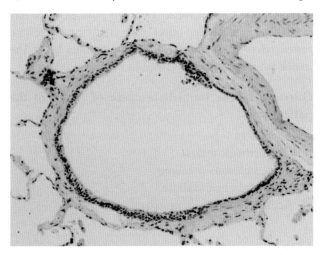

A. Alveolar duct
B. Bronchus
C. Alveolus
D. Bronchiole
E. Trachea

Question 2: **Which of the following statements is correct regarding pulmonary lobules?**

A. Pulmonary lobules consist of bronchus, alveolar duct, and alveoli
B. Bronchioles are characterized by the presence of cartilage and submucosal glands
C. Air-blood barrier is formed by squamous epithelium, endothelium, and basement membrane

D. Type I pneumocytes secrete surfactant
E. Type II pneumocytes form most of the respiratory surface of the lung

CASE 2

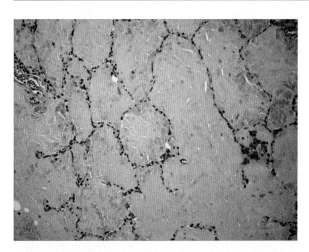

A 35-year-old Caucasian man presents with a 1-year history of progressive dyspnea on exertion with cough, which is productive of yellow sputum. He has smoked 15 packs of cigarettes for the past 15 years. Physical examination reveals cyanosis and bilateral inspiratory crackles. A chest radiograph reveals bilateral symmetrical alveolar opacities located in mid and lower lung zones. A microscopic appearance of wedge biopsy is shown here.

Question 1: **Which of the following conditions does this patient have?**

A. Pulmonary edema
B. Diffuse alveolar hemorrhage
C. Pneumocystis pneumonia
D. Pulmonary alveolar proteinosis
E. Pulmonary alveolar microlithiasis

CASE 3

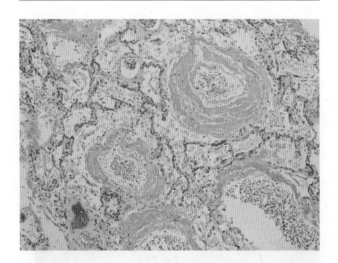

A 52-year-old woman was admitted for fever, cough, and respiratory distress. She had headache, cough, and mild dyspnea 5 days prior, which was diagnosed as influenza at local clinic and was treated with a cough suppressant. She had a temperature of 101.8°F, a heart rate of 131/min, a respiratory rate of 30/min, and a blood pressure of 142/60 mm Hg. Her oxygen saturation on room air was 89%. Pulmonary examination revealed dullness to percussion in the bases and coarse crackles could be heard bilaterally in all lung fields. Her chest radiograph at admission showed bilateral interstitial infiltrates. She was treated with a presumed diagnosis of community-acquired pneumonia. During the course of several hours, she developed severe shortness of breath and hypoxemia and was intubated. The patient died approximately 28 hours after admission. At autopsy, her lungs were enlarged and heavy.

Question 1: **A microscopic appearance of lung at autopsy is shown above. This pattern of pulmonary damage can be caused by all of the following conditions, EXCEPT:**

A. Narcotic overdose
B. Septic shock
C. Severe trauma
D. Oxygen toxicity
E. Pneumothorax

CASE 4

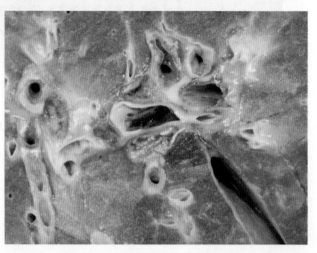

A 52-year-old man underwent open reduction and internal fixation for multiple lower leg fractures sustained in a road traffic accident. He had an uneventful surgery and was recovering well. On postoperative day 3, he developed sudden onset of severe dyspnea. Despite resuscitative measures, he died 30 minutes later. The major autopsy finding is shown in the figure.

Question 1: **The immediate cause of death in the patient was:**

A. Atelectasis
B. Hemorrhagic infarct
C. Acute pulmonary edema
D. Acute right heart failure
E. Acute pulmonary hemorrhage

CASE 5

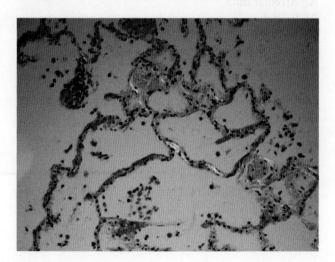

A 68-year-old man with a history of hypertension and diabetes presents with cough, dyspnea and lower limb edema for 3-month duration. On physical examination, his jugular vein is dilated and liver is palpable under the right costal margin. Chest auscultation reveals bilateral basal rales. High resolution computed tomography of the chest demonstrates diffuse reticulonodular pattern. A wedge biopsy from the right lower lobe is performed. The image shown (see previous page) demonstrates photomicrograph of a section from the lung after Congo red staining. Immunohistochemical studies reveal the deposition of monoclonal *kappa* light chains.

Question 1: **The most likely diagnosis is:**

A. Pulmonary interstitial fibrosis
B. Hyaline membrane disease
C. Amyloidosis, AA type
D. Pulmonary vasculitis
E. Amyloidosis, AL type

CASE 6

A 35-year-old woman presents with progressive dyspnea and a 5-kg weight loss over the past 3 years. She has no history of smoking. Physical examination shows an increase in the anteroposterior diameter of the chest. Auscultation shows decreased breath sounds in bilateral lung fields. A chest radiograph shows bilateral hyperlucent lungs, especially prominent in the upper lobes. Laboratory investigation reveals serum alpha-1-antitripsin level of 21 mg/mL (normal reference range 100–190 mg/dL).

Question 1: **Which of the following conditions is most likely to be present in her lungs?**

A. Centriacinar emphysema
B. Paraseptal emphysema
C. Interstitial emphysema
D. Panacinar emphysema
E. Irregular emphysema

CASE 7

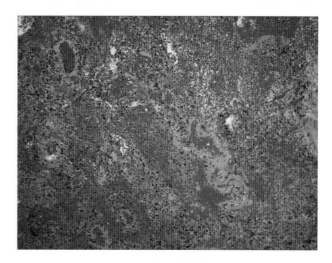

A 27-year-old previously healthy man presents to his physician with acute onset of hemoptysis. On physical examination, he has a temperature of 98.6°F and a blood pressure of 156/94 mm Hg. A chest radiograph shows bilateral fluffy infiltrates. A microscopic appearance of wedge biopsy is presented in the figure. Two days later, he has oliguria with a serum creatinine of 2.7 mg/dL.

Question 1: **Which of the following serologic tests is most likely to be positive in this patient?**

A. Anti-glomerular basement membrane antibody
B. Anti–double-stranded DNA antibody
C. Anti-Smith antibody
D. Anti-centromere antibody
E. Anti-ribonucleoprotein antibody

CASE 8

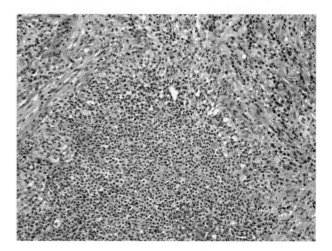

A 45-year-old man presents with malaise, mild fever, and hemoptysis for 2 weeks. He has been suffering from recurrent rhinorrhea, sinusitis, and occasional epistaxis for last 9 months and received antibiotic therapy without significant improvement. On physical examination, his temperature is 99.2°F. Auscultation reveals few crackles over both lungs. Laboratory studies show blood urea nitrogen of 33 mg/dL, creatinine 3.8 mg/dL, ALT 155U/L, AST 162U/L, and total bilirubin 1.2 mg/dL. The C-ANCA titer is 1:245. The microscopic appearance is shown on the previous page.

Question 1: **Which of the following is the most likely diagnosis?**

A. Eosinophilic granulomatosis with polyangiitis
B. Granulomatosis with polyangiitis
C. Hypersensitivity pneumonitis
D. Goodpasture syndrome
E. Sarcoidosis

CASE 9

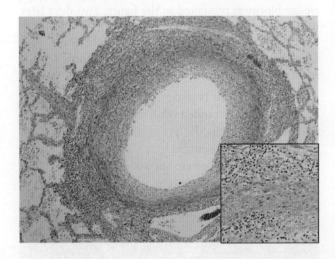

A 50-year-old man was admitted for fever, cough, and worsening of dyspnea for the past 2 months. He had 4-year history of dyspnea, wheezing, and sinusitis and was treated with inhaled bronchodilator drugs and steroids. Laboratory data showed white blood cell count of 22,000/mm^3 with eosinophilic count of 30%. His chest radiograph showed bilateral diffuse alveolar patches. A microscopic appearance of wedge lung biopsy is shown here.

Question 1: **Eosinophilic infiltrates in the lung characterize all of the following disorders EXCEPT:**

A. Loeffler's syndrome
B. Allergic bronchopulmonary aspergillosis
C. Hypersensitivity pneumonitis
D. Bronchial asthma
E. Eosinophilic granulomatosis with polyangiitis

CASE 10

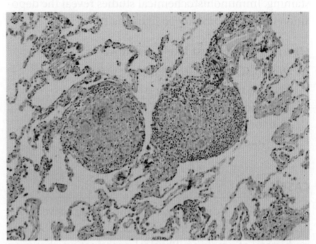

A 44-year-old woman presents with progressive dyspnea on exertion, lethargy, loss of appetite of 6-month duration, intermittent mild wheezing, and cough. She was treated by her primary physician with antibiotics for 3 weeks, without significant clinical improvement. She is a nonsmoker, but she is known to be breeding a budgerigar as hobby. On physical examination, her temperature is 99.7°F. There are scattered crepitations throughout both lung fields. A chest radiograph shows bilateral diffused micronodular densities. A transbronchial lung biopsy is performed and a microscopic appearance is shown in the figure.

Question 1: **Inhalation of which of the following materials is the most likely cause of this lesion?**

A. Coal dust
B. Asbestos
C. Silica
D. Talc
E. Bird dust

CASE 11

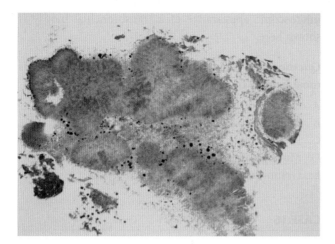

A 55-year-old alcoholic man presents with fever, cough, purulent sputum, and exertional breathlessness for 2 months. He had a gingival inflammation half a year ago and was treated locally. On physical examination, his temperature is 101.3°F. Respiratory system examination reveals right-sided crepitations. A chest radiograph shows multiple nodular opacities of right lower lobe. A microscopic appearance of transbronchial lung biopsy is shown here.

Question 1: **Which of the following organisms is most likely to be detected by culture?**

A. *Candida albicans*
B. *Mycobacterium tuberculosis*
C. *Nocardia asteroides*
D. *Actinomyces israelii*
E. *Aspergillus fumigatus*

CASE 12

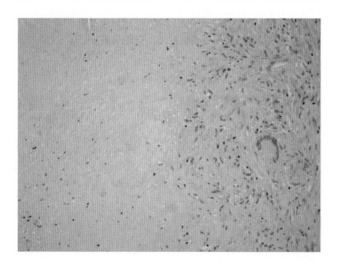

A 52-year-old homeless man presents with cough and weight loss for the past 3 months. A chest radiograph reveals a 3-cm nodule with cavity in the left upper lobe. The microscopic appearance of a lung biopsy of the nodule is shown in the figure.

Question 1: **Which special stain should be performed to confirm the diagnosis?**

A. Gomori methenamine silver (GMS) stain
B. Ziehl–Neelsen stain
C. Periodic acid-Schiff (PAS) stain
D. Gram stain
E. Giemsa stain

CASE 13

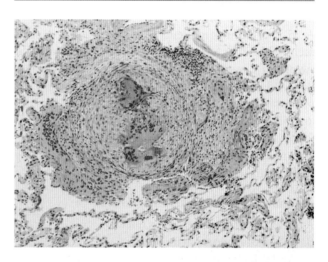

A 31-year-old African American man has had a non-productive cough and dyspnea on exertion for the past 3 weeks. He has smoked one pack of cigarettes a week for 10 years. On physical examination, his lungs are clear to auscultation and he has no palpable adenopathy. A chest radiograph shows reticulonodular opacities with prominent hilar and mediastinal lymphadenopathy. A transbronchial biopsy is performed and the microscopic appearance of the lesion is depicted here. Gomori methenamine silver (GMS) and acid-fast bacilli (AFB) stains are negative for microorganisms.

Question 1: **Which of the following conditions does the patient most likely have?**

A. Hypersensitivity pneumonia
B. M. tuberculosis infection
C. Langerhans cell histiocytosis
D. Sarcoidosis
E. Pulmonary histoplasmosis

CASE 14

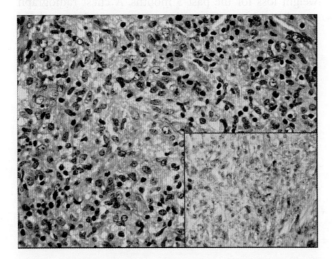

A 35-year-old man presents to the emergency department with chill, fever, dry cough, dyspnea, and night sweats for 2 weeks. He has a long history of HIV infection and is nonadherent to antiretroviral therapy. At presentation, his CD4 count is 145 cells//μL and his HIV load is 245,000 copies/mL. A chest radiograph reveals foci of consolidation with a cavity in the left upper lobe. The microscopic appearance of transbronchial lung biopsy with acid-fast bacilli (AFB) stain is shown here.

Question 1: **The most likely diagnosis is:**

A. *Mycobacterium tuberculosis* infection
B. Cytomegalovirus pneumonia
C. *Mycobacterium avium* complex infection
D. Sarcoidosis
E. *Pneumocystis jirovecii* infection

CASE 15

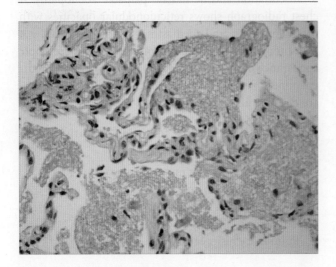

A 30-year-old previously healthy man presents with fever, nonproductive cough, and shortness of breath. A microscopic appearance of a transbronchial biopsy is shown here.

Question 1: **Which of the following diagnostic tests is most helpful in confirming the diagnosis?**

A. Gram stain
B. Acid-fast bacilli (AFB) stain
C. Prussian blue stain
D. Mucicarmine stain
E. Gomori methenamine silver (GMS) stain

CASE 16

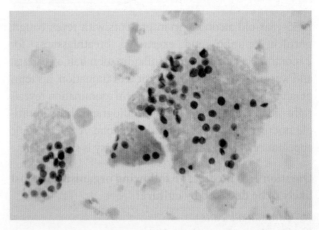

A 36-year-old woman has had insidious dyspnea, cough, and weight loss for 3 weeks. She reported occasional cough, wheezing, and fever during the last 4 years. Her chest radiograph shows bilateral diffuse interstitial infiltrate. Smear of bronchoalveolar lavage is stained with Gomori methenamine silver (GMS) stain. The high-power microscopic appearance is shown in the image.

Question 1: **The most likely underlying disease in this patient is:**

A. Systemic lupus erythematosus
B. Diabetes mellitus
C. Sarcoidosis
D. Pulmonary histoplasmosis
E. Acquired immunodeficiency syndrome

CASE 17

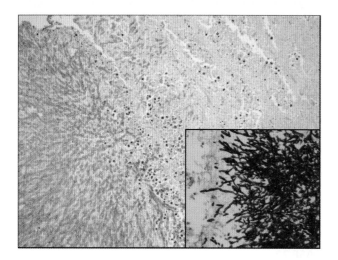

A 55-year-old woman presents with cough with purulent sputum, wheeze, and dyspnea for 5-day duration. She has had rheumatoid arthritis for 8 years and is taking prednisone and azathioprine for last 2 months. On physical examination, her temperature is 99.8°F with no alterations on pulmonary auscultation. A chest radiograph shows a suspicious subpleural mass in the left upper lobe. A microscopic appearance of wedge biopsy with Gomori methenamine silver (GMS) stain is shown here.

Question 1: **Which condition is probably present in her lungs?**

A. Acute invasive aspergillosis
B. *Candida* pneumonia
C. Pulmonary zygomycosis
D. Pulmonary histoplasmosis
E. Pulmonary cryptococcosis

CASE 18

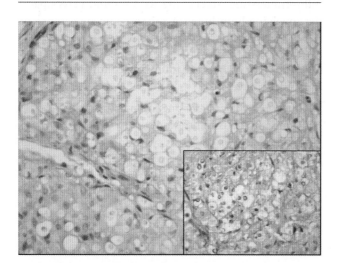

A 32-year-old man with human immunodeficiency virus (HIV) infection presents with fever, cough, and dyspnea, accompanied by neck rigidity for 2-week duration. A chest radiograph demonstrates a well-defined, 3.5-cm mass in upper right lobe. The microscopic appearance of transbronchial lung biopsy and mucicarmine stain (inset) is shown here.

Question 1: **What is the most likely diagnosis?**

A. Cytomegalovirus pneumonia
B. Adult respiratory distress syndrome
C. Pneumocystis jirovecii pneumonia
D. *Candida* pneumonia
E. Cryptococcal pneumonia

CASE 19

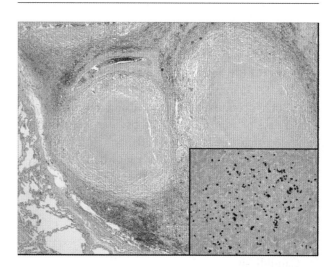

A 59-year-old farmer of South Ohio presents with low-grade evening fever, dry cough, and left chest pain for 5-month duration. He has no night sweats. Physical examination is unremarkable except for a temperature of 103.6°F. A chest radiograph reveals apical consolidation with cavities in the left upper lobe. A microscopic appearance of wedge biopsy with Gomori methenamine silver (GMS) stain (inset) is shown here.

Question 1: **Which of the following conditions does the patient most likely have?**

A. Pulmonary histoplasmosis
B. *Candida* pneumonia
C. Pulmonary cryptococcosis
D. Pulmonary coccidioidomycosis
E. Pneumocystis pneumonia

CASE 20

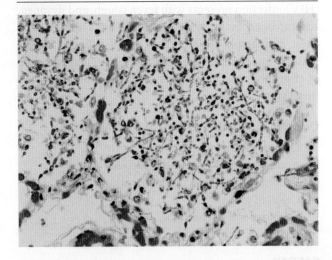

A 72-year-old woman was admitted for recurrent fall and syncope. She had a history of pancreatic ductal adenocarcinoma status post Whipple resection 6 months ago and was on chemotherapy. On physical examination, temperature was 101.8°F, heart rate was 114/min and blood pressure was 88/55 mm Hg. She was given fluids and antibiotics. But her condition deteriorated and she passed away after 3 days of admission. At autopsy, her lungs showed multiple patchy areas of consolidations. A microscopic appearance of pulmonary lesion is shown in the figure.

Question 1: **What is the most likely diagnosis?**

A. Cryptococcosis
B. Histoplasmosis
C. Aspergillosis
D. Candidiasis
E. Coccidioidomycosis

CASE 21

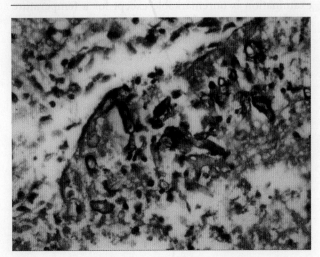

A 54-year-old diabetic woman presents with fever, cough, purulent sputum, and hemoptysis for 3 weeks and no improvement with antibiotics. A chest radiograph shows bilateral multiple cavitary nodules, ranging from 1 to 3 cm in diameter. A microscopic appearance of wedge biopsy with PAS stain is shown here.

Question 1: **Which of the following is the most likely diagnosis?**

A. *Candida* pneumonia
B. Pulmonary aspergillosis
C. Pulmonary zygomycosis
D. Pulmonary histoplasmosis
E. Pulmonary cryptococcosis

CASE 22

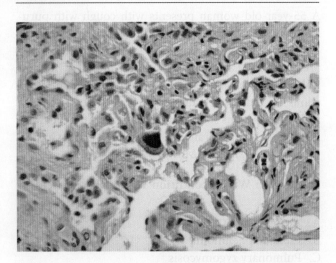

A 65-year-old man presents with fever, cough, and dyspnea. He has a history of chronic lymphocytic leukemia treated with systemic chemotherapy. He was noted to be hypoxic on room air. A chest radiograph reveals diffuse interstitial thickening with ground-glass opacities involving both lungs. A microscopic appearance of transbronchial biopsy is depicted here.

Question 1: **Which of the following conditions does he most likely have?**

A. *Pneumocystis jirovecii* pneumonia
B. Lymphomatous infiltration
C. Adult respiratory distress syndrome
D. Cytomegalovirus pneumonia
E. Atypical adenomatous hyperplasia

CASE 23

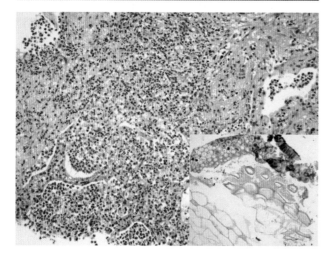

A 45-year-old man presents with shortness of breath, fever, and productive cough for the last 3 days. His sputum is thick and yellow. He has a history of chronic alcoholism and occasional heroin abuse. He last uses heroin 5 days prior to current admission. On physical examination, his temperature is 101.4°F. On auscultation, air entry is markedly reduced on the right lower base of lung. His chest x-ray shows complete consolidation of right lower lobe. A transbronchial biopsy is performed. A microscopic appearance of the lesion is shown here.

Question 1: **This patient may have the following type of pulmonary injury EXCEPT:**

A. Adult respiratory distress syndrome
B. Lipoid pneumonia
C. Pulmonary alveolar proteinosis
D. Organizing pneumonia
E. Empyema

CASE 24

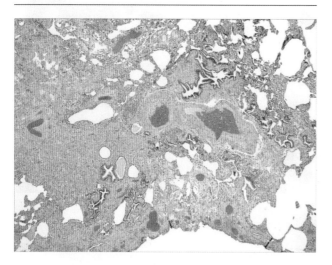

A 59-year-old man nonsmoker presents with nonproductive cough and progressive shortness of breath for the last 2 years. There have been no associated fevers or chills. Physical examination reveals end-expiratory wheezes and basilar crackles. Pulmonary function tests show a restrictive pattern. His chest CT scan shows bilateral reticular and ground-glass opacifications in the subpleural region. The microscopic appearance of wedge lung biopsy is shown here.

Question 1: **The histologic feature thought to be a key to the development of this condition is:**

A. Honeycomb change
B. Smooth muscle proliferation
C. Fatty accumulation
D. Vasculitis
E. Fibroblastic foci

CASE 25

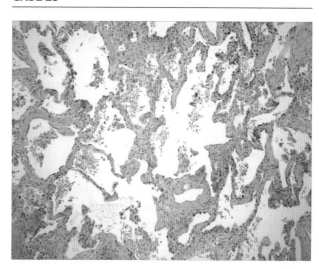

A 49-old-man with no significant past medical history presents with dry cough and exertional dyspnea for the past 5 months. He is a nonsmoker and has no history of occupational exposure. Physical examination of the chest on admission reveals bilateral middle-to-late inspiratory fine crackles in the middle and lower zones. Pulmonary function tests shows diffusion disturbance. His chest radiograph shows bilateral ground-glass opacities involving mainly the lower lobes. The microscopic appearance of wedge biopsy is shown here.

Question 1: **The following features are characteristics of this disorder EXCEPT:**

A. Most cases are idiopathic
B. It is divided into two patterns based on fibrosis
C. Histological feature is characterized by temporal uniformity

D. It may be a manifestation of collagen vascular disease

E. It is the most common cause of idiopathic interstitial pneumonia

CASE 26

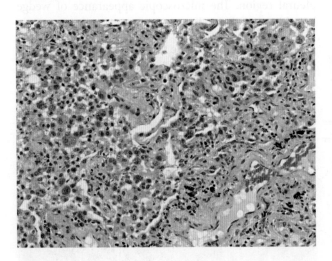

A 47-year-old man presents with increasing shortness of breath and dry cough for last 6 months. He has smoked 20 cigarettes daily for 25 years. There has no history of any known exposure to dust, drugs, or extrinsic allergens. Pulmonary function tests demonstrate a reduced diffusion capacity for carbon monoxide. A chest x-ray shows bilateral ground-glass opacity predominantly in the lower lung fields. A microscopic appearance of wedge lung biopsy is shown here.

Question 1: The following features are seen in patients with respiratory bronchiolitis (RB) and respiratory bronchiolitis-associated interstitial lung disease (RBILD) EXCEPT:

A. RB and RBILD are strongly associated with cigarette smoking

B. Accumulation of pigmented macrophages within the lumen of respiratory bronchiole and surrounding alveolar spaces is the main histologic feature

C. Patients with RBILD are usually older than those with DIP

D. RB, RBILD, and DIP are highly related

E. The prognosis of these disorders is favorable

CASE 27

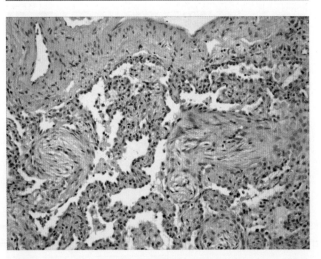

A 59-year-old woman presents with a 6-week history of progressive dyspnea, nonproductive cough, fever, and malaise. Her general practitioner treated her with a course of antibiotics with no improvement. Her chest radiograph shows bilateral multiple patchy alveolar opacities. The microscopic appearance of transbronchial biopsy is shown here.

Question 1: Which of the following conditions does she most likely have?

A. Bronchopneumonia

B. Usual interstitial pneumonia

C. Organizing pneumonia

D. Tuberculosis

E. Diffuse alveolar damage

CASE 28

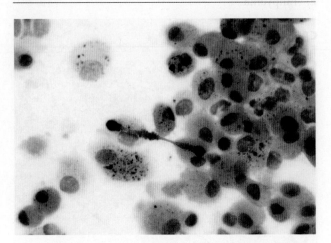

A 58-year-old man presents with chronic left chest pain of 6-month duration, associated with dyspnea on exertion. There is no history of cigarette smoking. He has been a carpenter for 40 years. On examination, his chest expansion is slightly reduced bilaterally. Crackles are heard in both lower zones. CT scan of the chest shows bilateral pleural thickening and calcification, mainly in the mid and lower zones. There are reticulonodular changes in the lung bases. A microscopic appearance of cytology of bronchoalveolar lavage fluid is shown here.

Question 1: **What condition is most likely present in his lung?**

A. Sarcoidosis
B. Berylliosis
C. Silicosis
D. Asbestosis
E. Byssinosis

CASE 29

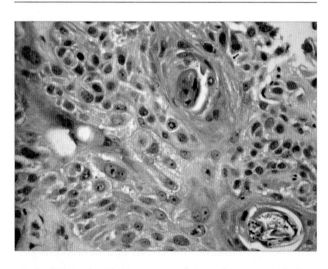

A 65-year-old man presents to his primary care physician with complaints of cough and 6-kg weight loss within the past 4 months. He is a chain smoker. Physical examination reveals finger clubbing. Chest radiograph reveals a 3.5-cm cavitary mass in the left hilar region. Laboratory studies are remarkable for a serum calcium level of 12.5 mg/dL, phosphorus concentration of 3.5 mg/dL, and albumin level of 3.6 g/dL. Bronchoscopy shows a lesion almost occluding the left mainstem bronchus. A biopsy is performed and a microscopic appearance of the lesion is shown here.

Question 1: **Which of the following is the most likely diagnosis?**

A. Small cell carcinoma
B. Squamous cell carcinoma
C. Adenocarcinoma
D. Adenocarcinoma in situ
E. Carcinoid tumor

CASE 30

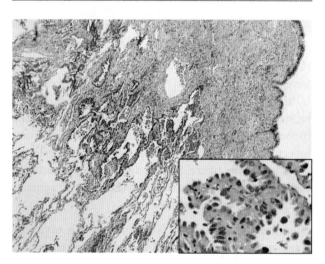

A 43-year-old man presents with cough and mucoid expectoration for 2 weeks. Chest x-ray reveals a 1.5-cm nodule in the right upper lobe in the subpleural location. Biopsy shows a well-differentiated adenocarcinoma. Subsequently, right upper lobectomy is performed. The microscopic image depicts a lesion which is found in the uninvolved lung parenchyma, away from the mass.

Question 1: **Which of the following is the most likely diagnosis?**

A. Atypical adenomatous hyperplasia (AAH)
B. Adenocarcinoma in situ (AIS)
C. Chronic bronchiolitis
D. Tumorlet
E. Invasive adenocarcinoma

CASE 31

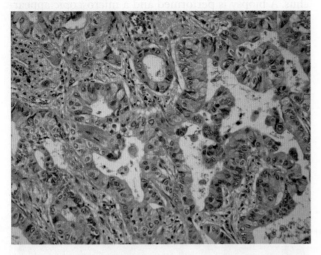

A 65-year-old woman presents with a 5-month history of nonproductive cough with loss of appetite, and 5-kg weight loss. She is a nonsmoker. Physical examination is unremarkable. Chest radiograph shows a subpleural mass in the left lower lobe. A fine-needle aspiration biopsy is performed and she undergoes a left lower lobectomy. The microscopic appearance of the lesion is shown in the figure. She receives therapy directed at epithelial growth factor receptor (EGFR) and remains symptom free for the next 5 years.

Question 1: **If the patient is diagnosed with advanced stage of this tumor, which of the following statements is true regarding molecular testing?**

A. Perform molecular testing for EGFR and ALK
B. Perform molecular testing for RET
C. Perform molecular testing for BRAF
D. Do not perform molecular tests
E. Perform molecular testing for cyclin D1

CASE 32

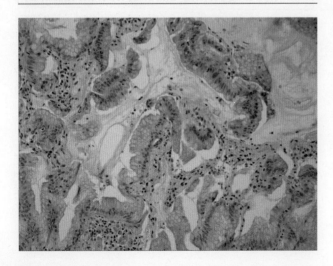

A 69-year-old man presents with history of chronic cough and expectoration of 7-month duration. Chest radiography reveals a 3.4 cm mass in left upper lobe. A CT-guided biopsy is performed. The image depicts microscopy of the lesion.

Question 1: **Which of the following is the most likely diagnosis?**

A. Adenocarcinoma in situ
B. Well-differentiated mucinous adenocarcinoma
C. Metastatic mucinous adenocarcinoma
D. Pulmonary hamartoma
E. Atypical adenomatous hyperplasia

CASE 33

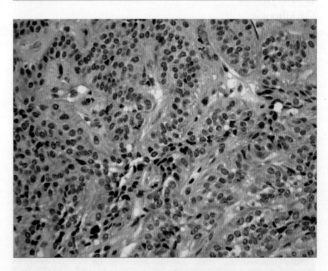

A 40-year-old man presents with a 3-week history of cough and hemoptysis. On physical examination, his temperature is 101.3°F. Chest x-ray shows consolidation of left upper lobe. His condition improves with antibiotic therapy. However, his cough and hemoptysis persist. Bronchoscopic examination shows an obstructive mass filling the bronchus of the left upper lobe. A left lobectomy is performed. Microscopic appearance of the tumor is depicted in the image.

Question 1: **Which of the following statements is true regarding this tumor?**

A. Necrosis and frequent mitoses are common findings
B. It is associated with cigarette smoking
C. Frequently presents with lymph nodal metastasis
D. Majority of the patients present with carcinoid syndrome
E. The tumor is of neuroendocrine cell origin

CASE 34

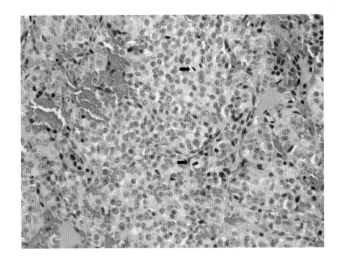

A 65-year-old man was being followed up on serial scans for a small nodule of left lung. Recently, there has been evidence of enlargement (1.5 cm). A biopsy was performed which was diagnosed as a carcinoid tumor. Subsequently he underwent left lower lobectomy. The photomicrograph represents the histologic appearance of the tumor.

Question 1: **What is the most likely diagnosis?**

A. Typical carcinoid tumor
B. Atypical carcinoid tumor
C. Small cell carcinoma
D. Adenocarcinoma
E. Squamous cell carcinoma

CASE 35

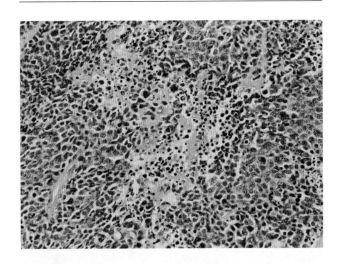

A 55-year-old man presents with truncal obesity, back pain, and easy bruisability for the past 6 months. On physical examination, he is afebrile, and his blood pressure is 160/95 mm Hg. A chest radiograph shows an ill-defined 5-cm mass involving the hilum of right lung. A biopsy is performed. Histology of the lesion is depicted in the figure. The patient was told that the lesion is not amenable to surgical resection.

Question 1: **Which of the following is the most likely diagnosis?**

A. Adenocarcinoma
B. Small cell carcinoma
C. Squamous cell carcinoma
D. Non-Hodgkin lymphoma
E. Carcinoid tumor

CASE 36

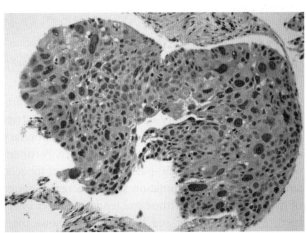

A 65-year-old man presents with fever, chills, cough, and productive sputum for the last 2 days. The patient complains of nonproductive cough for 6 months with occasional hemoptysis. He has lost 15 lb over the same period. He has smoked 50-pack-year cigarettes for the last 40 years. On physical examination, his temperature is 102.6°F. There is decreased breath sounds and dull percussion on the right upper zone. His chest x-ray shows consolidation of right upper lobe. The patient is treated with antibiotics for 2 weeks. A post-treatment chest x-ray reveals a 3-cm right hilar mass. A transbronchial biopsy is performed. The microscopic appearance of tumor is shown in the figure. Immunohistochemical studies reveal that tumor is positive for p63, p40, and cytokeratin 5/6 (CK5/6), but negative for CD45, TTF-1, calretinin, synaptophysin, and chromogranin.

Question 1: **What is the most likely diagnosis?**

A. Non-Hodgkin lymphoma
B. Poorly differentiated adenocarcinoma
C. Mesothelioma
D. Large cell neuroendocrine carcinoma
E. Poorly differentiated squamous cell carcinoma

CASE 37

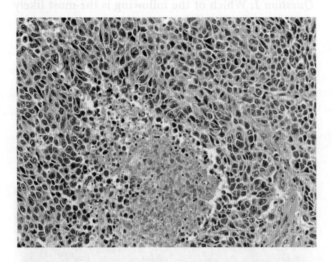

A 71-year-old man presents to the emergency department with a week history of lower back pain. He tries analgesics without much relief. He denies any pulmonary symptoms, or bowel or bladder incontinence. Pertinent social history includes a 50-pack-year history of tobacco smoking. Physical examination shows decreased range of motion of his back with severe tenderness over lower back. MRI of thoracic and lumbar spine shows marrow-replacing lesions at multiple vertebral levels with spinal cord sparing. Chest CT scan reveals a 2.1-cm lobulated soft tissue mass in the right lower lobe. A microscopic appearance of needle biopsy of vertebral lesion is presented in the figure. Immunohistochemical stains are positive for cytokeratin 7, thyroid transcription factor 1 (TTF-1), synaptophysin and CD56, but negative for cytokeratin 20, chromogranin, and p63.

Question 1: **What is the most likely diagnosis?**

A. Metastatic large cell neuroendocrine carcinoma of lung
B. Metastatic sarcomatoid carcinoma of lung
C. Metastatic small cell carcinoma of lung
D. Metastatic adenocarcinoma of lung
E. Metastatic squamous cell carcinoma of lung

CASE 38

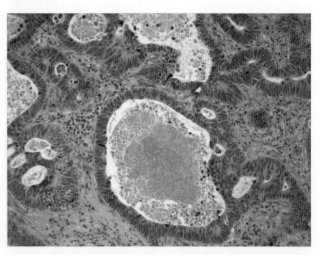

A 68-year-old man, current smoker, presents with cough and hemoptysis for the last 3 weeks. He also complains of several episodes of rectal bleeding over the last 2 years and changes in pattern of stools for the last 3 months. His chest CT scan shows multiple nodules in bilateral lungs, ranging from 1 to 5 cm. A microscopic appearance of lung lesion is shown in the figure.

Question 1: **Which combination of the following phenotypic markers is expressed on this tumor?**

A. TTF-1+, CDX-2−, CK7+, CK20−
B. Hep-1+, Arginase 1+, CK7−, CK20−
C. PSA+, PAP+, CK7−, CK20−
D. CDX2+, TTF-1−, CK7−, CK20+
E. P63+, P40+, CK5/6+, TTF-1−

CASE 39

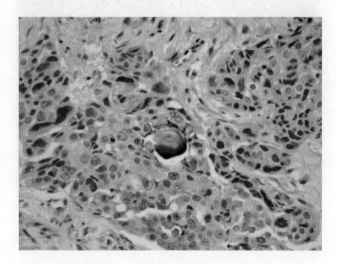

A 45-year-old woman presents with low-grade fever, cough, and sputum for 2 weeks. She has a history of stage IIA infiltrating ductal breast carcinoma and underwent a standard radical mastectomy 7 years ago. She was given six courses of adjuvant chemotherapy. Her chest radiograph shows multiple different-sized nodules in both lung fields. A transbronchial biopsy is performed. A microscopic appearance of the lesion is shown in the image. Immunohistochemical studies revealed: intense positivity for CK7, WT-1, and PAX, while the stains for GCDFP-15, mammaglobin, TTF-1, CDX-2, CK20, and p63 are negative.

Question 1: **Which of the following molecular tests is recommended for this patient?**

A. EGFR
B. K-ras
C. BRCA1/2
D. Her2/neu
E. ALK

CASE 40

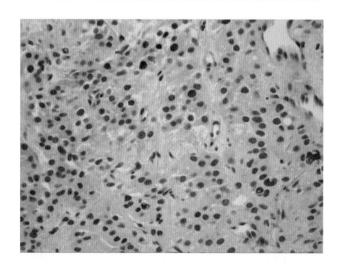

A 59-year-man with no significant past medical history presents with abnormal chest x-ray, found through a routine health examination. His chest radiograph shows bilateral multiple nodular lesions, ranging from 0.5 to 1.5 cm. A microscopic appearance of the lesion from transbronchial biopsy is shown in the figure. Immunohistochemical studies reveal that the lesion is positive for prostate-specific antigen (PSA) and prostatic acid phosphatase (PAP), but negative for TTF-1.

Question 1: **What is the most frequent metastatic site for this tumor?**

A. Liver
B. Lung
C. Brain
D. Adrenals
E. Bones

CASE 41

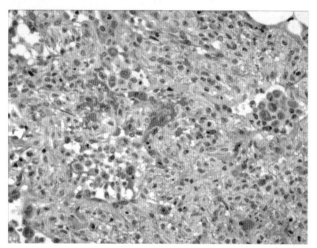

A 30-year-old man presents with exertional shortness of breath and nonproductive cough for 8-year duration. Dyspnea has been progressively increasing over past 2 years. He has a 10-year history of smoking approximately 1 pack per day. A chest radiograph demonstrates bilateral diffuse reticulonodular lesions. A microscopic appearance of lung biopsy is shown here. Immunohistochemical studies show the lesion is positive for S100 protein, CD1a and Langerin, but negative for keratins (CKAE1/3, cam 5.2) and melanin A.

Question 1: **The most likely diagnosis is:**

A. Langerhans cell histiocytosis
B. Usual interstitial pneumonia
C. Eosinophilic pneumonia
D. Metastatic carcinoma
E. Metastatic melanoma

CASE 42

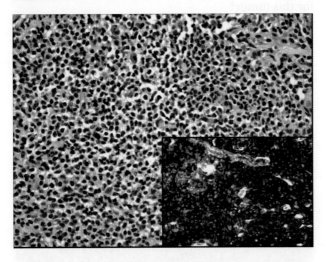

A 62-year-old man is found to have a 3-cm right lower lobe mass, while performing CT scan for chest injury sustained during a car accident. A transbronchial biopsy from the mass is present in the figure. Immunohistochemistry reveals that the neoplastic cells react positively for CD20 and bcl-2, but are negative for CD5, CD10, CD23, CD1a, and cyclin D1. Fluorescent in situ hybridization [FISH] study reveals a t(8;11) translocation.

Question 1: Which of the following is the most likely diagnosis?

A. Lymphoid interstitial pneumonia
B. Chronic lymphocytic leukemia/small lymphocytic lymphoma
C. Extranodal marginal zone lymphoma of bronchus-associated lymphoid tissue
D. Langerhans cell histiocytosis
E. Mantle cell lymphoma

CASE 43

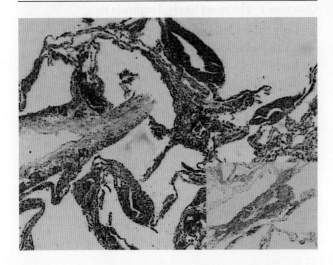

A 42-year-old woman presents with dry cough, exertional dyspnea, and fatigue. She had a 20-pack-year history of smoking but she quit 3 years ago. Her vitals are within normal limits. Physical examination demonstrates bilateral basal crepitations and diminished breath sounds. A computed tomography (CT) scan of the chest reveals bilateral diffuse cystic changes. A microscopic appearance of lung-wedge biopsy is shown here. Immunohistochemical studies reveal that the lesion is positive for smooth muscle actin (inset), HMB-45 and estrogen and progesterone receptors.

Question 1: All the following statements are correct regarding this lesion EXCEPT:

A. It is primarily seen in women of productive age.
B. It is associated with leiomyoma of uterus.
C. It can occur in patients with tuberous sclerosis complex.
D. It is associated with angiomyolipoma of kidney.
E. Patients may present with recurrent pneumothoraces.

CASE 44

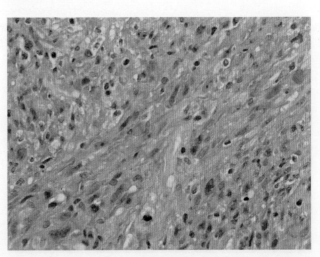

A 67-year-old man with a history of cigarette smoking for 40 years presents with cough and hemoptysis for 6 months. He also reports a 20-lb weight loss over the past few weeks. His past medical history is unremarkable. On examination, his vital signs were within normal limits. Chest auscultation reveals decreased breath sounds in the left apex. Chest computed tomography (CT) scan revealed a 5.5-cm lobulated mass occupying the left hilum. A microscopic appearance of lung biopsy is shown here. Immunohistochemical studies show the lesion is positive for TTF-1, pancytokeratin (AE1/3), epithelial membrane antigen (EMA), but negative for p63 and smooth muscle actin.

Question 1: Which of the following is the most likely diagnosis?

A. Primary pulmonary leiomyosarcoma
B. Primary pulmonary synovial sarcoma
C. Metastatic melanoma
D. Squamous cell carcinoma
E. Pulmonary sarcomatoid carcinoma

CASE 45

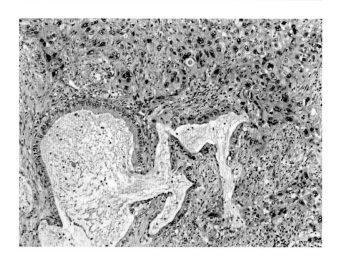

A 57-year-old woman with no smoking history presents with cough, chest pain and hemoptysis of 4-weeks duration. She has significant weight loss over past 6 months. On physical examination, she has mild anemia. Chest CT scan reveals a 3.5-cm irregularly demarcated cavitary mass in the lower lobe of the left lung. She undergoes a left lower lobectomy. The microscopic appearance of the lesion is shown in the figure.

Question 1: Which of the following is the most likely diagnosis?

A. Adenocarcinoma
B. Small cell carcinoma
C. Squamous cell carcinoma
D. Adenosquamous carcinoma
E. Mucoepidermoid carcinoma

CASE 46

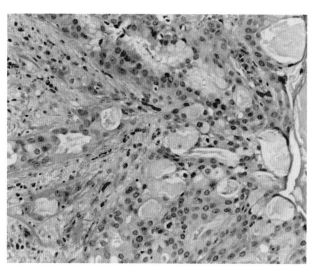

A 30-year-old woman with no smoking history is admitted with fever, chills, worsening cough, and purulent sputum for 1 week. She had an episode of right upper lobe pneumonia a year ago. She recovered after treatment with antibiotics drugs. However, she has had a chronic cough since then. She has no history of hemoptysis, night sweats, tuberculosis, or tuberculosis exposure. Her test for tuberculin is negative. Her physical examination is remarkable for reduced breath sound in the upper third of the right hemithorax. A chest radiograph shows right upper lobe collapse. Her chest CT scan demonstrates a 1.9-cm mass obstructing the right upper bronchus with associated atelectasis. However, a biopsy of the mass is nondiagnostic. The patient undergoes right upper lobe resection. The microscopic appearance of the lesion is shown in the figure.

Question 1: Which is the most likely diagnosis?

A. Squamous cell carcinoma
B. Carcinoid tumor
C. Mucoepidermoid carcinoma
D. Adenoid cystic carcinoma
E. Adenocarcinoma

Answers

CASE 1

Question 1: D. Bronchiole

The image shows a respiratory bronchiole in the center which is devoid of cartilage in the wall, and surrounded by alveoli.

Question 2: C. Air-blood barrier is formed by squamous epithelium, endothelium, and basement membrane

The lungs contain many branching airways, collectively known as the bronchial tree. Air enters the lungs through the primary bronchi, which branch into secondary, which branch into tertiary bronchi.[1] Tertiary bronchi divide into smaller bronchi, and then divide further into bronchioles. Trachea and bronchi have supporting cartilage which keeps the airways open. Bronchioles are airways less than 1 mm in diameter. Bronchioles lack cartilage and submucosal glands and contain more smooth muscle in their walls than the bronchi. Those features allow airflow regulation by altering the diameter of the bronchioles.

* *

Pulmonary lobule (or secondary pulmonary lobule) is grossly visible as polygonal-shaped segments bound by connective tissue (interlobular septa). Pulmonary lobules are approximately 1 to 3 cm in diameter and identifiable with high-resolution CT scan. Pulmonary lobule typically contains 3 to 5 terminal bronchioles and many alveolar ducts and alveoli. The functional unit of the lung is the acinus, where gases are exchanged with surrounding blood vessels. The acinus contains respiratory bronchioles, alveolar ducts, and alveoli. The alveoli consist of an epithelial layer and extracellular matrix surrounded by capillaries. Alveoli are lined by squamous (type I pneumocytes) and cuboidal (type II pneumocytes) epithelial cells and macrophages. The wall of an alveolus is primarily composed of simple squamous epithelium (type I cells). Gas exchange occurs easily across this very thin epithelium. Type II cells are the progenitor cells for type I cells and produce surfactant. Type II cell

hyperplasia represents a nonspecific marker of alveolar injury and repair. Air-blood barrier is the intervening structure between alveolar air and blood that is formed by the type I pneumocytes of the alveolar wall, the endothelial cells of the capillaries and the basement membrane between the two cells.

CASE 2

Question 1: D. Pulmonary alveolar proteinosis

The image depicts alveoli filled with eosinophilic granular material, consistent with pulmonary alveolar proteinosis (PAP), which is characterized by alveolar accumulation of surfactant composed of proteins and lipids (positive for PAS stain). The etiology of this disorder is largely unknown. It is thought that overproduction of surfactant by type II pneumocytes or defective surfactant clearance by macrophages contributes to this condition. PAP may be divided into three distinct types: congenital, secondary, and primary or autoimmune types. Congenital PAP results from mutations in the gene encoding surfactant or granulocyte-macrophage colony-stimulating factor (GM-CSF). Secondary PAP develops in association with conditions involving functional impairment or reduced numbers of alveolar macrophages. Such conditions include dust and chemical exposure, infections, immunodeficiency and hematologic malignancies. Primary or autoimmune PAP has been attributed to anti–GM-CSF antibodies that undermine macrophage function. Primary or autoimmune PAP accounts for 90% of all PAP cases. There is a male predominance with a usual age range of 30 to 50 years. The common presenting symptom is progressive exertional dyspnea of insidious onset and cough. The histologic hallmark of PAP is an intra-alveolar accumulation of eosinophilic proteinaceous granular material, highlighted by periodic acid-Schiff (PAS) stain. The main differential diagnosis includes pulmonary edema and *Pneumocystis jirovecii* pneumonia. Pulmonary edema is accumulation of fluid in alveolar spaces that lacks globular material and macrophages seen in

492

PAP. *Pneumocystis jirovecii* pneumonia shows intraalveolar vacuolated or foamy exudate that corresponds to the organisms, which can be demonstrated by Gomori methenamine silver (GMS) stain.[6] Diffuse alveolar hemorrhage is characterized by intra-alveolar accumulation of blood, while pulmonary alveolar microlithiasis reveals airspaces with innumerable tiny calcified bodies.[14]

CASE 3

Question 1: E. Pneumothorax
The image shows alveolar walls, lined by acellular eosinophilic material, consistent with hyaline membrane. Acute respiratory distress syndrome (ARDS) is a rapidly progressive disorder characterized by a severe inflammatory process causing diffuse alveolar damage and resulting in a variable degree of ventilation perfusion mismatch, severe hypoxemia, and poor-lung compliance. Diffuse alveolar damage is the pathologic hallmark of ARDS and is divided into three phases: exudative phase, proliferative phase, and fibrotic phase. The exudative phase occurs in the first week following the onset of respiratory failure. The changes in the exudative phase include congestion, interstitial and alveolar edema, and alveolar hyaline membrane formed by fibrin and necrotic cellular debris. The proliferative phase begins 1 week after the injury and is characterized by extensive proliferation of type II pneumocytes and fibroblasts. In some cases, there is progression into to the fibrotic phase, in which the lungs undergo extensive remodeling with dense fibrous tissue and end stage honeycomb fibrosis develops. Majority of the cases of ARDS in adults are associated with pulmonary or nonpulmonary sepsis. Other risk factors include those causing direct lung injury (oxygen toxicity, inhalation of toxins and irritant gases, aspiration of gastric contents, pulmonary contusion, etc.) and indirect lung injury (burns, trauma, hemorrhagic pancreatitis, complicated surgery, narcotic overdose, etc.). Pneumothorax causes compressive atelectasis of the lung but does not result in ARDS.

CASE 4

Question 1: D. Acute right heart failure
The image shows a thrombus in the main pulmonary artery. Acute right ventricular failure is the most common cause of sudden death among patients with acute pulmonary embolism (PE). PE is a blockage of the main arteries of the lung or its branches by a substance that

travels from elsewhere in the body through the blood stream. More than 90% of cases of PE are complications of deep vein thrombosis from the leg or pelvic veins. Emboli can also be composed of fat, air, or tumor tissue. When emboli block the main pulmonary arteries, PE can cause sudden death. Deep venous thrombosis following trauma and immobilization is associated with risk factors, such as major surgery and a past history of venous thrombosis. Inherited conditions, such as antithrombin, protein C and protein S deficiencies, or Factor V Leiden mutation, are other major predisposing risk factors.

CASE 5

Question 1: E. Amyloidosis, AL type
The image shows a section from the lung after Congo red staining, with characteristic birefringence, when observed under polarized light. The patient has pulmonary amyloidosis, AL type. Amyloid deposits were confirmed by the apple-green birefringence after staining with Congo red. Extensive deposits of amyloid were present in the pulmonary interstitium and vascular walls. Amyloidosis is a heterogeneous group of disorders associated with the deposition of protein in an abnormal fibrillar form. There are four major categories of systemic amyloidosis: (1) primary or immunoglobulin light-chain (AL) disease, (2) secondary or amyloid protein A (AA) disease, (3) hereditary or mutant transthyretin (ATTR) disease, and (4) dialysis-associated or β_2-microglobulin (β_2M) disease.[4] There are three patterns of pulmonary involvement: (1) tracheobronchial form with diffuse or focal thickening of the walls of the trachea and bronchi, (2) nodular parenchymal form with solitary or multiple nodules, and (3) diffuse interstitial pattern. Pulmonary interstitial fibrosis usually shows interstitial inflammation and fibrosis without amyloid deposition. Hyaline membrane disease is a respiratory disease of the newborn, especially in the premature infant, in which a membrane composed of proteins and dead cells lines the alveoli. Pulmonary vasculitis refers to inflammation and damage to blood vessels in the lung.

CASE 6

Question 1: D. Panacinar emphysema
Emphysema is a condition of the lung characterized by abnormal permanent enlargement of airspaces distal to the terminal bronchioles, accompanied by destruction of

their walls but without obvious fibrosis.[5] It is classified according to anatomical distribution of the lesion within the acini. Panacinar emphysema is a clinically distinct type of emphysema, most commonly due to hereditary alpha-1-antitrypsin (A1AT) deficiency. The main physiological function of A1AT, also known as a proteinase inhibitor, is to protect the lung tissue from the proteolytic enzymes. A1AT deficiency allows neutrophil elastase to degrade elastic fibers and connective tissue resulting in emphysematous change. This type of emphysema is characterized by uniform destruction and enlargement of the acini from the respiratory bronchioles to the terminal alveolar sacs. Centriacinar (centrilobular) emphysema is the most common form of emphysema. This type is frequently associated with long-term cigarette smoking and predominantly involves the upper and posterior portions of the lung. Centriacinar emphysema is characterized by destruction and enlargement of central or proximal parts of respiratory unit, formed by respiratory bronchioles, with sparing of the distal alveoli. Paraseptal (distal) emphysema involves mostly the distal acinus, but proximal portion of the acinus is normal. It occurs primarily adjacent to the pleura and connective tissue septa, especially in the upper lobe. This type produces apical bullae and may cause spontaneous pneumothorax in young adults. Interstitial emphysema is characterized by entry of air into the connective tissue of lung, mediastinum or subcutaneous tissue. Most patients have a history of mechanical ventilation. Irregular emphysema is the irregular involvement of acini and is associated with pulmonary scarring.

CASE 7

Question 1: A. Anti-glomerular basement membrane antibody

The biopsy of the lung shown in the image, demonstrates extensive intra-alveolar hemorrhage. This patient most likely has Goodpasture syndrome, which is defined as an autoimmune disorder in which circulating anti-glomerular basement membrane (GBM) antibodies reacts with the basement membrane of alveoli and glomeruli. Linear deposition of IgG along the basement membrane of the alveoli and glomeruli by immunofluorescence is characteristic of the disease. Typically, young male smokers are affected by the disease. In more than 90% of patients with Goodpasture syndrome, anti-GBM antibodies can be detected in the serum. Lung involvement usually consists of diffuse alveolar hemorrhage while the kidneys

typically show a rapidly progressive glomerulonephritis. The anti–double-stranded DNA antibody and anti-Smith antibody are markers for systemic lupus erythematosus (SLE). The anti-centromere antibody is a marker for CREST syndrome, while anti-ribonucleoprotein antibody is a marker for mixed connective tissue disease.

CASE 8

Question 1: B. Granulomatosis with polyangiitis

The biopsy of lung shows a collection of neutrophils surrounded by histiocytes. Granulomatosis with Polyangiitis (GPA), formerly called Wegener granulomatosis, is an uncommon systemic vasculitis of unknown etiology, characterized by necrotizing granulomatous inflammation, tissue necrosis, and variable degrees of vasculitis in small- and medium-sized blood vessels.[6] The disease is characterized by the classic triad of necrotizing granuloma of the upper and lower respiratory tract, focal necrotizing vasculitis of lung and pauci-immune segmental necrotizing glomerulonephritis. Sex distribution of GPA is equal and most of the patients present in the fifth decade, although the age ranges can extend to both extremes. Symptoms may either develop suddenly or gradually and the first symptoms usually involve the respiratory tract. Antineutrophil cytoplasmic antibodies (C-ANCA) with a cytoplasmic staining pattern by immunofluorescence are found in more than 90% of active patients. The most common histological features are necrotizing granulomatous inflammation and necrotizing vasculitis. The necrotizing granulomatous inflammation is characterized by large areas of geographic necrosis bounded by palisading histiocytes. Giant cells, either scattered or in loose clusters, are commonly seen. Necrotizing vasculitis in GPA typically involves small vessels, which are partly to completely replaced by an inflammatory infiltrate with varying proportion of neutrophils, eosinophils, and histiocytes. Eosinophilic granulomatosis with polyangiitis (EGPA) is associated with severe asthma, peripheral blood eosinophilia, and pulmonary infiltrates. It typically occurs in young adults. Vasculitis is characterized by fibrinoid necrosis with eosinophilic infiltrate and granulomatous inflammation. Hypersensitivity pneumonitis (HSP or HP) is an inflammation of the alveoli caused by hypersensitivity to inhaled organic dusts. The histological features are chronic interstitial inflammation with small non-necrotizing granulomas but lack necrotizing vasculitis. Renal and pulmonary diseases are the presenting features of Goodpasture syndrome, with intra-alveolar hemorrhage but without any necrotizing granulomatous inflammation and necrotizing vasculitis. Sarcoidosis is characterized by non-necrotizing granulomatous inflammation without definitive vasculitis.

CASE 9

Question 1: C. Hypersensitivity pneumonitis

The microscopic picture shows a medium-sized artery and surrounding pulmonary tissue are infiltrated by numerous eosinophils. Eosinophilic granulomatosis with polyangiitis (EGPA), formerly known as Churg–Strauss syndrome, is a rare systemic small-vessel necrotizing vasculitis, characterized by the triad of asthma, peripheral blood eosinophilia and vasculitis. It particularly involves pulmonary, gastrointestinal, neural, and cardiovascular systems. The pathogenesis of is largely unknown. The disease affects both sexes equally with the mean age of 50 years at diagnosis. The natural course can be described to follow three phases: (a) rhinosinusitis and asthma, (b) blood and tissue eosinophilia, and (c) eventually systemic vasculitis. Asthma and hypereosinophilia are present in most cases. Recurrent episodes of asthma may persist for years before the onset of the vasculitis. The histologic features include the combination of tissue infiltration by eosinophils, necrotizing vasculitis, and extravascular granulomas. Tissue eosinophilic infiltration is manifested by areas of eosinophilic pneumonia, in which large numbers of eosinophils and macrophages accumulate within alveolar spaces accompanied by eosinophilic infiltration of alveolar septa.[7] Vasculitis is characterized by intimal and medial infiltration by numerous eosinophils and other inflammatory cells. Necrotizing granulomas are often found in the adjacent parenchyma. The histologic differential diagnosis of EGPA in the lung includes disorders associated with a prominent eosinophil infiltrate and granulomatous inflammation. Granulomatosis with polyangiitis, formerly known as Wegener granulomatosis is characterized by necrotizing granulomatous inflammation surrounding vasculature, but tissue eosinophilia is not a prominent feature. Eosinophilic pneumonia, ABPA, and asthmatic bronchitis show tissue eosinophilia, but lack vasculitis and systemic involvement.

* *

Eosinophilic lung disease consists of a heterogeneous group of disorders characterized by accumulation of eosinophils in the alveolar spaces or interstitium and is often accompanied by blood eosinophilia. Eosinophilic lung disease can be classified as idiopathic or secondary to known causes. Secondary disorders include infections (parasitic, and fungal), drug/medication reactions, inhalant exposure (e.g., crack cocaine), allergic bronchopulmonary aspergillosis (ABPA), primary connective tissue disease (e.g., rheumatoid arthritis-related eosinophilic pneumonia), and primary malignancy (leukemias, lymphomas, and lung carcinoma). Loeffler's syndrome refers to simple pulmonary eosinophilia from any fungal, parasitic, or drug-induced causes. Allergic bronchopulmonary aspergillosis is a chronic eosinophilic syndrome associated with exposure to Aspergillus antigens. In bronchial asthma, the walls of the affected airways are infiltrated by eosinophils. EGPA is a small-vessel vasculitis defined as an eosinophil-rich and granulomatous inflammation involving the respiratory tract and associated with asthma and eosinophilia. Hypersensitivity pneumonitis (HSP or HP) is a diffuse interstitial granulomatous lung disease due to immunologic reaction to inhaled foreign substance, usually certain types of dust, fungus, or molds.[8] The histologic appearance of chronic HP is characterized by bronchocentric cellular interstitial pneumonia with poorly formed granulomas and organizing pneumonia. The inflammatory infiltrate consists mostly of lymphocytes with some plasma cells and histiocytes. Eosinophils are scant or absent.

CASE 10

Question 1: E. Bird dust

The biopsy of the lung shows patchy interstitial infiltrates of lymphocyte and plasma cells with poorly formed granulomas, which is suggestive of hypersensitivity pneumonitis (HP). HP comprises a group of allergic lung diseases caused by inhalation of various antigens contained in organic dusts. Farmer's lung (FL) (thermophilic actinomycetes) and bird fancier's lung (BFL) (avian proteins) remain the most prevalent forms of the disease. Bird fancier's lung is a form of HP resulting from airborne exposure to avian antigens present in the dry dust of the droppings and sometimes in the feathers of a variety of birds. Birds such as pigeons, budgerigars (parakeets), parrots, turtle doves, turkeys, and chickens have been implicated. HP represents a combination of immune complex-mediated (type III) and T cell–mediated, delayed (type IV) hypersensitivity reaction. The disease may present acutely or subacutely and such episodes usually resolve with cessation of the antigen exposure. Chronic disease may progress to irreversible form. HP is histologically characterized by small, indistinct, non-necrotizing granulomas, chronic inflammatory change in small airways and diffuse interstitial infiltrates of chronic inflammatory cells. The lesions are usually diffuse but more severe in the peribronchiolar areas. Bronchiolitis obliterans with intraluminal budding fibrosis or organizing pneumonia are often seen in localized areas. Granulomas may progress to fibrosis. The criteria required to make the diagnosis of HP are not clearly defined. The diagnosis can be suspected on the basis of a compatible temporal relationship between pulmonary symptoms and a history of environmental or occupational exposure. Bronchoalveolar lavage (BAL) analysis and compatible histological changes can support the diagnosis of HP. BAL analysis often shows a decreased CD4+/CD8+ ratio (less than 1.0). The majority of patients with HP have an excellent prognosis after cessation of antigen exposure. If the disease is not recognized at an early phase, fibrosis can develop. Coal dust inhalation can result focal interstitial pigment deposition. Exposure to asbestos may lead to foci of fibrosis in the walls of respiratory bronchioles accompanied by the presence of asbestos bodies. Silicosis is characterized by sharply circumscribed nodules of dense, whorled hyalinized collagen. Talcosis is typified by patchy granulomas and foci of interstitial fibrosis associated with abundant dust deposits.

CASE 11

Question 1: D. Actinomyces israelii

The image depicts high-power view of an actinomycotic abscess showing acute inflammation with "sulfur granule," composed of bacteria with branching filaments arranged in a radial pattern. Pulmonary actinomycosis is a rare disease with an occult onset and progressive chronic course. It is caused by *Actinomyces* sp, which are anaerobic gram-positive bacilli with beaded, branching, and filamentous morphology. The organism can also be stained by silver impregnation method like Gomori methenamine silver (GMS) stain. These bacteria are normally present in the human oral cavity. The disease usually develops as a result of aspiration of pathogens from oropharyngeal or gastrointestinal contents. Individuals with advanced dental caries are particularly predisposed. It usually affects males in the fourth and fifth decades of life. Pulmonary actinomycosis tends to occur in immunodeficiency states, malnutrition, diabetes

mellitus, cirrhosis, and after radiotherapy. The major differential diagnosis in lung biopsy specimens is with *Nocardia*, which are aerobic, gram-positive, weakly acid-fast bacilli with beaded and filamentous morphology. *Nocardia* does not form sulfur granules. *Candida* species are usually characterized by the presence of budding yeast forms and pseudohyphae. Caseating granulomatous inflammation is typical for *Mycobacterium Tuberculosis* infection.[9] *Aspergillus* species demonstrate fungal hyphae with septa and branching at 45-degree angles.

CASE 12

Question 1: B. Ziehl–Neelsen stain

The image is a necrotizing granuloma. It consists of pink, amorphous material in the center representing caseous necrosis, surrounded by a rim of epithelioid histiocytes and Langerhans giant cells. This inflammation is typical for *Mycobacterium Tuberculosis* infection. Ziehl–Neelsen stain was first described by two German physicians: Franz Ziehl and Friedrich Neelsen. It is a special stain used to identify acid-fast organisms. Gomori methenamine silver (GMS) and periodic acid-Schiff (PAS) stains are the two most common stains used to identify fungi in tissues and cytology specimens in the daily practice of pathology. Mycobacteria are negative for Gram stain. Giemsa stain is commonly used to look for *Helicobacter pylori* in tissue sections.

CASE 13

Question 1: D. Sarcoidosis

The image shows a discrete noncaseating granuloma consisting of clusters of epithelioid cells and giant cells occurring within sclerotic fibrosis. The presence of granuloma(s) is necessary to establish the diagnosis of sarcoidosis. However, the granulomas in sarcoidosis are nonspecific, which are not diagnostic of either sarcoidosis or any other granulomatous diseases. Among the diseases to be excluded are mycobacterial, fungal, and parasitic infections, chronic beryllium disease, and hypersensitivity pneumonitis. Special stains for organisms (acid-fast bacilli and silver stains) are routinely performed to exclude infection. The final diagnosis is usually made based on a combination of clinical and radiological findings and histological evidence of noncaseating granulomatous inflammation. In sarcoid granulomas, a variety of inclusions may be present, including

Schaumann's bodies, asteroid bodies, and birefringent crystals. These inclusions are nonspecific and not diagnostic of sarcoidosis. Hypersensitivity pneumonitis shows interstitial infiltrates of lymphocytes and plasma cells with poorly formed granulomas. A history of environmental or occupational exposure is usually present. Caseating granulomatous inflammation is typical for *Mycobacterium tuberculosis* infection and pulmonary histoplasmosis, which are positive for special stains (AFB and silver stains). Pulmonary Langerhans cell histiocytosis (PLCH) is characterized by proliferation and infiltration of Langerhans cells mixed with eosinophils without granulomatous inflammation.

CASE 14

Question 1: C. *Mycobacterium avium* complex infection

The image shows collection of epithelioid histiocytes forming a granuloma. Ziehl–Neelsen stain (inset) shows numerous acid-fast bacilli in the cytoplasm of histiocytes, which are typical for *Mycobacterium avium* complex (MAC) infection. MAC consists of *M. avium* and *M. intracellulare*, because these species are difficult to differentiate. These organisms are found in soil and water and in infected animals. Transmission is thought to be due to inhalation of environmentally derived airborne organisms, rather than person to person. Oral ingestion is generally considered more likely in the immunocompromised host. MAC is the most common cause of infection by nontuberculous mycobacteria (NTM) in patients with AIDS. Profound immunosuppression is the major risk for the development of disseminated MAC infection. Previous studies demonstrate that the median CD4 cell count is consistently less than 50 cells/mm^3 at the time that disseminated disease is diagnosed. MAC has been associated with pulmonary infections, osteomyelitis, tenosynovitis, synovitis, and disseminated disease. Histologically, the lungs show granulomatous inflammation with less tendency to caseate than with M. tuberculosis. In AIDS patient, the lungs show numerous macrophages in the alveolar spaces. Well-formed granulomas are usually absent. The histiocytes contain massive number of bacilli, which can be highlighted by acid-fast bacilli (AFB) stain. Caseating granulomatous inflammation is typical for *Mycobacterium Tuberculosis* infection. AFB stain shows rare acid-fast bacilli. Cytomegalovirus (CMV) pneumonia is characterized by the presence of cytomegalic cells with basophilic cytoplasmic inclusions

and a large nuclear inclusion surrounded by a halo. Sarcoidosis is a noncaseating granulomatous disease, in which a diagnosis requires exclusion of other causes of granulomatous inflammation.[10] *Pneumocystis* pneumonia is caused by the yeast-like fungus, which can be demonstrated by GMS stain.

CASE 15

Question 1: E. Gomori methenamine silver (GMS) stain

Microscopic picture shows intra-alveolar pink foamy exudates, in which the organisms appear as small "bubble" in a background of proteinaceous exudates, without any significant inflammation. This is the classical lesion of *Pneumocystis jirovecii* pneumonia. *Pneumocystis jirovecii* pneumonia is one of the most common opportunistic infections in patients with AIDS. Gomori methenamine silver (GMS) stain can demonstrate numerous *Pneumocystis jirovecii* cysts within exudates. Gram stain is useful for determining what bacterial organisms may be present. Acid-fast bacilli (AFB) stain is used to look for acid-fast bacilli, such as mycobacteria. Prussian blue stain is used to demonstrate iron in tissue section. Mucicarmine stain is used for the evaluation of mucins and cryptococcus.[11]

CASE 16

Question 1: E. Acquired immunodeficiency syndrome

Image shows Gomori methenamine silver (GMS) stain revealing round or oval cysts with a central dark dot. These are typical features of *Pneumocystis jirovecii*. Although *P. jirovecii* pneumonia can be seen with a variety of acquired and congenital immunodeficient states, it is most often associated with acquired immunodeficiency syndrome (AIDS). A stain pattern of *P. jirovecii* can be similar to that of the yeast form of *Histoplasma capsulatum*. The difference between those two organisms is that *P. jirovecii* does not have budding forms and is extracellular in location while *H. capsulatum* has budding forms and is intracellular in location. Patients with autoimmune disease, e.g., systemic lupus erythematosus, may develop a variety of infections if they are treated with immunosuppressive drugs. Patients with diabetes mellitus are prone to bacterial infection. Patients with sarcoidosis treated with corticosteroids may have opportunistic infections.

CASE 17

Question 1:A. Acute invasive aspergillosis

The image shows lung parenchyma with hemorrhagic necrosis. GMS stain (inset) demonstrates hyphae with septa and branching at 45-degree angles, characteristic of *Aspergillus* species. Aspergillosis is a major cause of morbidity and mortality in immunocompromised patients.[12] *Aspergillus* species are widespread in the environment and are commonly isolated from soil, plant debris, and indoor environment, including hospitals.[12] *Aspergillus fumigatus* is the most often isolated from the lungs of immunocompromised patients and is responsible for fatal invasive aspergillosis. The risk factors for invasive aspergillosis include neutropenia, hematopoietic stem-cell transplantation, solid-organ transplantation, prolonged therapy with high-dose corticosteroids, advanced AIDS, and chronic granulomatous disease. Invasive aspergillosis is typically angiocentric and produces hemorrhagic infarcts. Antifungals remain the mainstay of therapy for the patients with invasive aspergillosis. Amphotericin B is the first-line therapy; however, the overall response rate for amphotericin B is low (30–55% in all patient populations) and there is a high incidence of adverse events. The mortality rate for invasive pulmonary aspergillosis can be 50% to 90% with respiratory failure and massive hemoptysis as major complications. *Candida* species are usually differentiated from other fungal forms by the presence of budding yeast forms and pseudohyphae. The hyphae of *zygomycetes* and *aspergillus* are different in tissue section. The hyphae of *zygomycetes* are broad, non-septate, twisted or folded, and have a branching pattern with 90-degree angles. *Histoplasma* and *cryptococcus* are other yeast-form fungi.

CASE 18

Question 1: E. Cryptococcal pneumonia

The image shows abundant fungal yeasts with mucinous capsules, which are highlighted by mucicarmine stain (inset). *Cryptococcus neoformans* is an encapsulated, round-to-oval yeast measuring 4 to 6 microns with a surrounding polysaccharide capsule. Cryptococcus grows readily from soil contaminated with avian excreta, particularly those of pigeons. Pulmonary cryptococcosis is caused by inhalation of spores of cryptococcus neoformans. The infection is most often associated with HIV infection, but other conditions predisposing to cryptococcal infection includes

solid-organ transplantation, hematologic malignancy, chronic corticosteroid treatment, and sarcoidosis. Cryptococcal infection has two major clinical forms: pulmonary infection and cerebromeningeal infection. The natural history of pulmonary cryptococcosis is highly dependent on the immune status of the patient. In the immunocompetent patient, pulmonary cryptococcosis may be self-limited, that may resolve over a period of weeks to months without directed antifungal therapy. However, immunocompromised patients are more likely to develop disseminated cryptococcosis. A definitive diagnosis of cryptococcosis is made by fungal culture or by identification of the organisms within cells or tissue of bronchoalveolar lavage (BAL), transbronchial biopsy, or open lung biopsy. On routine H&E staining, cryptococcus neoformans is difficult to identify. On Gomori methenamine silver (GMS) and periodic acid-Schiff (PAS) staining, it can be recognized as oval shape yeasts with narrow-based budding. Serum cryptococcal antigen (CrAg) detection is highly sensitive for the diagnosis of disseminated cryptococcosis. Cytomegalovirus (CMV) pneumonia is characterized by the presence of cytomegalic cells with basophilic cytoplasmic inclusions and a large nuclear inclusion surrounded by a halo. Adult respiratory distress syndrome (ARDS) is characterized by alveolar hyaline membrane. *Pneumocystis jirovecii* pneumonia can be demonstrated by numerous intra-alveolar round or oval cysts by GMS stain. *Candida* sp are usually differentiated by the presence of budding yeast forms and pseudohyphae.

CASE 19

Question 1: A. Pulmonary histoplasmosis

Microscopic image shows necrotizing granulomatous inflammation containing oval yeasts, confirmed by GMS stain. Pulmonary histoplasmosis is an infection caused by dimorphic fungus *Histoplasma capsulatum*.[13] It is the most common pulmonary endemic fungal infection worldwide and the most common endemic mycosis in AIDS patients. It is endemic in the south-central United States, especially in the Ohio and Mississippi river valleys. Approximately 500,000 new cases of *H. capsulatum* infections are reported annually in the United States. *H. capsulatum* infection is acquired by inhaling mycelium spores from soil contaminated by bird or bat droppings. The severity of the initial infection depends largely on the amount of the inoculum and immune status of the host. Only 5% to 10% of infections cause symptoms. A self-limiting and often latent primary pulmonary involvement may result in coin lesions on chest radiography. Chronic progressive secondary lung disease is characterized by infiltrations and cavitations predominantly in the upper lung fields. In immunosuppressed patients, particularly those with AIDS, *H. capsulatum* behaves as an opportunist and can cause disseminated forms of disease in both initial and secondary infections. From an exudative inflammation to a granulomatous process, the histological reaction to *H. capsulatum* varies depending on the pattern of infection. In chronic infection, the most common reaction is a necrotizing granuloma. *H. capsulatum* are spherical to oval yeasts with narrow-based budding and are often situated in clusters due to the intracellular growth within histiocytes. *Candida* sp are oval budding yeasts with pseudohyphae. *Cryptococcus* sp are round budding yeasts with thick capsule. *Coccidioides* sp are large mature spherules with thick refractile wall filled with endospores. *H. capsulatum* can be differentiated from *Pneumocystis carinii* by the presence of budding yeast forms as well as the lack of an intra-alveolar location.

CASE 20

Question 1: D. Candidiasis

Image shows alveolar spaces filled with fungal yeasts and pseudohyphae, which are consistent with pulmonary candidiasis. Candidiasis is the most common opportunistic infection in immunocompromised patients. Among nine different species that are pathogenic in humans, *Candida albicans* is the most common. *C. albicans* is part of normal microflora of mouth and oropharynx, digestive tract, and vagina. Pulmonary candidiasis can be acquired by either hematogenous dissemination or aspiration from oropharynx. Pulmonary candidiasis is difficult to diagnose due to nonspecific radiological and culture findings. The presence of yeasts in alveolar lavage or sputum specimens is not specific and blood cultures may also be negative. Definitive diagnosis often rests on histopathologic evaluation of the specimen. On tissue sections, *Candida* sp are oval yeast-like cells 2 to 6 μm in diameter with narrow-based budding, pseudohyphae and occasionally true hyphae. *Cryptococcus* sp are round budding yeasts with thick capsule. *Histoplasma capsulatum* are spherical to oval yeasts with narrow-based budding and are often situated in clusters due to the intracellular growth within histiocytes. *Aspergillus* can be separated by the presence of septate hyphae with dichotomous acute angle branching. *Coccidioides* sp

are characterized by large mature spherules with thick refractile wall filled with endospores.

CASE 21

Question 1: C. Pulmonary zygomycosis

Lung-wedge biopsy shows a hemorrhagic cyst filled with thick wall broad nonseptate hyphae with right-angle branching. Zygomycosis is an uncommon fungal infection caused by the class Zygomycetes, order Mucorales, and Entomophthorales.[14] Mucorales (mucormycosis) is the most common type causing human infections and is specified by a rapid clinical course, significant tissue destruction, and invasion of blood vessels. Pulmonary zygomycosis is most prevalent in immunocompromised patients including those with neutropenia, hematologic malignancies, inadequately controlled diabetes mellitus and corticosteroid therapy. The clinical presentation is indistinguishable from that of invasive pulmonary aspergillosis. The diagnosis is made based on clinical manifestations, histopathological examinations, and fungal culture. Aspergillosis can be distinguished by its septate hyphae with acute angle branching at 45 degrees. *Candida* species are usually separated from other fungal forms by the presence of yeast-like cells and pseudohyphae. Histoplasmosis and cryptococcosis are other yeast forms of fungi.

CASE 22

Question 1: D. Cytomegalovirus pneumonia

Image shows cytopathic effects of cytomegalovirus (CMV) including cytomegaly, multiple small basophilic cytoplasmic inclusions, and a large nuclear inclusion surrounded by a halo. Immunohistochemistry for CMV reveals stains of the nuclear and cytoplasmic inclusions. CMV infection is a frequent complication of immunosuppressive states such as AIDS, transplant patients, and those who receive immunosuppressive therapy for cancer or immunologic disease. CMV is an important cause of morbidity and mortality in immunosuppressed patients. The diagnosis of CMV pneumonia is based on viral culture and pathologic evaluation of lung biopsies or bronchoalveolar lavage (BAL) specimens. There is no evidence of atypical lymphocytic proliferation and atypical alveolar cell proliferation. *Pneumocystis jirovecii* pneumonia can be demonstrated by numerous intra-alveolar round or oval cysts by GMS stain. Adult respiratory distress syndrome (ARDS) is characterized by alveolar hyaline membrane.

CASE 23

Question 1: C. Pulmonary alveolar proteinosis

The lung biopsy shows intra-alveolar neutrophil infiltration and fragments of vegetable material (inset), consistent with aspiration pneumonia. Aspiration results from the inhalation of the contents of the oral or upper gastrointestinal tract into the lung. Aspiration into the right lung and lower lobe is more common due to the larger caliber and more vertical orientation of the right mainstem bronchus. Aspiration in adults occurs mostly in patients with several predisposing conditions such as altered mental status (anesthesia, alcohol, or drug), dysphagia from neurologic disorders (dementia, Parkinson disease, multiple sclerosis, poststroke), Esophageal motility disorders (GERD, scleroderma, polymyositis), and oropharyngeal colonization (gingival dental sepsis). The most common pathogens implicated in causing aspiration pneumonia are *Staphylococcus aureus*, *Streptococcus pneumoniae*, anaerobes (*Bacteroides*, *Peptococcus*, *Fusobacterium* sp) and gram-negative bacilli. The anaerobes normally are found in the oral cavity and are readily aspirated. Aspiration into the lower respiratory tract can cause a wide variety of pulmonary injury including airway obstruction, pneumonia, organizing pneumonia, and abscess formation. Acute inflammation may extend to the pleural cavity and produce an empyema. Acute aspiration of gastric acid (Mendelson's syndrome) results in pulmonary edema, hemorrhage, and diffused alveolar damage, which is the clinical syndrome of adult respiratory distress. If the aspirated material has a high-lipid content, alveolar macrophages ingesting the lipids fill the alveolar space. The foamy macrophages and acute inflammation in alveolar spaces is known as lipoid pneumonia. Pulmonary alveolar proteinosis (PAP) is characterized by intra-alveolar accumulation of a granular appearing proteinaceous material. The etiology of PAP is unknown. PAP is unrelated to aspiration injury.

CASE 24

Question 1: E. Fibroblastic foci

Biopsy shows typical features of usual interstitial pneumonia (UIP) including subpleural interstitial fibrosis with alternating areas of normal lung. UIP is a morphological pattern of lung interstitial disease characterized by progressive fibrosis of both lungs. UIP is the most common idiopathic interstitial pneumonia, accounting for 50% to 60% of cases of idiopathic interstitial pneumonias (IIPs), but can also be seen in other etiologies including collagen vascular diseases, asbestosis, environmental, or drug exposures.[15] The incidence is estimated as 10.7 cases per 100,000 for males and 7.4 cases per 100,000 for females. Patients usually are between the ages of 40 and 70 years with insidious onset of nonproductive cough and dyspnea. The histopathologic features of UIP include patchy interstitial fibrosis with alternating areas of normal lung; scattered fibroblastic foci in the background of dense acellular collagen; architectural alteration due to chronic scarring or honeycomb change. The hallmark of UIP is temporal heterogeneity, in which fibrosis shows variation in time and there are areas of dense collagen with scattered fibroblastic foci. The transition from normal lung parenchyma to old remodeled lung parenchyma occurs through patchy areas of lung injury evidenced by fibroblastic foci. The remodeled lung is evident mainly in the subpleural and basilar regions. Additional features include smooth muscle hyperplasia, metaplastic bone formation, fatty accumulation in the visceral pleura, and mild to moderate interstitial chronic inflammation. Granulomas, vasculitis, microorganisms, or minerals, e.g., silica crystals and ferruginous bodies, are absent in idiopathic UIP. The outlook of UIP for long-term survival is poor. Most patients die of respiratory failure within 3 to 8 years of onset of symptoms. The mean survival is 2.8 to 3.6 years.

CASE 25

Question 1: E. It is the most common cause of idiopathic interstitial pneumonia

The biopsy of the lung in the image shows uniformly thickening of the alveolar walls by mild interstitial chronic inflammation and fibrosis. Nonspecific interstitial pneumonia (NSIP) is a form of interstitial lung disease with a histologic appearance that does not meet histologic criteria for usual interstitial pneumonia (UIP), diffuse interstitial pneumonia (DIP), respiratory bronchiolitis interstitial lung disease (RBILD), diffuse alveolar damage (DAD) or chronic obstructive pneumonia (COP).[16] NSIP is the second most common cause of idiopathic interstitial pneumonias (IIPs), accounting for 14% to 36% of cases. Most cases of NSIP are idiopathic. However, NSIP can be seen in patients with collagen vascular diseases, toxic environmental exposures, drugs, hypersensitivity pneumonitis, infection, and prior lung injury. NSIP is relatively common manifestation of collagen vascular disease and may precede the diagnosis of collagen vascular disease by months or even years. Therefore, clinical history, time course of disease, and radiographic findings should be correlated before a diagnosis of idiopathic NSIP is rendered. The pathogenesis of NSIP is unclear, although epithelial injury and immune activation have been implicated. The average age at the onset of disease ranges between 46 and 55 years with a slight female predominance. Patients with NSIP most commonly manifests as an insidious onset of shortness of breath over several months, often accompanied by a cough. Pathologically, NSIP is characterized by spatially and temporally uniform interstitial inflammation with varying degrees of fibrosis. NSIP has been divided into two categories based on the level of fibrosis. NSIP, cellular pattern consists of mild to moderate chronic interstitial inflammation, usually lymphocytes and a few plasma cells. The lungs are uniformly involved, but the distribution of the lesion may be patchy. Fibrotic NSIP is characterized by the presence of dense or loose interstitial fibrosis that is uniformly present (temporal uniformity). The prognosis for the cellular NSIP pattern is more favorable than fibrotic NSIP. Cellular NSIP have a 100% 5-year survival rate. Fibrotic NSIP have a 90% 5-year survival rate and 35% 10-year survival rate.

CASE 26

Question 1: C. Patients with RBILD are usually older than those with DIP

Image shows alveolar spaces filled with macrophages, with hyperplasia of type II pneumocytes. Desquamative interstitial pneumonitis (DIP) is an uncommon clinical and pathologic conditions characterized histologically by the presence of numerous macrophages filling the alveolar spaces without prominent fibrosis and honeycombing. DIP is often associated with cigarette smoking but can also been seen in connective tissue diseases.[17] The pathogenesis of DIP is unknown. The average age at onset of symptoms is between 40 and 50 years with a mean age of 42. DIP is more common in men with a male to female ratio of 2:1. The most frequent clinical features of DIP are the insidious onset of breathlessness during exercise and a persistent cough that is not always productive of sputum. Bibasilar crackles and cyanosis are frequently present, and clubbing is not unusual. The main histological feature of DIP is intra-alveolar macrophage accumulation with a diffuse distribution throughout the pulmonary acini. Those macrophages have abundant eosinophilic cytoplasm and often contain a finely granular light-brown pigment. The alveolar architecture is generally well maintained and interstitial fibrosis is usually mild. The prognosis for patients with DIP is much better than UIP, with an estimated 10-year survival of 70%. Smoking cessation and corticosteroid therapy have proven to be effective. Chronic hypersensitivity pneumonitis can be differentiated from DIP histologically by chronic interstitial inflammatory pneumonia with small poorly formed granulomas. UIP is characterized by patchy fibrosis that varies in intensity and age. In chronic eosinophilic pneumonia, the alveolar spaces are diffusely filled with eosinophils and plump eosinophilic macrophages. Langerhans cell histiocytosis consists of proliferation of CD1a positive Langerhans cells along small airways.

* *

Respiratory bronchiolitis (RB) is a histopathologic lesion of the small airways that occur commonly in cigarette smokers (smoker's bronchiolitis).[18] Respiratory bronchiolitis-associated interstitial lung disease (RBILD) is RB with clinical and radiographic characteristics of ILD. RB, RBILD, and DIP are highly related and represent different degrees of small airway and lung parenchymal reaction to cigarette smoking. RB is on the asymptomatic end of a spectrum that culminates in DIP. The pathogenesis of RBILD is unknown, but almost all patients are current or past heavy cigarette smokers.[19] Patients with RBILD are a decade younger than those with DIP, with a mean age of 36. There is no sex predilection. The most frequent presenting symptoms are the insidious onset of exertional breathlessness and cough. Bibasilar end-inspiratory crackles are present frequently but clubbing is rare. In RB, the chest radiograph usually is normal or of limited diagnostic value. Bronchial wall thickening and areas of ground-glass attenuation are frequent on chest radiography with patients in RBILD. The diagnosis of RBILD requires clinical-radiological-pathological correlation. The histopathology of RB and RBILD are identical. The main feature is the accumulation of finely pigmented macrophages within the lumen of the respiratory bronchiole and surrounding alveolar spaces.[18] The macrophages typically have glassy eosinophilic cytoplasm with fine brown granular pigmentation. Foamy macrophages are not a feature of these disorders. The wall of the bronchioles and surrounding alveoli may show mild chronic inflammation and fibrosis. The bronchiolar epithelial cells may show goblet cell hyperplasia. In addition, foci of centrilobular emphysema are commonly seen in patients with RB and RBILD. The prognosis of most patients with RBILD is favorable. Cessation of smoking is important in the resolution of these lesions.

CASE 27

Question 1: **C. Organizing pneumonia**
Image shows polypoid plugs of loose connective tissue protruding into the lumen of bronchiole, alveolar ducts, and spaces. Organizing pneumonia is a distinct entity characterized by the presence of intraluminal plugs (Masson bodies) of loose connective tissue within the bronchioles and alveolar ducts.[20] This pathological pattern has no etiologic specificities and may be encountered in a variety of lung disorders. Cryptogenic organizing pneumonia (COP) is the idiopathic form of organizing pneumonia of unknown etiology. Secondary organizing pneumonia can be seen in association with infections (viral, bacteria, and fungal), drug/medication reactions (amiodarone, gold, and methotrexate), primary connective tissue disease (rheumatoid arthritis, and systemic lupus erythematosus), and radiotherapy. Bronchopneumonia is marked by patchy acute (neutrophilic) suppurative exudates of the peribronchial and peribronchiolar lung parenchyma. Usual interstitial pneumonia (UIP) is a morphologic entity characterized by honeycomb fibrosis mostly in lower lobes with variation in time and intensity of fibrosis. Tuberculosis is marked by necrotizing (caseating) granulomatous inflammation. Diffuse alveolar damage (DAD) is a form of acute lung injury characterized by formation of hyaline membrane.[21]

CASE 28

Question 1: **D. Asbestosis**
Image shows an asbestos body characterized by dumbbell-shaped structure and with golden brown coating and a beaded translucent core. Asbestos is a term for a group of naturally occurring hydrated silicate fibers, which are ideal for a variety of construction and insulation purposes. Exposures to asbestos can occur in a variety of occupational settings, including mining, milling, and the manufacture and use of asbestos-containing products. Most patients with asbestos-related lung disease have a strong exposure history; however, disease can occur with minimal exposure. There is a correlation between the level of exposure and the severity of the disease for many asbestos-related lung disorders. Inhalation of asbestos fibers can result in a number of distinct pathologic

processes. Asbestosis is interstitial pulmonary fibrosis caused by inhaled asbestos dust. The interstitial pulmonary fibrosis is patchy and accentuated in the subpleural regions. In the most advanced cases, honeycomb fibrosis is present. The histologic diagnostic hallmark of asbestosis is the presence of asbestos bodies in association with interstitial fibrosis. Pleural-based abnormalities include diffuse visceral pleural fibrosis, hyaline parietal pleural plaques, benign pleural effusion, and malignant mesothelioma. In addition, asbestos exposure alone and in combination with cigarette smoking is associated with an increased incidence of lung carcinoma.

**

Sarcoidosis and berylliosis are marked by noncaseating granulomas. The histologic hallmark of silicosis is the silicotic nodule, which consists of a circumscribed nodule of dense, whorled hyalinized collagen with crystalline foreign material. Byssinosis is a pulmonary disease from exposure to cotton fibers.

CASE 29

Question 1: **B. Squamous cell carcinoma**
Image shows well-differentiated squamous cell carcinoma characterized by the presence of keratinization and intercellular bridges. Hypercalcemia and a central cavitary lung mass, which is seen in squamous cell carcinoma. SCC has a strong association with smoking; over 90% of SCCs occur in cigarette smokers. Arsenic is also strongly associated with SCC. Hypercalcemia in SCC is a paraneoplastic syndrome, due to production of parathyroid hormone-related protein.[22] Majority of the tumors arise centrally in the mainstream, lobar, or segmental bronchi. The mass is prone to undergo central necrosis, forming a cavitary mass. Histologically, it shows keratinization, pearl formation, and/or intercellular bridges. These features vary with degree of differentiation, being prominent in well-differentiated tumors, and absent in poorly differentiated tumors.[23,24] Squamous cell carcinomas are amenable to surgical resection. Stage for stage, survival rate for SCC is significantly better than for adenocarcinoma. Approximately 80% of patients with resected stage I SCC are alive at 5 years after diagnosis compared to approximately 70% of similarly staged adenocarcinomas. Small cell carcinomas are also known to produce paraneoplastic syndromes, which include Cushing syndrome, Lambert–Eaton syndrome, and syndrome of inappropriate antidiuretic hormone secretion (SIADH). Adenocarcinomas

are usually peripheral in location, and are not associated with paraneoplastic hypercalcemia.[25] Adenocarcinoma in situ is a peripheral lung tumor that can mimic pneumonia.

CASE 30

Question 1: A. Atypical adenomatous hyperplasia (AAH)

The center of the image shows a small focus of atypical alveolar cells, characterized by lepidic growth pattern with hobnail pattern. Atypical adenomatous hyperplasia (AAH) is considered to be a precursor lesion of adenocarcinoma. AAH is a solitary lesion in which atypical bronchioloalveolar polygonal cells proliferate along the alveolar septa in a lepidic fashion. The cells constituting AAH are apt to be mildly to moderately atypical with increased nuclear-cytoplasmic ratio, often possessing hyperchromatic nuclei and prominent nucleoli. Small indentations can be typically found between two neighboring cells (so-called hobnail phenomenon). Intranuclear inclusions are frequently seen. This size criterion is crucial in the diagnosis of AAH. AAH lesions reach a maximum diameter of ≤5 mm by definition. Adenocarcinoma in situ (AIS) is a lesion with an exclusively lepidic pattern of growth and without any invasive focus. The overall size of AIS is >5 mm and ≤3 cm by definition. Chronic bronchiolitis is characterized by a prominent lymphocytic infiltrate within and surrounding the walls of small airways. However, atypical bronchioalveolar proliferation is not part of chronic bronchiolitis. Tumorlet is a nodular proliferation of neuroendocrine cells with a diameter less than 5 mm. Invasive adenocarcinoma is a malignant epithelial tumor with glandular differentiation and/or mucin production, in which the neoplastic glands vary in size and shape and are often surrounded by desmoplastic stroma.

CASE 31

Question 1: A. Perform molecular testing for EGFR and ALK

Image shows invasive moderately differentiated adenocarcinoma with an acinar growth pattern, in which glands of different sizes and shapes embedded in fibrous tissue can be seen. Adenocarcinoma is the most common subtype of lung carcinoma, accounting for 40% or more of all primary lung carcinomas. This subtype is relatively more common in women and is also the most common subtype that develops in nonsmokers. More than two-thirds of cases arise in the periphery of the lung as a small subpleural nodule, often in a subpleural location, and often with an associated scar. The tumor is usually noncavitary. Histologically most common subtype of adenocarcinomas is the acinar variant, which features a glandular, tubular or solid growth pattern. The cytologic features range from very bland (well-differentiated) to highly anaplastic forms (poorly differentiated). Subtypes of adenocarcinoma include papillary, mucinous, enteric-like, clear cell, glassy cell, and adenocarcinoma in situ. Bronchial carcinoids are uncommon endobronchial neoplasms arising from the neuroendocrine cells. Small cell carcinomas are aggressive neoplasms arising from the neuroendocrine cells and are not amenable to surgical therapy. Squamous cell carcinomas are centrally occurring lung carcinomas often associated with smoking. Metastatic adenocarcinoma often shows multiple tumor nodules in bilateral lungs.

* *

Pulmonary adenocarcinomas consistently express the following immunohistochemical markers: Cytokeratin 7, TTF-1 (nuclear positivity), and Napsin-A. Thyroid transcription factor 1 (TTF-1) has been shown to be quite useful in differentiating primary pulmonary adenocarcinoma from lung metastases of adenocarcinomas from a variety of organs. It can also be used to identify metastatic pulmonary adenocarcinoma in distant sites. Synaptophysin and chromogranin are neuroendocrine cell markers that are usually positive in small cell lung carcinoma and carcinoid tumor. p63 immunoreactivity is positive in squamous cell carcinoma, while CD45 positivity is characteristic of lymphoma.

* *

Advent of targeted molecular therapies based on genetic mutations has made it mandatory to test for genetic mutations in lung carcinomas, particularly pulmonary adenocarcinomas. The most important of these are epidermal growth factor receptor (EGFR) and anaplastic lymphoma kinase (ALK). Activating mutations involving tyrosine kinase domain of EGFR gene have been identified in a subset of pulmonary adenocarcinomas, especially those adenocarcinoma with lepidic growth pattern and in "never smokers." Carcinomas with these mutations are more common in the Far East and almost never harbor activating *k-ras* mutation. Patients with advanced lung adenocarcinoma, harboring EGFR mutation respond to EGFR tyrosine kinase inhibitors (gefitinib, erlotinib). They have a much better prognosis than those receiving chemotherapy alone. EML4-ALK fusion gene resulting from an inversion on chromosome 2p has been identified in about 5% of pulmonary adenocarcinomas. This usually occurs exclusive of EGFR mutation. Patients with these ALK-rearrangements respond to inhibitors of ALK-kinase activity (crizotinib). Recently, US Food and Drug Administration (FDA) have approved crizotinib for the treatment of patients with locally advanced or metastatic adenocarcinoma that is positive for ALK by Fluorescent in situ Hybridization (FISH).

CASE 32

Question 1: B. Well-differentiated mucinous adenocarcinoma

The image depicts well-differentiated mucinous adenocarcinoma with a predominantly lepidic growth pattern. Immunohistochemistry of the tumor reveals positivity for CK7, Napsin-A, and TTF- 1, while being negative for CK20, p63, and CDX-2. This staining pattern confirms a lung primary. The newly proposed 2011 International Association for the Study of Lung Cancer (IASLC), American Thoracic Society (ATS), and European Respiratory Society (ERS) classification of lung adenocarcinoma recommends discontinuing the use of the term bronchioloalveolar carcinoma (BAC).[26] Historically, the term BAC was used to designate those lung adenocarcinoma that exhibited a predominantly lepidic growth pattern. The IASLC/ATS/ERS classification recommends that adenocarcinoma with lepidic predominant component should be classified as one of the following subtypes: (i) Adenocarcinoma in situ (AIS), (ii) Minimally invasive adenocarcinoma (MIA), and (iii) Lepidic predominant invasive adenocarcinoma.[26] AIS is defined as a <3 cm tumor with a pure lepidic pattern. MIA is defined as a <3 cm lepidic predominant tumor and <5 mm stromal invasion. Lepidic predominant invasive adenocarcinoma is defined as a tumor that is >3 cm in total size and/or >5 mm invasive size.[26,27] The classification also recommends that in small biopsies the diagnosis of AIS should not be made since the entire tumor is not available for evaluation. Hence the preferred nomenclature, as in the current case, is a well-differentiated mucinous carcinoma. Metastatic mucinous adenocarcinoma often shows multiple tumor nodules in bilateral lungs. Pulmonary hamartoma is a benign lesion by the presence of cartilage, adipose tissue and epithelial invaginations. Atypical adenomatous hyperplasia (AAH) is considered to be a precursor lesion with a diameter of ≤5 mm.

CASE 33

Question 1: E. The tumor is of neuroendocrine cell origin

The image depicts a carcinoid tumor characterized by uniform polygonal cells arranged in organoid, trabecular, or solid growth patterns. Carcinoid tumor is a well-differentiated neuroendocrine tumor. The neuroendocrine tumors of the lung are classified as: carcinoid tumorlets (<4 mm), carcinoids, atypical carcinoids, large cell neuroendocrine carcinomas, and small cell neuroendocrine carcinomas.[28] In contrast to higher grade neuroendocrine tumors, carcinoids do not show any convincing relationship with cigarette smoking. Central tumors often present with airway-related symptoms, such as wheezing, recurrent pneumonia and cough. Peripheral carcinoids are often asymptomatic and are discovered incidentally as pulmonary "coin lesions." Histologically, carcinoid tumors are characterized by uniform polygonal cells arranged in organoid, trabecular, or solid growth patterns. The tumor cells have regular, round to oval nuclei with finely granular chromatin (described as "salt and pepper") and moderate to abundant eosinophilic cytoplasm. Mitotic activity is low in typical carcinoid (<2 per 10 high-power fields). Necrosis should be absent. Peripheral carcinoids are morphologically similar to central carcinoids, except for often demonstrating spindled morphology. Immunohistochemically, most carcinoids show strong expression of neuroendocrine markers, such as chromogranin, and synaptophysin as well as epithelial markers (cytokeratin, epithelial membrane antigen). Electron microscopy demonstrates characteristic neurosecretory granules in the cytoplasm. Unlike small bowel carcinoids, they are rarely associated with carcinoid syndrome. Carcinoid tumors have low malignant potential. Only about 5% of patients present with lymph node metastasis and <5% of cases show distant metastatic disease.

CASE 34

Question 1: B. Atypical carcinoid tumor

Image shows a tumor composed of nests of atypical cells with "salt and pepper" nuclear chromatin. The tumor has a high mitotic rate (arrows) (>2 per 10 high-power fields). Atypical carcinoids are neuroendocrine tumors having a prognosis intermediate between typical carcinoid tumor and undifferentiated small cell and large cell neuroendocrine carcinomas. Atypical carcinoids have a mitotic rate between 2 and 10 per 10 high-power fields. Necrosis may be present, but to a limited degree. Typical carcinoids have a low mitotic rate (<2 per 10 high-power fields). Undifferentiated small and large cell neuroendocrine carcinomas have 10 or more mitoses per 10 high-power fields. The tumor cells are usually positive for neuroendocrine and epithelial markers. Atypical carcinoids show significantly greater malignant potential than classic carcinoids. About 25% of patients have lymph node metastasis at presentation and approximately 25% of patients are dead by 5 years after diagnosis. Adenocarcinoma is defined as a malignant epithelial neoplasm characterized by gland formation. Squamous cell carcinoma is typified by the presence of keratinization and intercellular bridges.

CASE 35

Question 1: B. Small cell carcinoma

The biopsy of the lesion shows characteristic of small cell carcinoma. This patient has features of Cushing syndrome, resulting from ectopic corticotropin production, which is one of the common complaints of small cell lung carcinoma (SCLC). SCLC accounts for about 10% of primary lung carcinomas. It has a very strong association with cigarette smoking. Majority of the patients present with a central mass with bulky hilar/mediastinal adenopathy. Apart from Cushing syndrome, SCLC is also associated with other paraneoplastic syndromes such as syndrome of inappropriate ADH secretion (SIADH), and Eaton-Lambert syndrome. Microscopically, SCLC is characterized by diffuse population of small "blue cells" (about two to three times larger than resting lymphocytes) with dark hyperchromatic nuclei and very scant cytoplasm. Crush artifacts and nuclear molding are often prominent. Mitotic figures are frequent. There is often prominent apoptosis and extensive confluent necrosis. Small cell carcinomas are aggressive tumors that tend to metastasize early. Surgery is not an option for these patients. Patients are usually treated with chemotherapy, however cure is never achieved. Adenocarcinoma is a peripheral neoplasm that does not produce paraneoplastic Cushing syndrome. Squamous cell carcinoma is a central tumor that also develops in smokers, but it is more likely to produce hypercalcemia as paraneoplastic syndrome. Non-Hodgkin lymphomas rarely occur in the lung, are not associated with smoking, and do not produce Cushing syndrome.[29]

CASE 36

Question 1: E. Poorly differentiated squamous cell carcinoma

The needle lung biopsy shows features of poorly differentiated carcinoma without obvious glandular or squamous differentiation. Immunohistochemical studies confirm squamous cell carcinoma by positive stains for p63, p40, and CK5/6. Squamous cell carcinoma are classified as well, moderately, and poorly differentiated, depending on the presence of either keratinization or intercellular bridges. The grading is a measurement of how closely the tumor cells resemble the parent tissue (organ of origin). Well-differentiated tumor cells closely resemble the tissue from the organ of origin, while poorly differentiated and undifferentiated tumor cells are disorganized and abnormal looking. Well-differentiated squamous cell carcinoma shows area of keratinization and easily identifiable intercellular bridges. Moderately differentiated squamous cell carcinoma may still shows area of either keratinization or intercellular bridges. Poorly differentiated squamous cell carcinoma lacks definitive evidence of squamous differentiation. Examination of poorly differentiated carcinoma using routine light microscopy alone is inadequate to assess these tumors optimally. Additional immunohistochemical studies are routinely performed. Squamous cell carcinoma usually shows positive staining for p63, p40, and CK 5/6, but negative staining for TTF-1. Non-Hodgkin lymphoma demonstrates positive staining for CD45, but negative staining for TTF-1, p63, p40, and CK5/6. Poorly differentiated adenocarcinomas stain positive for TTF-1, but negative for p63, p40, and CK5/6. Mesothelioma expresses calretinin and WT-1, and is negative for TTF-1, p63, p40, and CK5/6. Large cell neuroendocrine carcinoma is positive for neuroendocrine markers (synaptophysin, chromogranin, CD56), but negative staining for p63, p40, and CK5/6.

CASE 37

Question 1: A. Metastatic large cell neuroendocrine carcinoma of lung

The biopsy of the vertebral lesion shows sheet-like arrangement of large-sized tumor cells with prominent nucleoli and geographic necrosis, which are positive for TTF-1, synaptophysin and CD56. The findings are consistent with metastatic large cell neuroendocrine carcinoma of the lung. Large cell neuroendocrine carcinoma (LCNEC) is a poorly differentiated nonsmall cell carcinoma, which exhibits features of neuroendocrine differentiation. It accounts for approximately 1.6% to 3.1% of all lung cancers. Most patients with LCNECs are male and have a history of heavy smoking. The median age at presentation is 65 years. The tumors are more frequently present at peripheral locations, as opposed to typical and atypical carcinoid tumors, which are generally centrally located. Therefore, patients with LCNEC are less likely to present with symptoms such as cough or hemoptysis. The features of LCNEC on imaging studies are nonspecific and indistinguishable from other nonsmall cell carcinoma. Microscopically, LCNEC typically shows organized nesting, palisading, or rosette-like growth patterns with extensive coagulative necrosis. The neoplastic cells are large with moderate-to-abundant cytoplasm, fine chromatin, and prominent nucleoli. The mitotic rate is usually in excess of 10 per 10 high-power microscopic fields. All tumors show immunoreactivity for cytokeratin and at least one neuroendocrine marker such as chromogranin, CD56, or synaptophysin. Electron microscopy shows the presence of intracytoplasmic dense core granules. It is a highly aggressive tumor. It has a distant metastasize rate of 65% and poor prognosis even in early stages, with survival rates similar to small cell lung carcinomas (SCLCs). The life expectancy of stage IV LCNEC with distant metastasis is estimated at around 6 months.

**

Separation of LCNEC from nonsmall cell carcinomas such as sarcomatoid carcinoma, adenocarcinoma, and squamous cell carcinoma depends primarily on the presence or absence of neuroendocrine features by morphology, immunohistochemistry, or electron microcopy.

CASE 38

Question 1: D. CDX2+, TTF-1–, CK7–, CK20+

The tumor consists of irregular tubular or cribriform patterns of columnar cells with basophilic cytoplasm and elongated nuclei. Necrotic, exfoliated cells in the lumina of the glands can also be seen. The morphologic features are characteristics of metastatic colorectal adenocarcinoma. Colorectal adenocarcinoma is usually immunoreactive for CDX-2 and CK20 and is negative for CK7. CDX-2 is a homeobox gene related to Drosophila caudal gene that encodes a nuclear transcription factor. CDX-2

is a sensitive and specific marker for primary and metastatic colorectal adenocarcinomas. Majority of lung adenocarcinoma are immunoreactive for thyroid transcription factor 1 (TTF-1) and CK7 and are negative for CK20 and CDX-2. Prostatic adenocarcinoma is usually immunoreactive for prostate-specific antigen (PSA) and prostatic acid phosphatase (PAP) and is negative for CK7 and CK20. Primary and metastatic squamous cell carcinoma expresses p63, p40, and CK5/6, but is negative for TTF-1.

CASE 39

Question 1: C. BRCA1/2

The lung-needle biopsy demonstrates a few papillae lined by markedly pleomorphic cells with hyperchromatic nuclei. Psammoma bodies are evident. These morphologic features are highly suggestive of serous carcinoma of the ovary. A diagnosis is confirmed by immunoreactivity for Wilms tumor 1 (WT-1) and PAX8. WT-1 gene encodes a transcription factor that is necessary for the development of the kidneys and gonads (ovaries in females and testes in males). It is located in a region of chromosome 11 that is deleted in people with Wilms tumor, aniridia, genitourinary anomalies, and mental retardation syndrome, known by the acronym WAGR syndrome. Immunohistochemically, WT-1 is detected in the nucleus of tumor cells of Wilms tumor, mesothelioma, and ovarian serous carcinoma. PAX8 is a member of the paired box (PAX) family of transcription factors important in embryogenesis of the thyroid, Mullerian, and renal/upper urinary tracts. Immunohistochemically, PAX8 is detected in the nucleus of tumor cells of ovarian carcinoma, uterine carcinoma, thyroid carcinoma and renal cell carcinoma. Primary lung adenocarcinoma is usually immunoreactive for TTF-1 and CK7, but negative for WT-1, and PAX8. Metastatic breast carcinoma is usually immunoreactive for GCDFP-15, mammaglobin and CK7, but negative for WT-1 and PAX8. Metastatic colorectal adenocarcinoma is usually immunoreactive for CDX-2 and CK20, and negative for CK7, WT-1 and PAX-8. Primary and metastatic squamous cell carcinoma is immunoreactive for p63, but negative for TTF-1, WT-1, and PAX8.

**

The patient mostly likely has a hereditary breast and ovarian cancer syndrome (HBOC). HBOC is caused by a germline mutation in BRCA1 or BRCA2, and is characterized by an increased risk for breast cancer, ovarian cancer, and several other cancers. The lifetime risk for breast cancers in individuals with a mutation in BRCA1 or BRCA2 has been estimated between 40% and 80%. The lifetime risk for ovarian cancers in individuals with a mutation in BRCA1 or BRCA2 has been estimated between 11% and 40%. A diagnosis of HBOC is made following molecular genetic testing in an individual or family with a germline BRCA1 or BRCA2 mutation. Several molecular diagnostic markers, such as EGFR, *k-ras,* and ALK in tumor tissue demonstrate prognostic and predictive value in patients with nonsmall cell lung cancer (NSCLC). HER2/neu is an important marker for breast carcinoma and is generally associated with higher grade tumors that are more likely to metastasize, thereby portending a worse prognosis in the absence of therapy.

CASE 40

Question 1: E. Bones
The tumor shown in the image consists of crowded small acini with irregular contours and prominent nucleoli. Antibodies to PSA and PAP are highly specific for tumors of prostatic origin. The most common sites for metastatic prostatic adenocarcinoma are lymph nodes and bones. Only 10% of all prostatic adenocarcinomas yield lung metastases. Moreover, most patients with pulmonary metastases already have multiple lymph node and/or bone metastases. Only a few cases of pulmonary metastases without any other metastatic site have been reported in the literature. Although clinically apparent pulmonary metastasis occurs less frequently, microscopic evidence of pulmonary involvement is seen in up to 12% to 46% cases at autopsy. One study showed that hematogenous metastases were present in 35% of 1,589 patients with prostatic carcinoma at autopsy, with most frequent involvement being bone (90%), lung (46%), liver (25%), pleura (21%), and adrenals (13%).

CASE 41

Question 1: A. Langerhans cell histiocytosis
The image shows clusters of cells with grooved nuclei and presence of eosinophils in the vicinity. Pulmonary Langerhans cell histiocytosis (PLCH) is an unusual interstitial lung disease characterized by monoclonal proliferation and infiltration of Langerhans cells.[30] Langerhans cells are dendritic cells of bone marrow origin and function as antigen-presenting cells. PLCH is strongly associated with cigarette smoking. Affected patients are typically young adults who often present with cough and dyspnea. The early histologic lesion of PLCH consists of proliferation of Langerhans cells along small airways leading to formation of 1- to 5-mm nodules. Variable numbers of Langerhans cells, plasma cells, macrophages, lymphocytes, and eosinophils form loosely aggregated granulomas around distal bronchioles. Since these lesions often contain eosinophils, they are also called "eosinophilic granuloma." The Langerhans cells are characterized by moderate eosinophilic cytoplasm and prominently grooved nuclear membranes producing a coffee-bean appearance. Langerhans cells can be identified by immunohistochemical studies for S100 protein as well as CD1a and Langerin antigens. The peculiar small tennis racket-shaped granules are viewed on electron microscopy as Birbeck granules. Fibrotic cases of PLCH may be confused with usual interstitial pneumonia, but the fibrotic scars of PLCH are bronchiolocentric. In contrast to the interstitial cellular infiltration of PLCH, eosinophilic pneumonia consists of an intra-alveolar accumulation of eosinophils. Metastatic carcinoma is positive for keratins (CK AE1/3, CAM 5.2), but is negative for S100 protein, CD1a and Langerin. Metastatic melanoma is usually positive for S100 protein and melanin A, but is negative for CD1a and Langerin.

CASE 42

Question 1: C. Extranodal marginal zone lymphoma of bronchus-associated lymphoid tissue
The lung needle biopsy demonstrates a dense lymphoid infiltrate, composed of a monotonous population of small- to medium-sized lymphocytes having abundant clear cytoplasm, resulting in a monocytoid appearance. These features are highly suggestive of a lymphoid neoplasm. Immunoreactivity for CD20 shows predominantly a B-cell population, supporting a diagnosis of non-Hodgkin lymphoma. Negative immunoreactivity for CD5 and CD23 helps rule out chronic lymphocytic leukemia/small lymphocytic lymphoma, while negative staining for cyclin D1 help exclude mantle cell lymphoma. The absence of Langerhans cells with their unique convoluted nuclei and negative immunoreactivity for CD1a excludes the possibility of Langerhans cell histiocytosis. Presence of t (8; 11) confirms a diagnosis of extra nodal marginal zone lymphoma. Extranodal marginal zone lymphoma of bronchus-associated lymphoid tissue (BALToma) is the most common primary pulmonary

lymphoma, accounting for around 75% cases. Half of them are found incidentally on chest imaging. Nonspecific symptoms may be present, such as cough, chest pain, dyspnea, and fatigue. Most cases occur in adults, and there is no specific relationship to infection or autoimmune disorders. Histologically, the tumor is composed of a nodular or diffuse infiltrate of small lymphocytes, monocytoid cells with clear cytoplasm, and plasmacytoid cells. The tumor cells can also infiltrate the bronchial mucosa with production of "lymphoepithelial lesions," similar to MALToma at other body sites. The infiltrating cells are positive for CD19, CD20, and bcl-2, but negative for CD5, CD10, CD23, and cyclin D1.

CASE 43

Question 1: **B. It is associated with leiomyoma of uterus**
The micrograph of lung tissue shows cystic structures and smooth muscle proliferation infiltrating within septa, which is consistent with lymphangioleiomyomatosis (LAM). The inset shows characteristic immunoreactivity for smooth muscle actin. LAM is an uncommon disease that affects women primarily between 30 and 49 years of age. It is characterized by abnormal proliferation of smooth muscle cells and cystic destruction of the lung. LAM occurs sporadically or in association with tuberous sclerosis complex. Both types of LAM have demonstrated mutations in tumor suppressor genes: the hamartin gene (TSC1) on chromosome 9 (9q34) and the tuberin gene locus (TSC2) on chromosome 16 (16p13.3). Clinically, LAM is characterized by progressive dyspnea, recurrent pneumothoraces or chylothorax, and abdominal and thoracic lymphadenopathy. LAM is often associated with angiomyolipoma in the kidneys, and an increased frequency of meningioma. Grossly, the lungs are enlarged and diffusely cystic as in severe emphysema. The two key histologic features of LAM are cysts and proliferation of atypical smooth muscle cells (LAM cells). Cystic spaces are lined with hyperplastic type II pneumocytes. The LAM cells are round, oval or spindle-shaped, and grow in a haphazard arrangement. LAM cells infiltrate distal airways, which leads to airway narrowing, air trapping, formation of bullae, and pneumothoraces. Obstruction of lymphatics causes chylous effusions of the thorax and abdomen. LAM cells are immunohistochemically positive for smooth muscle markers (such as smooth muscle actin and desmin) and melanocytic markers (such as HMB-45

and Melan-A) as well as estrogen and progesterone receptors. LAM can be confused with benign metastatic leiomyoma (BML). BML usually occurs in women with a history of leiomyoma. BML tends to be nodular lesions in absence of thin-walled cysts. Immunohistochemistry for HMB-45 is negative for BML.

CASE 44

Question 1: **E. Pulmonary sarcomatoid carcinoma**
The biopsy of lung, as depicted in the image, shows tumor tissue composed of pleomorphic spindle cells, which are positive for TTF-1, pancytokeratin (AE1/3), and epithelial membrane antigen (EMA). The findings are consistent with pulmonary sarcomatoid carcinoma (PSC). PSC is a group of poorly differentiated nonsmall cell carcinomas (NSCLC) of the lung containing sarcoma-like differentiation (spindle and/or giant cell) or a component of sarcoma (malignant bone, cartilage, or skeletal muscle). PSC is very rare, accounting for about 1% of all lung malignancies. In 2004 WHO classification on lung cancers, PSC encompasses five different histological subtypes: spindle cell carcinoma, giant cell carcinoma, pleomorphic carcinoma, carcinosarcoma, and pulmonary blastoma. The use of immunohistochemical studies should help distinguish these tumors from true sarcomas. PSCs are stained to varying extent with antibodies to cytokeratins (i.e., AE1/3), CAM 5.2, epithelial membrane antigen (EMA), and carcinoembryonic antigen (CEA). These tumors have poorer prognosis than the other NSCLC subtypes because of greater aggressiveness, and frequent chemoresistance.

* *

The main differential diagnosis of PSC is centered on the exclusion of true sarcomas. Primary pulmonary leiomyosarcoma is characterized by malignant spindle cell proliferation, which expresses smooth muscle actin and desmin. Primary pulmonary synovial sarcoma may show overlapping morphology and immunohistochemical profile of PSC. Molecular studies for the presence of the SYT-SSX fusion transcript (classical of synovial sarcoma) may be necessary for such a distinction. Melanomas usually express S-100 protein and melanocytic differentiation markers that are typically negative in PSCs. Squamous cell carcinoma may show a spindle cell pattern, which is usually positive for p63, p40, and keratin 5/6.

CASE 45

Question 1: **D. Adenosquamous carcinoma**

Image shows a composite tumor, exhibiting poorly differentiated squamous cell carcinoma with dense, eosinophilic cytoplasm (top right) and adenocarcinoma (bottom left). The findings are consistent with adenosquamous carcinoma. Adenosquamous carcinoma is a morphologically mixed type of tumor, composed of adenocarcinoma and squamous cell carcinoma, in varying proportions, each representing ≥10% of the entire tumor. It accounts 0.4% to 4% of all lung cancers. The clinical, radiographic, and gross pathologic aspects of adenosquamous carcinoma are mostly similar to those of pure adenocarcinoma of the lung. Morphologically, adenosquamous carcinoma is characterized by the presence of unequivocal areas of squamous cell carcinoma and adenocarcinoma. Well or moderately differentiated squamous cell component usually shows keratinization, pearl formation, and/or intercellular bridges, which are absent in poorly differentiated squamous cell component. In adenocarcinomatous component, glandular or tubular differentiation is usually present. Adenosquamous carcionomas reveal positive immunostaining for markers indicating its separate components: p40, p63, and keratin 5/6 in squamous cell carcinoma component and TTF-1 and Napsin A in adenocarcinomatous component. The prognosis of adenosquamous carcinoma is worse than that of individuals with pure adenocarcinoma or squamous cell carcinoma. Adenosquamous cell carcinoma should be differentiated from squamous cell carcinoma, adenocarcinoma and high-grade mucoepidermoid carcinoma. Squamous cell carcinoma and adenocarcinoma may contain other minor components, which are <10%. High-grade mucoepidermoid carcinoma is composed of a random mixture of sheet like and glandular cells present as scattered goblet cells rather than tubular, acinar, papillary patterns, lacking individual cell keratinization and squamous pearl formation. In addition, foci of low-grade mucoepidermoid carcinoma are often present.

CASE 46

Question 1: **C. Mucoepidermoid carcinoma**

The image shows a malignant tumor composed of an admixture of squamous cells and mucus secreting cells, classical of mucoepidermoid carcinoma (MEC). It is a rare tumor of the lung that accounts for 0.1% to 0.2% of all pulmonary tumors. The World Health Organization (WHO) classifies pulmonary MEC as "salivary gland type" tumors along with adenoid cystic carcinoma and epimyoepithelial lung carcinomas. Pulmonary MEC has been divided into low-grade and high-grade categories. They can occur over a broad age range, including childhood. Most pulmonary MEC arise in the proximal bronchi. Symptoms are primarily those of bronchial irritation and obstruction, and include cough, hemoptysis, and postobstructive pneumonia. Symptoms are usually similar in both low-grade and high-grade tumors. Histologically, MEC is characterized by a combination of mucus-secreting, squamous, and intermediate cells. Low-grade MECs are comprised predominantly of glandular elements and mucin-secreting cells, while high-grade MEC consists largely of sheets or nests of squamoid and intermediate cells intermixed with smaller populations of mucus-secreting cells. Low-grade MEC is histologically distinguished from high-grade MEC based on the lack of cytologic atypia including nuclear pleomorphism and absence of significant mitotic activity and cellular necrosis. Histological grade is an important prognostic indicator, with high-grade MECs demonstrating a greater risk for metastases, tumor recurrence, and death. Surgical resection is the most effective treatment for pulmonary MEC. Complete tumor removal with nodal dissection, and preservation of functional parenchyma is the goal of therapy. Adjuvant radiotherapy is required in cases of unresectable tumors. Adjuvant chemotherapy is usually not necessary. However, tyrosine-kinase inhibitor Gefitinib has shown promising results in few cases with EGFR gene mutation. Patients with low-grade MECs have a generally excellent prognosis with a 5-year survival rate approaching 95%. In this population, adjuvant therapy is not indicated. In contrast, high-grade MECs carry a much poorer prognosis.

* *

Squamous cell carcinoma is characterized by the presence of tumor cells having varying degrees of squamous differentiation, and without any mucinous component. Carcinoid tumor is a neuroendocrine tumor, composed of islands of tumor cells having salt-and-pepper chromatin, and expressing markers of neuroendocrine differentiation. Adenoid cystic carcinoma is another salivary gland like tumor which has been described in the lung. This tumor is characterized by cribriform growth pattern with basaloid tumor cells and absence of a squamous component. Adenocarcinoma is a common lung carcinoma having varying degrees of glandular differentiation, and without a squamous component.

REFERENCES

1. Colby TV, Leslie KO, Yousem SA. Lungs. In: Mills SE, ed. *Histology for Pathologists*. 4th ed. Philadelphia, PA: Lippincott Williams & Wilkins; 2012:505–540.

2. Gilroy SA, Bennett NJ. Pneumocystis pneumonia. *Semin Respir Crit Care Med*. 2011;32:775–782.

3. Krause ML, Cartin-Ceba R, Specks U, et al. Update on diffuse alveolar hemorrhage and pulmonary vasculitis. *Immunol Allergy Clin North Am*. 2012;32:587–600.

4. Lachmann HJ, Hawkins PN. Amyloidosis and the lung. *Chron Respir Dis*. 2006;3:203–214.

5. Pipavath SN, Schmidt RA, Takasugi JE, et al. Chronic obstructive pulmonary disease: radiology-pathology correlation. *J Thorac Imaging*. 2009;24:171–180.

6. Yunt ZX, Frankel SK, Brown KK. Diagnosis and management of pulmonary vasculitis. *Ther Adv Respir Dis*. 2012;6:375–390.

7. Fernández Pérez ER, Olson AL, Frankel SK. Eosinophilic lung disease. *Med Clin North Am*. 2011;95:1163–1187.

8. Grunes D, Beasley MB. Hypersensitivity pneumonitis: a review and update of histologic findings. *J Clin Pathol*. 2013;66:888–895.

9. Hunter RL. Pathology of post primary tuberculosis of the lung: an illustrated critical review. *Tuberculosis*. 2011;91:497–509.

10. Heinle R, Chang C. Diagnostic criteria for sarcoidosis. *Autoimmun Rev*. 2014;13:383–387.

11. Brizendine KD, Baddley JW, Pappas PG. Pulmonary cryptococcosis. *Semin Respir Crit Care Med*. 2011;32:727–734.

12. Kousha M, Tadi R, Soubani AO. Pulmonary aspergillosis: a clinical review. *Eur Respir Rev*. 2011;20:156–174.

13. McKinsey DS, McKinsey JP. Pulmonary histoplasmosis. *Semin Respir Crit Care Med*. 2011;32:735–744.

14. Kauffman CA. Pulmonary fungal infections. *Respirology*. 2012;17:913–926.

15. Smith M, Dalurzo M, Panse P, et al. Usual interstitial pneumonia-pattern fibrosis in surgical lung biopsies. Clinical, radiological and histopathological clues to aetiology. *J Clin Pathol*. 2013;66:896–903.

16. Poletti V, Romagnoli M, Piciucchi S, et al. Current status of idiopathic nonspecific interstitial pneumonia. *Semin Respir Crit Care Med*. 2012;33:440–449.

17. Godbert B, Wissler M, Vignaud J. Desquamative interstitial pneumonia: an analytic review with an emphasis on aetiology. *Eur Respir Rev*. 2013;22:117–123.

18. Churg A, Müller NL, Wright JL. Respiratory bronchiolitis/interstitial lung disease: fibrosis, pulmonary function, and evolving concepts. *Arch Pathol Lab Med*. 2010;134:27–32.

19. Vassallo R. Diffuse Lung disease in cigarette smokers. *Semin Respir Crit Care Med*. 2012;33:533–542.

20. Beardsley B, Rassl D. Fibrosing organising pneumonia. *Postgrad Med J*. 2014;90:475–481.

21. Obadina ET, Torrealba JM, Kanne JP. Acute pulmonary injury: high-resolution CT and histopathological spectrum. *Br J Radiol*. 2013;86:20120614.

22. Kanaji N, Watanabe N, Kita N, et al. Paraneoplastic syndromes associated with lung cancer. *World J Clin Oncol*. 2014;10:197–223.

23. Kim L, Tsao MS. Tumour tissue sampling for lung cancer management in the era of personalised therapy: what is good enough for molecular testing? *Eur Respir J*. 2014;44:1970–2013.

24. Rezaei MK, Nolan NJ, Schwartz AM. Surgical pathology of lung cancer. *Semin Respir Crit Care Med*. 2013;34:770–786.

25. Petersen I. The new classification of lung adenocarcinoma. *Zentralbl Chir*. 2013;138 (Suppl 1):S16–S24.

26. Travis WD, Brambilla E, Noguchi M, et al. International Association for the Study of Lung Cancer/American Thoracic Society/European Respiratory Society: international multidisciplinary classification of lung adenocarcinoma: executive summary. *Proc Am Thorac Soc*. 2011;8:381–385.

27. Weichert W, Warth A. Early lung cancer with lepidic pattern: adenocarcinoma in situ, minimally invasive adenocarcinoma, and lepidic predominant adenocarcinoma. *Curr Opin Pulm Med*. 2014;20:309–316.

28. Travis WD. Pathology and diagnosis of neuroendocrine tumors: lung Neuroendocrine. *Thorac Surg Clin*. 2014;24:257–266.

29. William J, Variakojis D, Yeldandi A, et al. Lymphoproliferative neoplasms of the lung: a review. *Arch Pathol Lab Med*. 2013;137:382–391.

30. Suri HS, Yi ES, Nowakowski GS, et al. Pulmonary langerhans cell histiocytosis. *Orphanet J Rare Dis*. 2012;19:7–16.